Proceedings of the 17th Collegium Internationale Neuro-Psychopharmacologicum Congress

Proceedings of the 17th Collegium Internationale Neuro-Psychopharmacologicum Congress

Guest Editors

Itaru Yamashita
Professor of Psychiatry
Hokkaido University School of Medicine
Sapporo, Japan

Michio Toru
Professor of Neuropsychiatry
Tokyo Medical and Dental University
School of Medicine
Tokyo, Japan

Alec J. Coppen
Director of Medical Research Council Unit
MRC Neuropsychiatry Research Laboratory
Epsom, U.K.

Raven Press New York

Note

This volume was prepared from typed manuscripts in a camera-ready format to assure rapid publication in time for distribution at the 17th Collegium Internationale Neuro-Psychopharmacologicum. All regular issues of Clinical Neuropharmacology are formally typeset.

Library of Congress Catalogue Card No. 76-644724
ISBN 0-88167-732-9

Raven Press, 1185 Avenue of the Americas, New York, New York 10036

© 1990 by Raven Press Books, Ltd. All rights reserved. This book is protected by copyright. No part of it may be reproduced, stored in a retrieval system, or transmitted, in any form or by any means, electronic, mechanical, photocopying, recording, or otherwise, without the prior written permission of the publisher.
Raven Press cannot be held responsible for errors or for any consequences arising from the use of the information contained herein.

Made in the United States of America

PREFACE

This special issue of Clinical Neuropharmacology is devoted to the contributions presented at the 17th Collegium Internationale Neuro-Psychopharmacologicum (C.I.N.P.) Congress held in Kyoto, Japan, September 10–14, 1990.

These proceedings include short articles related to the communications presented in the plenary lectures and symposia. A book of abstracts has been published separately for non-oral and poster presentations. The C.I.N.P. Congress, as the international meeting of neuropsychopharmacologists, provides current understanding and new developments in the fields of neuropharmacology and psychopharmacology. One of the main goals of the Congress and of this volume is to integrate sessions between pharmacologists on one side and psychiatrists and neurologists on the other. The exchange of relevant information between basic scientists and clinical researchers is of fundamental importance in a rapidly growing research field such as neuropsychopharmacology.

In neuropharmacology, the program particularly emphasized the problems of dementia, including recent developments in the biological aspects and drug treatment of dementia and related conditions. Other main topics discussed in the symposia were the biology of drug addiction and alcoholism, and the evaluation of new strategies in Parkinson's disease and refractory epilepsy. Basic research in the molecular genetics of CNS diseases, intraneuronal calcium, amino acids, neuropeptides, eicosanoids, stress-induced neurochemical changes, primary cultured neurons, etc., have also been discussed in detail.

In the field of psychopharmacology, the mechanisms of action and the rational use of antidepressants, antipsychotics, lithium and other mood stabilizers, and anxiolytics have been widely reexamined. Extensive work has been focused on new drugs, such as atypical antipsychotics, reversible MAO-inhibitors, anxiolytics not acting at the benzodiazepine receptor, and antiepileptics that are effective as mood stabilizers. Biology and treatment of panic, post-traumatic stress, impulse control disorders, and anxiety states have been meaningfully reconsidered. Our understanding of molecular aspects of receptors and psychotropic drugs is rapidly expanding. Many new findings in brain imaging, biological markers, pharmacotherapy of postnatal and childhood disorders were presented and discussed.

We trust that from this volume the readers will find many exciting discoveries and ideas that challenge previous assumptions on the biological aspects of neurological and psychiatric disorders and on the mechanisms of many pharmacological agents.

The Editors

Clinical Neuropharmacology

A JOURNAL OF REVIEWS AND ORIGINAL INVESTIGATIONS IN THE
PHARMACOLOGY OF CENTRAL NERVOUS SYSTEM DYSFUNCTION

VOLUME 13, SUPPLEMENT 2, 1990

Proceedings of the 17th Collegium Internationale Neuro-Psychopharmacologicum Congress

September 10–14, 1990, Kyoto, Japan

CONTENTS

PLENARY LECTURES

PL-1	**Serotonin and Psychiatry** D. G. Grahame-Smith *(U.K.)*	1
PL-2	**The Course of Affective Disorders: Implications for Psychopharmacology** J. Angst *(Switzerland)*	3
PL-3	**The Adrenergic Receptors: Structure/Function and Regulation** Robert J. Lefkowitz *(U.S.A.)*	5
PL-4	**Presynaptic Receptors in Psychopharmacology** S. Z. Langer, A. M. Galzin, and S. Arbilla *(France)*	7
PL-5	**Movements of Calcium Ion in Cells and Neuronal Function** M. Endo *(Japan)*	9
PL-6	**The Brain as Regulator and Target of Hormones** Florian Holsboer *(F.R.G.)*	11

SYMPOSIA

Professor Ryo Takahashi Memorial Symposium: Monoaminergic Function in Affective Disorders
Chairs: Y. Shimazono and T. Kariya *(Japan)*

I1-1-1	**Animal Study on the Role of Serotonin in Depression** Haruo Nagayama *(Japan)*	13
I1-1-2	**Responsiveness of the 5-HT$_2$ Receptor Family in Affective Disorders** M. Mikuni, A. Kagaya, Y. Kuroda, F. Kato, and K. Takahashi *(Japan)*	15

11-1-3	Is Serotonergic Function Really Abnormal in Major Depression? H. Y. Meltzer, M. Schreiber, B. Bastani, and J. F. Nash *(U.S.A.)*	17
11-1-5	β-Phenylethylamine and Noradrenergic Function in Depression M. Nakagawara *(Japan)*	19

The Nature and Treatment of Therapy-Resistant Depression
Chairs: W. Pöldinger *(Switzerland)* and K. Sarai *(Japan)*

11-2-1	Oriental Medicine for Therapy Resistant Depression K. Sarai *(Japan)*	21
11-2-3	Treatment of Therapy-Resistant Depression K. Achté *(Finland)*	23
11-2-5	Bright Light and Sleep Deprivation as Adjuvant Therapies in Major Depression E. Holsboer-Trachsler, R. Stohler, M. Hatzinger, U. Gerhard, V. Hobi, and A. Wirz-Justice *(Switzerland)*	25
11-2-6	Serotonin-Functional Approach for Diagnosis and Treatment of Therapy Resistant Depressions W. Pöldinger *(Switzerland)*	27

Pathophysiology and Treatment of Obsessive–Compulsive Disorders
Chairs: D. L. Murphy *(U.S.A.)* and V. Gentil *(Brazil)*

11-3-1	Are There Cross-Cultural Differences in Obsessive Compulsive Disorder? Sumant Khanna *(India)*	29
11-3-2	When All Is Said and Done—An Update on Psychosurgical Intervention in Intractable Obsessive Compulsive Disorder P. Mindus and B. A. Meyerson *(Sweden)*	31
11-3-3	Phenomenology and Treatment of Obsessive Compulsive Disorder T. Nakazawa *(Japan)*	33
11-3-4	Childhood Onset Obsessive Compulsive Disorder H. L. Leonard, S. E. Swedo, M. Lenane, D. C. Rettew, and J. L. Rapoport *(U.S.A.)*	35
11-3-5	Brain Serotonergic Subsystems in Obsessive–Compulsive Disorder D. L. Murphy and T. A. Pigott *(U.S.A.)*	37

Three-Dimensional Structure of Psychotropic Drugs and Receptors
Chairs: S. G. Dahl *(Norway)* and R. Stroud *(U.S.A.)*

11-4-4	Mapping of Serotonine Receptor Recognition Sites Applied to Drug Design M. Hibert *(France)*	39
11-4-5	Molecular Structure and Dynamics of the Dopamine D_2 Receptor and Ligands S. G. Dahl, Ø. Edvardsen, and I. Sylte *(Norway)*	41

Parkinson's Disease: Etiology and Treatment
Chairs: P. Riederer *(F.R.G.)* and T. Nagatsu *(Japan)*

11-5-1	Biochemical and Pharmacological Aspects of Parkinson's Disease P. Riederer, K. Jellinger, E. Sofic, and W. Paulus *(F.R.G. and Austria)*	43

11-5-2	The Functioning of Tyrosine Hydroxylase in Parkinson's Disease T. Nagatsu *(Japan)*	45
11-5-3	MAO-B and COMT Inhibition: Enhanced Benefit in DOPA Therapy M. Da Prada *(Switzerland)*	47
11-5-4	Functional Studies on Monoaminergic Transmitter Release in Parkinsonism W. Wesemann, H.-W. Clement, and Chr. Grote *(F.R.G.)*	49
11-5-5	Iron Melanin and Dopamine Interaction: Relevance to Parkinson's Disease D. Ben-Shachar and M. B. H. Youdim *(Israel)*	51
11-5-6	Deprenyl (Selegiline) as Monotherapy in Early Parkinson's Disease I. Shoulson and the Parkinson Study Group *(U.S.A.)*	53
11-5-7	Dopamine Agonists in Parkinson's Disease: Present Status and New Trends R. Horowski, I. Runge, P.-A. Löschmann, L. Turski, and H. Wachtel *(F.R.G.)*	55

Nerve Growth Factor: Basic Research and Clinical Perspective
Chairs: E. M. Shooter *(U.S.A.)* and H. Hatanaka *(Japan)*

11-6-1	An Overview of Nerve Growth Factors: From Molecules to Memory E. M. Shooter *(U.S.A.)*	57
11-6-2	NGF-Mediated Promotion of Cell Survival in Culture from Postnatal Rat CNS Hiroshi Hatanaka *(Japan)*	59
11-6-3	Molecular and Cellular Mechanisms of Neuronal Death Caused by Nerve Growth Factor Deprivation T. Koike *(Japan)*	61
11-6-4	Emerging Pharmacology of Neurotrophic Factors F. Hefti *(U.S.A.)*	63
11-6-5	NGF Treatment Affects Behavioral Recovery Following Septal Lesions in Rats B. Will and V. Pallage *(France)*	65

Anxiolytics Not Acting at the Benzodiazepine Receptor
Chairs: O. Benkert *(F.R.G.)* and S. Miura *(Japan)*

11-7-1	Models of Anxiety: Noradrenergic, GABAergic and Serotonergic Pathways J. Traber *(F.R.G.)*	67
11-7-2	Anxiolytics Not Acting at the Benzodiazepine Receptors, The Present State I: Tricyclic Antidepressants, MAO-Inhibitors and Neuroleptics R. Buller and O. Benkert *(F.R.G.)*	69
11-7-3	The Present State. II: Beta Blockers Peter Tyrer *(U.K.)*	71
11-7-4	The Future 1: 5-HT Agonists and $5-HT_2$ Antagonists: Buspirone, Ipsapirone, Gepirone, Ritanserin M. Murasaki and S. Miura *(Japan)*	73
11-7-5	5-HT Re-Uptake Blockers as Anxiolytics T. R. Insel, J. T. Winslow, and D. L. Murphy *(U.S.A.)*	75
11-7-6	Non Benzodiazepine Anxiolytics and Hypnotics Acting at the Benzodiazepine GABA Macromolecular Complex: Alpidem, Zolpidem, Suriclone, Zopiclone J. C. Bisserbe and J. P. Boulenger *(France)*	77

Fundamental Brain Imaging 1: PET and SPECT
Chairs: G. Sedvall *(Sweden)* and T. Yamasaki *(Japan)*

11-8-1 PET and SPECT as Experimental Tools in Clinical Neuropsychopharmacology 79
G. Sedvall, L. Farde, H. Hall, C. Halldin, A.-L. Nordström, and H. Nybäck *(Sweden)*

11-8-2 Differential Effects of Clozapine and Thiothixene on Regional Glucose Metabolism Assessed by PET in Schizophrenics 81
S. G. Potkin, M. S. Buchsbaum, J. F. Marshall, C. Heh, J. Singer, J. Costa, J. Wu, and W. E. Bunney, Jr. *(U.S.A.)*

11-8-3 PET Analysis of Glucose Metabolism in Schizophrenic Patients Before and During Drug Treatment 83
F.-A. Wiesel *(Sweden)*

11-8-4 Dopamine Receptor Elevations in Drug Naive Schizophrenia and Bipolar Affective Illness Measured by C-11 NMSP PET Studies: Update and Methodological Considerations 85
D. F. Wong, L. Tune, G. Pearlson, T. Young, E. Shaya, C. Ross, R. F. Dannals, A. A. Wilson, H. T. Ravert, J. Links, H. N. Wagner, Jr., and A. Gjedde *(U.S.A. and Canada)*

11-8-5 Comparison of Methods Used with [^{11}C]Raclopride and [^{11}C]NMSP for the PET-Determination of Central D2-Dopamine Receptors 87
L. Farde, A.-L. Nordström, L. Eriksson, C. Halldin, and G. Sedvall *(Sweden)*

11-8-7 Summary (Fundamental Brain Imaging 1: PET & SPECT) 89
T. Yamasaki *(Japan)*

5-HT as a Target for Antidepressants
Chairs: J. J. López-Ibor *(Spain)* and S. M. Stahl *(U.S.A.)*

11-9-1 Neuroendocrine Markers of Serotonin Responsivity in Depression 91
Stephen M. Stahl *(U.S.A.)*

11-9-2 Pharmacology of 5-HT$_{1A}$ Agonists 93
D. G. Spencer, Jr., J. De Vry, R. Schreiber, and J. Traber *(F.R.G.)*

11-9-3 Preliminary Studies of 5HT$_{1A}$ Agonists in Depression 95
N. M. Kurtz, J. Keppel-Hesselink, M. Beneke, and A. H. Heller *(U.S.A., The Netherlands, and F.R.G.)*

11-9-5 Potential Effectiveness of Drugs with an Affinity for 5-HT$_{1A}$ Receptors in Obsessive Compulsive Disorder 97
S. A. Montgomery, D. Baldwin, N. Fineberg, and D. Montgomery *(U.K.)*

11-9-6 5-HT Reuptake Inhibition in the Elderly 99
I. Karlsson *(Sweden)*

11-9-7 Pharmaco-Vigilance of a 5-HT$_{1A}$ Agonist (Buspirone) 101
J. J. López-Ibor, Jr., J. Honorato, C. Ballús, V. Conde, J. Giner, J. Guimón, and A. Rodriguez *(Spain)*

Sleep, Hypnotics, and Daily Activity
Chairs: T. Roth *(U.S.A.)* and Y. Hishikawa *(Japan)*

11-10-1 The Relation of Hypnotics to Sleep and Waking Function 103
T. Roth *(U.S.A.)*

11-10-2	**Amnestic Properties of Sedatives/Hypnotics** I. Hindmarch *(U.K.)*	105
11-10-3	**Daily Activity and Persistent Sleep–Wake Schedule Disorders** T. Ohta and T. Iwata *(Japan)*	106
11-10-4	**Effects of Zopiclone on Subjective Evaluation of Day-Time Sleepiness and on Psychomotor and Physical Performances in Athletes** M. Billiard, M. Tafti, and A. Besset *(France)*	108
11-10-5	**Hypnotic-Induced Decrement and Enhancement of Memory** Wallace B. Mendelson *(U.S.A.)*	109
11-10-6	**Effects of Zopiclone and Other Hypnotics on the Transient Change in Sleep–Wake Schedule** O. Kanno, H. Watanabe, and H. Kazamatsuri *(Japan)*	111

Biological Basis and Treatment of Anxiety States
Chairs: M. Lader *(U.K.)* and A. Mori *(Japan)*

11-11-1	**GABA and Noradrenergic Mechanisms in Anxiety** D. J. Nutt, P. Glue, C. W. Lawson, and S. Wilson *(U.K.)*	113
11-11-2	**Serotonergic Mechanisms in Anxiety** Arlene S. Eison and Michael S. Eison *(U.S.A.)*	115
11-11-3	**Target Receptors for Anxiolytic Drugs: The Relevance of Animal Models** D. J. Sanger, B. Zivkovic, and S. Z. Langer *(France)*	117
11-11-4	**Drug Models of Anxiety** T. W. Uhde *(U.S.A.)*	119
11-11-5	**From Laboratory to Clinic** Malcolm Lader *(U.K.)*	120

Dopamine D1 and D2 Receptors: Molecular, Pharmacological and Clinical Aspects
Chairs: S. O. Ögren *(Sweden)* and H. Beckmann *(F.R.G.)*

11-12-1	**Molecular Characterization of the Receptors for Dopamine** Marc C. Caron, Allen Dearry, Jay A. Gingrich, Pierre Falardeau, Robert T. Fremeau, Jr., Michael D. Bates, and Susan E. Senogles *(U.S.A.)*	122
11-12-2	**Multiple D2 Dopamine Receptors** Philip Seeman *(Canada)*	124
11-12-3	**Intramembrane Regulation of Dopamine D2 Receptors by Neuropeptide Receptors and Excitatory Amino Acid Receptors. Relevance for Schizophrenia** K. Fuxe, L. F. Agnati, G. Von Euler, S. Tanganelli, W. O'Connor, P. Osborne, T. Antonelli, and U. Ungerstedt *(Sweden and Italy)*	126
11-12-4	**Dopamine Receptors and Their Coupling to Ion Channels** R. A. North, M. G. Lacey, N. Uchimura, and N. Mercuri *(U.S.A.)*	128
11-12-5	**Role of D-1 and D-2 Receptors in Behaviour** S. O. Ögren *(Sweden)*	130
11-12-6	**Clinical Significance of D1 and D2 Receptors** H. Beckmann *(F.R.G.)*	132

Tardive Dyskinesia and Other Adverse Side-Effects of Neuroleptics
Chairs: J. L. Waddington *(Ireland)* and H. Kazamatsuri *(Japan)*

11-13-1 Prospective Studies of Tardive Dyskinesia Development — 134
J. M. Kane, M. Woerner, B. Saltz, J. Lieberman, and K. Bergmann *(U.S.A.)*

11-13-2 Antecedents of Vulnerability to Tardive Dyskinesia and Cerebral MRI in Schizophrenia — 135
J. L. Waddington, E. O'Callaghan, C. Larkin, O. Redmond, J. Stack, and J. T. Ennis *(Ireland)*

11-13-3 Transcultural Aspects of Tardive Dyskinesia — 137
H. Kazamatsuri *(Japan)*

11-13-4 PET Studies of Dopamine Receptor Occupancy in Relation to Neuroleptic Side Effects — 139
A.-L. Nordström, L. Farde, F.-A. Wiesel, and G. Sedvall *(Sweden)*

11-13-5 Neuroleptic-Induced Parkinsonism in Schizophrenia — 141
W. F. Hoffman, L. C. Ballard, G. A. Keepers, T. E. Hansen, and D. E. Casey *(U.S.A.)*

11-13-6 Neuroleptic Malignant Syndrome — 143
G. M. Simpson and S. Gratz *(U.S.A.)*

Implications of New Knowledge About Affective Disorders for Their Treatment: A Critical Reappraisal of Findings of WHO Network of Research Centers
Chairs: N. Sartorius *(Switzerland)* and I. Yamashita *(Japan)*

11-14-1 Advances in the Treatment of Depression — 145
P. Kielholz *(Switzerland)*

11-14-2 Current Problems of Psychoneuroimmunology — 146
M. E. Vartanian and G. I. Kolyaskina *(U.S.S.R.)*

11-14-3 Advances in Membrane Research — 148
Leonid Prilipko *(Switzerland)*

11-14-4 Advances in Genetic Research in Psychiatry — 150
J. Mendlewicz *(Belgium)*

11-14-5 Biological Markers: Past and Future — 152
I. Yamashita and T. Koyama *(Japan)*

Neurochemical Mechanisms in Cerebral Ischemia
Chairs: C. G. Wasterlain *(U.S.A.)* and K. Kogure *(Japan)*

11-15-1 Pharmacological Modification of Post-Ischemic Brain Cell Injury — 154
Kyuya Kogure and Hiroyuki Kato *(Japan)*

11-15-2 Components of Hypoxic Neuronal Injury in Hippocampal Slices Which Are Independent of Calcium Influx — 156
J. E. Parsons, R. A. Wallis, and C. G. Wasterlain *(U.S.A.)*

11-15-3 Mechanisms of Drug Actions Against Neuronal Damage Caused by Ischemia — 158
J. Krieglstein, C. Backhauss, C. Karkoutly, J. Prehn, and M. Seif el Nasr *(F.R.G.)*

11-15-4 The Pharmacology of NMDA Receptors in Relation to Neuronal Degeneration — 160
A. C. Foster, C. L. Willis, M. H. M. Bakker, and R. Tridgett *(U.K.)*

11-15-5   Non-NMDA Antagonists Protect Against Delayed Neuronal Cell Death Induced
          by Cerebral Ischemia   162
          T. Honore, M. J. Sheardown, A. J. Hansen, K. Eskesen, and N. Diemer
          (Denmark)

Brain Imaging 2: Alternative Techniques
Chairs: D. R. Weinberger *(U.S.A.)* and B. Saletu *(Austria)*

11-16-1   Morphometric Studies of Brain Anatomy with MRI in Normal Monozygotic Twins
          and Monozygotic Twins Discordant for Schizophrenia   164
          D. R. Weinberger, R. Suddath, M. Casanova, G. W. Christison, and E. F. Torrey
          (U.S.A.)

11-16-2   EEG Mapping in Diagnosis and Treatment of Dementia: On Relations to
          Computed Tomography and Psychometry   166
          B. Saletu, E. Paulus, P. Anderer, P. K. Fischhof, and L. Wicke *(Austria)*

11-16-3   Effects of Typical and Atypical Neuroleptics on *In Vivo* Brain Glucose Metabolism
          Evaluated by PET   168
          David Pickar, William E. Semple, Paul Andreason, Richard R. Owen,
          P. Eric Konicki, Thomas Nordahl, and Robert M. Cohen *(U.S.A.)*

11-16-4   MRI-SPECT and PET-EEG Findings on Brain Dysfunction in Schizophrenia   170
          W. Guenther *(F.R.G.)*

11-16-6   Quantitative Receptor Mapping in Postmortem Human Brain as It Relates to In
          Vivo Neuroimaging   172
          J. E. Kleinman *(U.S.A.)*

New Drug Treatment for Schizophrenia
Chairs: E. C. Johnstone *(U.K.)* and K. Inanaga *(Japan)*

12-1-1   L-DOPA in Very Impaired Schizophrenic Patients   174
          D. G. C. Owens, P. E. Harrison-Read, and E. C. Johnstone *(U.K.)*

12-1-2   Effects of Mianserin on Negative Symptoms in Schizophrenia   176
          Y. Mizuki *(Japan)*

12-1-3   Dopamine Autoreceptor Agonists in the Treatment of Positive and Negative
          Schizophrenia   178
          O. Benkert, H. Wetzel, and K. Wiedemann *(F.R.G.)*

12-1-5   Treatment of a New Benzamide Derivative Emonapride (YM-09151) for
          Schizophrenia   180
          Y. Kudo *(Japan)*

12-1-6   Serotonin 5-HT$_2$ Receptor Blockers in Schizophrenia   182
          Y. G. Gelders, S. L. E. Heylen, G. Vanden Bussche, A. J. M. Reyntjens, and
          P. A. J. Janssen *(Belgium)*

Affective Disorders of Later Life: Diagnostic and Treatment Issues
Chairs: G. D. Burrows *(Australia)* and I. J. Heuser *(F.R.G.)*

12-2-2   Depression and Suicide in Late Life   184
          M. Shimizu *(Japan)*

12-2-3	Neuroendocrineimmune Regulation of Aging Joseph Meites *(U.S.A.)*	186
12-2-4	Limbic Hypothalamic Pituitary Adrenal-Axis Dysfunction in Elderly Depressed Patients I. J. Heuser, H.-J. Wark, D. Borchardt, and L. Hermle *(F.R.G.)*	188
12-2-5	Pharmacokinetic Aspects of Antidepressant Treatment in Late Life T. R. Norman and G. D. Burrows *(Australia)*	190

New Reversible MAO Inhibitors: Basic and Clinical Aspects
Chairs: M. Youdim *(Israel)* and R. Amrein *(Switzerland)*

12-3-2	MAO Inhibitors, Old and New: Similarities and Differences B. A. Callingham *(U.K.)*	192
12-3-3	Preclinical Profile of Moclobemide M. Da Prada *(Switzerland)*	194
12-3-4	Newer Aspects of the Selective, Reversible Inhibitor of MAO-A, Brofaromine P. C. Waldmeier, J. Kraetz, and L. Maitre *(Switzerland)*	196
12-3-5	Moclobemide: Drug and Alcohol Interactions A. J. Puech and I. Berlin *(France)*	198
12-3-6	Overview of Clinical Investigations with Brofaromine J. A. Snaith *(Switzerland)*	200
12-3-7	Clinical Overview on Moclobemide J. W. G. Tiller *(Australia)*	202
12-3-8	Reversible MAO Inhibitors in Comparison to Established Antidepressants R. L. Borison *(U.S.A.)*	204

Lithium and Other Mood-Stabilizing Agents: Basic Aspects
Chairs: R. Belmaker *(Israel)* and T. Furukawa *(Japan)*

12-4-1	Serotonergic and Dopaminergic Neuronal Change, Including Receptor Changes, After Chronic Lithium T. Koyama, Y. Odagaki, A. Muraki, and I. Yamashita *(Japan)*	205
12-4-2	GABA Receptor Alterations After Chronic Lithium—In Comparison with Carbamazepine and Sodium Valproate N. Motohashi *(Japan)*	207
12-4-3	Mechanisms of Lithium in Modulation of Aminergic Receptor Functions Arne Geisler and Arne Mørk *(Denmark)*	209
12-4-4	Intracerebroventricular Inositol Does Not Reverse High Dose Lithium Toxicity in Rats O. Kofman and R. H. Belmaker *(Israel)*	211
12-4-5	Augmentation of 5-HT Neurotransmission by Lithium C. de Montigny and P. Blier *(Canada)*	213
12-4-6	Potential Targets for the Action of Lithium in the Brain: Muscarinic Receptor Regulation R. H. Lenox and J. Ellis *(U.S.A.)*	215

Excitatory Amino Acids in Neuro-Psychiatry
Chairs: C. W. Cotman *(U.S.A.)* and P. Laduron *(France)*

12-5-1 Organization and Plasticity of Excitatory Amino Acid Receptors in the Rodent and Human Brain — 217
C. W. Cotman, J. W. Geddes, and J. Ulas *(U.S.A.)*

12-5-2 The Glutamate Receptor Gene Family — 219
S. Heinemann, B. Bettler, J. Boulter, E. Deneris, R. Duvoisin, G. Gasic, M. Hartley, I. Hermans-Borgmeyer, M. Hollmann, D. Johnson, A. O'Shea-Greenfield, R. Papke, and S. Rogers *(U.S.A.)*

12-5-3 Glutamate Channel Kinetics Underlie the Slow EPSC in Hippocampal Neurons — 220
G. L. Westbrook, R. A. J. Lester, J. D. Clements, and C. E. Jahr *(U.S.A.)*

12-5-4 Activity and Excitatory Amino Acid Receptors in the Developing and Regenerating Visual System — 222
Ronald L. Meyer *(U.S.A.)*

12-5-5 Links Between Synaptic Plasticity and Behavior — 224
C. A. Barnes, C. A. Erickson, and B. L. McNaughton *(U.S.A.)*

Multiple 5-HT Receptors
Chairs: E. G. Anderson *(U.S.A.)* and E. M. Sellers *(Canada)*

12-6-1 Serotonin Receptors — 226
M. B. Tyers *(U.K.)*

12-6-2 Clinical Effects of 5HT-1A Partial Agonists, Buspirone and Gepirone, in the Treatment of Depression — 228
D. S. Robinson, R. E. Gammans, R. C. Shrotriya, S. W. Jenkins, J. J. Andary, D. R. Alms, and M. E. Messina *(U.S.A.)*

12-6-3 The 5-HT$_2$ Receptors: What Do They Do? Possible Roles in Affective Disorders — 230
J. E. Leysen *(Belgium)*

12-6-4 Serotonin and Cognition — 232
J. M. Barnes, N. M. Barnes, B. Costall, A. M. Domeney, M. E. Kelly, and R. J. Naylor *(U.K.)*

12-6-5 Role of 5-HT Receptors in Addictive Disorders — 234
E. M. Sellers, M. B. Sobell, and G. A. Higgins *(Canada)*

12-6-6 Clinical Importance of Multiple Serotonin Receptors: Summary and Future Directions — 236
Edmund G. Anderson *(U.S.A.)*

Mode of Action of Antidepressants (1): New Findings and New Profiles
Chairs: G. Racagni *(Italy)* and L. Maitre *(Switzerland)*

12-7-1 5-HT-1A Receptor-Mediated Effects of Antidepressants: Relation to G Protein Function — 237
M. E. Newman and B. Lerer *(Israel)*

12-7-2 Protein Phosphorylation After Acute and Chronic Antidepressant Treatment — 239
N. Brunello, J. Perez, D. Tinelli, E. Bianchi, and G. Racagni *(Italy)*

12-7-3	**Electrophysiological Studies with Antidepressant Drugs in Hippocampal Slices from the Rat** Helmut L. Haas and Susanne Birnstiel *(F.R.G.)*	241
12-7-4	**Monoamine Hypotheses of Depression: Is Levoprotiline the Stumbling-Block?** P. C. Waldmeier and L. Maître *(Switzerland)*	243
12-7-5	**Corticotropin-Releasing Factor (CRF) and Depression: Behavioral, Hormonal and Receptor Changes in Rats Following Chronic Administration of CRF** M. E. Abreu, L. H. Conti, D. G. Costello, and S. J. Enna *(U.S.A.)*	245

Psychopharmacology of Impulse Control Disorders
Chairs: M. Linnoila *(U.S.A.)* and A. J. Bond *(U.K.)*

12-8-1	**Rodent Models of Aggressive Behaviour and Serotonergic Drugs** B. Olivier and J. Mos *(Holland)*	247
12-8-2	**Serotonergic Mechanisms and Impulsive Aggression in Vervet Monkeys** Michael J. Raleigh and Michael T. McGuire *(U.S.A.)*	249
12-8-3	**Pharmacological Manipulation of Aggressiveness and Impulsiveness in Healthy Volunteers** A. J. Bond *(U.K.)*	251
12-8-4	**Suicidal Behavior and Serotonin** L. Träskman-Bendz, C. Alling, G. Regnéll, P. Simonsson, and R. Öhman *(Sweden)*	253
12-8-5	**Violent Behavior, Serotonin and Glucose Metabolism** M. Virkkunen and M. Linnoila *(Finland and U.S.A.)*	255

Atypical Antipsychotic Drugs: Clinical Advantages
Chairs: H. Y. Meltzer *(U.S.A.)* and H. Hippius *(F.R.G.)*

12-9-1	**Drug Treatment of Schizophrenia: Current Concepts** D. Naber and H. Hippius *(F.R.G.)*	257
12-9-2	**Clinical Efficacy of Clozapine in the Treatment of Schizophrenia** H. Y. Meltzer, L. D. Alphs, B. Bastani, L. F. Ramirez, and K. Kwon *(U.S.A.)*	259
12-9-3	**Side Effects of Clozapine and Their Management** L. D. Alphs, H. Y. Meltzer, B. Bastani, and L. F. Ramirez *(U.S.A.)*	261
12-9-4	**Current Views on Tardive Dyskinesia** J. Gerlach *(Denmark)*	263
12-9-5	**Mechanism of Action of Atypical Antipsychotics** P. L. Herrling *(Switzerland)*	265

Neuro-Regulation of Sleep and Rhythms
Chairs: F. W. Turek *(U.S.A.)* and A. Steiger *(F.R.G.)*

12-10-1	**Pharmacological and Non-pharmacological Manipulation of Circadian Rhythms** F. W. Turek, C. Wickland, and O. Van Reeth *(U.S.A. and Belgium)*	267
12-10-3	**The Two-Process Model of Sleep Regulation: Simulating Ultradian Sleep Dynamics and Effects of Hypnotics** A. A. Borbély and P. Achermann *(Switzerland)*	269

12-10-4	Dose-Related Suppression of REM Sleep by the Serotonin-1 Agonist Eltoprazine J. Quattrochi, D. Binder, A. Mamelak, J. Williams, and J. A. Hobson *(U.S.A.)*	271
12-10-5	Sleep–EEG Data as It Relates to the Cholinergic–Aminergic Imbalance Theory of Affective Disorders D. Riemann and M. Berger *(F.R.G.)*	273
12-10-6	Sleep–EEG and Nocturnal Hormonal Secretion in Depressed Patients and Under Psychoactive Drugs A. Steiger, U. von Bardeleben, C. Lauer, B. Rothe, and F. Holsboer *(F.R.G.)*	275

Antidepressants: Selective 5-HT Reuptake Inhibitors
Chairs: B. E. Leonard *(Ireland)* and F. S. Abuzzahab *(U.S.A.)*

12-11-1	The Unanswered Questions in the Use of Selective Serotonin Reuptake Inhibitors F. S. Abuzzahab, Sr. *(U.S.A.)*	277
12-11-2	$5HT_2$ Receptor Sensitivity After Chronic Administration of Sertraline and Other Selective Serotonin Uptake Inhibitors Elaine Sanders-Bush *(U.S.A.)*	279
12-11-3	The Neuronal Transport of Serotonin as a Target of Action of Antidepressant Drugs S. Z. Langer, H. Esnaud, and D. Graham *(France)*	281
12-11-4	The Clinical Pharmacology and Pharmacokinetic Aspects of Selective Serotonin Uptake Inhibitors Louis Lemberger *(U.S.A.)*	283
12-11-5	Clinical Efficacy of 5-HT Uptake Inhibitors Stuart A. Montgomery *(U.K.)*	285
12-11-6	The Effect of Serotonin Reuptake Inhibitors on Some Peripheral Markers of the Serotonergic System in Depressed Patients B. E. Leonard *(Ireland)*	287

Lithium and Other Mood-Stabilizing Agents: Clinical Research
Chairs: N. Johnson *(U.K.)* and T. Ohkuma *(Japan)*

12-12-1	Dosage Schedules in the Treatment of Mood Disorders with Lithium P. Plenge, E. T. Mellerup, H. V. Jensen, K. Olafsson, A. Bille, and J. Andersen *(Denmark)*	289
12-12-2	The Relation Between Antimanic and Prophylactic Action of Lithium A. Koukopoulos, D. Reginaldi, A. Tundo, and L. Tondo *(Italy)*	291
12-12-3	The Treatment of Affective Disorders with Carbamazepine A. Kishimoto *(Japan)*	293
12-12-4	Pharmacokinetics of Carbamazepine in the Treatment of Mood Disorders Martin J. Brodie *(Scotland)*	295
12-12-5	Valproate-Treatment of Psychotic Disorders in Comparison with Carbamazepine-Therapy H. M. Emrich and M. Dose *(F.R.G.)*	297
12-12-6	Antimanic Effect of Zotepine, a New Thiepin Derivative—Acute and Long-Term Treatment T. Harada *(Japan)*	299

Neuropharmacology of Excitatory Amino Acids
Chairs: A. Horita *(U.S.A.)* and T. Shibuya *(Japan)*

12-13-2	**Endogenous Excitotoxins and Neuropsychiatric Disorders** John W. Olney *(U.S.A.)*	301
12-13-3	**Mechanisms of Phencyclidine (PCP)-N-Methyl-D-Aspartate (NMDA) Receptor Interaction: Implications for Psychiatric Disorders** Stephen R. Zukin and Daniel C. Javitt *(U.S.A.)*	303
12-13-4	**Modulation of NMDA Receptors by ACh in the Central Nervous System** N. Akaike and N. Tateishi *(Japan)*	305
12-13-5	**Relation Between an Excitatory Amino Acid, Acetylcholine and Ca Channel in the Cerebellar Granule Cell** Y. Wanatabe and T. Shibuya *(Japan)*	307
12-13-6	**Exogenous Excitatory Amino Acids (EAAs) in Neurodegenerative Disorders** P. S. Spencer, C. Allen, R. Allen, G. Kisby, A. C. Ludolph, S. M. Ross, and D. N. Roy *(U.S.A.)*	309

Biological Markers in Relatives of Psychiatrically Ill Patients
Chairs: J.-C. Kreig *(F.R.G.)* and P. S. Holzman *(U.S.A.)*

12-14-1	**Neuropsychological Indicators of the Vulnerability to Schizophrenia** W. Maier, Ch. Hain, and F. Rist *(F.R.G.)*	311
12-14-2	**Variable Expressivity of the Phenotype in the Relatives of Schizophrenic Patients** Philip S. Holzman *(U.S.A.)*	313
12-14-3	**^{3}H-Spiperone Binding Capacity in Lymphocytes: A Family Study** B. Bondy, M. Ackenheil, R. R. Engel, M. Ertl, G. Minelli, C. Mundt, and G. Schleuning *(F.R.G.)*	315
12-14-4	**Psychometric, Polysomnographic, and Neuroendocrine Findings in Subjects at High Risk for Psychiatric Disorders** J.-C. Kreig, C. J. Lauer, and F. Holsboer *(F.R.G.)*	317

Mode of Action of Antidepressants (2): How Has Basic Research Helped the Clinician to Treat Depression?
Chairs: E. Richelson *(U.S.A.)* and G. Yagi *(Japan)*

12-15-1	**Aging Effect on Response to Nortriptyline in Depressed Patients** S. Kanba, K. Matsumoto, and G. Yagi *(Japan)*	319
12-15-2	**Central Noradrenergic Function in Depression and Antidepressants** O. Tajima and K. Kamijima *(Japan)*	321
12-15-3	**Clinical Significance of Receptor Effects of Antidepressants** E. Richelson *(U.S.A.)*	323
12-15-4	**From Rat 5-HT Neurons to the Strategy of Lithium Augmentation in Refractory Depression** C. de Montigny *(Canada)*	325
12-15-5	**The Selective Serotonin Reuptake Inhibitors** J. P. Feighner and W. F. Boyer *(U.S.A.)*	327

Biology and Psychopharmacology of Post-Traumatic Stress Disorder
Chairs: J. Davidson *(U.S.A.)* and B. Lerer *(Israel)*

12-16-1	**Psychoendocrinology and Pharmacotherapy of PTSD** E. L. Giller, Jr., R. T. Kosten, R. Yehuda, B. D. Perry, S. Southwick, and J. W. Mason *(U.S.A.)*	329
12-16-2	**Response to Tricyclic Therapy in PTSD** J. Davidson, H. Kudler, R. Stein, L. Ericksen, and R. Smith *(U.S.A.)*	331
12-16-3	**Posttraumatic Stress Disorder and Major Depression: An Integrated Perspective** B. Lerer, A. Dolev, A. Bleich, and R. P. Ebstein *(Israel)*	332
12-16-4	**Psycho-Neuro-Physiologic Characteristics of Combat Veterans with Posttraumatic Stress Disorder** A. Bleich, Y. Attias, Y. Dagan, P. Lavie, A. Shalev, and B. Lerer *(Israel)*	334
12-16-5	**Behavior Therapy and Psychophysiological Assessment of PTSD: Controlled Trials** Terence M. Keane *(U.S.A.)*	336
12-16-6	**Dreams' Repression in Adjusted Holocaust Survivors** Peretz Lavie and Hanna Kaminer *(Israel)*	338

Panic Disorders: Conflict and Consensus
Chairs: L. L. Judd *(U.S.A.)* and M. Roth *(U.K.)*

13-1-1	**Etiology, Diagnosis, and Course of Panic Disorder** R. M. A. Hirschfeld *(U.S.A.)*	340
13-1-2	**Family Genetic Studies in Panic Disorder** Myrna M. Weissman *(U.S.A.)*	342
13-1-5	**Psychological Treatments of Panic Disorder** David M. Clark and Michael Gelder *(U.K.)*	344
13-1-6	**Emerging Consensus for Treatment of Panic Disorder** L. L. Judd and A. H. Rosenfeld *(U.S.A.)*	346

New Theories and Research in Schizophrenia
Chairs: W. E. Bunney, Jr. *(U.S.A.)* and M. Toru *(Japan)*

13-2-1	**Psychosis and the Genetics of Brain Asymmetry** T. J. Crow *(U.K.)*	348
13-2-2	**Possible Neurotransmitter Imbalances in Schizophrenia** A. Carlsson and M. Carlsson *(Sweden)*	350
13-2-3	**Possible Involvement of Neuropeptides in Chronic Schizophrenia** H. Shibuya *(Japan)*	352
13-2-4	**Functional Subtyping of Schizophrenic Patients** E. R. John, L. Prichep, J. Volavka, J. Brodie, K. Alper, and R. Cancro *(U.S.A.)*	354
13-2-5	**Testing Neural Models of Schizophrenia with Positron Emission Tomography** M. S. Buchsbaum, R. Haier, M. Katz, R. Tafalla, S. Lottenberg, S. Potkin, and W. E. Bunney, Jr. *(U.S.A.)*	356

Advances in Basic Research and Treatment of Refractory Epilepsy
Chairs: D. Schmidt *(F.R.G.)* and M. Seino *(Japan)*

13-3-1   Basic Mechanisms of Refractory Epilepsies   358
B. S. Meldrum *(U.K.)*

13-3-2   Diagnostic Evaluation of Uncontrolled Epilepsy   360
William H. Theodore *(U.S.A.)*

13-3-3   Single or Polytherapy for Refractory Epilepsy   362
A. Sengoku *(Japan)*

13-3-4   Methodological Requirements for Clinical Trials in Refractory Epilepsies—Our Experience in Zonisamide   364
K. Yagi and M. Seino *(Japan)*

13-3-5   New Drugs for Refractory Epilepsies   366
D. Schmidt and S. Ried *(F.R.G.)*

Biology of Drug Addiction
Chairs: A. Herz *(F.R.G.)* and H. Kaneto *(Japan)*

13-4-1   The Nature of Addiction, with Special Reference to Alcohol   368
H. Kalant *(Canada)*

13-4-2   Neurochemistry of Opioid Addiction   370
A. Herz, R. Bals-Kubik, R. Spanagel, and T. S. Shippenberg *(F.R.G.)*

13-4-3   The Involvement of Endorphins in Drug Selfadministration   372
J. M. Van Ree, M. Kornet, and N. Ramsey *(The Netherlands)*

13-4-4   Cocaine Abuse and Dependence: Pharmacological Explorations and Interventions   374
Jerome H. Jaffe *(U.S.A.)*

13-4-5   Is It Possible to Dissociate Morphine Analgesia, Tolerance and Dependence?   376
H. Kaneto *(Japan)*

Stress-Induced Neurochemical Changes and Their Pharmacological Implications
Chairs: G. Biggio *(Italy)* and M. Tanaka *(Japan)*

13-5-1   Stress-Induced Changes in Brain Noradrenergic System and Emotions: Neurochemical Mechanism of Anxiolytic Drugs   378
M. Tanaka, Y. Yoshida, H. Yokoo, T. Tanaka, and A. Tsuda *(Japan)*

13-5-2   Central Dopamine Involvement in Stress-Induced Gastric Pathology   380
G. B. Glavin *(Canada)*

13-5-3   The Impact of Stress and Injury on Central Dopaminergic Activity   382
Michael J. Zigmond, Kristen A. Keefe, Gretchen L. Snyder, Edward M. Stricker, and Elizabeth D. Abercrombie *(U.S.A.)*

13-5-4   The Action of Stress on GABAergic Transmission   384
A. Concas, M. Serra, E. Sanna, and G. Biggio *(Italy)*

13-5-5   Dopamine and Neuropeptides Interactions in Sleep Deprivation   386
W. Fratta, P. Fadda, M. C. Martellotta, and G. L. Gessa *(Italy)*

13-5-6   CNS Targets for ACTH: Their Potential Role in Stress Responses   388
J. A. D. M. Tonnaer, W. J. Florijn, T. de Boer, and D. H. G. Versteeg *(The Netherlands)*

New Trends in the GABA$_B$ Receptor Field
Chairs: N. G. Bowery *(U.K.)* and H.-R. Olpe *(Switzerland)*

13-6-1   **GABA$_B$ Receptors in Brain Function**   390
N. G. Bowery *(U.K.)*

13-6-2   **Partial Purification of γ-Aminobutyric Acid$_B$ Receptor from Bovine Brain**   392
Y. Ohmori and K. Kuriyama *(Japan)*

13-6-3   **GABA$_B$ Receptors in the Hippocampus: Actions on Pre- and Postsynaptic Sites**   394
B. H. Gähwiler, D. A. Brown, T. Knöpfel, and S. M. Thompson *(Switzerland and U.K.)*

13-6-4   **The Role of GABA-B Receptors in the Control of Neuronal Excitability**   396
H.-R. Olpe, G. Karlsson, M. W. Steinmann, C. Kolb, F. Brugger, M. F. Pozza, and A. Hausdorf *(Switzerland)*

13-6-5   **GABA-B Receptors: From Neurotransmission to Behaviour**   398
H. Bittiger, R. Bernasconi, F. Brugger, W. Froestl, R. Hall, G. Karlsson, K. Klebs, H.-R. Olpe, M. F. Pozza, M. W. Steinmann, and H. Van Riezen *(Switzerland and U.K.)*

13-6-6   **Intrathecal Baclofen in the Treatment of Spinal Spasticity**   400
R. D. Penn, J. S. Kroin, and J. M. Magolan *(U.S.A.)*

Molecular Genetics in Basic Neuropsychopharmacology
Chairs: P. Seeburg *(F.R.G.)* and S. Nakanishi *(Japan)*

13-7-2   **Gene Transfer into Neural Crest Derived Post Mitotic Cells**   402
A. L. Boutillier, F. Barthel, B. A. Demeneix, and J. P. Loeffler *(France)*

13-7-4   **Molecular Studies of NMDA Receptors**   404
R. S. Zukin, R. Haring, L. Kushner, J. Lerma, and M. V. L. Bennett *(U.S.A.)*

13-7-5   **Spider Toxins as Probes for Glutamate Receptor**   406
N. Kawai, T. Nakajima, and T. Takenawa *(Japan)*

13-7-6   **The Structure and Function of Na$^+$ and Cl$^-$-Coupled GABA Transporter(s)**   408
B. I. Kanner, R. Radian, A. Bendahan, S. Keynan, N. Mabjeesh, A. Shouffani, J. Guastella, H. A. Lester, N. Davidson, H. Nelson, and N. Nelson *(Israel and U.S.A.)*

Basic and Clinical Approach to Dementia Syndromes
Chairs: C. G. Gottfries *(Sweden)* and T. Nishimura *(Japan)*

13-8-1   **Intermediary Metabolism Disturbance in AD/SDAT and Its Relation to Molecular Events**   410
S. Hoyer *(F.R.G.)*

13-8-2   **Neurotransmitter Changes in Early- and Late-Onset Alzheimer-Type Dementia**   412
H. Arai and R. Iizuka *(Japan)*

13-8-3   **Neurochemical Changes in Grey and White Matter and Neuroendocrine Disturbances in Dementia Disorders**   414
C. G. Gottfries *(Sweden)*

13-8-4   **Cytoskeletal Aberration in Alzheimer's Disease Fibroblasts**   416
T. Nishimura and M. Takeda *(Japan)*

13-8-5	The Neurotransmitter Bases for Depression and Dementia in Alzheimer's Disease V. Chan-Palay *(Switzerland)*	418
13-8-7	The Use of a 5-Hydroxytryptamine Reuptake Blocker (Citalopram) as an Emotional Stabilizer in Dementia Syndromes A. L. Nyth and C. G. Gottfries *(Sweden)*	420

Long-Term Treatment of Panic Disorders
Chairs: G. Klerman and D. F. Klein *(U.S.A.)*

13-9-1	Course and Outcome in Panic Disorder M. B. Keller *(U.S.A.)*	422
13-9-2	The Pathophysiology of Spontaneous Panic as Related to Respiratory Dyscontrol Donald F. Klein *(U.S.A.)*	424

Relapse, Prediction, and Maintenance Treatment of Schizophrenia
Chairs: D. P. van Kammen *(U.S.A.)* and M. Murasaki *(Japan)*

13-10-1	Intermittent vs. Maintenance Medication in Schizophrenia: Two Year Results M. I. Herz, W. M. Glazer, M. A. Mostert, M. A. Sheard, and H. V. Szymanski *(U.S.A.)*	426
13-10-2	Indication and Informed Consent for Neuroleptic Longterm Treatment in Schizophrenia H. Helmchen *(F.R.G.)*	428
13-10-3	The Clinical Significance of a Plasma Haloperidol and Fluphenazine Level T. Van Putten, S. R. Marder, W. C. Wirshing et al. *(U.S.A.)*	430
13-10-4	Clinical and Biological Predictors of Relapse in Schizophrenia S. R. Marder, T. Van Putten, M. Aravagiri, W. C. Wirshing, K. Johnson-Cronk, and M. Lebell *(U.S.A.)*	432
13-10-5	Prediction of Relapse in Schizophrenia J. Lieberman, J. Kane, M. Woerner, J. Alvir, M. Borenstein, and H. Novacenko *(U.S.A.)*	434
13-10-6	Prediction of Relapse Following Neuroleptic Withdrawal: The Role of Noradrenaline D. P. van Kammen, J. Peters, J. Yao, D. Mc Adam, A. Mouton, and W. Breeding *(U.S.A.)*	436

Regulation of Intraneuronal Calcium in Psychopharmacology
Chairs: A. C. Dolphin *(U.K.)* and N. Akaike *(Japan)*

13-11-1	Novel Ca^{2+} Currents in Mammalian CNS Neurons N. Akaike and K. Takahashi *(Japan)*	438
13-11-2	Muscarinic Receptors, Phosphoinositide Metabolism and Intracellular Calcium in Neuronal Cells S. R. Nahorski, D. G. Lambert, R. J. H. Wojcikiewicz, S. Safrany, and E. M. Whitham *(U.K.)*	440
13-11-3	Spatially Organized Intracellular Ca^{2+} Signals in Response to Different Secretagogues in Adrenal Chromaffin Cells T. R. Cheek, T. R. Jackson, R. B. Moreton, A. J. O'Sullivan, R. D. Burgoyne, and M. J. Berridge *(U.K.)*	442

13-11-4 Intracellular Ca^{2+} Stores in Non-Muscle Cells: An Overview 444
Susan Treves, Francesco Zorzato, Paola Chiozzi, Monica De Mattei,
Francesco Michelangeli, Antonello Villa, Paola Podini, Tomohide Satoh,
Jacopo Meldolesi, and Tullio Pozzan *(Italy)*

13-11-5 Pharmacological Analysis of Neuronal Calcium Channels: Interaction with G
Proteins, Second Messengers and Calcium Channel Ligands 446
A. C. Dolphin, E. Huston, R. H. Scott, and J. F. Wootton *(U.K. and U.S.A.)*

13-11-6 Role of Extrecellualr Calcium in Excitotoxic Injury of Cultured Cortical Neurons 448
D. W. Choi, J. H. Weiss, and D. M. Hartley *(U.S.A.)*

Assessment of Reinforcing Properties of Drugs: A Determinant of Abuse Liability
Chairs: N. Ator *(U.S.A.)* and T. Yanagita *(Japan)*

13-12-1 Enhancement of Reinforcing Efficacy by Development of Physical Dependence 450
K. Takada, Y. Wakasa, and T. Yanagita *(Japan)*

13-12-2 Genetic Approaches to the Analysis of Addiction Processes 452
Frank R. George *(U.S.A.)*

13-12-3 Individual Differences in Drug Preference in Humans 454
H. de Wit *(U.S.A.)*

13-12-4 Behavioral and Pharmacological Strategies for Reducing Drug Abuse 456
M. E. Carroll *(U.S.A.)*

Brain Circuitry Computer Reconstruction
Chairs: S. H. Koslow *(U.S.A.)* and A. I. Leshner *(U.S.A.)*

13-13-1 Brain Circuitry Computer Reconstruction: Human Brain Project 458
Stephen H. Koslow and Alan I. Leshner *(U.S.A.)*

13-13-2 Structure–Function Correlation of the Living Human Brain with MRI and PET: A
Means of Anatomical and Functional Localization 460
J. C. Mazziotta, D. Valentino, C. A. Pelizzari, G. T. Chen, and F. Bookstein
(U.S.A.)

13-13-3 Visualizing the 3-D Structure, Function of Brain 462
Arthur W. Toga *(U.S.A.)*

13-13-4 Multimodal 3D Imaging of EEG and MRI 464
Michael W. Torello *(U.S.A.)*

Benzodiazepine Dependence: Basic and Clinical Studies
Chairs: C. R. Schuster *(U.S.A.)* and N. Kato *(Japan)*

13-14-1 Approach to Benzodiazepine Dependence Studies Through Ligand Receptor
Binding In Vivo 466
Osamu Inoue and Toshiro Yamasaki *(Japan)*

13-14-2 Effects of Benzodiazepine and Nonbenzodiazepine Hypnotics on the Hippocampal
Rhythmic Activity in Cats 468
N. Yamaguchi, Y. Kiyota, Y. Kubota, H. Kido, H. Sakamoto, and N. Akiyama
(Japan)

13-14-3	Discriminative Stimulus and Reinforcing Effects of Benzodiazepines in Normal Human Volunteers C. E. Johanson *(U.S.A.)*	470
13-14-4	Preclinical and Clinical Studies of the Abuse and Dependence Potential of Benzodiazepines and Other Sedatives Roland R. Griffiths *(U.S.A.)*	472
13-14-5	Benzodiazepine Dependence and the Management of Withdrawal J. Guy Edwards, Timothy Cantopher, and Stefano Olivieri *(U.K.)*	474
13-14-6	International Regulation of Benzodiazepines Inayat Khan *(Switzerland)*	476

Molecular Genetics in Clinical Neuropsychopharmacology
Chairs: J. Mendlewicz *(Belgium)* and K. Mikoshiba *(Japan)*

13-15-2	Molecular Genetics of Affective Disorders J. Mendlewicz, D. Hirsch, and C. Van Broeckhoven *(Belgium)*	478
13-15-4	Linkage Studies on Chromosome 11q in Schizophrenia D. H. R. Blackwood, W. J. Muir, D. M. St. Clair, A. Hubbard, D. Baillie, and M. Walker *(Scotland)*	480
13-15-5	Molecular Genetics of Familial Alzheimer's Disease C. Van Broeckhoven, H. Backhovens, G. Van Camp, P. Stinissen, W. Van Hul, A. Lofgren, M. Cruts, A. Wehnert, G. de Winter, A. Vandenberghe, M. Bruyland, J. Gheuens, and J.-J. Martin *(Belgium)*	482
13-15-6	Molecular Genetic Research in Neurodegenerative Disease Katsuhiko Mikoshiba *(Japan)*	484

Pharmacological Treatment of Alzheimer's Disease
Chairs: G. Toffano *(Italy)* and T. Nabeshima *(Japan)*

13-16-2	Neuropathological and Behavioral Changes in Alzheimer's Disease Peter J. Whitehouse *(U.S.A.)*	486
13-16-3	NGF and Alzheimer's Disease. Perspectives from Basic Research G. Vantini, M. Fusco, L. Cavicchioli, G. Toffano, and A. Leon *(Italy)*	488
13-16-4	Tetrahydroaminoacridine in Alzheimer's Disease Leon J. Thal *(U.S.A.)*	490
13-16-5	Preclinical Pharmacology of Phosphatidylserine G. Pepeu, M. G. Vannucchi, and F. Casamenti *(Italy)*	492
13-16-6	Clinical Trials with Phosphatidylserine (PS) L. Amaducci, L. Bracco, and A. Lippi *(Italy)*	494

What's Treatable in Dementia?
Chairs: R. J. Ancill *(Canada)* and K. Hasegawa *(Japan)*

14-1-1	The Treatment of Depression in Dementia R. J. Ancill *(Canada)*	496
14-1-2	Aggression in Dementia P. V. Rabins *(U.S.A.)*	498

14-1-4	**The Pharmacological Management of Cognitive Impairment in the Demented Patient** M. S. J. Pathy *(U.K.)*	500
14-1-5	**Methodological Problems in Clinical Research in Dementia** A. Clarke *(U.K.)*	502

Alcoholism: Experimental and Clinical Studies
Chairs: R. G. Lister *(U.S.A.)* and K. Kuriyama *(Japan)*

14-2-1	**Alcohol and Anxiety** R. G. Lister *(U.S.A.)*	504
14-2-2	**Alcohol-Induced Alterations in the Function of Cerebral GABA$_A$ Receptor Complex** T. Hashimoto, T. Ueha, H. Mizutani, and K. Kuriyama *(Japan)*	506
14-2-3	**Alcohol and Anxiety: Ethopharmacological Approaches** R. J. Blanchard and D. C. Blanchard *(U.S.A.)*	508
14-2-4	**Drug Treatment of Anxiety in Alcohol Withdrawal** S. E. File, A. Zharkovsky, and P. K. Hitchcott *(U.K.)*	510
14-2-5	**Alcohol and Anxiety: A Clinical Perspective** David T. George and Markku Linnoila *(U.S.A.)*	512

Influence of Hypothalamo-Pituitary-Gonadal Axis on Brain and Behavior
Chairs: U. Halbreich *(U.S.A.)* and C. Hiemke *(F.R.G.)*

14-3-1	**Actions of Sex Hormones on the Brain** C. Hiemke and M. Banger *(F.R.G.)*	514
14-3-2	**Sensitivity to Hypothalamic Neurons to Oxytocin In Vitro: Relevance to Estrogen Induction of Lordosis Behavior** L.-M. Kow and D. W. Pfaff *(U.S.A.)*	516
14-3-4	**Hormonal Control of Socio-Sexual Approach Behavior** B. J. Meyerson *(Sweden)*	518
14-3-5	**Gonadal Hormones, Ovulation and Symptom Formation** T. Bäckström *(Sweden)*	520
14-3-6	**Influence of Gonadal Hormones on Cognitive Function in Women** E. Hampson *(Canada)*	522
14-3-7	**Gonadal Hormones, Serotonin, Noradrenaline and Mood** U. Halbreich, N. Rojansky, S. Carson, J. Piletz, and A. Halaris *(U.S.A.)*	524

Postnatal Mental Illness
Chairs: M. Sandler *(U.K.)* and T. Ban *(U.S.A.)*

14-4-1	**Neuroendocrine and Psychosocial Mechanisms in Post-Partum Psychosis** R. Kumar, A. Wieck, M. Marks, I. C. Campbell, and S. A. Checkley *(U.K.)*	526
14-4-2	**Clinical Clues to the Aetiology of Puerperal Psychosis** Ian Brockington *(U.K.)*	528
14-4-3	**Do Biochemical Factors Play a Part in Postnatal Depression?** Vivette Glover, Patricia Hannah, and Merton Sandler *(U.K.)*	530

14-4-5	Endocrine Studies of the Maternity Blues T. Okano and J. Nomura *(Japan)*	532

Trans-Ethnic Psychopharmacology
Chairs: D. Moussaoui *(Morocco)* and S. Takahashi *(Japan)*

14-5-1	Pharmacoanthropology in Psychiatry W. Kalow and T. Inaba *(Canada)*	534
14-5-3	Measurement of Haloperidol Reductase Activity in Red Blood Cells from the Japanese Psychiatric Patients S. Takahashi, T. Someya, M. Shibasaki, N. Ishida, T. Kato, and T. Noguchi *(Japan)*	536
14-5-4	Ethnic Comparison of Haloperidol and Reduced Haloperidol Plasma Levels: Chinese Versus Non-Chinese W. H. Chang, M. W. Jann, H. G. Hwu, T. Y. Chen, E. K. Yeh, C. P. Chien, L. Ereshefsky, S. R. Saklad, and A. L. Richards *(R.O.C. and U.S.A.)*	538
14-5-5	Clomipramine Plasma Levels in Maghrebian and French Depressed Patients D. Moussaoui, H. Loo, G. Ferrey, M. F. Poirier, N. Aymard, N. Kadri, and A. Squalli *(Morocco and France)*	540

Neurobehavioral Toxicology and Teratology
Chairs: V. Cuomo *(Italy)* and T. Fujii *(Japan)*

14-6-1	Problems in Laboratory Experimentation in Neurobehavioral Toxicology and Teratology Hugh A. Tilson *(U.S.A.)*	541
14-6-2	Functional Behavioural Assessment of Changes in CNS Regulatory Systems After Early Drug or Chemical Exposure G. Bignami and E. Alleva *(Italy)*	543
14-6-3	Neurobehavioral Toxicity of Immunoactive Drugs J. Elsner and G. Zbinden *(Switzerland)*	545
14-6-4	Functional Alterations Produced by Developmental Exposure to Hormones T. Fujii and M. Horinaka *(Japan)*	547
14-6-5	Neurobehavioral Changes Produced by Developmental Exposure to Psychotropic Drugs V. Cuomo, R. Cagiano, M. A. de Salvia, C. Lacomba, and G. Renna *(Italy)*	549

Benzodiazepine Receptor Function
Chairs: H. Möhler *(Switzerland)* and S. Paul *(U.S.A.)*

14-7-1	Molecular Pharmacology of the GABA/Benzodiazepine Receptor Complex H. Möhler, P. Malherbe, and G. J. Richards *(Switzerland)*	551
14-7-3	Allosteric Modulation of $GABA_A$ Receptors: Participation of Multiple Signals A. Guidotti *(U.S.A.)*	553
14-7-5	Pharmacological Profiles of Non-Benzodiazepine Ligands for Central Benzodiazepine Receptors C. R. Gardner *(U.K.)*	555

14-7-6	**Pharmacological Profile of a Novel Benzodiazepine Inverse Agonist, S-135, as a Memory Enhancer** Kazuo Kawasaki and Akira Matsushita *(Japan)*	557

Clinical Utility of Drug Monitoring in Psychiatry
Chairs: L. F. Gram *(Denmark)* and B. Müller-Oerlinghausen *(F.R.G.)*

14-8-1	**Significance of Genetic Polymorphism and Selective P450 Interactions in Psychopharmacology** L. F. Gram, K. Brøsen, E. Skjelbo, and S. Sindrup *(Denmark)*	559
14-8-2	**Monitoring Neuroleptic Drug Levels: Time for Introduction into Clinical Routine?** D. L. Garver *(U.S.A.)*	561
14-8-3	**Predicting Therapeutic Outcome from Early Pharmacokinetic Measurements of Neuroleptics** W. Gaebel, B. Müller-Oerlinghausen, and J. Schley *(F.R.G.)*	563
14-8-4	**Therapeutic Drug Monitoring of Antidepressants in Practice** Sheldon H. Preskorn *(U.S.A.)*	565
14-8-5	**The Role of Pharmacokinetics and Drug Level Monitoring in the Clinical Development of New Psychotropic Drugs** Paolo Lucio Morselli *(France)*	567
14-8-6	**Future Utilization of Pharmacokinetic Information in Psychiatry** B. Müller-Oerlinghausen *(F.R.G.)*	569

Drugs That May Enhance Cognitive Function
Chairs: L. Angelucci *(Italy)* and S. Tadokoro *(Japan)*

14-9-1	**Aspects of Animal Experiments for Evaluation of Cognitive Enhancers** H. Kuribara and S. Tadokoro *(Japan)*	571
14-9-2	**Long Term Treatment with Acetyl-L-Carnitine Reduces Age-Dependent Impairment of Cognition** L. Angelucci, O. Ghirardi, M. T. Ramacci, and A. Imperato *(Italy)*	573
14-9-3	**Pharmaco-EEG and Brain Mapping in Cognitive Enhancing Drugs** B. Saletu, J. Grünberger, and P. Anderer *(Austria)*	575
14-9-4	**New Cholinesterase Inhibitors for Treatment of Alzheimer Disease** Ezio Giacobini and Robert Becker *(U.S.A.)*	577
14-9-5	**Nicotine as a Cognitive Enhancer** D. M. Warburton *(U.K.)*	579
14-9-6	**Neuronal Phospholipid Abnormalities in Alzheimer's Disease: Therapeutic Opportunities** J. H. Growdon, I. Lopez Gonzalez-Coviella, J. K. Blusztajn, and R. J. Wurtman *(U.S.A.)*	581

Stimulant-Induced Psychoses: Relationship to Sensitization
Chairs: R. M. Post *(U.S.A.)* and M. Sato *(Japan)*

14-10-1	**Evolution of Amphetamine Psychoses, Concept and Course** M. Sato *(Japan)*	583

14-10-2	Mechanisms of Stimulant and Stress Sensitization: Where to Look Seymour M. Antelman and Anthony R. Caggiula *(U.S.A.)*	585
14-10-3	Mechanism of Methamphetamine-Induced Behavioral Sensitization K. Akiyama, T. Hamamura, H. Ujike, A. Kanzaki, and S. Otsuki *(Japan)*	587
14-10-4	Cocaine-Induced Psychosis: Comparison with Amphetamine E. H. Ellinwood and T. Lee *(U.S.A.)*	589
14-10-5	Mechanisms of Cocaine-Induced Sensitization P. W. Kalivas, P. Duffy, and J. D. Steketee *(U.S.A.)*	591
14-10-6	Anatomy and Pharmacology of Cocaine-Induced Behavioral Sensitization R. M. Post, S. R. B. Weiss, and A. Pert *(U.S.A.)*	593

Neuropeptides in Neuropsychopharmacology
Chairs: S. J. Watson *(U.S.A.)* and T. Matsuo *(Japan)*

14-11-1	Corticotropin-Releasing Factor: Preclinical and Clinical Studies C. B. Nemeroff, G. Bissette, M. J. Owens, M. A. Vargas, C. Pihoker, K. R. R. Krishnan, S. T. Cain, and C. Banki *(U.S.A. and Hungary)*	595
14-11-2	Neural Circuits Mediating Inhibition of the Hypothalamo-Pituitary-Adrenocortical Axis J. P. Herman and S. J. Watson *(U.S.A.)*	597
14-11-3	Neurotensin Involvement in the Action of Antipsychotic Drugs and the Pathogenesis of Schizophrenia G. Bissette, B. Levant, and C. B. Nemeroff *(U.S.A.)*	599
14-11-4	The Relationship Between Structural Brain Imaging, Limbic HPA Activity and CSF CRF and Catecholamine Metabolites in Affective Disorders and Schizophrenia S. C. Risch, R. J. Lewine, R. D. Jewart, N. H. Kalin, M. Stipetic, E. D. Risby, M. B. Eccard, J. Caudle, W. E. Pollard, and M. Brummer *(U.S.A.)*	601
14-11-5	The Role of CRH Systems in Mediating Psychopathology: Animal Models N. H. Kalin, L. K. Takahashi, and S. E. Shelton *(U.S.A.)*	603
14-11-6	Interleukin-1 Receptors in the Brain-Endocrine-Immune Axis Errol B. De Souza, Toshihiro Takao, and Daniel E. Tracey *(U.S.A.)*	605

Psychopharmacology of Childhood Disorder
Chairs: M. Campbell *(U.S.A.)* and H. Naruse *(Japan)*

14-12-1	Controlled Studies of the Pharmacology of Child and Adolescent Mood Disorders N. D. Ryan *(U.S.A.)*	607
14-12-2	Alprazolam Effects in Children and Adolescents with Anxiety Disorders J. G. Simeon, H. B. Ferguson, V. Knott, N. Roberts, C. Dubois, and D. Wiggins *(Canada)*	609
14-12-3	New Pharmacotherapies in Infantile Autism H. Naruse, M. Takesada, T. Hayashi, Y. Nakane, and K. Yamazaki *(Japan)*	611
14-12-4	Pharmacotherapy of Behavior Disorders R. Klein *(U.S.A.)*	613
14-12-5	Lithium in Aggressive Children with Conduct Disorder M. Campbell, A. M. Small, M. V. Padron-Gayol, J. J. Locascio, V. Kafantaris, and J. E. Overall *(U.S.A.)*	615

14-12-6 Controlled Study of Lithium for Mood and Substance Dependency Disorders in Adolescence   617
B. Geller, J. S. Williams, T. B. Cooper, and D. L. Graham *(U.S.A.)*

Neuroleptics in Low-Dosage as Therapy in Non-Psychotic Psychiatric Diseases
Chairs: W. Pöldinger *(Switzerland)* and S. Sieberns *(F.R.G.)*

14-13-1 Low Dose Neuroleptics for Nonpsychotic Diseases in Psychiatry   619
W. Pöldinger *(Switzerland)*

14-13-2 Preferential Dopamine Autoreceptor Blockade: A Possible Pharmacotherapeutic Principle in Antidepressant Therapy   621
A. Carlsson *(Sweden)*

14-13-3 Indications for a Low-Dose Neuroleptic Therapy in Non-Psychotic Psychiatric Diseases   623
H. J. Möller *(F.R.G.)*

14-13-4 Neuroleptics in the Treatment of Anxiety   625
K. Achté *(Finland)*

14-13-5 Low Dose Neuroleptanxiolysis in Anxiety States   627
K. Heinrich and E. Lehmann *(F.R.G.)*

14-13-6 Flupenthixol-Decanoat Versus Fluspirilen in Anxious-Depressive Syndromes: A Double-Blind Comparison   629
M. Osterheider *(F.R.G.)*

14-13-7 Efficacy and Tolerability of Flupenthixol-Depot in the Treatment of Depressive and Psychosomatic Disorders: A Multicenter Trial in General Practice   631
G. Budde *(F.R.G.)*

Primary Cultured Neurones in Neuropharmacological Studies
Chairs: L. Hertz *(Canada)* and R. Kato *(Japan)*

14-14-1 CNS 5-HT Neurons and Glial S-100$_B$ 633
Efrain C. Azmitia and Patricia M. Whitaker-Azmitia *(U.S.A.)*

14-14-2 Analysis of Molecular Mechanisms Underlying Up-Regulation at Cerebral Muscarinic Receptor Using Primary Cultured Cerebral Cortical Neurons   635
S. Ohkuma and K. Kuriyama *(Japan)*

14-14-3 Dynamic Aspects of Inositol Polyphosphate Metabolism in Cultured Adrenal Chromaffin Cells   637
Nobuyuki Sasakawa, Toshio Nakaki, and Ryuichi Kato *(Japan)*

14-14-4 Associative Cooperativity Between Excitatory Amino Acid (EAA) Receptors to Trigger Arachidonic Acid Release from Striatal Neurons in Culture   639
J. Bockaert, J. P. Pin, K. Oomagari, M. Sebben, and A. Dumuis *(France and Japan)*

14-14-5 Mechanisms of Drug Protection Against Neurotoxicity in Neuronal Cell Cultures   641
P. J. Pauwels and J. E. Leysen *(Belgium)*

14-14-6 Monoamine Oxidase (MAO) Activity and Monoamine Effects in Cerebellar Neurons and Astrocytes   643
L. Peng, X. M. Li, P. H. Yu, B. H. Juurlink, E. Hertz, A. V. Juorio, and L. Hertz *(Canada)*

Biochemical and Functional Aspects of Eicosanoids in the CNS
Chairs: R. Paoletti *(Italy)* and O. Hayaishi *(Japan)*

14-15-2   Further Studies on Sleep–Wake Regulation by Prostaglandins D_2 and E_2 645
Osamu Hayaishi *(Japan)*

14-15-3   Functional Sites of Cyclooxygenase Products in the CNS   647
Y. Watanabe, Yu. Watanabe, K. Matsumura, H. Onoe, P. G. Gillberg,
Y. Koyama, S. Tsubokura, and O. Hayaishi *(Japan and Sweden)*

14-15-4   Lipoxygenase Metabolites as Mediators of Synaptic Modulation   649
A. Volterra *(U.S.A.)*

14-15-5   Lipoxygenation of Arachidonic Acid (AA) in Retina   651
Nicolas G. Bazan *(U.S.A.)*

14-15-6   Prostaglandin—Hypothalamic-Pituitary-Adrenal Axis Interaction   653
A. A. Mathé, M. Thorén, N. H. Kalin, S. Shelton, P. Bergman, and C. Stenfors
(U.S.A.)

The Proper Conduct of Psychotropic Drug Evaluation
Chairs: S. Montgomery *(U.K.)* and M. Kurihara *(Japan)*

14-16-1   Guidelines to Ensure Antipanic Drugs Are Effective   655
H. G. M. Westenberg and J. A. Den Boer *(The Netherlands)*

14-16-2   Guidelines for Investigating Antidysthymic and Antidepressant Drugs Must Take
Epidemiological Data into Account   657
J. Angst *(Switzerland)*

14-16-4   Guidelines for the Evaluation of Brief Depressions and the Separation from Major
Depression   659
S. A. Montgomery, D. Montgomery, and D. Baldwin *(U.K.)*

14-16-5   Methodology and Application of Long-Term Efficacy Studies for Long-Term
Illnesses   661
J. M. Danion and S. Montgomery *(France and U.K.)*

ADDRESS LIST   663
AUTHOR INDEX   681

Proceedings of the
17th Collegium Internationale
Neuro-Psychopharmacologicum
Congress

SEROTONIN AND PSYCHIATRY

D.G. GRAHAME-SMITH
MRC Unit and University Department of Clinical
Pharmacology, Radcliffe Infirmary, Oxford, OX2 6HE, U.K.

5-HT is a signalling molecule with the CNS. Its signal may result in a very quick response, e.g. ion channel opening, or in a slow response, e.g. a second messenger cascade culminating in gene expression, or in responses with intermediate latencies. The molecular functions of 5-HT are therefore extremely versatile. This versatility is extended by the occurrence of neuroadaptive responses which change the way 5-HT acts.

In recent years there has been an explosion in the number of recognised specific 5-HT subtypes. At first they were characterised by binding, biochemical and behavioural studies and now their separate existence has been proven by genetic cloning techniques. The multiplicity of 5-HT receptors and the evolving knowledge of their functions in the control of the activity of 5-HT systems themselves and other neurotransmitter systems, promises to be immensely beneficial in the therapy of mental illness.

At a level of increased complexity it is apparent that from three groups of raphe nuclei in the pons/medulla, eminate different types of 5-HT neurone. They project to many areas of the brain and spinal cord. They have been shown to have different anatomies and functions, though their commonality is the release of 5-HT. Different 5-HT neurones may innervate the same brain area presumably exerting different effects. There is therefore ample scope for separate 5-HT systems to influence in different ways multiple areas of the brain involved in psychological, cognitive, sensory, autonomic, neuroendocrine and emotional function. Personally, I begin to see that it is possible for drugs affecting 5-HT function to be effective in a diverse range of mental illnesses: manic-depressive disease, anxiety, obsessional states, alcoholism, eating disorders, Alzheimers disease, agressivity, and maybe schizophrenia.

We are able now to manipulate with drugs many aspects of 5-HT function: synthesis, storage, release, and action at receptor level and beyond in the ensuing cascades. Since drugs act at a molecular level some newer concepts of influencing 5-HT function will be reviewed examining particularly, the $5-HT_{1A}$ anxiolytics, lithium, antidepressants and ECT. The potential for manipulating various aspects of 5-HT function by interfering with calcium and potassium channel function will be discussed.

There is another world of serotonin in Psychiatry, outside this molecular one. I shall attempt to analyse the types of evidence adduced for the intrinsic involvement of 5-HT in manic-depressive illness, in anxiety, obsessive-compulsive disorder, alcoholism and eating disorders. So far this evidence is indirect and far from watertight. Nevertheless, the actions of drugs with specific actions of 5-HT, many _in vivo_ and _in vitro_ biochemical studies in man, and the results of 5-HT-related neuroendocrine challenge tests, do provide an impressive body of evidence that abnormalities of 5-HT function are involved in the "causation" of some mental syndromes, particularly depression.

A new and controversial hypothesis will be put forward to invoke more specifically abnormalities of 5-HT-linked neuronal ion channel function in the causation of depression and its treatment with lithium, antidepressants and ECT.

THE COURSE OF AFFECTIVE DISORDERS: IMPLICATIONS FOR PSYCHOPHARMACOLOGY

J. ANGST
Psychiatric University Hospital Zurich, Research Department, Zurich, Switzerland

A correct treatment of patients with affective disorders requires a solid knowledge of the course for the following reasons: choice of drug, selection of suitable patients for long-term prophylactic medication, termination of the treatment of an episode or a prophylaxis, unwanted effects from ECT or drugs on the natural history of affective disorder (e.g. recurrence, re-hospitalization, switch from depression to hypomania, rapid cycling, etc.)

Important elements describing course and natural history are: age of onset, length and amplitude of episodes and cycles, change of psychopathology, outcome in terms of recovery, chronicity, organic brain syndromes and suicide. Prospective studies on the course provide us with descriptive and predictive models of the natural history of affective disorders of psychiatric patients, patients from primary care facilities and community samples.

The course is a fundamental classifier for affective disorder, for the distinction of subgroups of the bipolar and unipolar depressive spectra, the schizo-affective spectrum, and the definition of monophasic, oligophasic, polyphasic depression, rapid cyclers, continuous recurrent and chronic course patterns, and finally, seasonal affective disorder. The course can also be used as a validator of psychiatric classification if the latter is clearly independent.

Community studies suggest the existence of a broad spectrum of minor and major affective syndromes. The bipolar spectrum embraces hyperthymic personality traits or mild hypomanic mood swings (m), severe manic episodes (M), preponderant manic bipolar disorder (Md), nuclear bipolar manic disorder with severe mania and depression (MD), bipolar II disorder (mD) of Dunner et al. (1), cyclothymia (md). In a similar way depressive syndromes can be classified by severity into minor and major ones.

The subgroups are defined by their course pattern: major depressive disorder (single-episode, recurrent, chronic), dysthymia and recurrent brief depression all belong to the same unipolar depressive spectrum. Some groups differ in sex ratio, age of onset, and recurrence rates: bipolar episodes manifest earlier, are briefer, and show much higher recurrence but probably lower suicide rates than unipolar depression. Life-table analyses show a linear distribution of suicide over lifetime (no increase, no decrease).

The female-male ratio is higher in major depression than in recurrent brief depression and it is higher in bipolar II than in bipolar I disorders. Recurrence and outcome, including suicide rates, do not show sex differences.

Recent findings suggest that ECT can switch unipolar depression to bipolar disorder, furthermore ECT is associated with an increase of rates of hospitalization as shown by Winokur and Kadrmas (2). Antidepressant drugs can deteriorate recurrence of bipolar disorders in some cases, but a drug-induced switch from depression to hypomania is still unproven.

There is good evidence of a reduction of suicide attempts with a long-term prophylactic medication. Up to now there is no data, but hope for a preventive effect on suicide.

More detailed reviews were given by the author on the course of depressive illness (3) and of schizo-affective psychoses (4).

REFERENCES

1. Dunner, D.L., Fleiss, J.L., Fieve, R.R.: The course of development of mania in patients with recurrent depression. Am. J. Psychiatr. 133: 905-908, 1976.
2. Winokur, G., Kadrmas, A.: Convulsive therapy and the course of bipolar illness, 1940-1949. Convuls. Therapy 4: 126-132, 1988.
3. Angst, J.: Clinical course of affective disorders. In: Depressive illness: Prediction of course and outcome, edited by T. Helgason and R.J. Daly, Springer Verlag, Berlin, pp. 1-44, 1988.
4. Angst, J.: The course of schizoaffective disorders. In: Schizoaffective psychoses, edited by A. Marneros, M.T.Tsuang, Springer Verlag, Berlin, pp.63-93, 1986.

The Adrenergic Receptors: Structure/Function and Regulation

Robert J. Lefkowitz, M.D., Duke University Medical Center, Durham, NC, USA

Receptors which recognize and initiate the actions of catecholamines such as adrenaline and noradrenaline are known as adrenergic receptors. Based on pharmacological criteria, several distinct types of adrenergic receptors have been classified. Biochemically, these are coupled through guanine nucleotide regulatory proteins to several cellular effector systems such as adenylate cyclase and phospholipase C. Moreover, the adrenergic receptors are prototypic for a wider family of receptor molecules all of which are coupled through guanine nucleotide regulatory proteins to various biochemical effector enzymes, ion channels, etc. Our group has extensively characterized all of the known members of the adrenergic receptor family as well as several closely related receptors. The genes for each of these have been cloned and the deduced sequences shown to be closely related not only one to another but to

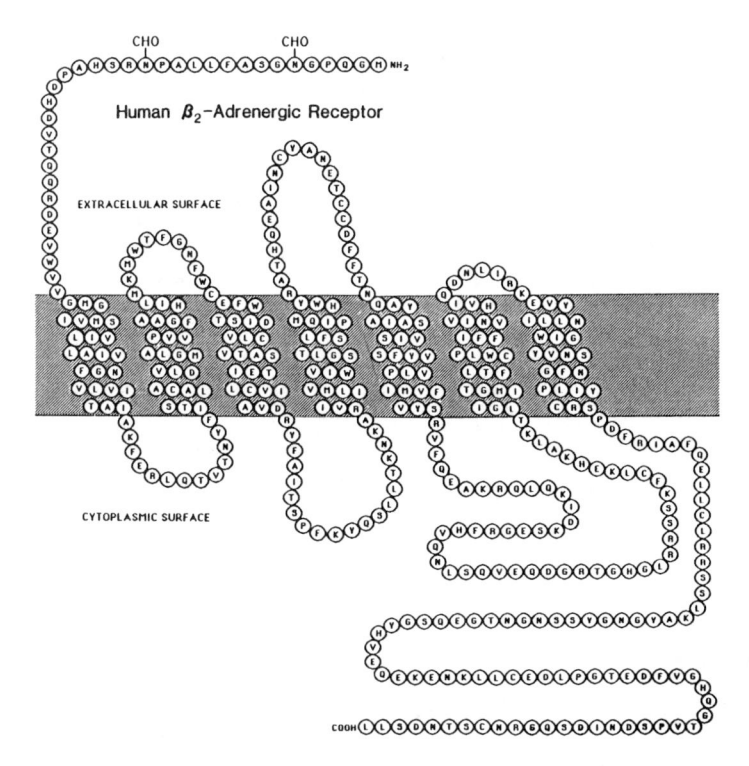

Fig. 1: Structure of the human β_2-adrenergic receptor as it may be organized within the plasma membrane.

the visual receptor rhodopsin and to several other receptors such as the muscarinic cholinergic receptors (1,2). All of these receptors have a characteristic seven membrane spanning domain topography (Fig. 1).

The function of the receptors is controlled by various means. One important mechanism is covalent modification by phosphorylation on cytoplasmic domains (3). In addition to the cyclic AMP dependent protein kinase, a cyclic AMP independent kinase, which we have termed βARK, (for beta-adrenergic receptor kinase) is involved in this regulation. The role of βARK in mediating aspects of rapid agonist-induced desensitization of the receptor has been shown in several ways including: a) demonstration that in vitro phosphorylation of the receptor by βARK decreases its function under appropriate experimental conditions; b) demonstration that site directed mutagenesis of the receptor so as to remove the sites of phosphorylation of the enzyme leads to marked attenuation of the desensitization process and c) by the development of inhibitors of βARK which have been shown, in permeabilized cell systems, to markedly attenuate the desensitization process. Such inhibitors of regulatory enzymes which normally lead to desensitization may ultimately provide a novel class of therapeutic agents which may serve to prolong and augment the therapeutic efficacy of many different classes of pharmacological agents by preventing rapid desensitization to their actions.

REFERENCES

1. Dohlman, H.G., Caron, M.G., and Lefkowitz, R.J. A family of receptors coupled to guanine nucleotide regulatory proteins. Biochemistry 26:2657-2664, 1987.
2. Lefkowitz, R.J. and Caron, M.G. Adrenergic Receptors. J. Biol. Chem. 263:4993-4996, 1988.
3. Benovic, J.L., Bouvier, M., Caron, M.G. and Lefkowitz, R.J. Regulation of adenylyl cyclase-coupled β-adrenergic receptors. Ann. Rev. Cell Biol. 4:405-428, 1988.

PRESYNAPTIC RECEPTORS IN PSYCHOPHARMACOLOGY

S.Z. LANGER, A.M. GALZIN and S. ARBILLA
Department of Biology, Synthélabo Recherche (L.E.R.S., 58, rue de la Glacière, 75013 Paris, France

The concept of presynaptic receptors modulating the release of neurotransmitters has arisen from studies on peripheral noradrenergic neurons (1), and has now been extended to the central nervous system for several neurotransmitters, such as noradrenaline, serotonin, acetylcholine and dopamine (2). It is possible to differentiate between presynaptic inhibitory autoreceptors, acted upon by transmitters which can regulate their own release and in some cases their synthesis, and presynaptic heteroreceptors sensitive to endogenous compounds other than the neuron's own transmitter. In addition to the presynaptic receptors modulating transmitter release, presynaptic recognition sites associated with the transporter at the level of the nerve terminal were characterized in serotoninergic, noradrenergic and dopaminergic neurons (3). These presynaptic sites associated with the transporter system differ pharmacologically from the presynaptic autoreceptors which modulate the release of transmitters.

Table 1 : PRESYNAPTIC RECEPTORS CONTROLLING NEUROTRANSMISSION

NEUROTRANSMITTER RELEASE	PRESYNAPTIC RECEPTOR INHIBITORY	FACILITATORY
NORADRENALINE (NA)	α_2-adrenergic μ and δ opiate D_2-dopaminergic	$GABA_A$-ω complex
DOPAMINE (DA)	D_2-dopaminergic	M_2-muscarinic
ACETYLCHOLINE (Ach)	M_2-muscarinic D_2-dopaminergic μ and δ opiate	-
SEROTONIN (5HT)	$5HT_1$* α_2-adrenergic D_1-dopaminergic	$5HT_3$ $GABA_A$-ω complex

* $5HT_{1B}$ in rat and mouse ; $5HT_{1D}$ in man, both in nerve terminals ; $5HT_{1A}$ in neuronal cell bodies.

In table 1 are shown the different presynaptic receptors involved in the modulation of monoamines and Ach release in the central nervous system.

Presynaptic autoreceptors which inhibit NA, DA, Ach and 5HT release as well as the $5HT_3$ facilitatory autoreceptor are acted upon by their own neurotransmitter. Blockade of α_2-adrenergic, D_2-dopaminergic, M_2-muscarinic and $5HT_1$ inhibitory receptors increases the release of the respective neurotransmitters while blockade of $5HT_3$ facilitatory autoreceptor inhibits 5HT release. A physiological role has also been established for the presynaptic D_2-dopamine heteroreceptor modulating Ach release, and in some brain regions for the α_2-adrenergic heteroreceptor modulating 5HT release. The facilitatory M_2-muscarinic receptor modulating DA release also seems to play a physiological role. Presynaptic autoreceptor D_2-agonists may be useful in schizophrenia while α_2-adrenoceptor antagonists and $5HT_1$-autoreceptor antagonists may be potential antidepressants.

The physiological role of the $GABA_A-\omega$ (BZ) complex at modulating NA and 5HT release remains an open question because of the lack of effects of flumazenil on its own. However activation of ω-receptors by agonists facilitates transmitter release indicating the physiological involvement of GABA.

On the other hand, it is well established that opiate receptor agonists can inhibit NA and Ach release, while D_2 agonists inhibit NA release and D_1 agonists inhibit 5HT release. However selective blockade of these presynaptic heteroreceptors does not result in changes of transmitter release indicating that these receptors are not physiologically activated.

Presynaptic transporter systems for monoamines represent the main physiological mechanism of inactivation of the released transmitters. Their blockade result in an increase in the availability of neurotransmitters in the synaptic gap and is linked to antidepressant effects.

CONCLUSION

Presynaptic receptors modulating transmitter release represent potential pharmacological targets for new drugs. The development of drugs with selectivity for these presynaptic modulatory receptors may offer a new approach in the treatment by correcting altered neurotransmission implicated in the pathology of some psychiatric disorders.

REFERENCES

1. Langer, S.Z. Presynaptic regulation of catecholamine release. Biochem. Pharmacol. 23:1793-1800, 1974.
2. Langer, S.Z. Presynaptic regulation of the release of catecholamines. Pharmacol. Rev., 32:337-362, 1981.
3. Langer, S.Z. Presynaptic regulation of monoaminergic neurons. In: Psychopharmacology: A Generation of Progress, H.Y. Meltzer, ed, pp. 151-157. Raven Press, New York.

MOVEMENTS OF CALCIUM ION IN CELLS AND NEURONAL FUNCTION

M. ENDO
Department of Pharmacology, Faculty of Medicine, University of Tokyo, Bunkyo-ku, Tokyo, Japan

It has been well known that besides triggering exocytotic release of neurotransmitters, calcium ion may also play an important role in a number of functional processes in nerve cells especially in those to lead to modulations or adaptations in their functions. In these relatively long-term functions calcium ion acts as an intracellular second messenger and initiates a cascade of complex reactions, with or without interacting with other second messengers such as cyclic nucleotides, diacylglycerol or inositol trisphosphate in complex ways, sometimes collaboratively and sometimes antagonistically.

Calcium ion thus regulates functions of ion channels, various biochemical reactions and cytoskeletal structures. These effects of calcium ion are initiated by binding of calcium ion to the calcium-receptive protein in the reaction sysytem. In some cases, calcium-receptive proteins themselves are the member proteins responsible for the functions, and conformational changes of the receptive proteins induced by calcium ion directly lead to performance of the respective function, as in the case of contraction of striated muscles. In other cases, the effect of calcium ion is exerted indirectly through the phosphorylation or dephosphorylation of the functional proteins. The regulation of protein phosphorylation by calcium ion could be achieved again either directly by calcium-dependent protein kinases or phosphatases, or indirectly by altering the level of other second messengers such as cyclic nucleotides or diacylglycerol which regulate phosphorylation. In any cases, the magnitude of the reactions is determined primarily by the extent and duration of elevation in calcium ion concentration at the site of the calcium-receptive protein of the reaction system.

The elevation of calcium ion concentration in the cytoplasm is brought about either by influx of calcium ion from the extracellular medium or by release of calcium ion from intracellular calcium stores. In both cases, movement of calcium ion occurs passively, along the electrochemical potential gradient, through calcium channels in the plasma membrane or in the membrane of the intracellular calcium store, most probably endoplasmic reticulum. The calcium channels in the plasma membrane are entirely different from channels in the membrane of the calcium store. Furthermore, in each membrane there exist more than one types of calcium channels. Therefore, properties of calcium ion mobilization can be understood only after elucidating how openings of these calcium channels are regulated.

The removal of elevated caclium ion is made in the reverse direction, namely, by extruding it to the extracellular medium or by taking it up to the intracellular calcium store. The movement of calcium ion in these processes is against the electrochemical potential gradient and requires energy-supplied active transport. Again, different kinds of calcium pumps operate in the plasma and the store membranes, and in the plasma membrane sodium-calcium exchange system, which, combined with the sodium pump, constitutes a secondary active calcium transport mechanism, also functions for extrusion of calcium ion.

In this talk, I shall primarily describe the mechanisms of calcium mobilization, especially those of calcium release from intracellular stores, based mainly on our studies on muscle cells, in the belief that the essential processes are the same, at least qualitatively, in nerve cells as well.

There are at least two types of calcium release channels in the membrane of calcium stores, calcium-induced calcium release (CICR) channel and inositol trisphosphate-induced calcium release (IICR) channel. CICR channels in the sarcoplasmic reticulum of striated muscles have been well characterized. They are activated by a micromolar level of calcium ion, but at higher concentrations approaching a millimolar level an inhibitory effect of calcium ion on CICR also becomes apparent. Caffeine enhances CICR in such a way that in the presence of the drug lower concentrations of calcium ion are required to activate the CICR channel, and maximal channel activity at the optimal calcium ion concentration is increased. Magnesium ion has an exactly opposite effect; it reduces the calcium-sensitivity as well as the maximal activity of the CICR channel. All the adenine derivatives, typically ATP, increases the open probability of the CICR channel without altering its calcium-sensitivity. Procaine, tetracaine and some (but not all) other local anesthetics inhibits CICR. A plant alkaloid, ryanodine, specifically acts on the CICR channel; it binds the channel only when the channel is open, and fixes the channel in an open state. Utilizing this specific binding, the CICR channel protein from skeletal muscle has been isolated in several laboratories and sequenced by Numa's group.

IICR channels have some similar features to those of CICR channels. Thus, they are similarly affected by calcium ion, adenine derivatives and procaine. However, unlike CICR IICR can be activated by inositol trisphosphate in the complete absence of calcium ion, but the IICR channel activity is strongly enhanced by a submicromolar level of calcium ion, while micromolar level of calcium ion exerts an inhibitory action as well. Also unlike CICR, IICR is not affected by magnesium ion, caffeine or ryanodine, but inhibited by heparin. IICR channel protein from cerebellum has also been sequenced by Mikoshiba's group.

These calcium release channels may be heterogeneously distributed among intracellular calcium stores. IICR channels are thought to respond to inositol trisphosphate produced by agonist-receptor interaction, while the physiological function of CICR channels in many cells are still not clear except in striated muscles, where CICR channels are thought to be the physiological calcium release channels although the mode of physiological channel opening is quite different from CICR itself, even in cardiac muscle.

Calcium channels in the surface membrane are not uniform either, consisting of different types of voltage-dependent calcium channels and of so-called receptor-operated calcium channels. The spatial and temporal distribution of calcium ion in the cells as a result of activities of these various calcium channels in the plasma and the store membranes as well as of calcium extrusion or uptake activity together with its functional implications will also be discussed.

THE BRAIN AS REGULATOR AND TARGET OF HORMONES
Florian Holsboer
Max-Planck-Institute for Psychiatry, Munich, F.R.G.

Any kind of behavioral change is reflecting altered function of the brain. Sensory inputs are transformed into neural activity and - according to the meaning it has for the individual -processed into physiological events. Depending upon an individual's genetic disposition, personal past history and command of coping devices the adaptive demand ("stress") will trigger differential internal bodily strains. The qualitative and quantitative nature of these internal strains is critical for development and course of illness. Given that a cognitive input is recognized as potentially stressful in the cerebral cortex, the brain stem and limbic system will be individually activated. Within the latter brain structure, the hippocampus and particularly the hypothalamus regulate the neuroendocrine, autonomic, nervous and neuroimmune systems. In turn, the affected peripheral endocrine glands and immune tissues produce compounds that feed back to the brain in a differentiated mode. In addition to these functional pathways linking the brain to peripheral organs and tissues, there is now ample evidence for a direct two-way communication between the immune and endocrine systems.

Within this conceptual framework investigating the physiological aspect of stress and in particular the limbic hypothalamic-pituitary-adrenocortical-(LHPA)system is of particular promise. In response to a cognitive or non-cognitive stressor this neuroendocrine system is activated. The key hormone to achieve this activation is corticotropin-releasing hormone (CRH), which controls peripherally circulating levels of ACTH and cortisol. CRH is not only involved in the endocrine adaptation to stress, but also in some of the stress related behavioral changes, such as disturbed sleep, loss of appetite and sexual drive, anxiety and altered locomotor activity. Recent clinical studies now support that several symptoms of major depression are mediated by CRH and other neuropeptides involved in fine-tuning of CRH effects. The immunological implication of central CRH overproduction is a peripheral decrease of natural killer cell cytotoxicity. The hypothesis of a central CRH excess as one possible cause for depression opens a new territory of possible treatments for affective illness. A first step into this development is to study why the hypersecretion of corticosteroids or the synthetic analogue dexamethasone fails to successfully feedback on CRH biosynthesis and release.

This brings us to the issue how the brain changes its physiologic function while overexposed to corticosteroids. A binary receptor system - mineralo- and glucocorticoid receptors - is involved in differential control of brain functions, regulating endocrine and non-endocrine behavior. At the cellular level cytosolic corticosteroid receptors are activated by their ligands and enhance or suppress transcription of many genes including those, which code for peptides thought to be involved in overt behavior or immune defense. The interplay between CRH, cortisol and interleukin-1ß is among the best studied examples of this kind.

The activation of the pituitary-adrenocortical hormone secretion triggered by brain circuits is nonspecific for precipitation of any particular disease. What clinically results from LHPA hyperactivity depends on an individual's vulnerability resulting from the genetic "blueprint" and the shaping of brain circuitry by environmental and experiential influences. Although it remains unresolved how cognitive processes are transduced into physiologic events, most evidence points to the limbic system as the locus where final steps of transduction from mental stress into neuroendocrine response patterns.

ANIMAL STUDY ON THE ROLE OF SEROTONIN IN DEPRESSION

HARUO NAGAYAMA
Department of Neuropsychiatry, Medical College of Oita,
Oita 879-56, Japan

The serotonin (5-HT) deficiency theory still has considerable influence on the understanding of depression despite the numerous contradictions. We conducted a series of experiments to clarify the role of 5-HT in depression.

1. Study Using a Tetrabenazine (TBZ)-Induced Model
Using TBZ-induced behavioral depression (BD) in rats, we obtained the following results:
1) 5-HT decrease and 5-hydroxyindole acetic acid (5-HIAA) increase in the brain coincided with the occurrence of TBZ-induced BD. Changes in norepinephrine and dopamine levels, however, did not coincide with the development of BD.
2) PCPA shortened the duration of TBZ-induced BD.
3) Concomitant administration of TBZ and 5-hydroxytryptophan (5-HTP) at doses too low to produce BD when used alone produced BD and an increase in 5-HIAA in the brain.

2. Pharmaco-behavioral Study Using a 5-HTP-Induced Model
Rats were trained to push a pedal continuously by operant conditioning. Following IP administration of L-5-HTP 25 mg/kg, the pedalling activity decreased significantly for several hours. Various drugs were administered one hour before 5-HTP administration.
1) Methysergide blocked 5-HTP-induced BD and led to behavior normalization during both acute and chronic administration. By contrast, fluoxetine increased 5-HTP-induced BD.
2) After chronic administration of various antidepressants, 5-HTP was administered according to the above method. Mianserine, desipramine, doxepine, imipramine, and trazodone all blocked 5-HTP-induced BD at comparable clinical doses. Generally, their blocking activities increased with time. In contrast, chlorpromazine demonstrated no effect on 5-HTP-induced BD. These results suggest that the antidepressants normalize behavior by blocking postsynaptic 5-HT receptors when excessive transmission of 5-HT receptors is induced by 5-HTP at the synapse. One possible mechanism responsible for this blocking of postsynaptic 5-HT receptors is primary, direct blocking by antidepressants. Another possible mechanism is blocking of the re-uptake of 5-HT, which increases 5-HT at the synaptic cleft, thereby secondarily decreasing the sensitivity of post synaptic 5-HT receptors. However, there was a positive correlation between the

blocking effects of antidepressants at both day 1 and week 3 after the start of administration. In other words, no inverse relation was noted as suggested by the latter theory. Clomipramine and zimelidine demonstrated no effect on BD during both acute and chronic administration. Fluoxetine, on the other hand, increased BD substantially. There was a significant positive correlation between the IC50 of re-uptake blocking rates of antidepressants and the blockade percentage of BD by these drugs. Namely, the weaker the drug's ability to block re-uptake of 5-HT, the greater its blocking effect on 5-HTP-induced BD. These findings suggest that antidepressants directly block the postsynaptic 5-HT receptors, thus resulting in normalization of behavior.

3. Biochemical Study Using the 5-HTP-Induced Model
Chronic administration of mianserine for 21 days resulted in a substantial increase in the Bmax of 5-HT1A receptors in the frontal cerebral cortex of rats. A similar phenomenon was observed for amitriptyline, desipramine, doxepine, and trazodone. These results suggest that chronic blocking of postsynaptic 5-HT1A receptors by antidepressants increases the number of these receptors. However, the degree of inhibition of forskolin-induced adenylate cyclase by 8-OH-DPAT was not affected by chronic administration of antidepressants. Further investigations are necessary on the functional role of 5-HT1A receptors in the pathogenesis of depression.
Chronic administration of mianserine produced no changes in the number of 5-HT1B receptors, the levels of 5-HT, 5-HTP, and 5-HIAA, or the metabolic turnover of 5-HT in the brain. The only change noted was a decrease in the number of 5HT2 receptor-binding sites in the frontal cerebral cortex. At present we are investigating its functional role in the development of depression.

4. Hypothesis of Excessive Transmission of 5-HT
Our data suggests that BD used in our model of depression resulted from excessive transmission of 5-HT at the synaptic cleft. Many antidepressants seem to relieve BD and eventually normalize behavior by blocking this phenomenon postsynaptically. Then, their antidepressant effects in humans may be produced by inhibiting postsynaptic transmission of 5-HT in the brain. This in turn suggests that excessive transmission of the 5-HT system plays a pathogenic role in at least several subtypes of human depression.

Acknowledgment: The first half of this report presents the results of collaborative research with Prof. Ryo Takahashi.

Responsiveness of the 5-HT$_2$ Receptor Family in Affective Disorders

M. Mikuni, A. Kagaya, Y. Kuroda, F. Kato and K. Takahashi
Division of Mental Disorder Research, National Institute of
Neuroscience, N.C.N.P., Kodaira, Tokyo, 187, Japan

Ryo Takahashi has proposed as great result of collabolation with M.H. Aprison and his colleagues that there develops a compensatory supersensitivity of postsynaptic receptor in depressed patients, due to chronic low levels of 5-HT function. Endocrinological study and platelet study on 5-HT receptor function in affective disorders may permit the investigation of receptor function in living persons. It is well-known that H.Y. Meltzer and his colleagues postulated increased hypothalamic 5-HT$_2$ receptor function in depressed patients based on the finding of an increased cortisol respose to 5-HTP in depressed patients.

In this preliminary work, we have determined 5-HT(100uM) stimulated inositol monophosphate accumulation for 15min or Ca spike amplitude 15sec after 5-HT(10uM) stimulation in platelets from unmedicated depressed patients(mean age was 42, mean Hamilton rating score was 24), compared with normal controls (mean age was 38) as a mean of assessing 5-HT$_2$ receptor function. We have also investigated whether a lowering the metabolism of 5-HT by subchronic treatment with para-chlorophenylalanine(PCPA, 300mg/kg for the first 5 days, then 100mg/kg for the following 5 days, ip; or 100mg/kg for 10 days, ip) enhances postsynaptic 5-HT receptor-mediated phosphoinositide hydrolysis in rat hippocampal slices. Next question is which receptor subtype plays a role in 5-HT agonist stimulated corticosterone secretion, since 5-HT$_2$ and 5-HT$_{1c}$ receptors exhibit striking conservation of amino acid sequence and also modulate similar intracellular signaling pathways. We tried to investigate the effect of 5-HT$_{1c}$ agonist and 5-HT$_2$ antagonist, m-chlorophenylpiperazine(m-CPP,3mg/kg,sc) challenged at the light phase in a 24-h light-dark cycle on blood corticosterone level of rat. We have also investigated whether subchronic administration of tricyclic antidepressants agents(7-9mg/kg,po) alter blood corticosterone levels 1h after m-CPP challenging.

RESULTS AND DISCUSSION

The inositol monophosphate accumulation at 100uM 5-HT was significantly increased in platelets from unmedicated patients with major depression as compared to control subjects(150 ± 7% of basal for depressed patients, 132 ± 3% for controls)(1). The spike amplitude of Ca ion induced by 10uM 5-HT was also increased in platelets from another group of unmedicated depressed patients, compared with normal controls(128 ± 6nM over basal for depressed patients, 109 ± 6nM over basal for controls), although the basal level of Ca ion in platelets were unchanged in both depressed patients and controls(73 ± 4nM). These results indicate that responsiveness of 5-HT$_2$ receptor coupled with an effector system is increased in platelets from depressed patients, although the recent findings concerning the density of 5-HT$_2$ receptor binding in platelets from depressed patients are inconsistent(2)(3).

10-day treatment with high dose of PCPA resulted in a significant increase(225% of basal) in the response of inositol monophosphate accumulation to 5-HT via both 5-HT$_2$ and 5-HT$_{1c}$ receptor in rat hippocampal slices(4), whereas low dose of PCPA had no significant effect upon the 5-HT(100uM) response as compared to vehicle(173% for low dose of PCPA, 173% for vehicle). High dose of PCPA caused 98% reduction in the level of 5-HT and 42% reduction in NE content with no significant difference from low dose of PCPA in the cerebral cortex. It is not clear what factor makes the difference between the effct of high and low dose of PCPA on 5-HT induced inositol monophosphate accumulation, but it is unlikely to be due to the difference of amines and their metabolites levels. Lowering the level of 5-HT in brain may not be enough to produce the enhancement of 5-HT induced inositol monophosphate accumulation.

m-CPP produced a remarkable increase in blood corticosterone levels to 17 times than vehicle. This increase was completely blocked by an equipotent 5-HT$_{1c}$ and 5-HT$_2$ antagonist,mianserin(3mg/kg) or ritanserin(1mg/kg) pretreatment. However, spiperone(3mg/kg), ketanserin(1mg/kg) or propranolol(20mg/kg) did not affect the m-CPP induced increase in blood corticosterone levels. These results indicate that the response of blood corticosterone release to m-CPP is mediated by 5-HT$_{1c}$ receptors, and are consistent with the recent report that 5-HT$_2$ and 5-HT$_{1c}$ agonist, MK-212 activates 5-HT$_{1c}$ receptor to produce ACTH secretion. Subchronic administration of desipramine(7mg/kg, po) was able to reduce the m-CPP stimulated corticostrone secretion to 60%, significantly as compared to controls. Imipramine, or clomipramine(9mg/kg, po) also produce the same tendency to reduce the m-CPP response to 75% of controls, but not significant(5). It is, therefore, indicated that 5-HT$_{1c}$ receptor-mediated effector system may be reduced by subchronic treatment with tricyclic antidepressant agents.

In conclusion, it is clear that hyperresponsiveness of 5-HT$_2$ receptors is present in platelets from major depressive patients. However, it may now be possible to begin to consider that 5-HT$_{1c}$ receptors may also play a role in the pathogenesis of affective disorders as well as 5-HT$_2$ receptors.

REFERENCE

1. Mikuni, M. et al.:Soc for Neurosci Abstr 15(1):pp673 (1989)
2. Biegon, A. et al.:Life Sci. 41:2485-2492 (1987)
3. Cowen, P.J. et al.:J.Affect. Dis. 13:45-50 (1987)
4. Kusumi, I. et al.:J. Neural Transm. 80: (in press)
5. Kato, F. et al.:Life Sci (submitted)

IS SEROTONERGIC FUNCTION REALLY ABNORMAL IN MAJOR DEPRESSION?

H.Y. MELTZER, M. SCHREIBER, B. BASTANI AND J.F. NASH
Department of Psychiatry, Case Western Reserve University School of Medicine, Cleveland, OH, U.S.A.

There are numerous lines of evidence which suggest an abnormality of serotonin (5-HT) in major depression (5). Broadly speaking, they fall into two categories: basic and clinical. Basic research indicates that the mechanism of action of antidepressant drugs, ECT and lithium is, at least in part, via their ability to enhance serotonergic activity. Clinical studies involving: dietary tryptophan manipulation, plasma tryptophan levels, CSF 5-hydroxyindoleacetic acid (5-HIAA), platelet $5-HT_2$ and imipramine binding sites and 5-HT uptake, neuroendocrine challenge studies, postmortem studies of 5-HT receptors, and consideration of the effect of enhancing serotonergic function on the treatment of depression, are consistent with decreased 5-HT as a factor in depression.

In aggregate, these lines of research provide compelling evidence for the 5-HT hypothesis of depression. The evidence, in particular, for an abnormality of $5-HT_2$ receptors in the brain (1) and platelets of depressed patients (2), seems to be particularly robust. However, the cortisol response to MK-212, a $5-HT_2/5-HT_{1C}$ agonist is not significantly different in depressed patients compared to normal controls (Meltzer et al., unpublished results). Nevertheless, there is mixed evidence for a decrease in the 5-hydroxytryptophan-induced increase in cortisol secretion, which also appears to be $5-HT_2/5-HT_{1C}$ mediated (4,6)].

Results will be presented on CSF 5-HIAA and homovanillac acid levels which indicate only a weak relationship to severity of depression.

Plasma tryptophan, total and free, levels were measured in unmedicated depressed patients and were within normal limits. Plasma tryptophan was significantly lower in females but did not differ in normal and depressed females. We have previously reported evidence for a decreased availablity of tryptophan following a tryptophan load in some depressed patients (3), which could contribute to decreased 5-HT synthesis.

There is, however, some evidence not consistent with the hypothesis of decreased serotonergic activity in depression. Tianeptine, a drug which promotes the reuptake of 5-HT from the synapse, has been reported to be an effective antidepressant. Fluoxetine and other specific 5-HT uptake blockers are no more effective than typical antidepressant drugs in treating major depression, although they are more effective in treating obsessive-compulsive disorder. Nevertheless, neuroendocrine evidence will be presented which indicates that suggest these agents are more effective than the typical antidepressant drugs in promoting both pre- and postsynaptic serotonergic activity (Meltzer, H.Y., unpublished data). This includes the effect of postsynaptic 5-HT$_2$/5-HT$_{1C}$ receptor stimulation. However, it may be that this augmentation by the 5-HT blockers does not occur for other types of 5-HT receptors.

Serotonin is but one of many neurotransmitters and neuromodulators implicated in depression. The possibility of an interaction between 5-HT and the catecholaminergic system, in particular, seems most attractive.

Specific subtypes of depression, e.g., psychotic depression, or only specific symptoms of depression, e.g., sleep disturbance and anorexia, may be related to serotonergic dysfunction rather than all aspects of major depression. New methods to study serotonergic function in man, e.g., PET studies of tryptophan metabolism and specific 5-HT receptor subtypes are needed to definitively test the 5-HT hypothesis of major depression. Attention to the interaction of specific 5-HT receptor subtypes with each other also appears to be of particular importance.

REFERENCES:

1. Arora, R.C., and Meltzer, H.Y. (1989): Life Sci., 44:725-734.
2. Arora, R.C., and Meltzer, H.Y. (1989): Am. J. Psychiatry, 146: 730-736.
3. Koyama, T., and Meltzer, H.Y. (1986): In New Results in Depression, H. Hippius et al., eds., pp. 169-188. Springer-Verlag, Berlin.
4. Maes, M., et al., (1987): J. Aff. Dis., 13:23-30.
5. Meltzer, H.Y., and Lowy, M.T. (1987): In Psychopharmacology, The Third Generation of Progress, H.Y. Meltzer, ed., pp. 513-526 Raven Press, New York.
6. Meltzer, H.Y., et al., (1984): Arch. Gen. Psychiatry 41:379-387.

β-PHENYLETHYLAMINE AND NORADRENERGIC FUNCTION IN DEPRESSION

M.NAKAGAWARA

Neuropsychiatry, Yamanashi Medical College, Tamaho, Yamanashi, Japan

β-Phenylethylamine (PEA), an endogenous monoamine that resembles amphetamine in its chemical structure, has been identified in the human brain. Although PEA is present in much smaller amounts than noradrenaline, the mode of action of PEA as a neuromodulator is of special interest (3). Recently, there has been growing clinical evidence to suggest that PEA plays a role in affective disorders (2). The levels of free 3-methoxy, 4-hydroxyphenylethylene glycol (MHPG) in plasma is also useful for evaluating the role of brain noradrenergic systems, and has been employed as an index of noradrenergic function in depression. Desmethylimipramine (DMI) induced growth hormone (GH) secretion is mediated by alpha-2 post synaptic adrenoceptors, and a blunted GH response to DMI has been reported in depression (1). In the present study, a new sensitive method for determination of PEA in human plasma was investigated, and then the plasma levels of PEA and MHPG were determined in patients with depression. The GH responses to DMI were also measured.

SUBJECTS AND METHODS

The depressive patients and healthy subjects who participated in the study gave voluntary written informed consent. Blood samples for the determination of PEA and MHPG were drawn between 11:00AM and 12:00AM. Blood for DMI stimulation test were drawn 30 min before and 120 min after a single oral loading dose of 50 mg DMI. PEA, MHPG and GH were analysed by capillary gas spectrometry, high performance liquid chromatography and radioimmunoassay, respectively.

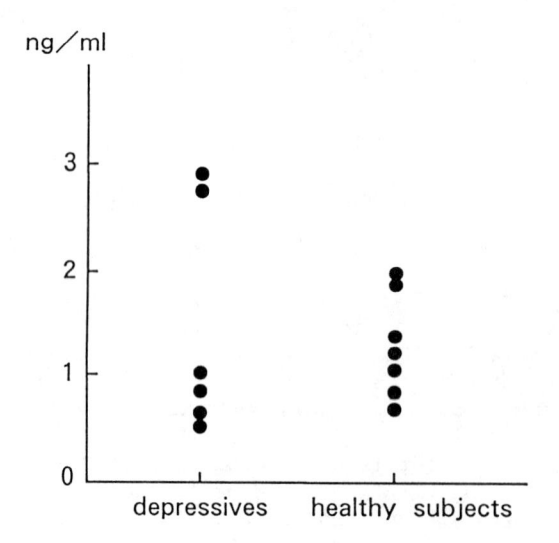

Fig.1: Plasma levels of β-phenylethylamine in depressive patients

RESULTS AND DISCUSSION

The depressive patients were divided into groups with high and low PEA levels (Fig.1). Blunted response of GH after DMI, and higher MHPG levels in plasma, were shown in the patients with low levels of plasma PEA. On the other hand, a normal GH response to DMI and low plasma levels of MHPG were found in the other group of depressive patients. These results suggest that biochemically, two different subgroups may exist in depression.

ACKNOWLEDGEMENTS: I am deeply grateful to Prof. Tetsuhiko Kariya (Dept. of Neuropsychiatry, Yamanashi Medical College) for helpful suggestions. I thank Dr. Kunihiko Shioe, Dr. Yoshio Sato, Dr. Masami Hirano, Mrs Chisato Shimizu (Dept. of Neuropsychiatry, Yamanashi Medical College) and Mrs Akiko Watanabe (Dept. of Neuropsychiatry, Tokyo Medical and Dental University) for their invaluable assistance.

REFERENCES

1. Matussek,N. (1988): In Neuroendocrinology of mood, K.Fuxe, D.Ganten, D.Pfaff eds., pp 141-182. Springer, Berlin.
2. Nakagawara,M. (1986): Jap. J. Psychopharmacol., 6:295
3. Yoshimoto,S. et al (1987): Psychiat. Res., 21:229-236.

ORIENTAL MEDICINE FOR THERAPY RESISTENT DEPRESSION

K.SARAI
Sarai Clinic and Department of Neurology and Psychiatry
Hiroshima University School of Medicine, Hiroshima, Japan

The cause of depression is unknown and modern medical treatment is still imperfect. In our everyday practice we find some depressive patients whose course is prolonged inspite of several changes of combination of antidepressnts with other drugs. Usually they are apt to complain some physical symptoms persistently like hypochondria,which is no more used in western medicine nowadays though. This state is called "post-depressive neurotic state". In this state modern drugs are no more effective for such hypochondriacal symptoms. In this state we can use oriental herbal medicines as a supplemental treatment. Oriental traditional medicine has different doctrine from western medicine, and for those who are unfamiliar with oriental medicine, it seems old-fashioned and idealistic. However, the technique of observation for treatment is specific and more precise than western medicine. Besides herbal medicines have some effects to harmonize autonomic dysfunction, and these medicines have scarcely side effects. For these reason oriental herb medicines are still usable.

In these days herb medicines which we use are based on traditional Chinese formulas and manifactured into granule (usual dosage: 2.5g three times daily) According to GMP. The following application of herb medicines to some symptoms of therapy resistent depression would be discussed in detail.

1. YOKKAN-SAN for sleeplessness according to bad dream

Nowadays we do not have a suitable drugs for bad dream except YOKKAN-SAN. YOKKAN-SAN consists of SOJUTU,BUKURYO, SENKYU,TOKI, CHOTO,SAIKO and KANZO. Generally these herbs have sedative effects for central nervous system. Among them CHOTO was selected and examined by radio-receptor assay using H^{35}-HT and cerebral cortex of rat brain, which revealed that CHOTO was a kind of antagonist of serotonin. According to a physiological examination using intestine of guinea pig, CHOTO was recognized as a partial agonist of serotonin. Recently central serotonin is thought to have some relation to affects, especially aggression and others, which might have some relationship to bad dream.

2. CHOTO-SAN for a kind of headache

Usual headache of depression is treatable by antidepressants, anxiolytics and other drugs, however a kind of headache is therapy resistant. In this case, especially for morning headache of old aged, CHOTO-SAN is preferably prescribed. CHOTO-SAN consists of CHOTO,CHIMPI,HANGE,BAKUMON-TO,BUKURYO,NINJIN,KIKKA,SEKKO,SHOKYO and KANZO. We suppose that this kind of headache may have relation to serotonin. CHOTO has anti-serotonergic action and other herbs have central sedative effects.

3. HANGE-KOBOKU-TO for esophageal functional stenosis

Esophageal functional stenosis had been called "globus hystericus", however, Dr. Chitani named it "globus melancholicus" , because this phenomenon appeared mostly in depression, which was also reported on New England J. Med. in 1987. In old China they also recognized it as "spirit of a plum stone in esophagus". For this symptom antidepressants are not so effective, and HANGE-KOBOKU-TO usually prescribes. HANGE-KOBOKU-TO consists of HANGE,KOBOKU,BUKURYO,SOYO and SHOKYO. The efficacy of this drug is almost 60%, however the mechanism of action is still unknown.

4. SAIKO-KA-RYUKOTU-BOREI-TO for anxiety and depressive symptoms

Some depressive patients are too sensitive to usual antidepressants, and they can not tolerate such drugs, then they are treated by sulpiride and benzodiazepines. When their efficacies are not enough, SAIKO-KA-RYUKOTU-BOREI-TO is prescribed thereafter. This drug is effective for anxious ,agitated and depressive state (even manic state). According to animal experiments, this drug increase norepinephrine in hippocampus ($p<0.01$) and 5-hydroxyindole acetic acid in hypothalamuth ($p<0.05$), and decrease serotonin in forebrain cortex($p<0.05$) and dopamine in forebrain cortex ($p\ 0.05$) in chronic administration. Concerning the receptor related behavior of serotonin 2 (wet dog shake), this drug has same effet of imipramine in acute administration, but not in chronic administration.

5. RYOKEI-JUTUKAN-TO for dizziness

Middle aged depressed women with dizziness are apt to be therapy resistant by antidepressants, and RYOKEI-JUTUKAN-TO is effective for these patients, and this drug has antiedematous effect.

Other herb medicines for depression exist.

TREATMENT OF THERAPY-RESISTANT DEPRESSION

K. ACHTE
Department of Psychiatry, University of Helsinki, Finland

According to Kielholz (3), 60 to 70% of patients suffering from severe depression are cured by drug therapy and supportive psychotherapy within one to two months. If the patient is not cured within two to three months, the drug must be changed. According to Kielholz, about 15% of patients can still be helped at this stage. If the patient is not cured after two courses of different anti-depressants, the depression is therapy-resistant. It is estimated that 15 to 20% of all depressive patients are resistant to therapy. They are often hospitalized. A thorough physical examination should be conducted for such patients to exclude any organic disease such as malignancies.

Electroconvulsive therapy (ECT) is often the most efficious treatment for therapy-resistant depression, and it also spares the patient (1) It is usually applied under general anaesthesia, unilaterally to the non-dominant hemisphere to prevent memory disorders. At least 50% of the cases of therapy-resistant depression respond to ECT (4).

In addition to ECT, monoamine exidase (MAO) inhibitors have been increasingly used for the treatment of depression. It is assumed that in sufficient doses (often 100 to 250 mg a day) MAO inhibitors may be effective in any kind of depression.

Thyroid hormone can be used for the treatment of therapy-resistant depression in combination with tricyclic antidepressants. In addition to the DST test, the DRH test is a useful aid in the assesment of depression. Abnormal DRH response is considered to be indicative of the beneficial effect of the thyroid hormone used in combination with antidepressants in therapy-resistant depression, i.e. depression resistant to conventional forms of therapy. A number of other biochemical tests intended for the assessment of depression are being developed. They may improve the accuracy of diagnosis. Thyroxin 0.1 to 0.5 mg is a suitable dose for intensifying the effect of tricyclic antidepressants. The effect is seen within two weeks. If no effect is achieved, the drug should be discontinued. Side effects resemble the symptoms of hyperthyroidism. Cardiac insufficiency and stenocardia are contraindications to thyroxin. Favourable results have been achieved by the use of thyroxin alone in some therapy-resistant depressions (2).

If the patient does not respond to the combination of tricyclic antidepressants and thyroid hormone, the combination of a tricyclic antidepressant and lithium may be useful. As a matter of fact, this combination is very often used in the treatment of unipolar and bipolar therapy-resistant depression. Sometimes small doses of neuroleptics can be used to support the therapy, particularly in the evening if the patient suffers from sleep disorders.

The "Newcastle coctail" contains, in addition to lithium and chlorimipramine, tryprophan 2 to 3 mg a day. The effect of the medication should become manifest within three weeks. If no effect is achieved, the treatment should be discontinued. In rare cases the combination of tricyclic antidepressants and lithium can cause a state of confusion. Small doses of lithium increase serotonergic activity, and blood concentrations of 0.2 to 0.4 mEq/l may be sufficient to intensify the effect of the usual antidepressants.

Some of the patients who do not respond to the combination of tricyclic antidepressants and lithium respond within six weeks to the combination therapy with lithium, tricyclic antidepressant and carbamazepine.

In prolonged and severe therapy-resistant depressions in women, good results have been achieved by combining large oestrogen doses (up to 25 mg of conjugated oestrogens p.o. a day for three months) with antidepressants.

A new trend in the treatment of therapy-resistant depression is to advance the sleep-wakefulness cycle. This is combined with the use of tricyclic antidepressants. Sleeping time is shifted to 6 p.m. - 2 a.m. The condition may be connected after two weeks or develop into hypomania. The response lasts longer than in sleep deprivation therapy. When a response is achieved, the sleeping time is gradually shifted back to normal, half an hour per 24-hour day.

Sleep deprivation is best implemented so that the patient "skips one night", i.e. stays awake all night and the following day and then goes to bed at the usual time. The patient stays awake for 38 to 40 hours. Medication may well be continued during sleep deprivation excluding, of course, hypnotics.

Light therapy has also been tried recently but there is no clear evidence of its efficacy (SAD syndrome). A placebo effect may be involved.

REFERENCES

1. Achté, K., Alanen, Y.O. and Tienari, P. (1990):Psykiatria 1. 6th edit. WSOY, Porvoo-Helsinki-Juva.
2. Helmchen, H. (1990): Therapy resistance in depression. Paper presented in the International Symposium of the P.T.D. Committee, 29th and 30th January 1990, St. Moritz.
3. Kielholz, P. (1971): Diagnosen und Therapie der Depression für den Praktiker. 3. Auflage. J.F. Lehmanns Verlag, München.
4. Mandel, M.R. (1978): Indications for electroconvulsive therapy in treatment of depression. In Massachusetts General Hospital Handbook of General Hospital Psychiatry, T.P. Hackett and N.H. Cassem, eds., pp. 226-230. C.V. Mosby Co, St. Louis, Mo.

BRIGHT LIGHT AND SLEEP DEPRIVATION AS ADJUVANT THERAPIES IN MAJOR DEPRESSION

E. HOLSBOER-TRACHSLER, R. STOHLER, M. HATZINGER, U. GERHARD, V. HOBI AND A. WIRZ-JUSTICE
Psychiatric University Clinic, 4025 Basel, Switzerland

Therapy resistant depressive patients, when carefully evaluated, can be more correctly described as depressives who are difficult to treat. Unclear diagnoses, inadequate dosage and length of treatment are often the reasons behind a so called therapy resistance. Strategies that have proved to be useful for depressives who are difficult to treat are infusion therapy (1) or combinations of different drugs (7). Lithium alone (5,2) or combined with carbamazepine is recommended as the treatment of choice for "rapid cyclers". Non-pharmacological modalities such as sleep deprivation (4) and light (6) can be considered as practical adjuvant therapies.

SUBJECTS AND METHOD

We are studying the effect of adjuvant non-pharmacological therapeutic modalities on the time course of tricyclic antidepressants in hospitalised major depression. 15 patients with major depression (DSM III-R) were randomly assigned to treatment with either: 1. trimipramine (200 mg/d) alone; 2. trimipramine with partial sleep deprivation (PSD) in the second half of the night (3x / week 2, 1x /weeks 3-6); or 3. trimipramine with light therapy (6-8 pm 5000 lux; 5x / week 2, 3x / weeks 3-6). Severity of depression was estimated by the Hamilton Rating Scale (HRS-17-items) weekly (1-6). A cognitive psychomotor performance test battery (7) was applied during the baseline drug treatment (day 5), after addition of 3 PSD or 5 days of light (day 14), and at the end of the study (day 42).

RESULTS

All patients improved; HRS score at onset 23.8 ± 4.9; at the end of 6 weeks 10.4 ± 7 ($p < 0.01$). At the end of the second week of drug treatment, after adjuvant intensive PSD and light therapy, marked improvement occured in all cognitive psychomotor tests. In contrast, improvement in the group treated only with trimipramine was slight. At the completion of the study, improvement was greatest in patients treated with trimipramine and PSD. Trimipramine alone also resulted in improvement. However on the regimen of 3 x / week adjuvant light treatment the initial improvement in cognitive psychomotor performance was not maintained, although reaction time was further improved.

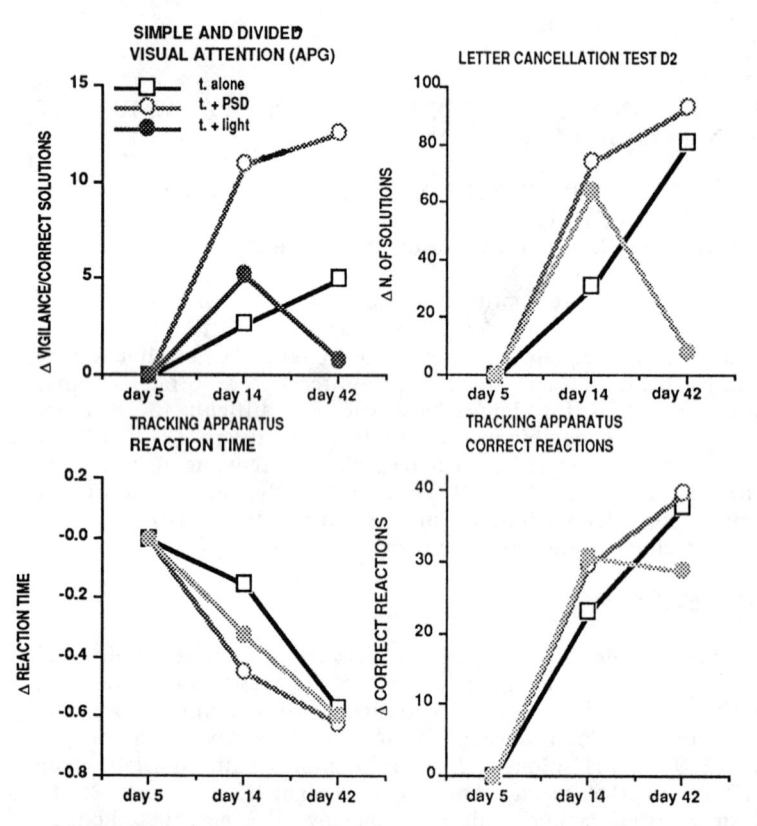

DISCUSSION
These results indicate that additional chronobiological intervention rapidly improved cognitive psychomotor performance before marked changes in Hamilton depression scores appeared. In severe depressives who are difficult to treat neuropsychological tests could help to give more objective information than traditional rating scales.

REFERENCES
1. Gastpar, M., Gildsdorf, U., Baumann, P.: Comparison of oral and intravenous treatment of depressive states, a preliminary WHO collaborative study. Proc. IV; WORLD Congr. biolog. Psychiat., Philadelphia, 1985.
2. Gross, C.C., J.B. Weilberg, J.B., Gastfriend, D.R.: Adjunct Low Dose Lithium Carbonate in Treatment-Resistant Depression: A Placebo-Controlled Study. J. Clin. Psychopharmacol. 8/2: 120-124, 1988.
3. Hobi, V. et al.: A New Device for Testing Cognitive-Psychomotor Functions. Blutalkohol 25: 97-115, 1988.
4. Holsboer-Trachsler, E., Wiedemann, K., Holsboer, F.: Serial Partial Sleep Deprivation in Depression - Clinical Effects and Dexamethasone Suppression Test Results. Neuropsychobiology 19: 73-78, 1988.
5. Kissling, W.: Lithium as an antidepressant. Int. J. Neurosc. 31-120, 1988.
6. Kripke, D.F.: Therapeutic effects of bright light in depressed patients. Annals New York Academy of Sciences 453: 270-281, 1985.
7. Wager, S.G., Klein, D.F.: Drug Therapy Strategies for Treatment-Resistant Depression. Psychopharmacol. Bull,1: 69-74, 1988.

SEROTONIN - FUNCTIONAL APPROACH FOR DIAGNOSIS AND TREATMENT OF THERAPY RESISTANT DEPRESSIONS

W. Pöldinger
Psychiatric University Clinic, CH-4025 Basel/Switzerland

The problem of therapy resistant depressions lies in the increasing difficulty of treating depressions. This has led to new diagnostic concepts as e.g. the syndrome of a serotonin deficit. H.M. van Praag titles one of his papers in 1988 "serotonin dysfunctions among psychic diseases: Functional vs. nosologic interpretation". He has pleaded for over twenty years for a reevaluation of the syndrome in psychiatry (3). Late he coined the term of a "functional psychopathology" (van Praag et al., 1975). In this context the studies on serotonin metabolism among suicidal patients deserve mentioning, which point at a shortage of serotonin, as well as similar disturbances among patients with aggression directed toward others. Anxiety is a further psychopathological dimension of serotonin research; a field in which serotonin reuptake inhibitors have proven their efficacy, mainly for panic disorders. Also in the context of the psychopharmacological treatment of obsessions and compulsions a participation of the serotonin metabolism should be considered. Van Praag (2) points at the fact that the functional point of view is a potential explanation for the "unspecifity" of certain compounds which is hard to grasp. In my opinion the 5-HT research in psychiatry illustrates clearly the relevance and feasibility of the functional approach in psychopathology. In this perspective 5-HT seems to be less of a "neurotransmitter for all cases" (van Kammen, 1987), but rather to announce a new age for the biological research in psychiatry. In table 1 the symptoms of the syndrome of the serotonin shortage are listed: In this context one might - borrowing from F. Freyhan's concept of the target syndromes first proposed in 1957 - speak now of "functional target syndromes" (1). This fits with the fact that antidepressants can be used in a variety of indications well beyond the depressions.

Table 1
The syndrome of a serotonin shortage
- states of depression
- states of anxiety
- sleep disorders
- eating and drinking disorders
- states of aggression and self-aggression
- obsessive-compulsive symptoms
- functional ANS disorders
- psychomatic disorders
- states of pain

REFERENCES

1. Pöldinger, W.: Die alte Neurasthenie und neue funktionelle Konzepte. TW Neurologie/Psychiatrie: Sonderheft "Angst, Aggression, Selbstaggression", 1989.
2. Praag, H.M. van (ed.): Serotonine disturbance in psychiatric disorders: functional versus nosological interpretation. Adv. Biol. Psychiatry, vol 17. Karger Basel, 1988.
3. Praag, H.M. van, Leijnse, B.: Neubewertung des Syndromes. Skizze einer funktionellen Pathologie. Psychiatria Neur. Neurochir. 68: 50-66, 1965.

ARE THERE CROSS-CULTURAL DIFFERENCES IN OBSESSIVE COMPULSIVE DISORDER ?

Sumant Khanna

Department of Psychiatry, National Institute of Mental Health and Neurosciences, Bangalore, India.

Obsessive Compulsive Disorder (OCD) is now being recognised in almost all countries all over the world. Within the spectrum of trans-cultural psychiatry there is a need to determine whether there are differences in the presentation of the disorder across cultures. In a biological framework it is important to recognise whether the clinical manifestation is associated with the same biological observations and from the point of view of therapy whether similar strategies are efficacious.

In the current study findings about the clinical profile, biology and therapy of OCD from our centre (1-6) will be compared with observations from other centres.

Clinically, OCD in India is as prevalent in hospital settings as in other countries. It has a slightly later age of onset as compared to the West, but females have a later age of onset as reported by other workers. There is a slight excess of males in the clinical population, probably due to their disproportionate use of health facilities. Patients are more likely to present with obsessive fears and convictions involving sex and religion. Washers and checkers seem to be similar across cultures.

Biologically similar patterns of CSF amines and responses to clonidine, dexamethasone and mCPP have been recognised in work done at our centre and other parts of the world. Patients who have different profiles from those commonly seen in other centres did not differ significantly in their biological profiles.

A recently completed trial of clomipramine has shown its superior efficacy over nortryptiline. Open trials have also suggested similar findings.

These findings suggest that [1] Obsessive Compulsive Disorder is present universally, [2] Culture may have a pathoplastic effect on its clinical presentation, [3] In spite of the clinical presentation, there are no differences in the biological abnormalities in Obsessive Compulsive Disorder across cultures and [4] Similar therapeutic strategies are effective in both settings. These observations suggest that biological and therapeutic observations in OCD are generalisable.

REFERENCES

1. Khanna, S.: Biological correlates of obsessive compulsive disorder. Ind. J. Psychol. Med. 11:59-68 , 1988.
2. Khanna, S. and Channabasavanna, S.M.: Towards a classification of compulsions in obsessive compulsive disorder. Psychopathology 20:23-28 , 1987.
3. Khanna, S. and Channabasavanna, S.M.: Phenomenology of obsessions in obsessive compulsive disorder. Psychopathology 21:12-18 , 1988.
4. Khanna, S. and Channabasavanna, S.M.: Clomipramine in resistant obsessive compulsive disorder. Ind. J. Psychiat. 30:375-379 , 1988.
5. Khanna, S., Kaliaperumal, V.G. and Channabasavanna, S.M.: Clusters of phenomenology in obsessive compulsive disorder. Br. J. Psychiat. 156:51-54 , 1990.
6. Khanna, S., Rajendra, P.N. and Channabasavanna, S.M.: Socio- demographic variables in obsessive compulsive disorder in India. Int. J. Soc. Psychiat. 32/3:47-54 , 1986.

WHEN ALL IS SAID AND DONE - AN UPDATE ON PSYCHOSURGICAL INTERVENTION IN INTRACTABLE OBSESSIVE COMPULSIVE DISORDER

P Mindus (1,2), B A Meyerson (2)
Departments of Psychology and Psychiatry (1), and Neurosurgery (2), Karolinska Hospital, P O Box 60 500, S-104 01 Stockholm, Sweden

Obsessive compulsive disorder (OCD) is notorious for its chronicity, severity and resistance to treatment. It has recently been estimated that 20-30 % of OCD patients are refractory to conventional therapy, and 9 % are reported to suffer from illnesses with a chronic, deteriorative course. These patients represent potential candidates for psychosurgery.

To date, over 450 patients with OCD undergoing psychosurgery have been reported in the literature, a probable underestimation of the true rate. Although different authors have used the same or different techniques for the production of lesions placed in the same or different limbic or paralimbic targets, strikingly similar results are reported, with clinically and statistically significant improvements in two thirds of the patients. These are remarkable results given the chronicity and severity of the cases treated, in whom all available conventional therapeutic options had been exhausted. Prospective, independent studies show that negative effects on personality and intellectual functions, which followed upon the older, extensive interventions, are not to be expected after modern stereotactic procedures.

Whereas the efficacy of psychosurgery in severe OCD is well established, the underlying therapeutic mechanisms remain unknown. There is increasing evidence to show that OCD patients have brain dysfunction and/or pathology, although the precise location, nature and aetiological significance of the lesions are unknown. Recently advanced hypotheses on pathogenetic mechanisms all assume an imbalance between certain cortical and subcortical structures in OCD.

This paper first gives an overview of the three most established psychosurgical procedures in OCD: cingulotomy, limbic leucotomy and capsulotomy. Our experiences with the latter procedure - in use regularly at the Karolinska Institute since1970 - will be reviewed, followed by reports from ongoing prospective, multidisciplinary studies using, inter al, magnetic resonance and positron emission tomography. The paper closes with a discussion on both how psychosurgery might exert its action and help elucidate the underlying pathogenetic mechanisms in severe OCD.

PHENOMENOLOGY AND TREATMENT OF OBSESSIVE COMPULSIVE DISORDER

T. Nakazawa
Saiseikai Central Hospital and Hasegawa Hospital
Tokyo, JAPAN

Obsession and anxiety are recognized as biologically relative. Anxiety is evidenced with a skin potential reflex and a component of baseline deflection on photoelectric finger plethysmogram, indicating the first for trait anxiety and the latter for state anxiety. However, these two markers for anxiety are not applicable for obsession. In order to examine obsession it is appropriate to examine performance on a task of various complexity.

1. Reaction time on psychomotor task: Tapping

To study the relationship between the task complexity and obsessive compulsive disorder (OCD), a pattern input unit (apparatus) consisting of three different tapping tasks of complexity was employed in our experiment. CYCLE 1 (the simplest task) required subjects to tap the fixation spot located in the center of a tablet; CYCLE 2 to tap 2 spots displaying 2 points in 10 cm distance and in a 45° inclination; and CYCLE 3 to tap 2 spots as indicated for CYCLE 2, but with an increased complexity of reverse prism (Fig. 1).

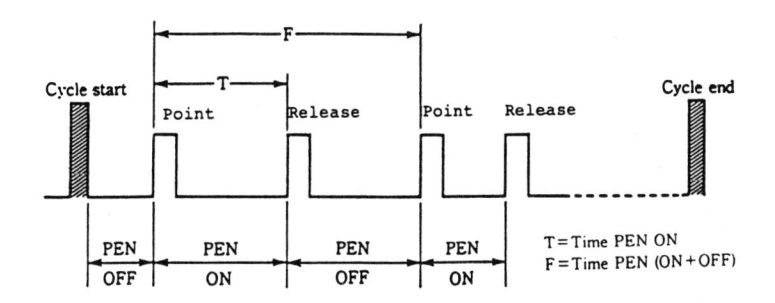

Fig. 1: Measurement of tapping

In our experiment groups of OCD (15 cases), DSM III Schizophrenia paranoid type (15 cases), and the healthy controls (21 persons) were subjected to this tapping test. The results revealed that OCD group and paranoid Schizophrenia group showed a very similar reaction pattern, although some characteristics peculiar to OCD were suggested (Table 1).

(1) Differences in standard deviation (SD) obtained in the number of tapping and coefficient of variation (CV) in activity were minimal.
(2) Regarding the total tapping number, in the performance of CYCLE 1 no difference was observed between the OCD and the healthy control group. In CYCLES 2 and 3, no difference between OCD and Schizophrenia group was observed.

TABLE 1: COMPARISON OF TAPPING INTERVAL(F) AND POINTING TIME(T) BY MEANS AND STANDARD DEVIATION (mSec)

		INTERVAL(F)			POINTING TIME(T)		
	CYCLE	1	2	3	1	2	3
Control	X	180.1	428.2	1771.0	52.3	84.4	278.7
	SD	30.1	142.7	675.1	21.1	35.1	148.1
Schizo phrenia	X	269.4	610.9	5000.9	82.2	133.8	665.7
	SD	164.7	188.7	3028.8	53.6	58.2	529.4
OCD	X	193.9	607.9	6198.1	43.6	127.6	1232.2
	SD	24.6	115.9	3969.7	9.5	27.7	1285.2

(3) A remarkable delayed pointing time was evidenced in accordance with an increased complexity.
(4) Accuracy rate (evaluated as accurate when the pen was tapped on the spot within 2 mm distance from an indicated point for both one and two tappings) obtained in OCD group indicated that accurate and consistent performance (CYCLE 3) under complex task of space conversion condition was conducted in OCD compared to Schizophrenia group showing decreased accuracy.
(5) In the depression group (12 cases) a consistency in activity rhythm was well maintained in the CYCLE 1 compared to other groups. However, the total number of tapping was small and an error rate in CYCLE 3 testing remarkably increased.

2. Selective reaction time and clomipramine

In other experiment subjects were required to indicate high-Hz tone after hearing both high and low-Hz tone at random in a different interval, as quickly as possible by pressing a botton for only high-Hz tone, and the reaction time was measured. No difference in reaction time after continuous high-Hz tone and intermittent high and low-Hz tone was observed in OCD group. On the other hand, a delay in reaction time and individual variation were clearly indicated in paranoid Schizophrenia. After long-term administration of clomipramine to OCD group the same experimental procedure was taken. Reduced reaction time was observed, but no significant difference due to high and low-Hz tones was reported. Thus, the results suggest that OCD is a group having characteristics of consistency and a salient accuracy, which provide OCD a life controlled by a constant rhythm based on their own clock acquired.

In addition, the results of dichotic listening method for examining the linguistic obsession conducted in Japan will be presented.

CHILDHOOD ONSET OBSESSIVE COMPULSIVE DISORDER

H.L.LEONARD, S.E.SWEDO, M.LENANE, D.C.RETTEW, and J.L.RAPOPORT,
Child Psychiatry Branch, National Institute of Mental Health, Bldg 10,
Room 6N240, 9000 Rockville Pike, Bethesda, Md, 20892

Obsessive compulsive disorder (OCD) has been estimated to have a point prevalence rate of 0.8% in children and adolescents (3). One-half to one-third of adult OCD patients have an onset of their illness in childhood or adolescence (8). At the National Institute of Mental Health (NIMH), seventy consecutive child and adolescent OCD patients were prospectively studied (11). The 23 girls and 47 boys had a mean age of onset of 10.1 ($\pm$3.52) years, with a mean age at presentation of 13.7 ($\pm$2.67) years. Boys had an earlier (prepubertal) mean age of onset of 9.6 ($\pm$3.8) years compared to that of 11.0 ($\pm$2.7) for girls (pubertal). The clinical presentation of the illness was very similiar to that seen in adults. Washing rituals were the most common, having been reported in 60 of 70 cases (85%). Other frequently reported rituals included repeating (51%), checking (46%), counting (18%), ordering/arranging (17%), and hoarding (11%). Co-morbid DSM-III diagnoses were common, and only 18 of the 70 (26%) had no psychiatric diagnosis other than OCD at the time of initial presentation. The most frequently coexisting Axis I diagnoses were major depression (26%), simple phobia (17%), overanxious disorder (16%), adjustment disorder with depressed mood (13%), oppositional disorder (11%), and attention deficit disorder (10%) (11).

Although the etiology of OCD is still unknown, brain imaging and pharmacological studies have led scientists to propose a frontal lobe-limbic-basal ganglia model and a "serotonin hypothesis of OCD"(9). Adult OCD patients with childhood onset of their symptoms had a decreased caudate volume on computerized tomography (7) and altered patterns of glucose utilization on positron emission tomography scans when compared to normal controls (10). Children and adolescents have a pharmacologic response similiar to that of the adult OCD patients when treated with serotonin reuptake blockers (6). A genetic component for OCD is consistent with our findings that 20% of the first degree relatives of the OCD probands met diagnostic criteria for OCD, which is far greater than the 2% expected rate for the general population (5).

Two controlled double-blind crossover treatment trials of clomipramine have shown it to be specifically effective in children and adolescents with severe primary OCD and superior to both placebo (2) and desipramine (6). Dosages of clomipramine targeting 3 mg/kg/day were used. Fluoxetine, although approved only for use as an adult antidepressant, has been effective for OCD in small open trials in pediatric cases.

Long-term follow-up studies have consisted of small clinical samples and have reported a mixed prognosis. Flament et al (4) evaluated 25 (93%) of 27 OCD patients initially treated in a clomipramine controlled study, and found that 17 (68%) still met diagnostic criteria 2-7 years later. Two year follow-up evaluation of 40 recent OCD patients treated at the NIMH found that 10 (25%) had no OCD symptoms, 22 (55%) had only mild symptoms, and 8 (20%) had moderate to severe symptomatology. Two-thirds of the patients in each symptom group were on medication for their OCD at the time of re-evaluation. The only follow-up study of an epidemiologic sample found that of the 16 OCD adolescents (of 5108 screened) initially diagnosed with OCD, 5 (31%) still met criteria for OCD and 4 (25%) had "subclinical OCD" at 2 year followup (1). Preliminary results from a double-blind desipramine substitution of 10 OCD children and adolescents maintained on clomipramine found that 9(90%) of the patients relapsed during the desipramine substitution. Questions concerning the long-term prognosis and the necessity for ongoing pharmacologic maintenance require further research attention.

REFERENCES

1. Berg CZ, et al: Childhood Obsessive Compulsive Disorder: A two-year prospective follow-up of a community sample. J Child & Adolesc Psychiatry, 28:528-533, 1989.
2. Flament MF, et al: Clomipramine treatment of childhood compulsive disorder. Arch Gen Psychiatry 42:977-983, 1985.
3. Flament MF, et al: Obsessive compulsive disorder in adolescence: An epidemiological study. J Am Acad Child Adolesc Psychiatry 27:764-771, 1988.
4. Flament MF, et al: Childhood obsessive compulsive disorder: a prospective follow-up study.J Child Psychol&Psychiat, 27:289-295,1990.
5. Lenane M, et al: Psychiatric disorders in first degree relatives of children and adolescents with obsessive compulsive disorder. J American Academy of Child and Adolesc Psychiatry, in press.
6. Leonard HL, et al: Treatment of obsessive compulsive disorder with clomipramine and desipramine in children and adolescents: A double-blind crossover comparison. Arch Gen Psychiatry, 46:1088-1092,1989.
7. Luxenburg JS, et al: Neuroanatomic abnormalities in obsessive-compulsive disorder detected with quantitative x-ray computed tomography. Am. J of Psychiatry, 145:1089-1093, 1988.
8. Rapoport JL: Annotation, child obsessive-compulsive disorder. J Child Psychol Psychiatry 27: 285-289, 1986.
9. Rapoport JL: Neurobiology of Obsessive Compulsive Disorder. J Amer Med Assoc, 260:2888-2890, 1989.
10. Swedo SE, et al: Cerebral glucose metabolism in chiildhood-onset obsessive compulsive disorder. Archives Gen Psychiatry, 46:518-523, 1989.
11. Swedo SE, et al: Obsessive Compulsive Disorder in children and adolescents, Clinical Phenomenology of 70 consecutive cases. Archives Gen Psychiat 46:335-341, 1989.

BRAIN SEROTONERGIC SUBSYSTEMS IN OBSESSIVE-COMPULSIVE DISORDER

D.L. MURPHY and T.A. PIGOTT
Laboratory of Clinical Science, National Institute of Mental Health Intramural Research Program, Bethesda, MD, U.S.A.

Our research group and others have been systematically evaluating the possible involvement of brain serotonin in different neuropsychiatric disorders, including obsessive-compulsive disorder (OCD) (1). At the present, the evidence linking central nervous system serotonergic alterations to OCD and to medication-induced therapeutic changes in OCD patients seems quite compelling (3). This paper provides an update of recent studies supporting earlier data linking a serotonin subsystem dysregulation to OCD, which is ameliorated by medications with serotonin-selective actions (1-5).

On the basis of consistent results in a series of small controlled trials and a recent large, multicenter study, clomipramine is now the most well-established pharmacologic therapy for OCD. It's mode of action had for some time been suggested to be related to its partially selective actions as a serotonin uptake inhibitor. This hypothesis has been supported by evidence that more highly selective serotonin uptake inhibitors like fluvoxamine and fluoxetine appear effective in OCD compared to placebo. A recent controlled study from our group comparing 32 OCD patients treated with both clomipramine (210 mg/d) and fluoxetine (80 mg/d) for 10-week periods demonstrated similar efficacy for both agents (5).

In studies with single doses of serotonergic agonists, antagonists, and several non-serotonergic anxiogenic agents, as well as longer term administration of some of these agents, evidence pointing towards serotonin subsystems being differentially affected in OCD patients has begun to emerge. For instance, exaggerated anxiogenic and other behavioral responses, including OCD symptom exacerbations, which are elicited by oral administration of the serotonin agonist, m-chlorophenylpiperazine (m-CPP) were originally found to be attenuated during successful clomipramine treatment of OCD patients [reviewed in (3)] and have now, similarly, been found to be negligible when m-CPP is administered to patients receiving fluoxetine (2; Pigott et al., unpublished data); a down-regulation of a hyper-responsive serotonergic subsystem has been postulated (2,3).

Studies of phenylpiperazines in animal models of anxiety suggest a hippocampal 5-HT$_{1C}$ receptor-mediated action for anxiety-related actions of m-CPP (6). Of interest, single doses of the partial 5-HT$_{1A}$ agonists, ipsapirone and buspirone, do not produce anxiogenic responses or OCD symptom exacerbation in OCD patients (Lesch, K.P., personal communication; Pigott et al., unpublished data), while longer-term administration of buspirone studied in a controlled crossover comparison with clomipramine led to therapeutic benefit in OCD (4). The serotonergic specificity of the behavioral effects of m-CPP in OCD patients studied before and during treatment with serotonin uptake inhibiting medications is suggested by comparison studies using agents (lactate, yohimbine, carbon dioxide) which are anxiogenic in other psychiatric patients populations, but which were not found to elicit either greater anxiety responses or OCD symptom exacerbations in OCD patients compared to controls [reviewed in (3)].

REFERENCES

1. Coccaro, E.F., and Murphy, D.L. Serotonin in Major Psychiatric Disorders. American Psychiatric Presss, Washington, DC, in press.
2. Hollander, E. et al. Repeat m-CPP challenge during fluoxetine treatment in obsessive compulsive disorder. Abstract, Annual Meeting of the Amer. Psychiatric Assoc., 1989, p. 189.
3. Murphy, D.L. et al. Obsessive-compulsive disorder as a 5-HT subsystem-related behavioural disorder. Br. J. Psychiatry 155:15-24, 1989.
4. Pato, M.T. et al. Clomipramine vs buspirone in OCD: A controlled trial. Abstract, Annual Meeting of the Amer. Psychiatric Assoc., 1989.
5. Pigott, T.A. et al. A controlled comparison of clomipramine and fluoxetine in the treatment of obsessive-compulsive disorder: Behavioral and biological results. Arch. Gen. Psychiatry, in press.
6. Whitton, P. and Curzon, G. Anxiogenic-like effect of infusing 1-(3-chlorophenyl)piperazine (mCPP) into the hippocampus. Psychopharmacology 100:138-140, 1990.

MAPPING OF SEROTONINE RECEPTOR RECOGNITION SITES APPLIED TO DRUG DESIGN

M. HIBERT
Merrell Dow Research Institute, B.P. 447 R/9, 16, rue d'Ankara, 67009 Strasbourg, France

The existence of numerous functional 5-HT receptor subtypes has been established on the basis of structure-activity relationship studies, ligand binding, second messenger, pharmacological and molecular biological data (1,2). Until we could define reliable three-dimensional models of the different receptor subtypes based on their primary sequence, we use the receptor mapping technique to assist drug design.

METHODS AND RESULTS

The multitude of conceptual and technical limitations to the receptor mapping approach could be very discouraging and might even inhibit the use of this approach. However, even the oversimplified models which have been used have proven to be not only useful for *a posteriori* rationalization, but also as powerful predictive tools in facilitating the design of original and selective receptor ligands potentially useful in the clinic.

Using four weakly active and non-selective 5-HT$_{1A}$ receptor antagonists or partial agonists (spiperone, methiothepin, propranolol, buspirone), we were able to define a pharmacophore and a three-dimensional map of the 5-HT$_{1A}$ recognition site (Fig. 1a). This model has been used to design compounds belonging to novel chemical classes and successfully predict their high potency and stereospecificity. Their selectivity has been rationally optimised after comparison of the 5-HT$_{1A}$ and α_1-adrenoceptor maps (3).

Our studies have led to the rapid design of MDL 73005, a highly active and selective 5-HT$_{1A}$ receptor ligand with anxiolytic properties (4).

MDL 73005

Similarly, models of the 5-HT$_{1B}$, 5-HT$_{1C}$, 5-HT$_{1D}$, 5-HT$_2$ and 5-HT$_3$ recognition sites have been defined (Fig. 1b,c) and used to modulate the selectivity of some ligands (5).

Finally, using this receptor mapping approach, the structural requirements of the different 5-HT receptor subtypes have been compared. This study indicates that there is a high degree of homology in the 5-HT binding domain of the different receptors but also clear differences in the local environment of the bound endogenous ligand.

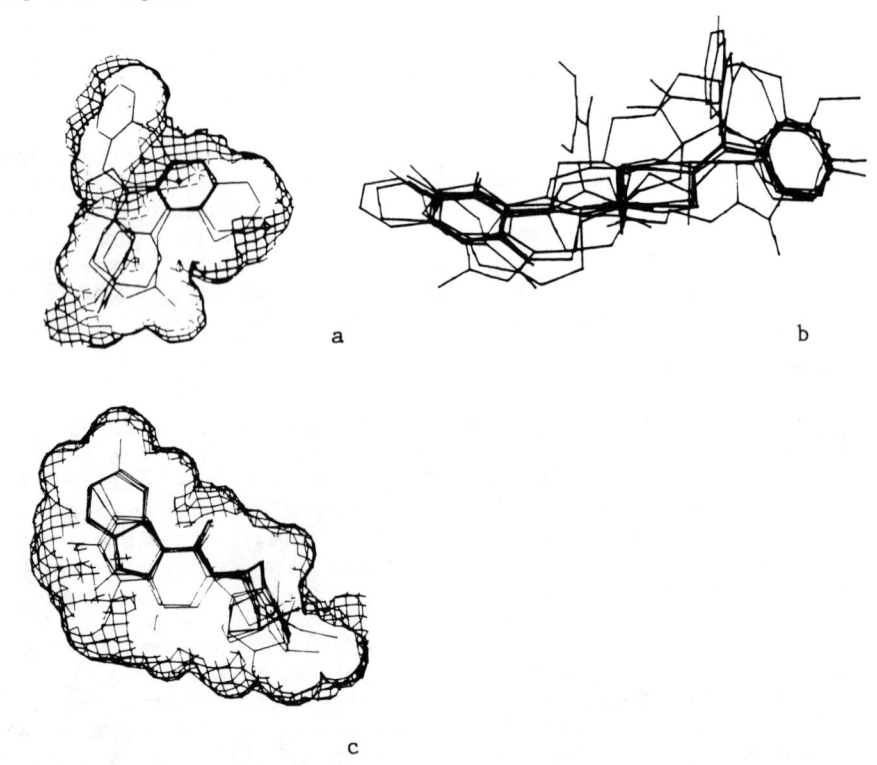

Fig. 1: Maps of the 5-HT$_{1A}$ (a), 5-HT$_2$ (b) and 5-HT$_3$ (c) antagonist recognition sites.

REFERENCES

1. Hibert, M.F., Mir, A.K. and Fozard, J.R. 5-HT receptors. Comprehensive Medicinal Chemistry. C. Hansch ed., Pergamon Press, Oxford. Chapter 12, 1990.
2. Hartig, P.R. Molecular biology of 5-HT receptors. Trends Pharmacol. Sci. 10: 64-69, 1989.
3. Hibert, M.F. et al. Graphics computer-aided receptor mapping as a predictive tool for drug design: development of potent selective and stereospecific ligands for the 5-HT$_{1A}$ receptor. J. Med. Chem. 31: 1087-1093, 1988.
4. Moser, P. et al. Characterization of MDL 73005EF as a 5-HT$_{1A}$ selective ligand and its effects in animal models of anxiety. Br. J. Pharmacol. 99: 343-349, 1990.
5. Hibert et al. J. Med. Chem., in press.

MOLECULAR STRUCTURE AND DYNAMICS OF THE DOPAMINE D_2 RECEPTOR AND LIGANDS

S.G. DAHL, Ø. EDVARDSEN and I. SYLTE

Department of Pharmacology, Institute of Medical Biology, University of Tromsø, N-9001 Tromsø, Norway

Information about the detailed three dimensional structure of the D_2 receptor molecule would add to our knowledge of how neuroleptic drugs work, and might be useful in development of new antipsychotic drugs. While the amino acid sequences are known for more than 10000 proteins, only some 300 three dimensional protein structures have been reported. The primary structure of several neurotransmitter receptors have been determined from cloning experiments, but any of their three dimensional structures have not yet been reported.

The detailed molecular mechanisms of interaction between neuroleptics and dopamine receptors are therefore not known. Several computational and crystallographic studies of dopamine receptor agonists and antagonists have been performed in order to determine three dimensional pharmacophoric patterns. However, such studies have usually been based upon static concepts of molecular structure. The method of molecular dynamics simulations, which combines a molecular mechanical force field with Newton's equations of motion for a molecular system, has provided new insight into the molecular motions and functioning of biologically active molecules.

MOLECULAR STRUCTURE AND DYNAMICS OF D_2 RECEPTOR LIGANDS

The AMBER (Assisted Model Building with Energy Refinement) programs (1) were used for calculations of three dimensional molecular structures and electrostatic potentials, and for molecular dynamics simulations. The MIDAS (Molecular Interactive Display and Simulation) programs (2) were used for molecular graphics with an Evans and Sutherland PS390 computer graphics system. The three dimensional structures, low-energy conformations and molecular dynamics of dopamine and a series of tricyclic neuroleptics of the phenothiazine and thioxanthene classes were examined. Various side chain conformations were observed during the molecular dynamics simulations. The motions between different side chain conformations followed quite unexpected trajectories, often with twisting of the whole molecule such that most of its mass was kept in place, rather than rotating around single bonds. The tricyclic ring systems showed unexpected flexibility, with variations between 103° and 175° in the angle between the phenyl rings.

STRUCTURE OF D_2 RECEPTORS

Specific binding of ligands to macromolecules usually involves enclosure of most of the ligand molecule by a binding pocket. Electrostatic interactions may contribute to the stabilization of such complexes, and molecular electrostatic potentials (3) may provide useful information about mechanisms of ligand-receptor interactions. The peptide chains of G protein coupled receptors contain 7 transmembrane stretches of residues. Binding sites for agonists and antagonists on β_2-adrenergic receptors are located within the putative transmembrane regions (4). These residues are present in corresponding positions in the rat D_2 receptor and in all other G protein coupled neurotransmitter receptors which have been sequenced. It was therefore postulated that they represent common agonist and antagonist binding sites for this class of receptors.

The molecular structure of dopamine and the amino acid sequence of the rat dopamine D2 receptor (5), were used to construct a three dimensional model of the receptor. It was postulated that the seven helixes form a hydrophilic core which contains the ligand binding sites, by a clockwise arrangement with the most polar side of each helix surface towards the center of the receptor molecule.

Molecular dynamics simulations demonstrated that unlike the static structures in a crystal, both dopamine, neuroleptic drugs and the receptor molecule must be considered as flexible entities which have considerable freedom to move in the biophase. In approaching the postulated endogenous binding site on the D_2 receptor, the dopamine molecule moved between several different conformations within a few picoseconds. This demonstrates the importance of the dynamic aspect for understanding mechanisms of drug-receptor interactions at the molecular level.

REFERENCES

1. Weiner, S.J., Kollman, P.A. Nguyen D.T. and Case, D.A.: An all atom force field for simulations of proteins and nucleic acids. J. Comput. Chem. 7:230-252, 1986.
2. Ferrin, T.E., Huang, C.C., Jarvis, L.E. and Langridge, R.: The MIDAS database system. J. Mol. Graphics 6:2-12, 1988, ibid 13-27.
3. Singh, U.C. and Kollman, P.A.: An approach to computing electrostatic charges for molecules. J. Comp. Chem. 5:129-145, 1984.
4. Dixon, R.A.F., Sigal, I.S., Rands, E. et al.: Ligand binding to the β-adrenergic receptor involves its rhodopsin-like core. Nature 326:73-77, 1987.
5. Bunzow, J.R., Van Tol, H.H.M., Grandy, D. K., et al.: Cloning and expression of a rat D_2 dopamine receptor cDNA. Nature 336: 783-787, 1988.

BIOCHEMICAL AND PHARMACOLOGICAL ASPECTS OF PARKINSON'S DISEASE P. Riederer*, K. Jellinger**, E. Sofic*, W. Paulus** * Clinical Neurochemistry, Dept. Psychiatry, University Würzburg, FRG and **L. Boltzmann Inst. Clin. Neurobiology, Lainz-Hospital, Vienna, Austria

The major hallmark in the pathology of Parkinson's disease (PD) is a depigmentation of substantia nigra pars compacta (SNZC) and a significant loss of dopamine (DA) in the nigro-striatal fibres. However, the cause of this degeneration is unknown. More recently iron has been suggested to play a role in the pathophysiology of PD on the basis of increased iron (1,2) and especially iron (III) (2,3,7) in SNZC the time course being related to the progression of the disease (3) thus correlating with the time course of the rate of depigmentation (4) and that of glutathione (GSH) (3). Under conditions of impaired radical scavenging mechanisms (3 for review) oxygen-derived radicals may contribute to cause PD (5). The iron-melanin interaction promotes lipid peroxidation as final neurotoxic event (6). We have focused this aspect by measuring iron, iron II and iron III in the SN as well as in its subareas SNZC and SNZR by biochemical (table) as well as histochemical methods (table).

RESULTS

The biochemical studies show that the increase of iron and iron III is only significant in cases with a loss of striatal DA > 80 % (7). In milder cases, ie. with a loss of DA < 65% the increase of iron is only marginal (table). The histochemical data are in line with such an assumption as they demonstrate a significant increase of iron III in progressed PD and a further increase in PD plus dementia. There is also evidence that melanin containing (and nonpigmented neurons) contain iron III only in rare occasions, while practically all iron III is seen in microglia, macrophages and in or around small vessel walls.

TABLE: SEMIQUANTITATIVE EVALUATION OF Fe^{++} IN PD AND CONTROLS USING BERLINE BLUE REACTION ON PARAFFIN SECTIONS

	SNZC	SNZR
Controls (7)	0,71 ± 0,48	1,71 ± 0,75
PD (7)	1,78 ± 0,56+	1,85 ± 0,47
PD+(PD+DAT) (13)	1,96 ± 0,48+	2,04 ± 0,48

means and s.d. +p< 0,05 Kruskal-Wallis-Test
PD age: 64-82 yrs (76,8); Controls age: 57-76 (67); diagnosis after histological examination; Perl's stain in paraffin sections according Gomari:
Am. J. Pathol. 12,655 (1936); semiquant. assessment (0 no iron; 1+ very few deposits visible, 2+ moderate deposits, 3+ large number or iron deposits visible)

TABLE: IRON II, IRON III AND DOPAMINE IN SNZC AND SNZR

	N	Fe II	Fe III	Fe total	dopamine
PD	SNZC (15)	116	116	116	29
	SNZR (15)	84	117	95	38

means as % of 9 controls () number of regions; Controls: age 76,2 ± 5,4 PD: age 75,5± 7,8; duration of PD: 6,5 ± 3,1 yrs; SN nerve cell loss 3,26 in a four point rating (Jellinger K., In: Calne D.B. (ed) Handbook of Exp. Pharmacol., Springer Verlag 1989); Lewy bodies in all 15 cases; ALZ lesions in 8 cases measurements: DA: HPLC-electrochemical detection according to E. Sofic, Thesis Univ. Vienna, Austria 1986; iron, iron II and iron III (Sofic et al., J. Neural Transm. 74:199-205,1988)

CONCLUSION
These data demonstrate that the proposed iron-melanin interaction may occur only outside of degenerating neurons, i.e. when melanin is washed out. If at all, iron seems to play an important pathologic role in glial tissue only, where it might contribute to the generation of endo- or exotoxins that can be taken up by dopaminergic neurons. In late phases of PD the unknown trigger of PD might be accelerated by this mechanisms as well as by an N-methly-D-aspartate-dependent enhanced Ca^{++} influx finally leading to multiple neuronal intoxications.

REFERENCES
1. Riederer, P., Umek, H.: L-Dopa-Substitution der Parkinson-Krankheit. Geschichte-Gegenwart-Zukunft. Springer Verlag, Wien-New York, 1985
2. Riederer, P., Sofic, E., Rausch, W.D., Schmidt, B., Reynolds, G.P., Jellinger, K., Youdim, M.B.H.: Transition Metals, Ferritin, Glutathione, and Ascorbic Acid in Parkinsonian Brains. J. Neurochem. 52:515-520, 1989
3. Riederer, P., Rausch, W.D., Schmidt, B., Kruzik, P., Konradi, C., Sofic, E., Danielczyk, W., Fischer, M., Ogris, E.: Biochemical Fundamentals of Parkinson's Disease. Mt. Sinai J. Med. 55 (1):21-28, 1988
4. Jellinger, K.: Pathology of Parkinson's Syndrome. In: Calne, D.B. (ed) Handbook of Experimental Pharmacology, Vol. 88. Springer-Verlag Berlin Heidelberg, pp, 47-112,1989
5. Cohen, G.: The Pathobiology of Parkinson's Disease: Biochemical Aspects of Dopamine Neuron Senescence. J. Neural Transm., Suppl. 19:89-103, 1983
6. Ben-Shachar, D., Riederer, P., Youdim, M.B.H.: Iron-Melanin Interaction and Lipid Peroxidation: Implications for Parkinson's Disease. PNAS, in press, 1990
7. Sofic, E., Riederer, P., Heinsen, H., Beckmann, H., Reynolds, G.P., Hebenstreit, G., Youdim, M.B.H.: Increased iron (III) and total iron content in post mortem substantia nigra of parkinsonian brain. J. Neural Transm. 74:199-205, 1988

THE FUNCTIONING OF TYROSINE HYDROXYLASE IN PARKINSON'S DISEASE

T. NAGATSU
Department of Biochemistry, Nagoya University School of Medicine, Nagoya 466 Japan

The characteristic biochemical changes in Parkinson's disease are the decreases in dopamine (DA) and the synthesizing enzyme, tyrosine hydroxylase (TH) (10) in the nigro-striatal DA neurons. The cell loss of DA neurons by unidentified causes is thought to result in the decreases in both DA and TH protein and activity. However, the decrease in TH activity in DA neurons even without cell loss could also reduce DA. TH activity *in vivo* could be reduced by the decreases in TH protein, in TH phosphorylation and in the biopterin cofactor. We examined the functioning of tyrosine hydroxylase both in postmortem parkinsonian brains, in the brains from 1-methyl-4-phenyl-1,2,3,6-tetrahydropyridine (MPTP)-treated mice, and in PC12h cells cultured in the presence of MPTP or the active metabolite, 1-methyl-4-phenylpyridinium ion (MPP$^+$) and in the presence of N-methyl-isoquinolinium ion (N-MeIQ$^+$), a probable endogenous neurotoxin.

MATERIALS AND METHODS

TH activity was measured by high-performance liquid chromatography with electrochemical detection [Nagatsu, et al., 1979 (11)]. TH protein content was measured by an enzyme immunoassay [Mogi, et al., 1984 (7)]. PC12h cells were cultured, as described by Naoi, et al., 1988 (13).

RESULTS AND DISCUSSION

Changes in TH in parkinsonian brains

Both TH protein content and TH activity (V_{max}) in the caudate nucleus, putamen, and substantia nigra of parkinsonian patients were decreased in parallel as compared with those of the age-matched control brains [Mogi, et al., 1988 (9); Rausch, et al., 1988 (18)]. In contract, TH homospecific activity (activity per enzyme protein) was significantly increased in the parkinsonian brains [Mogi, et al., 1988 (9)]. The results indicate that the decrease of TH activity in parkinsonian brains is due to the decrease of TH protein content as a result of cell death. The increase in the homospecific activity of residual TH in parkinsonian brains suggests such molecular changes in TH molecules as result in a compensatory increase in TH activity. We showed four types of human TH (types 1-4) to be produced by alternative mRNA splicing from a single gene [Kaneda, et al., 1987 (3); Kobayashi, et al., 1988 (6)]. Types 1-4 TH mRNA were found in the human brains, and the ratios of the four types were changed in the process of aging [Kaneda, et al., 1990 (4)]. These TH changes during aging appear to be accelerated in the parkinsonian brains. Different forms of TH could also change the regulation of the activity by phosphorylation and dephosphorylation. Narabayashi, et al., 1986 (15) reported a case of juvenile parkinsonism with decreased TH activity (V_{max}), but without cell loss of DA neurons in the substantia nigra. These results may indicate that reduced TH protein and activity also reduce DA even without cell loss.

Changes in TH in MPTP-treated mice and in PC12h cells in culture

MPTP produces early and late changes of TH in C57 BL mice *in vivo* and in rat pheochromocytoma PC12h cells in culture. MPTP inhibits *in vivo* TH activity in minutes after the subcutaneous administration to mice [Hirata and Nagatsu, 1986 (2)]. This inhibition may be due to DA released acutely into cytoplasm from the synaptic vesicles, due to inhibition of phosphorylation [Kiuchi, et al., 1988 (5)], and due to inhibition of biopterin cofactor synthesis. *In vitro* TH activity (V_{max}) is then reduced by inactivation without change in the TH protein content, probably due to dephosphorylation [Ozaki, et al., 1988 (17)].

At later stage in MPTP-treated mice, TH activity is decreased in parallel with the decrease in TH protein content. This decrease may be due to decreased TH protein synthesis. At least after 7 days' continuous administration of MPTP to mice the homospecific activity of TH did not change [Mogi, et al., 1987 (8)]. As reported above, the homospecific activity of TH in parkinsonian human brains was increased. Another difference in TH in the brains of MPTP-treated mice from TH in parkinsonian brains is that the decreased TH protein and activity are recovered to normal levels at least in young mice.

An endogenous MPTP-like substance of the parkinsonian brain, tetrahydroisoquinoline (TIQ) [Niwa, et al., 1987 (16)] produces parkinsonism in primates with decreased DA and TH in the nigrostriatal region. However, TIQ does not cause cell death [Nagatsu and Yoshida, 1988 (12) ; Yoshida, et al., 1990 (21)]. Both MPP^+ and $N-MeIQ^+$, a probable endogenous neurotoxin produced from TIQ, inhibits also TH and decreases DA in PC12h cells [Naoi, et al., 1988, 1989 (13, 14)].

TH activity and DA content in the striatum were reduced more markedly when cyclosporin A, an immune suppressor, was administered to mice together with MPTP. The cumulative effect of cyclosporin A on the MPTP-induced lesion in DA neurons may be ascribed to its effect on the immune system or may be dependent on its effect directly on the toxicity of MPTP [Hagihara, et al., 1989 (1)].

The nonneuronal cells transfected with human type 2 TH were used to produce L-DOPA for intracerebral grafting in animal models of parkinsonism [Uchida, et al., 1989, 1990 (19, 20)].

REFERENCES

1. Hagihara, M., et al., (1989): Neurochem. Int., 15: 249-254.
2. Hirata, Y. and Nagatsu, T. (1986): Neurosci. Lett., 68: 245-248.
3. Kaneda, N., et al., (1987) : Biochem. Biophys. Res. Commun., 146: 971-975.
4. Kaneda, N., et al., (1990): In Aging of the Brain: Cellular and Molecular Aspects of Brain Aging and Alzheimer's Disease: T. Nagatsu, Y. Ihara, S. Kohsaka, and R. Katzman, eds. in press. Japan Scientific Societies Press, Tokyo.
5. Kiuchi, K., et al., (1988): Neurosci. Lett., 89: 209-215.
6. Kobayashi, K., et al., (1988): J. Biochem., 103: 907-912.
7. Mogi, M., et al., (1984): Anal. Biochem., 138: 125-132.
8. Mogi, M., et al., (1987): Neurosci. Lett., 80: 213 218.
9. Mogi, M., et al., (1988): J. Neural Trasm., 72: 77-81.
10. Nagatsu, T., et al., (1964): J. Biol. Chem., 239: 2910-2917.
11. Nagatsu, T., et al., (1979): J. Chromatogr., 163: 247-252.
12. Nagatsu, T. and Yoshida, M. (1988): Neurosci. Lett., 87: 178-182.
13. Naoi, M., et al., (1988): Life Sci., 43: 1485-1491.
14. Naoi, M., et al., (1989): Neurochem. Int., 15: 315-320.
15. Narabayashi, H., et al., (1986): In Handbook of Clinical Neurology vol. 5, P.J. Vinken, G.W. Bruyn, and H.L. Klawans, eds. pp.157-165. Elsevier, Amsterdam.
16. Niwa, T., et al., (1987): Biochem. Biophys. Res. Commun., 144: 1084-1089.
17. Ozaki, N., et al., (1988): Neurosci. Lett., 85: 228-232.
18. Rausch, W. -D., et al., (1988) : J. Neurochem., 50: 202-208.
19. Uchida, K., et al., (1989): J. Neurochem., 53: 728-732.
20. Uchida, K., et al., (1990): Neurosci. Lett., 109: 282-286.
21. Yoshida, M., et al. (1990): In Alzheimer's and Parkinson's Diseases: Basic and Therapeutic Strategies, T. Nagatsu, A. Fisher, and M. Yoshida, eds. in press. Plenum Press, New York.

MAO-B AND COMT INHIBITION: ENHANCED BENEFIT IN DOPA THERAPY

M. Da Prada
Pharmaceutical Research Department, F. Hoffmann-La Roche Ltd, CH-4002 Basel, Switzerland

Although MADOPAR® and SINEMET® are still the mainstay drug treatments available for Parkinson's disease (PD), fluctuations in response, frequent dosing due to the short plasma half-life of L-DOPA and erratic pharmacokinetics, all cause problems in the management of these patients. Part of these problems are probably due to short half-life of cerebral dopamine (DA) which is rapidly deaminated by monoamine oxidase type B (MAO-B) and/or to the conversion of levodopa (DOPA) into 3-O-methyldopa (3-OMD) by the enzyme catechol-O-methyltranserase (COMT). In the following, the preclinical neurochemical characteristics of recently discovered reversible and highly selective inhibitors of MAO-B and COMT are summarized. These novel compounds, i.e. the MAO-B inhibitor Ro 19-6327 (N-[2-aminoethyl]-5-chloro-2-pyridine carboxamide HCl) and the COMT inhibitor Ro 40-7592 (3,4-dihydroxy-4'-methyl-5-nitrobenzophenone), are expected to offer innovative and safe approaches in the management of PD.

Ro 19-6327   Ro 40-7592

Ro 19-6327: A NOVEL, REVERSIBLE HIGHLY SELECTIVE MAO-B INHIBITOR

To date, (-)-deprenyl (selegiline) is the sole MAO-B inhibitor used clinically, as adjunct to DOPA and peripheral amino acid decarboxylase (AADC) inhibitors (e.g. MADOPAR® or SINEMET®), to improve symptom fluctuations in PD. Moreover, it was recently suggested that an early selegiline therapy could delay the requirement for antiparkinsonian medication possibly by slowing the degenerative process underlying PD. However, selegiline at relatively low doses (20 mg daily) and under long-term therapy does not only inhibit MAO-B but also, to some extent, MAO-A with the risk of hypertensive crises (cheese-effect) (1). Ro 19-6327 belongs to a new chemical class of non-toxic, mechanism-based, fully reversible, and highly selective MAO-B inhibitors both *in vitro* and *ex vivo*. In the rat brain *ex vivo*, the ED_{50} values (µmol/kg p.o. 2 h) obtained using phenylethylamine (PEA) and 5-hydroxytryptamine (5-HT) as substrates were: Ro 19-6327 0.2 and > 1000 vs selegiline 4.3 and > 500. In the rat MAO-B inhibition by Ro 19-6327 is short-lasting (12-24 h). Ro 19-6327, did not affect mean arterial blood pressure (MAP) even at high doses and did not potentiate the tyramine-induced increase in MAP in freely moving rats. In black mice, Ro 19-6327 prevented the 1-methyl-4-phenyl-1,2,5,6-tetrahydropyridine (MPTP)-induced depletion of brain dopamine in the striatal tissue. In healthy subjects, Ro 19-6327 is well tolerated even at the high dose of 200 mg and completely inhibits platelet MAO-B for 24 h after the dose of 100 mg.

REVERSIBLE AND SPECIFIC INHIBITION OF THE COMT IN THE CNS AND IN THE EXTRACEREBRAL TISSUE BY Ro 40-7592

To date, no peripherally and centrally active COMT inhibitors are available for clinical trials. It is well known that DOPA combined with peripheral AADC inhibitors is largely converted into 3-OMD. Once DOPA has reached the peripheral circulation it can still be converted into 3-OMD, mainly in the liver and in the kidney, but also in various other peripheral organs. Unlike DOPA, 3-OMD has a long plasma half-life of about 15 h. Therefore, 3-OMD accumulates in plasma during prolonged administration of DOPA and may interfere with the active transport of the latter into the brain, by competing with the same saturable transport system. Ro 40-7592 is a competitive (K_i= 30 nM) inhibitor of COMT of intermediate duration of action, very potent *in vitro* (rat liver IC_{50}= 36 nM) and *ex vivo* (ED_{50} for rat liver and kidney: 2.7 and 1.2 mg/kg p.o. 1 h). A reliable assessment of the COMT inhibitory effect by Ro 40-7592 was obtained by measuring the decrease of O-methylated catechol derivatives, e.g. 3-OMD, HVA and MOPEG, 2 h after Ro 40-7592 (30 mg/kg p.o.) and control values were attained about 16 h after dosing (3).

CONCLUSION

Ro 19-6327 due to its highly selective inhibitory effect on MAO-B is an excellent tool to assess whether complete and selective MAO-B inhibition protects dopaminergic neurones from age-associated degeneration, possibly by reducing the formation of free radicals or the conversion of MPTP-like compounds into neurotoxins in the CNS (2). The increased bioavailability and plasma half-life of DOPA and the reduced formation of 3-OMD by the coadministration of Ro 40-7592 with Madopar® offers a unique approach to a more rational therapy of PD.

REFERENCES

1. Bieck, P.R. and Antonin, K.H., (1989): J. Neural Transm., Suppl. 28:21-31, 1989.
2. Da Prada, M. et al. (1988): In Progress in Catecholamine Research Part B: Central Aspects, pp. 359-363. Alan R. Liss, Inc, New York.
3. Zürcher, G. et al. (1990): In Adv. Neurol. (9th Intern. Symposium on Parkinson's Disease, Jerusalem, June 5-9, 1988) (in press).

FUNCTIONAL STUDIES ON MONOAMINERGIC TRANSMITTER RELEASE IN PARKINSONISM

W. WESEMANN, H.-W. CLEMENT and CHR. GROTE
Department of Neurochemistry, Institute of Physiological Chemistry, Philipps University, D-3550 Marburg/Lahn, F.R.G.

Classical analytical methods, such as HPLC, for the study of neurotransmitter metabolism provide information only on the total content of a given transmitter (metabolite) in a distinct brain region or nucleus. However, to get an insight into the neuronal activity, it is necessary to assay neurotransmitter release. Pulse voltammetry introduced into neurobiology by Buda et al., 1981 (1) allows to estimate monoaminergic neurotransmitter activity in vivo by measuring the extraneuronal serotonin (5-HT) and catecholamine (metabolites) concentration.

In the Parkinson syndrome aside from the well-known reduction of the dopaminergic (DA) system also serotoninergic functions may be involved in secondary symptoms and in side-effects observed in DOPA therapy such as hyperthermia, sleep disturbances, depression, the "on-off" phenomenon, and the "restless leg" syndrome.

SUBJECT AND METHOD

The aim of the present study was to analyze by in vivo voltammetry the effect of drugs used in the therapy of M. Parkinson (transmitter precursors, MAO inhibitors, NMDA receptor antagonists), of the DA antagonist haloperidol, and of neurotoxins (6-hydroxydopamine = 6=OH-DA, 1-methyl-4-phenyl-1,2,3,6-tetrahydropyridine = MPTP, 1-methyl-4-phenylpyridinium ion = MPP^+) on extraneuronal DA and 5-HT (metabolite) concentration as a measure of the neuronal activity of aminergic transmitter systems. Carbon fibre electrodes were implanted into the striatum of Wistar rats, 250-300 g. Because of the small diameter (12 µm) of these electrodes, the lesion of the brain tissue was kept to a minimum. With exception of the experiments with memantine, in all studies 3.4-dihydroxyphenylacetic acid (DOPAC) and 5-hydroxyindoleacetic acid (5-HIAA) were taken as a measure for aminergic neuronal activity.

RESULTS AND DISCUSSION

<u>Neurotransmitter precursors</u>. In untreated rats, L-DOPA (200 mg/kg i.p.), the major drug in the treatment of M. Parkinson, increases extracellular DOPAC in the striatum. The same DOPA dose reduces extracellular 5-HIAA in the striatum by about 30%. Though tryptophan does not affect 5-HT release as measured by extraneuronal 5-HIAA concentration in the nucleus raphe dorsalis and in the striatum, this substance reduces striatal DOPAC. The direct precursor of 5-HT, 5-hydroxytryptophan, increases striatal 5-HIAA and reduces DOPAC levels. Hence, the Parkinson therapy with DOPA interferes with the serotoninergic system which is in accordance with the clinical observation that precursors of 5-HT may ameliorate side-effects of the DOPA therapy.

Inhibitors of monoamine oxidase (MAO). The MAO inhibitor deprenyl was the only inhibitor showing "pure" MAO B inhibition whereas pargyline in accordance with its activity as MAO A and MAO B inhibitor, reduced both, DOPAC and 5-HIAA levels. However, in contradistinction to our assumption, the specific MAO A inhibitor clorgyline decreased DOPAC more rapidly as compared to 5-HIAA.

Agonists and antagonists. Apomorphine as a DA agonist reduced in the concentration of 50 and 500 µg/kg i.p. extraneuronal DOPAC. This finding suggests that despite of the concentration-dependent D 1 and D 2 receptor activation, the presynaptic inhibition of DA release can be demonstrated by in vivo pulse voltammetry at both apomorphine concentrations. The antiparkinsonian and antispastic drug memantine (20 mg/kg i.p.), which blocks the NMDA receptor (2) enhances striatal DA release. The D2 antagonist haloperidol (0.5 mg/kg i.p.) increases extraneuronal DOPAC concentration. This observation agrees with the well-known mode of action of the compound.

Neurotoxins. As a model of M. Parkinson the effect of neurotoxins on monoaminergic metabolism in the striatum was studied. The neurotoxins 6-OH-DA, MPTP, and MPP^+ were unilaterally applied to the substantia nigra pars compacta and the catechol and 5-hydroxyindole signals were registered ipsi- and contralaterally in the striatum. Four weeks after unilateral lesion of the substantia nigra (SN) with 8 µg 6-OH-DA no catechol peak was obtained at the lesioned side whereas the contralateral catechol signal appeared to be normal. Though lower concentrations (50 µg) of MPTP totally abolished the DOPAC signal in acute experiments, higher doses (175 µg) of this toxin were necessary to attain a continual DOPAC decrease which could be demonstrated even after 3 weeks. MPP^+, as the active MPTP metabolite, induced in small (10 µg) and high doses (30 µg) a lasting reduction of extraneuronal catecholes. If neurotoxin treatment was followed by administration of 200 mg/kg i.p. DOPA, a catechol peak is obtained at the lesioned and the unlesioned side. In agreement with the aforementioned findings with untreated rats, the precursor DOPA reduced also in lesioned rats the 5-HT release.

SUMMARY

Activation of the DA system reduces 5-HT neurotransmitter activity and vice versa. Hence, side effects observed in the treatment of parkinsonian patients with DOPA may be caused by a reduction of the serotoninergic system.

REFERENCES

1. Buda, et al. (1981) In vivo electrochemical detection of catechols in several dopaminergic brain regions of anaesthetized rats. Eur. J. Pharmacol. 73: 61-68.
2. Kornhuber et al. (1989) [^{3}H]MK-801 binding sites in postmortem human frontal cortex. Eur. J. Pharmacol. 162, 483-490.

IRON MELANIN AND DOPAMINE INTERACTION: RELEVANCE TO PARKINSON'S DISEASE

D. BEN-SHACHAR and M.B.H. YOUDIM.
Department of Pharmacology, Faculty of Medicine and Rappaport Medical Research Center, Technion, Haifa, Israel.

The mechanism of degeneration of the melanized dopaminergic neurons in the substantia nigra (SN) in Parkinson's disease (PD) is unknown. The involvement of toxic hydroxyl free radicals which promote lipid peroxidation and thereby cell destruction has been suggested (1). Recent postmortem studies of Parkinsonian brains revealed a selective and highly significant increase of iron which catalyzes the formation of free hydroxyl radicals in the SN (2). Melanin is considered to be an effective radical scavenger in the SN, yet under certain conditions such as increased Fe^{+3} levels, melanin can induce the formation of oxygen radicals (3), probably by reducing Fe^{+3} to Fe^{+2}. The ability of melanin to bind iron and their combined effect on lipid peroxidation may have relevancy to the degenerative processes in PD.

METHODS:

Dopamine-melanin (DA-mel) was synthesized by a modified procedure of Das et al. (4). The specific binding of 20 various concentrations (0.5-400nM) of $^{59}FeCl_3$ (14.28 Ci/mg) to 3ug of DA-mel was assayed in the presence or absence of 10ug $FeCl_3$. The reaction mixture, 0.25 ml of 5mM Tris HCl buffer (final pH-6.5) was incubated at 37°C for 2 hrs. The reaction was terminated by adding 2 ml of cold buffer and filtering the mixture through GF/B filters. Radioactivity was counted in a liquid scintilation spectrometer. Lipid peroxidation in cortex homogenates was assayed by measuring malondialdehyde (MAD) formation (1,5).

TABLE 1: EQUILIBRIUM CONSTANTS FOR $^{59}FeCl_3$ BINDING SITES TO DA-MELANIN

	KD (nM)	Bmax (pmol/mg melanin)
HIGH	13±1.61	1.13±0.15
LOW	200±40	17.63±1.3

TABLE 2: EFFECT OF COMPOUNDS ON $^{59}FeCl_3$ BINDING TO DA-MELANIN

COMPOUND	% OF TOTAL BINDING
5uM MPTP	100
5uM MPP+	100
5uM DA	135
60nM DFO	50

RESULTS

Scatchard analysis of the saturation curve of the specific binding of $^{59}FeCl_3$ to DA-mel revealed both a high and a low affinity binding site (Table 1). Binding of iron to DA-mel was potentiated by dopamine and inhibited by the iron chelator, desferioxamine (DFO). Neither MPTP nor MPP had any effect on the binding of iron to melanin (Table 2). Basal lipid peroxidation, as measured by MDA formation, was promoted by iron salts and reduced by 3.0 and 12ug melanin. However, 12ug of melanin potentiated lipid peroxidation produced by iron. Lipid peroxidation was inhibited by DFO as well as by dopamine (Fig. 1).

Fig. 1: Iron induced ($FeCl - 10^{-4}M$) lipid peroxidation in rat cerebral cortex as indicated by MDA formation in the presence of 3ug DA-melanin (Mel), $10^{-4}M$ desferioxamine (DFO) and $10^{-4}M$ dopamine (DA). Results over respective basal levels are expressed.

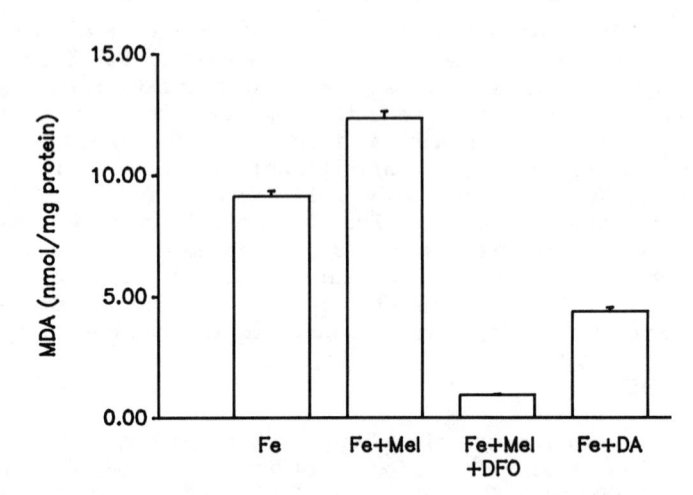

DISCUSSION

The ability of melanin to bind iron in a high affinity manner corresponds to its being an effective radical scavenger. The binding of iron to melanin is potentiated in the presence of dopamine in a concentration dependent manner. In Parkinsonian SN iron, and especially the Fe^{+3} form, is significantly elevated and the ratio of $Fe^{+2}:Fe^{+3}$ changes from 3:1 in controls to 1:1 (2). The diminished levels of endogenous H_2O_2 scavengers, ascorbate and GSH in Parkinsonian SN (2) predicts a significant accumulation of H_2O_2 generated from deamination and auto-oxidation of dopamine. The elevated levels of H_2O_2 and free iron in the Parkinsonian SN with melanin serving as a catalyst for conversion of Fe^{+3} to Fe^{+2} are ideal conditions for generating free cytotoxic radicals. The decrease in dopamine levels due to the degeneration of dopaminergic neurons in PD further intensifies this process.

REFERENCES

1. Dexter, D.T. et al., (1989): J. Neurochem. 53:381-389.
2. Riederer, P. et al., (1989): J. Neuorchem. 52:515-520.
3. Pilas, B. et al., (1988): Free Radical Biol 4:285-293.
4. Das, K.C. et al., (1986): J. Neurochem. 40:601-605.
5. Rehncrona, S. et al. (1980): J. Neurochem. 34:1630-1638.

DEPRENYL (SELEGILINE) AS MONOTHERAPY IN EARLY PARKINSON'S DISEASE

I. SHOULSON and the PARKINSON STUDY GROUP
Department of Neurology, University of Rochester Medical Center, Rochester, NY, U.S.A.

The progressive nigral degeneration of Parkinson's disease (PD) has been associated with oxidative-mediated events including increased monoamine oxidase (MAO) and free-radical generation [1]. Between September 1987 and November 1988, 800 patients with early, untreated PD were enrolled in the multi-center, placebo-controlled, double-blind trial "Deprenyl and Tocopherol Antioxidative Therapy of Parkinsonism" (DATATOP). Subjects were assigned by a 2 X 2 factorial design to receive deprenyl (10 mg/day), tocopherol (2000 IU/day), a combination of both drugs, or placebo, and followed regularly to determine the onset of disability requiring levodopa therapy (primary end point).

After 12 ± 5 months (mean $\pm$ sd) of follow-up, independent monitoring prompted a preliminary analysis. The 401 subjects who received deprenyl and the 399 subjects who did not receive deprenyl did not differ significantly with respect to any base-line variable. However, subjects treated with deprenyl experienced a 57% reduction in the risk of reaching the primary end point ($p < 10^{-10}$) and a 50% reduction in the risk of ceasing full-time employment ($p = 0.01$). Adverse effects of deprenyl were minor and infrequent [2].

The average rate of clinical decline as measured by the Unified Parkinson's Disease Rating Scale [1] was approximately 50% slower in subjects who received deprenyl compared to subjects who did not. While statistically significant symptomatic improvement was observed among deprenyl-treated subjects at 1 month and 3 months after base line, the extent of benefit was slight and unlikely of any clinical consequence [2].

The mechanisms underlying the beneficial effects of deprenyl are unclear. Deprenyl may have ameliorated PD by its dopaminergic action, through its methamphetamine and amphetamine metabolites, or by antidepressant activity. While these mechanisms may explain some of the benefit, neither our multi-center trial nor the independent study of Tetrud and Langston [3] support the notion that deprenyl monotherapy in early PD is attended by a robust symptomatic effect. The modest symptomatic effects that we observed after 1 and 3 months of therapy did not account for the long-term reduction in the rate of reaching the primary end point of disability.

The DATATOP study has been modified on the basis of our preliminary findings. All subjects who did not reach the end point of disability requiring levodopa were withdrawn from experimental treatments for two months, then administered active deprenyl 10 mg/day. Either active tocopherol (2000 IU/day) or placebo has been re-started in accordance with original treatment assignment. The blindness of all original treatment assignments has been maintained as subjects are followed until end point is reached for up to an additional 18 months of observation. If deprenyl only exerts symptomatic (dopaminergic) effects, then clinical worsening during the 2-month withdrawal phase is expected to occur disproportionately among subjects who were previously taking active deprenyl. Furthermore, subjects newly administered deprenyl should soon show benefits and "catch up" to subjects who were previously taken active deprenyl. If deprenyl predominantly exerts protective effects, then subjects previously taking active deprenyl, compared with subjects newly administered deprenyl, should continue to maintain their benefits with respect to the end point of disability.

Our preliminary findings support a recommendation for the treatment of otherwise untreated patients in the early stages of PD with deprenyl 10 mg/day. A lower dosage may be as effective or more effective since deprenyl acts as an irreversible inhibitor of the type-B monoamine oxidase. Caution should be taken in all deprenyl-treated patients since l-deprenyl is metabolized to the l-isomers of methamphetamine and amphetamine. Although we found deprenyl to be relatively safe as monotherapy in early PD, deprenyl in combination with levodopa or other dopaminergic agents may potentiate dopaminergic toxicity. Our modified trial is expected to address: 1) the extent that beneficial effects of deprenyl are related to symptomatic (dopaminergic) and/or protective (anti-neurotoxic) mechanisms, 2) the longer-term duration of deprenyl's effects, before and after levodopa therapy is required, 3) the independent and interactive effects of tocopherol, 4) the effect of experimental treatments on lifespan of our patients, and 5) the economic impact of these interventions.

ACKNOWLEDGEMENT

This research is supported by the United States Public Health Service grant NS 24778, administered by the National Institutes of Neurological Diseases and Stroke of the National Institutes of Health.

REFERENCES

1. Parkinson Study Group, (1989): DATATOP: A multi-center controlled clinical trial in early Parkinson's disease, Arch. Neurol. 46:1052-1060.

2. Parkinson Study Group, (1989): Effect of deprenyl on the progression of disability in early Parkinson's disease. New England Journal of Medicine 321:1364-1371.

3. Tetrud JW, Langston JW, (1989): The effect of deprenyl (selegiline) on the natural history of Parkinson's disease. Science 245:519-522.

Dopamine Agonists in Parkinson's Disease: Present Status and New Trends

R. Horowski, I. Runge, P.-A. Löschmann, L. Turski, H. Wachtel
Schering Research Labs. Berlin/Bergkamen, W.-Germany

I. Effects on Symptoms of Parkinson's Disease (PD) due to dopamine deficiency: They can be treated either by the dopamine (DA) precursor drug levodopa or by DA agonists which replace DA at the postsynaptic receptors. Classic DA agonists and related drugs (apomorphine, piribedil, PHNO) activate all DA receptors in a similar way whilst ergot-derived drugs (bromocriptine) and especially 8-α-aminoergolines (lisuride, terguride) seem to be more active on "empty" DA receptors and may have state-dependent partial agonist properties (1). Lisuride can also be used for parenteral applications. However, levodopa still is the "gold standard" and basis of therapy preferred by many patients in spite of its complicated kinetic and metabolic pattern. Reasons for this may include: 1. Peripheral decarboxylase inhibitors reduce peripheral DA-related side effects, and, therefore, DA agonists should be combined with the peripheral DA antagonist domperidone for comparison, 2. levodopa-derived DA activates both D_2 and D_1 receptors (which are claimed to act in a synergistic way) whilst DA agonists are weaker on D_1, or are only partial agonists/antagonists (D_1 agonism: dopamine > apomorphine > pergolide $\geq$ lisuride >> bromocriptine). In complete DA depletion, apomorphine and lisuride still restore mobility (whilst bromocriptine needs additional D_1 activation) but the majority of patients with PD who have continuous s.c. lisuride or apomorphine infusion still require at least a small dose of additional levodopa. 3. Levodopa is concentrated and activated within the DA neurons and released probably with the nerve impulse flow; thus over-stimulation of DA systems is reduced by such a "buffering" mechanism, and there is less autoreceptor activation, and finally, 4. levodopa also is a noradrenaline (NA) precursor drug (at least in NA depletion such as it occurs in PD) whilst apomorphine has no agonist and some ergot DA agonists even have antagonistic properties.

II. Improvement of levodopa-induced motor fluctuations (which are caused by longterm levodopa administration and are often very disabling) is a main indication for the addition of DA agonists to therapy. Levodopa dosage can be reduced and both dyskinesias (possibly a result of receptor overstimulation) and "wearing off" (a result of short levodopa half-life when neuronal "buffering" declines with progressive disease) improve by the addition of ergoline DA agonists whilst anti-akinetic effects are maintained (as shown recently, e.g., in the case of lisuride (2)). Regarding these longterm motor complications of levodopa therapy, DA agonists are superior because with longterm DA agonist monotherapy in responders, those side effects have not been observed. The improvement caused by DA agonists may be due to partial agonist properties (as is quite obvious with the pronounced partial agonist terguride (3) which has clear antidyskinetic effects without worsening motor function), presynaptic "stabilization" and more continuous receptor occupancy and activation, as is supported by the beneficial results of continuous s.c. infusion of lisuride in these patients (4). These results demonstrate that fluctuations are not related to progressive degeneration of the whole system but that kinetic factors are of great relevance. If continuous DA stimulation can be achieved with less technical problems, and if mental side effects can be controlled, this strategy of constant DA activation clearly needs further investigation of potential beneficial effects on fluctuations or the progression of the disease itself.

III. Early combination of DA agonists with levodopa prevents or postpones motor fluctuations, as shown in a controlled, randomized, prospective study with lisuride at an average dose of 1 mg/day (5), where levodopa could be reduced by 30 % with similar motor improvements as in the levodopa monotherapy group, but with significantly less fluctuations after 5 years' therapy (~ 10 % vs. ~ 60 %). Patients on lisuride monotherapy, too, had an extremely low incidence of fluctuations, but most of them needed additional levodopa over the years for full clinical effect. Further addition of the MAO B inhibitor deprenyl permitted a further reduction in the dose of levodopa, but an evaluation after 3 years did not demonstrate other differences regarding therapeutic efficacy, fluctuations, and disease progression (as judged from CURS ratings). The postponement of levodopa-induced fluctuations by lisuride does not seem to be caused just by dose-reduction, but additional mechanisms (presynaptic "stabilization", better receptor kinetics) are most probably involved.

IV. The influence of DA agonists on the progression of PD is not known (in contrast to animal studies, where the number of surviving rats can be increased, as observed, e.g., for levodopa, lisuride, and deprenyl). In PD, DA cells with special vulnerability (e.g. by mitochondrial complex I deficit) or specific affinity for toxins (e.g. by melanine or receptors) and under the influence of a general aging of the system may be killed by exo- or endotoxins (MPTP, Mn^{++}, toxic metabolites, quinones, peroxide, CO, or others). It is conceivable that, if a critical threshold is reached, the surviving cells show enhanced metabolic turnover (mediated by feedback-loops and, possibly, excitatory amino acids) and that, thereby, a vicious circle is induced with further endotoxin production, exhaustion of cell energy and of radical scavengers, subsequent Ca^{++} influx, and, finally, cell death which maintains the progression of the disease. With such a sequence of events, DA agonists by means of their presynaptic effects may again interfere in a positive way and thus influence the disease. Furthermore, new additional therapeutic strategies might be combined with DA agonists; however, large longterm studies will be necessary to investigate this further, and new techniques of quantification (e.g. PET methods) will become necessary.

Bibliography

1. Horowski, R. (1988):
   Funct. Neurol., III: 459-470
2. Rabey, J. M., Streifler, M., Treves, T., Korczyn, A. D. (1989):
   In: Parkinsonism and Aging, (Aging, Vol. 36),
   D.B. Calne et al., eds., pp. 261-267,
   Raven Press, New York
3. Wachtel, H., Dorow, R. (1983):
   Life Sci., 32: 421-432
4. Obeso, J.A., Horowski, R., Marsden, C.D. (1988):
   Continuous Dopaminergic Stimulation in
   Parkinson's Disease, J. NeuralTransm.,Suppl. 27,
   Springer, Wien New York
5. Rinne, U.K. (1989):
   Neurology, 39: 336-339

AN OVERVIEW OF NERVE GROWTH FACTORS: FROM MOLECULES TO MEMORY

E. M. SHOOTER
Department of Neurobiology, Stanford University School of Medicine, Stanford, CA 94305-5401, U.S.A.

Nerve growth factor (NGF) is the first member of a class of proteins, the neurotrophic factors or neurotrophins, which play an important role in the regulation of neuronal cell death during development, in maintaining the differentiated state of these neurons and in aiding in their recovery from injury or ageing. Although much of the early work on NGF was carried out on two populations of peripheral neurons, the sympathetic and some sensory neurons, the more recent discovery of an NGF-dependent group of neurons in the CNS has directed attention to the ability of NGF to rescue these basal forebrain cholinergic neurons after either acute injury or degeneration in ageing. The structures of two additional members of the NGF family have recently been described, those of BDNF and NT-3. While both proteins show significant homology to NGF, BDNF, at least, has a different neuronal specificity to NGF, interacting, with the central rather than peripheral projections of sensory neurons, including those in the nodose ganglion which are unaffected by NGF, and retinal ganglion cells. It is possible, therefore, that the NGF family of neurotrophic factors will regulate survival, maintenance and regeneration of several major CNS as well as PNS populations.

The ability of NGF to determine neuronal survival in development depends on the establishment of a retrograde flow of NGF from the target, across the nerve terminal, up the axon to the neuronal cell body. Those neurons which establish this flow survive, those that do no degenerate. NGF mRNA and protein appear in the target only at the time that the growing nerve fibers reach the target; however NGF synthesis does not depend on the interaction between the fiber and the target. While NGF mRNA levels increase steadily over several days to reach an equilibrium value NGF protein levels first peak and then decline as retrograde flow commences. Once established this retrograde flow must be maintained if the neurons are to reach and maintain their fully differentiated state. The flow is initiated by the binding of NGF to specific NGF receptors in the nerve terminal and their internalization in membrane bound vesicles. The later are transported along microtubules to deliver intact, biologically active NGF to the cell body. After acidification of the cytoplasm of the vesicles the NGF is transferred to the lysosomes for degradation, while a significant fraction of the receptors are probably recycled. The neuronal degradation of NGF is quite rapid and plays no part in its mechanism of action. This is not yet clear whether the initial signal transduction mechanism induced by NGF acts only at the level of the NGF receptor in the nerve terminal or during retrograde flow or in both places.

The growing fibers of trigeminal ganglion sensory neurons display very low levels of NGF receptor until they contact their target. At this stage NGF receptor levels increase in parallel with the increase in NGF levels in the target suggesting that NGF regulates expression of its own receptor. This has been directly demonstrated in adult sensory neurons and in PC12 pheochromocytoma cells. Although a cut or crush of a rat sciatic nerve interrupts the retrograde flow of NGF from the targets of sensory and sympathetic fibers, the proximal segments of these nerves and their cell bodies in large part survive and regenerate. This is due again in part, to the rapid synthesis and secretion of NGF by the Schwann cells at and distal to the site of injury and the consequent establishment of the retrograde flow. The replacement of the target source of NGF by the Schwann cell production is incomplete as judged by the reduced level of the retrograde flow of NGF in the regenerating fibers and by the loss of 20-30% of the sensory and sympathetic neurons providing fibers to the injured nerve. However infusion of additional NGF at the time of injury rescues the neurons which would otherwise degenerate. The induction of NGF in the Schwann cells occurs in two phases. The first is very rapid, occurring within minutes of injury, and reaching a maximum after 6h and then declining slowly. The nature of the inductive signal for this phase is unknown. The second phase of induction prevents NGF levels from falling too low, reaches a maximum after 3 or so days and is mediated by interleukin-1 released by invading macrophage. As the nerve fibers regenerate and the macrophage slowly leave the injured nerve NGF levels in the nerve return to normal, very low values. Surprisingly the Schwann cells also express NGF receptors of the low affinity type in a process mediated through loss of contact between the Schwann cells and the axonal-myelin membranes. As the nerve fibers regenerate and are again ensheathed by the Schwann cells the NGF receptor is down regulated. The role of these glial cell NGF receptors may be to concentrate NGF on the surface of the cells to make the NGF more readily available for advancing growth cones. These two different modes of regulation of the NGF receptor, by NGF for the receptors in neurons and by axonal contact for the receptors in Schwann cells clearly play key roles in the ability of NGF to promote survival and regeneration in peripheral neurons.

NGF-MEDIATED PROMOTION OF CELL SURVIVAL IN CULTURE FROM POSTNATAL RAT CNS.

Hiroshi HATANAKA
Division of Protein Biosynthesis, Institute for Protein Research, Osaka University, Suita-shi, Osaka, Japan.

Basal forebrain cholinergic neurons are thought to play an indispensable role in the functional neuronal pathways of learning and memory. Some correlations between death of these neurons and senile dementia of the Alzheimer type have been pointed out. NGF, one of the well-characterized neurotrophic factors, has been known to play an important role in neuronal differentiation and cell survival of basal forebrain cholinergic neurons (1).

In the present communication, we will demonstrate the establishment of a primary neuronal cell culture technique (2) from the postnatal rat CNS to study the NGF response to the cholinergic neurons, as shown in Fig. 1. We have appeared that, during the early postnatal day, the action of NGF changes from the induction of choline acetyltransferase activity to the promotion of cholinergic neuronal cell survival in septal cholinergic neurons in culture (3). NGF appeared to support cell survival of basal forebrain

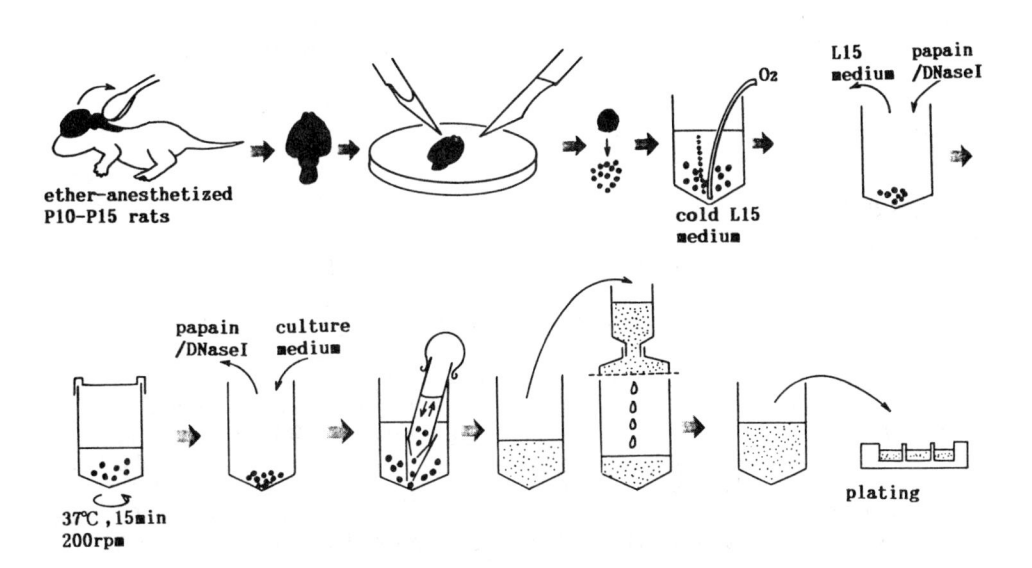

Fig. 1. Cell culture method for postnatal rat CNS neurons.

cholinergic neurons obtained from P11-P15 rat septum (3,4), the vertical limb of the diagonal band of Broca (3) and the nucleus basalis of Meynert (5,6). The role of NGF appeared to change from a differentiation factor to a survival-promoting factor during the early postnatal period, which is just coincident with the period of completion of the septal projection to the hippocampal formation.

RESULTS

The present established neuronal culture method has the following unique characteristics:

i) We were able to demonstrate that the survival effect by NGF on cultured rat cholinergic neurons was not dependent on plating cell density (7), contrary to the previous report which has described that NGF-dependent cell survival occurred only under low-density culture conditions, but not under high-density conditions, by using the septal cultures obtained from fetal (E17) and newborn (to P2) rat brain.

ii) A sufficient supply of oxygen during the preparation of dissociated cells from postnatal rat brain tissue is necessary for their viability in culture (7). And also, we found better cell survival of postnatal rat CNS neurons in culture in a 50% oxygen atmosphere during cultivation in a CO_2 incubator than with normal air.

iii) Postnatal neurons could be labeled retrogradely in vivo with fluorescent latex microspheres before culture. We found that the survival of retrogradely labeled neurons projecting to the hippocampus from septal neurons was promoted by the addition of NGF in culture (8).

iv) Postnatal CNS neurons consists of various types of cells as well as different cell size. We purified the magnocellular basal forebrain cholinergic neurons by the method of elutriation centrifugation.

v) Postnatal P4 rat septal cholinergic neurons cultured for 5 days were successfully transplanted to a denervated host hippocampus in one of 3 cases (9).

REFERENCES

1. Hatanaka, H. Tanpakushitsu Kakusan Kouso **35**: 365-379, 1990.
2. Hatanaka, H. and Tsukui, H. Exp. Med. **6**: 1211-1217, 1988.
3. Hatanaka, H. et al. Dev. Brain Res. **39**: 85-95, 1988.
4. Hatanaka, H. et al. Neurosci. Lett. **79**: 85-90, 1987.
5. Hatanaka, H. et al. Neurosci. Lett. **90**: 63-68, 1988.
6. Takei, N. et al. J. Neurochem. **53**: 1405-1410, 1989.
7. Hatanaka, H. et al. Neurosci. Res. in press, 1990.
8. Arimatsu, Y. et al. Dev. Brain Res. **45**: 297-301, 1989.
9. Hisanaga, K. et al. Brain Res. **475**: 349-355, 1988.

MOLECULAR AND CELLULAR MECHANISMS OF NEURONAL DEATH CAUSED BY NERVE GROWTH FACTOR DEPRIVATION

T. KOIKE
Department of Natural Science, Saga Medical School,
Nabeshima-machi, Saga 840-01, Japan.

There is ample evidence emphasizing the role of trophic factors in the development of neuron-target relationships so that only a restricted number of neurons will survive during the development of the nervous system (5). Developing sympathetic and embryonic sensory neurons established in the presence of nerve growth factor (NGF) die in vitro upon acute deprivation of NGF (1,4). This in vitro approach mimics the physiological situation in which neurons die during development or after axotomy when trophic factor support becomes insufficient. During development, however, sympathetic and sensory neurons become independent of NGF for survival both in vivo and in vitro: trophic deprivation does not cause immediate death of these neurons but results in neuronal atrophy and involution associated with depression of synaptic responses (5). Search for factors in controlling neuronal death and atrophy is yet to be pursued.

There is also evidence that afferent inputs, which cause membrane depolarization of the corresponding neurons, may control neuronal death in vivo. We have found that depolarizing agents including high K+ medium and cholinergic agonists prevent death of developing sympathetic neurons upon acute withdrawal of NGF (2). Evidence has been gathered that Ca2+ influx through dihydropyridine (DHP)-sensitive L-type Ca2+ channels plays a major role in the high K+ saving, whereas the depolarizing agents, choline and carbamylcholine, acting through nicotinic cholinergic receptors, exert their effects through activation of Ca2+ release from intracellular stores. In either case prevention of the death of NGF-deprived cells is associated with an increase of cytoplasmic free Ca2+ of sympathetic neurons. Indeed, fluorescence digital imaging technique using fura-2 as a probe has revealed that chronic exposure to high K+ medium results in an increase of cytoplasmic free Ca2+ from 110±11nM to 233±21nM, and the basal level of cytoplasmic Ca2+ of these neurons is increased to 225±16nM upon advancing aging in

Fig. 1:
A proposed scheme for cell death and atrophy of sympathetic neurons as a function of aging in vitro.

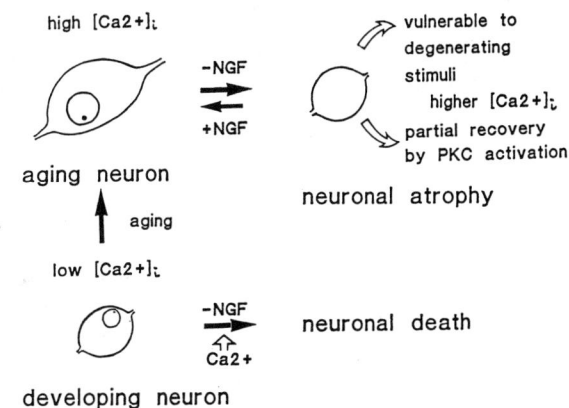

vitro (3). We hypothesize that aging neurons do not die upon acute deprivation of NGF because of high levels of the basal cytoplasmic Ca2+ which may inhibit the expression of death program in aging neurons (Fig. 1). These neurons, however, slowly become atrophic; this process is reversible and activation of Protein Kinase C partially facilitates recovery from atrophic conditions (unpublished). We speculate that these atrophic neurons may be extremely vulnerable to external degenerating stimuli.

Molecular mechanisms as to why neurons die in response to acute deprivation of NGF are unknown. Martin et al. (4) have found that neuronal death is prevented by cycloheximide, which indicates that new protein synthesis is necessary for this process or this drug stabilizes labile mRNA. To approach this we are currently utilizing PC12 cells as a model system. Indeed, PC12 cells respond to acute withdrawal of NGF by a decrease in ATP content (Fig. 2) or release of Adenylate Kinase activity (6) only when they have been treated with NGF. Thus, we are now

Fig. 2:
Alterations of ATP content of PC12 cells induced by acute withdrawal of NGF. The cells have been treated with NGF for various periods of time as indicated.

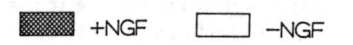

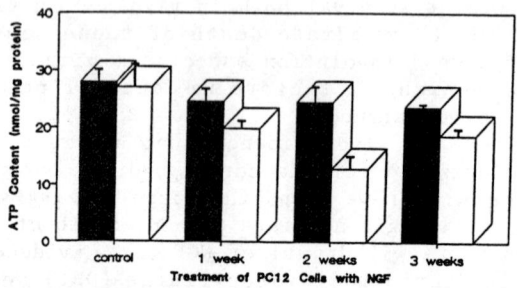

▓▓▓ +NGF   ☐ −NGF

in a position to address the question of whether or not cascade of gene activity is associated with neuronal death caused by acute withdrawal of NGF as has been postulated for addition of NGF to naive PC12 cells. We would also like to ask the question as to how quickly the message of NGF receptor will be degraded in response to trophic deprivation.

REFERENCES
1. Eichler, M.E. and Rich, K.M.: Death of sensory neurons after acute withdrawal of nerve growth factor in dissociated cell cultures. Brain Res. 482;340-346, 1989.
2. Koike, T. et al.: Role of Ca2+ channels in the ability of membrane depolarization to prevent neuronal death induced by trophic-factor deprivation: evidence that levels of internal Ca2+ determine nerve growth factor dependence of sympathetic ganglion cells. Proc. Natl. Acad. Sci. U.S.A. 86:6421-6425, 1989.
3. Koike, T. and Tanaka, S.: Nerve growth factor dependence of cultured sympathetic neurons is determined by cytoplasmic free calcium. J. Cell. Biochem. in press.
4. Martin, D.P. et al.: Inhibitors of protein synthesis and RNA synthesis prevent neuronal cell death caused by nerve growth factor deprivation. J. Cell Biol. 106:829-844, 1988.
5. Purves, D.: Body and Brain. Harvard Univ. Press, MA, U.S.A., 1988.
6. Tanaka, S. and Koike, T.: Degenerative responses of differentiated PC12 cells upon acute deprivation of nerve growth factor. Bull. Japan. Biochem. Soc., 61:1112, 1989.

EMERGING PHARMACOLOGY OF NEUROTROPHIC FACTORS

F. HEFTI
Andrus Gerontology Center, University of Southern California, Los Angeles, CA, U.S.A.

Currently used drugs to treat neurological disorders influence mechanisms related to neuronal impulse flow and transmission at the synapse. They do not affect the structural features of the central nervous system and there are no compounds reliably able to promote regeneration, plasticity and maintencance of structural integrity of selected neuronal systems. The discovery of neurotrophic factors may lead to such a new, structurally oriented neuropharmacology. Neurobiological research carried out in recent years revealed that proteins called neurotrophic factors influence development, maintenance of function, and regeneration of neurons. Nerve growth factor (NGF) is the first and best characterized among this group of molecules. Several other neurotrophic factors have been characterized with actions on neurons other than those responsive to NGF. The spectrum of actions will determine the therapeutic usefulness of individual neurotrophic factors.

NGF and Alzheimer's disease

Alzheimer's disease is associated with a loss of cholinergic neurons of the basal forebrain located and a large body of evidence supports the view that these cholinergic neurons are involved in functions related to cognition and memory. These cholinergic neurons respond to NGF during their entire life-span. In animals, NGF administration reverses age-related degenerative changes of cholinergic neurons and NGF-induced hypertrophy increases their resistance to experimental insults. Behavioral studies suggests that hypertrophy elevates the ability of cholinergic neurons to influence their postsynaptic neurons. Based on these considerations, it can be anticipated that NGF administration would attenuate the rate of degeneration of cholinergic neurons surviving in Alzheimer brains and improve their functional performance. Accordingly, NGF treatment may attenuate the deterioration of those aberrant behaviors which are a consequence of the cholinergic deficit. Possible detrimental actions of NGF have to be ruled out before the start of actual clinical trials (1.).

Neurotrophic factors other than NGF

Neurotrophic factors occur in miminal quantities making their isolation a difficult task. Brain-derived neurotrophic factor (BDNF) and ciliary neurotrophic factor (CNTF) have been purified, characterized, and corresponding cDNAs have been cloned. The sequence of BDNF is closely related to that of NGF suggesting the existence of other related neurotrophic molecules. Many other factors have been partially purified. Some putative neurotrophic factors turned out to be identical to previously characterized growth factors, in particular to basic fibroblast growth factor (bFGF). Furthermore, other previously characterized growth factors, including insulin-like growth factors (IGFs) and transforming growth factor-α (TGFs) were found to exert trophic actions on neurons.

Pharmacology of neurotrophic factors

There are several strategies which could be pursued to pharmacologically exploit neurotrophic factor mechanisms. Neurotrophic factors can be administered directly to the brain. Intracerbral administration is necessary, since these proteins do not cross the blood-brain barrier. Sufficient quantities of well characterized neurotrophic factors are a prerequisite for pharmacological and toxicological studies. The scarcity of natural molecules will make it necessary to produce recombinant proteins. A successful demonstration that intraventricular infusion of a neurotrophic factor is clinically effective is likely to stimulate research into alternative methods of administration. It seems possible to develop slow-releasing intracerebral implants. Slow-releasing polymers could be implanted in a simple neurosurgical session and pose less risk than intraventricular pumps. Grafting of brain tissue replacing degenerated cells is frequently proposed as a potential approach to treat brain dysfunction. Such techniques are not limited to natural cells but can include genetically modified cells which selectively secrete a desired neurotrophic factor.

Rather than administering entire trophic factor molecules, it may be possible to use active fragments or molecules mimicking the active sites of neurotrophic factors. Studies with peptide fragments and modified peptides will provide a basis for molecular modeling studies attempting to replace peptides with non-peptide effectors. While this approach has the potential to lead to trophic factor agonists which can be administered systemically, it has to be pointed out the systemic administration of such active molecules may substantially elevate the possibility of undesired side-effects.

A feasible approach to influence neurotrophic actions may be to search for ways to specifically manipulate the synthesis of endogenous neurotrophic factors. At the present time, the mechanisms controlling the selective expression of their genes are poorly understood.

Given the multitude of system affected by neurotrophic factors one has to direct awareness to the possibility that pharmacological use of growth factors and trophic agents may be detrimental to neuronal function, contrary to the beneficial role implied by the term "trophic". Such detrimental actions have to be considered and ruled out before clinically using trophic molecules. Neurotrophic agents may, by promoting the function of selective neuronal systems, alter the balance among various systems within neuronal networks. Trophic agents may induce the formation of aberrant synaptic connections which may disrupt normal signal flow. They may induce the expression of abnormal proteins by neuronal and non neuronal cells and stimulate pathological proliferation of non-neuronal cells.

The pharmacology of neurotrophic factors has been the topic of recent more detailed reviews (1,2).

References
1. Phelps, et al. (1989) Neurobiol. Aging 10:205-207.
2. Hefti, et al. (1989) Neurobiol. Aging 10:515-533.
3. Hefti, F. and Schneider, S. (1990): In Cognitive Disorders: Pathophysiology and Treatment, E.R. Gamzu, W.H. Moos and L.J. thal, eds., Marcel Dekker, Inc. New York.

NGF TREATMENT AFFECTS BEHAVIORAL RECOVERY FOLLOWING SEPTAL LESIONS IN RATS.

B. WILL and V. PALLAGE
Département de Neurophysiologie et Biologie des Comportements
Centre de Neurochimie du CNRS, 12 rue Goethe - 67000 STRASBOURG - FRANCE

Since the early seventies, there have been several reports that nerve growth factor (NGF) treatment of adult animals with brain lesions and aged animals alleviates lesion- as well as aging-induced impairments (e.g. 3,5). However, some "negative" effets (no NGF effect or even NGF-induced behavioral impairments) also have been reported (see 5). The reason for these discrepant findings is not clear but may involve the scarcity of knowledge concerning NGF neurotrophic effects on CNS neurons and the variety of experimental paradigms used to assess its effects. The object of this report is to clarify this issue, particularly with regard to animals with septo-hippocampal damage.

METHOD

In a series of experiments conducted on female rats which sustained electrolytic medial septal lesions at 30 days of age, we assessed the behavioral effects of a single intrahippocampal injection of 2.5 S NGF (10 ug/rat) given at the time of lesion surgery at several postoperative periods. Behavioral performances were measured in a test battery including 8-arm radial maze learning.

RESULTS

NGF was found to facilitate the behavioral recovery of rats with septal lesions. In contrast to suggestions in recent NGF literature, a single injection of the protein was sufficient to significantly alleviate some behavioral deficits in a long lasting fashion (table 1).

The beneficial effect of NGF on behavioral sparing and/or recovery was dependent on the size of the septal lesion since it was observed only in rats with small sized lesions (table 1).

The sympathetic sprouting into the cholinergically deafferented hippocampus may depend on the levels of endogenous NGF which was shown to accumulate in the hippocampus following medial septum lesions (e.g. 1). However, we were unable to find any evidence of an effect of a single intrahippocampal exogenous NGF administration on sympathetic sprouting (see also 4). Even if exogenous NGF would have affected sympathetic sprouting, this effect did not prevent the protein from facilitating behavioral recovery. Furthermore, superior cervical ganglionectomy (SCGx) did not significantly affect the behavioral effects of NGF treatment (table 1).

Table 1 : Radial maze performance

LESION SIZE

	Small	Large	Medium	Medium + SCGx
Sham		26 (5)	50 (13)	38 (6)
SL.NGF	38 (9)	162 (26)	111 (25)	106 (14)
SL.T.NGF			117 (30)	183 (56)
SL	150 (28)	193 (26)	181 (44)	209 (62)
SL.T			164 (27)	251 (90)

Total errors (mean + s.e.m. in parentheses) over 20 daily trials, five months after surgery. SL = septal lesion ; T = Transplant ; SCGx = superior cervical ganglionectomy.

When added to cholinergic-rich grafts (embyronic septal cell suspensions injected into the dorsal hippocampus), NGF increased the size of the grafts (see 2), especially when given in conjunction with ganglionectomy (table 2).

Table 2 : Graft volume

No NGF and no SCGx	=	6.2 (2.7)
No NGF and SCGx	=	6.5 (1.6)
NGF and no SCGx	=	10.3 (2.1)
NGF and SCGx	=	30.9 (8.3)

mean (mm3) and s.e.m. (in parentheses)

DISCUSSION

These data are supportive of the findings of most others interested in the effects of NGF on functional sparing and/or recovery after damage to the forebrain cholinergic neurons. Our data may help to understand some of the discrepant data reported thus far. One interpretation of these data is that 1) no NGF effects on behavioral recovery may be observed when the number of spared cholinergic neurons able to exploit the neurotrophic factor is insufficient to trigger the behavioral functions under study and 2) deleterious NGF-induced effects may be found when NGF is added to cholinergic-rich grafts, perhaps because of the compression of the host stucture produced by the "oversized" transplants.

REFERENCES

1. Collins, F., and Crutcher, K.A. (1989): Brain Res., 490:355-360.
2. Eriksdotter-Nilsson, M. (1989): Neurosci., 30:755-766.
3. Hefti, F. et al. (1989): Neurobiol. Aging, 10:515-533.
4. Saffran, B.N., and Crutcher, K.A. (1989): Soc. Neurosci. Abstracts , 15(1):91.
5. Will B. et al. (1988): In Pharmacological Approaches to the Treatment of Brain and Spinal Cord Injury, D.G. Stein and B.A. Sabel, eds., pp. 339-359. Plenum Publishing Corporation, New York.

MODELS OF ANXIETY: NORADRENERGIC, GABAERGIC AND SEROTONERGIC PATHWAYS

J. TRABER
Institute for Neurobiology, Troponwerke, Cologne, FRG

Since the early sixties the benzodiazepines (BZ) have been the drugs of choice for the treatment of anxiety disorders. The primary target for the BZ are benzodiazepine receptors allosterically linked to the $GABA_A$ receptor/chloride channel complex. In the presence of the BZ anxiolytics, the dose-response curve for the GABA-induced change in chloride conductance is shifted to the left with no change in the maximal response. Hence, BZ should enhance $GABA_A$ receptor function only at synapses where the GABA concentration is insufficient to open all available chloride channels (1). The fact that BZ are ineffective unless the receptor complex is activated by GABA suggests an BZ induced enhancement of $GABA_A$ receptor function only at GABAergic synapses and not at extrasynaptic sites (1). This kind of fine tuning of GABAergic transmission may lead to the selective anxiolytic actions of the BZ as compared to GABA mimetic drugs such as muscimol. The latter drugs (over)stimulate $GABA_A$ sites regardless of their functional state and their neuroanatomical locations and are no useful anxiolytics (2).

Besides the GABAergic, the locus coeruleus (LC) noradrenergic system is a neural substrate for excessive arousal or fear that might be involved in pathological anxiety (3). Electrical stimulation or increase of LC neuronal firing via, e.g., blockade of somatodendritic α_2 adrenoceptors by drugs such as yohimbine leads to a state of anxiety and dysphoria. Reduction of the functional activity of the LC via, e.g., α_2-adrenoceptor activation by drugs such as clonidine, reduces anxiety. BZ anxiolytics - via $GABA_A$ receptors - also depress spontaneous LC neuronal activity. This common net-effect on noradrenergic activity has been used to explain their common anti-anxiety effects. LC hyperactivity has also been implicated in the induction of panic states by sodium lactate and CO_2 (3) and thereby in the psychopathology of this condition. Not consistent with this hypothesis, carbamazepine, which does have antipanic effects, <u>increases</u> LC activity after acute administration (3).

Other anxiolytic drugs not blocking LC neuronal activity are the novel anti-anxiety agents buspirone (B), gepirone (G) and ipsapirone (I) (3, 4). These compounds have in common to interact more (I, G) or less (B) specifically with a newly discovered subtype of high affinity brain 5-HT receptors ($5-HT_{1A}$) by which the anxiolytic effects seem to be mediated (4). The brain serotoninergic system has also been implicated in the psychopathology of anxiety and in the mechanism of action of the benzodiazepines (4). B, G and I directly modulate 5-HT activity in such parts of the brain believed to be involved in the control of anxiety (septohippocampal system innervated by the raphe nuclei serotoninergic neurons; 5). These compounds are full agonists at the level of the raphe nuclei $5-HT_{1A}$ somatodendritic autoreceptor as measured electrophysiologically by the inhibition of spontaneous raphe cell firing. At the postsynaptic level, the drugs have differential intrinsic activities and are partial agonists in inhibiting the 5-HT$_{1A}$ receptor coupled forskolin stimulated adenylate cyclase in hippocampal tissue. B, G and I are active in a wide range of animal models of anxiety (4). Regioselective intracranial application and lesion experiments suggest a role for both presynaptic somatodendritic as well as postsynaptic 5-HT$_{1A}$ receptors (6).

Taken together, it seems that (at least) the three neurotransmitter systems mentioned participate in a complex interactive way in the mechanisms of anxiety.

REFERENCES

1. Enna, S.J., and Möhler, H. (1987): In *Psychopharmacology: The Third Generation of Progress*, H.Y. Meltzer, ed., pp. 265-272. Raven Press, New York.

2. Lloyd, K.G., and Morselli, P.L. (1987): In *Psychopharmacology: The Third Generation of Progress*, H.Y. Meltzer, ed., pp. 183-195. Raven Press, New York.

3. Redmond, D.E., jr. (1987): In *Psychopharmacology: The Third Generation of Progress*, H.Y. Meltzer, ed., pp. 967-975. Raven Press, New York.

4. Traber, J., and Glaser, T. (1987): *Trends Pharmacol. Sci.*, 8:432-437.

5. Gray, J.A. (1982): *The Neuropsychology of Anxiety.* Oxford Univ. Press, New York.

6. De Vry, J., et al., (1982): In *New Concepts in Anxiety*, M. Briley and S.E. File, eds., in press, MacMillan Press, London.

ANXIOLYTICS NOT ACTING AT THE BENZODIAZEPINE RECEPTORS THE PRESENT STATE I: TRICYCLIC ANTIDEPRESSANTS, MAO-INHIBITORS AND NEUROLEPTICS

R. BULLER and O. BENKERT

Department of Psychiatry (Head: Prof. O. Benkert), University of Mainz, Mainz, Federal Republic of Germany

The past decade has seen a considerable progress in the treatment of anxiety. Changes in the classification of anxiety disorders which are now incorporated in the DSM-III-R (APA, 1987) (1) have been influenced by developments in pharmacotherapy. The identification of panic disorder and agoraphobia with panic attacks as conditions which are responsive to continuous imipramine treatment (Klein, 1964) (2) started an intensive research on the efficacy of antidepressants in the treatment of anxiety syndromes.

Until then the term "anxiolysis" had been understood as a synonym for treatment with benzodiazepines. However, by now a number of antidepressants (tricyclics and MAO-inhibitors) are known to be efficacious in panic disorder. Some tricyclic antidepressants are also useful in obsessive compulsive disorder and possibly in generalized anxiety disorder. In social phobia MAOI may be effective (Noyes, 1987) (3).

The possibility of inducing drug dependence has caused physicians to reduce the number of benzodiazepine prescriptions. Problems with the safety and the side-effect profile of classic antidepressants have also stimulated the search for additional therapeutic strategies. One possible alternative in the treatment of anxiety and other psychosomatic disorders which is now widely applied in West Germany is the use of low-dosed depot neuroleptics like Fluspirilene once a week (Schmidt, 1989) (4). However, this practice may bear a risk of causing tardive dykinesia. Data to support the safety and efficacy of such a therapeutic scheme and to explain the mechanism by which neuroleptics act in anxiety disorders are still sparse.

With continuing new developments in the pharmaco-therapy of anxiety disorders research will try to disentangle the different ways in which drugs have an effect on neurotransmitter systems that play an important role in anxiety. On the other side, diagnostic conventions may also have to undergo changes in order to help identify drug-responsive conditions. Finally, terms like "antidepressant" or "anxiolytic" seem outdated because the indication for the use of these substances is now much wider.

For patients with different kinds of anxiety and anxiety disorders various therapeutic alternatives have been identified. The search for other treatments that offer greater safety will continue. However, because of their fast action and their low toxicity benzodiazepines - when used with care - will probably keep an important place among the anti-anxiety drugs.

REFERENCES

1. American Psychiatric Association (1987): Diagnostic and statistical manual of mental disorders, third edition, revised DSM-III-R. American Psychiatric Association, Washington, D.C.

2. Klein, D.F. (1964): Delineation of two drug-responsive anxiety syndromes. Psychopharmacologia 5:397-385.

3. Noyes, R. (1987) Drug treatment of anxiety disorders: update 1987. J. Affective Dis., 13:95-98

4. Schmidt, L.G. (1989): Utilization and safety of Fluspirilene in nonpsychotic outpatients. Pharmacopsychiat., 22:188-191.

THE PRESENT STATE. II: BETA BLOCKERS

PETER TYRER
ST. CHARLES' HOSPITAL, LONDON, W10 6DZ

Although beta-blocking drugs have been used for the treatment of anxiety for over 20 years adequate research data are available on only about 500 patients. These suggest that beta-blockers in relatively low dosage (e.g.<120mg propranolol or equivalent per day) are effective in the short-term treatment of anxiety of moderate severity, including anxiety associated with acute stress reactions as well as in generalised anxiety disorder. There is also evidence that phobic anxiety, particularly that associated with public speaking and playing musical instruments, can be helped by beta-blocking drugs. The drugs are particularly effective in treating the bodily symptoms of anxiety mediated through adrenergic beta-receptor stimulation; blushing, palpitations and awareness of fast heartbeat, and shaking. These benefits are most marked in acute dosage and begin within an hour of drug ingestion. Some recent studies also suggest that in somewhat higher dosage (between 120 and 240mg of propranolol or equivalent per day) beta-blockers are effective in treating more severe generalised anxiety with delay in the onset of action between two and four weeks[1]. No important differences have been noted between beta blockers with regard to anxiolytic effects, except that those acting selectively on the ß1 or ß2-receptor are less effective.

In longer term therapy the symptoms improved by beta-blockers cover a wide range; the likely mechanism is that beta-blockade of beta-mediated symptoms peripherally, reduces anxiety centrally by feedback, and so other anxiety symptoms are improved simultaneously. However, the possibility of beta-blocking drugs acting on anxiety through central beta-receptors cannot be discounted, particularly in view of evidence that improvement is often delayed and requires higher dosage. Beta-blockers are probably not effective in more severe anxiety, including panic disorder, but adequate data are limited. In comparison with other anti-anxiety drugs beta-blockers are generally less effective than benzodiazepines in particular. However, they have the advantage of not producing pharmacological dependence. They also do not impair sensori-motor functioning and this allows their use in situations where concentration and vigilance are necessary such as driving and operating machinery. In less severe generalised anxiety, during which the subject continues to work and take on responsibility, there are definite advantages in taking beta-blockers and their use may often be preferred to the more traditional sedative-hypnotic drugs. There is also evidence that beta-blocking drugs taken in combination with benzodiazepines allow lower dosage of benzodiazepines to be used. When these drugs are effective there is no evidence that tolerance develops and if necessary treatment can be given long-term.

It is concluded that beta-blocking drugs have a definite place in the treatment of pathological anxiety. The precise indication for their use remained undefined but acute stress and generalised anxiety are the key treatment groups.

Reference:

Tyrer, P. (1988): Drugs, 36, 773-83.

THE FUTURE 1: 5-HT AGONISTS AND 5-HT$_2$ ANYAGONISTS: BUSPIRONE, IPSAPIRONE, GEPIRONE, RITANSERIN

M. Murasaki and S. Miura
Department of Psychiatry, Kitasato University School of Medicine
Sagamihara, Japan

In 1950, meprobamate was synthesized as a tranquilizer and quickly became one of the best seller drugs all over the world. However, the era of meprobamate had rapidly ceased because of the development of tolerance and severe withdrawal symptoms. In stead of meprobamate, chlordiazepoxide was introduced in 1960 as much safer tranquilizer, followed by diazepam, oxazepam and other benzodiazepine(BZ) derivatives. Among many BZs, diazepam had continued to keep the position of the most frequently prescribed drug in the world for a long time. Nowadays, almost all psychiatrists and physicians are well satisfied with the anxiolytic effect of BZs, however, recently undesired side-effects such as the impairments of psychomotor function including memory disturbance and low dose dependence have been focused.

A new anxioselective anxiolytic, buspirone which is structurally unrelated to BZ and does not bind to BZ receptors, has been lunched, followed by ipsapirone, gepirone and SM-3997. These compounds are called azapirones. The main mechanism of these drugs is considered due to the great affinity for serotonin receptors, binding both presynaptic and postsynaptic serotonin(5-HT$_{1A}$) receptors. It acts on as an agonist at the presynaptic 5-HT$_{1A}$ receptors that inhibit serotonergic neuron firing, and as a partial agonist when bound to the postsynaptic 5-HT$_{1A}$ receptors that relay information from presynaptic to postsynaptic cells. The newest concept of the mechanism of buspirone is referred to the midbrain serotonin normalizer(1). With serotonin deficit diseases such as depression, the agonistic properties of buspirone will normalize serotonergic neurotransmission. However, with serotonergic excess disease such as anxiety, buspirone will be a functional antagonist, reducing serotonertic activity. The partial agonist properties of buspirone therefore allow it to normalize serotonin neurotransmission-excess disease(1).

The efficacy of buspirone has been established in many parallel-group controlled clinical trial. Buspirone is generally found to be superior to placebo and as effective as standard BZs such as diazepam, lorazepam and alprazolam in treating patients with general anxiety disorders without imparing psychomotor performance and without evidence of dependence or abuse potential(2). There is no evidence that relief of anxiety is qualitatively different with buspirone compared with diazepam and regular treatment of diazepam for 6 weeks leads to a significant risk of pharmacological dependence that is not present with buspirone(3). As obviously shown in Table 1, buspirone showed the good effect for the patients who had never had previous BZ experience, however, a great resistance to the antianxiety effect of buspirone had been approved in patients with history of BZ use. Those patients previously on BZs responded less well to buspirone, and the drug failed to reduce BZ withdrawal symptoms.

Thus, the efficacy and the safety of buspirone have been approved for the treatment of anxiety disorders, but some drawbacks are revealed as follows; 1) the rate of efficacy onset is slower than BZs, therefore, an acute or transient effect is not expected, 2) buspirone is significantly less effective than BZ in chronically anxious patients most of whom had previously taken BZs, and 3) buspirone has some unpleasant side-effects such as dizziness, nausea, headche, light-headedness, fatigue and nervousness more frequently than placebo.

Finally, the trends of buspirone prescription in the countries where buspirone has already approved as an anxiolytic, are overviewed. In West Germany where buspirone has firstly approved in 1985, the rate of buspirone prescription is the lowest among the anxiolyitcs and there is no trend of increase. In the United States, France and the United Kingdom, the frequency of buspirone prescription is gradually increasing to about 10% among the anxiolytics. Although the speed of increase of buspirone prescription is much slower in comparison with that of BZs in early 1960s, the steady increase has been recognized except West germany.

If the hypothesis that azapirones function as the midbrain serotonin normalizer, is correct, these compounds have a bright future, because they are effective for the treatment of both anxiety disorders and depression.

TABLE 1: Effect of buspirone on neuroses (uncontrolled clinical stadies in Japan)

	Nishizono et al (1988)		Okada et al (1988)		Kudo et al (1989)	
previous BZ treatment improvement rate (%)	no n=73	yes n=28	no n=54	yes n=28	no n=58	yes n=23
marked improvement	15.1	3.6	19.0	0	16.7	7.1
more than moderate improvement	53.4	35.7	62.1	8.7	48.1	28.6
more than slight improvement	83.6	57.1	88.0	26.1	72.2	60.7
aggravation rate(%)	4.1	14.3	5.6	17.4	5.6	25.0

REFERENCES

1. Eison, M.S.: Azapirones: clinical uses of serotonin partial agonists. Family Practice Recertification. 11(Suppl): 8-16, 1989.
2. Goa, K.L. and Ward, A.: Buspirone. Drugs. 32: 114-129, 1986.
3. Murphy, S.M., Owen, R. and Tyrer, P.: Comparative assessment of efficacy and withdrawal symptoms after 6 and 12 week's treatment with diazepam or buspirone. Br. J. Psychiatry. 154: 520-534, 1989.

5-HT RE-UPTAKE BLOCKERS AS ANXIOLYTICS

T. R. INSEL, J. T. WINSLOW, D. L. MURPHY
Laboratory of Clinical Science, NIMH, Poolesville,
MD, USA

Subjective reports, psychophysiologic studies, and new cerebral imaging techniques have all suggested that anxiety is a heterogeneous affect. It is not surprising then that the various forms of clinical anxiety respond differentially to pharmacologic treatments. The 5-HT re-uptake inhibitors have recently been shown to be specifically effective for reducing the symptoms of one particular anxiety disorder, obsessive-compulsive disorder (OCD). In several double-blind studies (1), the 5-HT re-uptake inhibitors clomipramine, fluvoxamine, and fluoxetine have all been shown to be anti-obsessional, while less potent 5-HT re-uptake inhibitors such as desipramine, imipramine, and nortriptyline appear no more effective than placebo. In direct comparisons, clomipramine and fluvoxamine both appear more effective than desipramine for the relief of OCD symptoms (including anxiety). Moreover, the decrease in OCD symptoms during treatment with clomipramine correlates highly with changes in CSF 5-HIAA (2) and platelet serotonin content (3). Patients improved with long-term clomipramine treatment show a partial relapse when administered the serotonin antagonist metergoline (4). Although the available data suggest that potent 5-HT re-uptake blockers are anti-obsessional and that these anti-obsessional effects are mediated via a serotonergic mechanism, these compounds may not be acting as anxiolytics. OCD is a complex disorder which involves a family of cognitive and behavioral symptoms, only some of which resemble anxiety.

The 5-HT re-uptake inhibitors also reduce the symptoms of other anxiety disorders, such as panic disorder and school phobia(5). However, these more classical anxiolytic effects are shared by several other tricyclic antidepressants which are not 5-HT re-uptake inhibitors, such as desipramine and nortriptyline as well as the benzodiazepines. Still, there are additional reasons to consider a role for serotonin in the pharmacologic modulation of anxiety symptoms in OCD and panic disorder. The serotonin agonist, m-CPP when administered orally, appears to increase anxiety symptoms in both OCD and panic disorder patients, but not in healthy controls. At least in the OCD patients, this response to m-CPP decreases after treatment with 5-HT reuptake inhibitors (Zohar et al., 1988).

We have recently embarked on a series of studies using 5-HT reuptake blockers in a novel animal model of anxiety. In the first 2-3 weeks postnatal, rat pups give ultrasonic calls when they are socially isolated. These distress calls have been compared to human separation distress and may represent a primitive form of anxiety. These calls are blocked by non-sedating doses of benzodiazepines (7) and altered by central administration of corticotropin-releasing factor (8). The 5-HT re-uptake inhibitors appear extremely potent in this model (Fig. 1). Clomipramine (5.0 mg/kg), citalopram (1.0 mg/kg), and paroxetine (1.0 mg/kg) decrease and by contrast, the catecholamine uptake inhibitors desipramine (5.0mg/kg), mazindol (0.5 mg/kg), and nortriptyline (1.0mg/kg), increase the number of calls during a 2 minute isolation test. The importance of 5-HT for the mediation of separation distress is further apparent in studies with the 5-HT neurotoxin MDMA. When MDMA (10 mg/kg) is administered either once or twice daily on postnatal days 1-4, treated pups show a dose-dependent depletion of 5-HT (but not NE or DA) associated with a progressive loss of the isolation call (Winslow & Insel, 1990). In other animal models of anxiety, such as the elevated plus maze, the 5-HT re-uptake inhibitors do not appear anxiolytic (9).

Serotonin has long been associated with the benzodiazepine-GABA system. One hypothesis for this relationship has suggested that benzodiazepine receptors may be pre-synaptic on 5-HT terminals, altering either release or re-uptake of 5-HT. With MDMA lesions of 5-HT terminals, we have recently addressed this question in the Rhesus monkey brain. MDMA decreases ^{3}H-paroxetine binding more than 60% in cortex and hippocampus, demonstrating a loss of 5-HT terminals in these regions (10). In adjacent sections, ^{3}H-flunitrazepam binding appears unaffected in the same regions, demonstrating conservation of benzodiazepine receptors. These studies in the primate brain suggest that benzodiazepine receptors are not located on 5-HT terminals. It therefore appears that the putative anxiolytic effects of the 5-HT drugs may not share a final common pathway with the benzodiazepines.

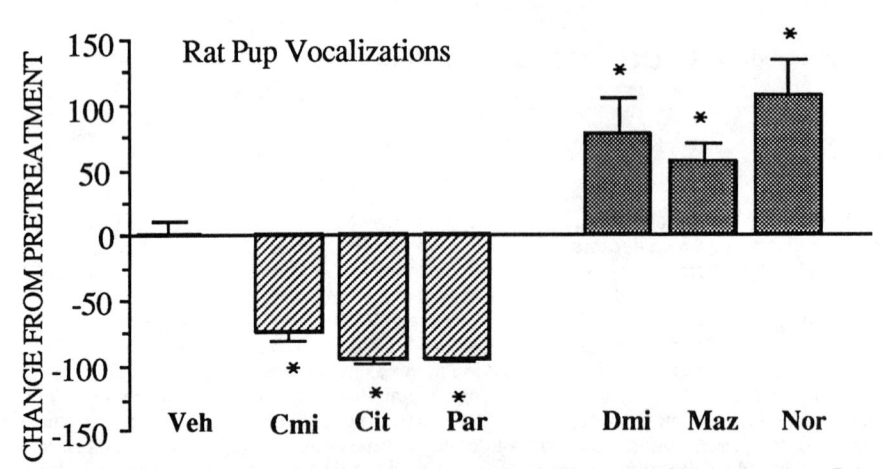

Fig. 1 Changes in the rate of ultrasonic vocalization during a 2 min. test of social isolation. Drugs were administered subcut. 30 min. before testing. * signifies p < .05 for difference from vehicle (Veh) administration. Cmi = clomipramine, Cit = citalopram, Par = paroxetine, Dmi = desipramine, Maz = mazindol, Nor = nortriptyline

REFERENCES
1. Zohar, J. and Insel, T.R.: Obsessive-compulsive disorder: Psychobiological approaches to diagnosis, treatment, and pathophysiology. Biol. Psychiat. 22:667-687, 1987.
2. Thoren, P., Asberg, M., Bertilsson, L. et al.: Clomipramine treatment of obsessive-compulsive disorder. II. Biochemical aspects. Arch. Gen. Psychiat. 37:1289-1294, 1980.
3. Flament, M.F., Rapoport, J.L., Murphy, D.L. et al.: Biochemical changes during clomipramine treatment of childhood obsessive-compulsive disorder. Arch. of Gen. Psychiat. 44:219-225, 1987.
4. Benkelfat, C., Murphy, D.L., Zohar, J. et al.: Clomipramine in obsessive-compulsive disorder: Further evidence for a serotonergic mechanism of action. Arch. Gen. Psychiat. 46:23-28, 1989.
5. Den Boer, J.A., Westenberg, H.G.M., Kamerbeek, W.D.J. et al.: Effect of serotonin uptake inhibitors in anxiety disorders: A double-blind comparison of clomipramine and fluvoxamine. Int. Clin. Psychopharmacol. 2:21, 1987.
6. Zohar, J., Insel, T.R., Zohar-Kadouch, R.C. et al.: Serotonergic responsivity in obsessive-compulsive disorder: Effects of chronic clomipramine treatment. Arch. Gen. Psychiat. 45:167-172, 1988.
7. Insel, T.R., Hill, J.L. and Mayor, R.B.: Rat pup ultrasonic isoltion calls: Possible mediation by the benzodiazepine receptor complex. Pharmacol. Biochem. Beh. 24:1263-1267, 1986.
8. Insel, T.R. and Harbaugh, C.R.: Central administration of corticotropin releasing factor alters rat pup isolation calls. Pharmacol. Biochem. Beh. 32:197-201, 1989.
9. Chopin, P. and Briley, M.: Animal models of anxiety: The effect of compounds that modify 5-HT neurotransmission . TIPS 8:383-388, 1987.
10. Insel, T.R., Battaglia, G., Johannessen, J.N. et al.: 3,4-Methylenedioxymethamphetamine ("Ecstasy") selectively destroys brain serotonin terminals in rhesus monkeys. J. Pharmacol. Exp. Ther. 249(3):713-720, 1989.

NON BENZODIAZEPINE ANXIOLYTICS AND HYPNOTICS ACTING AT THE BENZODIAZEPINE GABA MACROMOLECULAR COMPLEX : ALPIDEM, ZOLPIDEM, SURICLONE, ZOPICLONE.

J.C. Bisserbe and J.P. Boulenger
INSERM U. 320, Centre Esquirol, C.H.U. Côte de Nacre, 14033 Caen Cedex, France

Benzodiazepines (BZD) have been the treatment of choice for anxiety disorders and sleep disorders since their introduction in 1960. At this time they represented a major significant advance over the older sedative-hypnotics such as barbiturates and meprobamate which they rendered obsolescent. In 1977 the discovery of high-affinity binding sites in rodent and human brain was a major step in the understanding of the mechanism of action of anxiolytic compounds. It has been established that BZD interact at a supramolecular complex including the BZD receptor (BZR) the GABA receptor (GABAR) and a chloride channel. Anxiolytic BZDs enhance the efficiency of GABA in opening the chloride ionophore. This biochemical action could be the basis of the different pharmacological properties of BZD (4). Since the discovery of the BZR many non BZD compounds acting at the BZR have been found (3). Some of these compounds possess only a part of the BZD pharmacological profile (partial agonists), some antagonize BZD (antagonists), others like β-carbolines produce the opposite effect (inverse agonists). In addition, some of these new compounds (tracazolate, imidazopyridines) have enabled the pharmacological characterization of two subtypes of central BZR called BZR 1 and BZR 2 or alternatively $\omega 1$ and $\omega 2$ (7). These new developments have led to the expectation of clinically selective agents that would be devoid of the untoward effects of classical BZD : drowsiness, potentiation of depressants, psychomotor and memory impairment and dependance.

The cyclopyrrolones zopiclone and suriclone were the first non BZDs discovered to act at the BZR-GABAR - chloride ionophore supramolecular complex. Although biochemical data indicated that cyclopyrrolones bind to a site linked allosterically to BZR, these compounds have demonstrated a similar pharmacological profile to classic anxiolytic BZDs (3, 12). Zopiclone marketed as an hypnotic in doses of 7.5 mg has a half-life of 5 - 6 hours, with no active metabolites. Its clinical profile is close to BZD : increase in total sleep time and reduction of sleep awakening. Zopiclone (7.5 mg) does not share the BZD action on sleep structure increase in slow wave sleep (stage 3, 4) and a limited effect on REM sleep has been reported (1). In addition after-sleep residual effects after a single dose of 7.5 mg seem to be absent, effects on memory have been reported but lasted less than six hours

(2, 13). Zopiclone is devoid of respiratory depressant effects (11). Suriclone has shown clinical efficacy in generalized anxiety for dosages ranging from 0.6 mg/day to 2 mg/day (5, 8). The evaluation of cyclopyrrolone dependence liability would need a larger experience. Avalaible data in use in alcoholic patients on withdrawal of treatment in control subjects and insomniacs are not presently suggestive of dependence potentials.

Imidazopyridines alpidem and zolpidem differentiate from classic BZDs in their specific affinity for BZR1 resulting in a different pharmacological profile (14). Zolpidem marketed as a hypnotic has strong sedative properties. Clinical trials have demonstrated the efficacy of 10 mg of zolpidem in sleep induction, sleep maintenance and sleep duration without residual effects (9). Sleep structure alterations appeared to be limited (6). Nine hours after 10 mg of zolpidem no effects on attention, memory or motor performance were observed (6). Alpidem compared to placebo has demonstrated clinical efficacy in generalized anxiety (150 to 225 mg/day) and in anxiety prior to surgical operations. In comparative clinical trials the anxiolytic effect of alpidem was comparable to BZD with equivalent sedative side effects (10).

In summary, new agents acting at BZRs, either on a specific receptor subtype or with a partial agonist type of action have led to the hope of a selective clinical action of anxiolytics devoid of unwanted effects. Further clinical experience is needed to test these expectations.

1. Billiard M. et al. (1987) : Sleep 10 suppl 1: 27-34.
2. Broadhurst A., Cushnaghan R.C. (1987) : Sleep 10 suppl 1:48-53.
3. Gardner C.(1988) : Drug Development Res., 12: 1-28.
4. Haefely W. (1985) : In Psychopharmacology 2 , part 1 : Preclinical Psychopharmacology, Grahame-Smith D.G., P.J. Cowen, (Eds.), pp 92-181. Excerpta Medica, Amsterdam.
5. Hakim C. (1984) Clin. Neuropharm. 7 (suppl): 628-629
6. Hermann et al. (1988) : In Imidazopyridines in Sleep Disorders, Sauvanet P, Langer S.Z., Morselli P.L.,(Eds.), pp 97-110.LERS Monograph series 6, Raven Press.
7. Langer S.Z., Arbilla S.(1988) : Pharm. Biochem.& Behaviour, 29 : 763-766.
8. Lapierre Y.D. Oyewumi K.L. (1983) : Prog.Neuro-Psychopharm & Biol Psychiatry, 7 : 805-807.
9. Monti J.M. (1989) Eur. J. Clin. Pharmacol., 36 : 461-466.
10. Musch B. et al. (1988) Pharm. Biochem.& Behaviour, 29 : 803-806.
11. Ranlow P.J., Nielsen S.P.(1987) : Sleep, 10 suppl 1: 40-47.
12. Trifiletti R.R.& Snyder S.H. (1984) : Mol. Pharm. 26 : 458-469.
13. Warot et al. (1987) : Fundam. Clin. Pharm.1 : 145-152.
14. Zivkovic et al. (1988) : In Imidazopyridines in Sleep Disorders, Sauvanet P, Langer S.Z., Morselli P.L., (Eds.), pp 97-110.LERS Monograph series 6, Raven Press.

PET and SPEC as Experimental Tools in Clinical Neuropsychopharmacology

G. Sedvall, L. Farde, H. Hall, C. Halldin, A.-L. Nordström, H. Nybäck, Department of Psychiatry and Psychology, Karolinska Institute, Stockholm, Sweden

The development of neuroreceptor ligands binding with high affinity and selectivity to central neuroreceptors offers the possibility to use PET and SPEC to study binding characteristics in the living human brain. This demands several critical characteristics of such compounds, including a rapid and chemical labelling procedure, suitable in vivo kinetics as well as metabolic properties precluding the interferrence of labelled metabolites with the calculation of binding variables.

For the dopamine-D_2 receptor subtypes butyrophenone and substituted bensamide derivatives have been developed as in vivo ligands. Such compounds labelled with carbon 11, flourine 18 or iodine 123 have demonstrated useful properties for developing routine procedures allowing determination of in vivo affinities as well as receptor densities in the human brain.

The recent interest in D_1 dopamine receptor functions in schizophrenia and for the mechanism of action of antipsychotic drugs has also stimulated the development of useful ligands for D_1 dopamine receptors. ^{11}C-labelled SCH23390 and SCH39166 has recently been developed for D_1 dopamine receptor studies.

These ligands for D_1 and D_2 dopamine receptors can also be used as experimental tools for determining the quantitative degree of in vivo dopamine receptor occupancy in relation to treatment with potential antipsychotic drugs believed to interfere with dopamine receptor subtypes. Such studies indicated the quantitative as well as qualitative differences between chemically different types of antipsychotic drugs with regard to the relative interaction with D_1 and D_2 dopamine receptors in the living human brain. All potentially useful antipsychotic drugs induced a highly significant degree of D_2 dopamine receptor occupancy in relation to administration of clinical doses. Substituted bensamides as sulpiride and raclopride did not induce any significant interaction with D_1 dopamine receptor binding. On the other hand the unconventional antipsychotic drug clozapine as well as the phenothiazine derivative thioridazine, and some tioxanthene derivatives also induced a significant degree of D_1 dopamine receptor occupancy in addition to the occupancy of D_2 dopamine receptors. The relative effect on D_1 dopamine receptors was most marked for the unconventional antipsychotic drug clozapine.

Also for central benzodiazepine receptors PET techniques have been developed using ^{11}C Ro15-1788 as the ligand. Also with this ligand benzodiazepine receptor occupancy could be determined by studying the blockade of ligand binding or its displacement from central benzodiazepine receptor sites in relation to clinical treatment with high doses of benzodiazepine derivatives.

Recently the exploration of ligand binding to central nicotinic acetylcholine receptors has been explored by examining the in vivo binding of ^{11}C nicotine in healthy human volunteers using PET. Also the binding of this ligand could be demonstrated to be displacable by administration of high doses of nonlabelled nicotine.

The recent development of high resolution PET cameras (5 mm in all three dimensions) and the use of such neuroreceptor ligands will allow the detailed analysis of the penetration of various types of compounds into the human central nervous system. This procedure also offers the possibility to study the kinetics of these compounds in different brain compartments. The methods will also be useful for quantification of receptor characteristics as B_{max} and affinity in the living human brain. Another advantage of such techniques is the possibility of measuring the relative degree of receptor occupancy in relation to treatment with clinically interesting psychoactive compounds.

REFERENCES

Högberg, Thomas et al. Syntheses of [^{123}I]-, [^{125}I]- and unlabelled (S)-3-iodo-5,6-dimethoxy-N-[(1-ethyl-2pyrrolidinyl)methyl]salicylamide (NCQ 298), selective ligands for the study of dopamine D_2 receptors. Acta Pharm. Nord. 1(2) 1990, 53-60.

Sedvall, Göran. PET imaging of dopamine receptors in human basal ganglia: relevance to mental illness. TINS 1990. In press.

Sedvall, Göran et al. The future of psychopharmacology and positron emission tomography. In: Proc of the XVIth CINP Congress. Neuropsychopharmacology. WE Bunney, H Hippius, G Laakman & M Schmauss (Eds). Springer Verlag, Berlin.1990.

DIFFERENTIAL EFFECTS OF CLOZAPINE & THIOTHIXENE ON REGIONAL GLUCOSE
METABOLISM ASSESSED BY PET IN SCHIZOPHRENICS

S.G. POTKIN[*], M.S. BUCHSBAUM[*], J.F. MARSHALL[**], C. HEH[*], J. SINGER[***],
J. COSTA[****], J. Wu[*], W.E. BUNNEY, JR.[*],
[*]Psychiatry, [**]Psychobiology, University of California, Irvine, CA; [***]Sandoz
Pharmaceuticals, [****]Metropolitan State Hospital, Norwalk, CA

The dopamine hypothesis of schizophrenia derives much of its support from in-vitro animal studies in which antipsychotic drugs bind to the D2 receptors of the dopamine-rich basal ganglia with an affinity correlated with their clinical potency (Creese et al., 1976). PET can be used as a tool to study the mechanisms of action of antipsychotic drugs in humans. Using PET, Farde et al. (1988, 1989) demonstrated that clinically effective doses of a series of chemically distinct atypical and typical neuroleptic drugs occupy 65% to 85% of the D2 receptors in the putamen of schizophrenics. In contrast, clinically effective doses of clozapine occupied only 40% to 65% of these D2 receptors, thus reinforcing animal studies suggesting that the non-D2 actions of clozapine contribute to its antipsychotic action. In quantitative autoradiographic studies, clozapine actions can clearly be differentiated from typical neuroleptics: clozapine upregulates D1 but not D2, and down-regulates S2 receptors; in contrast, haloperidol upregulates D2 and has no effect on D1 or S2 receptors (O'Dell et al., 1990). Human autoradiographic studies demonstrate a regional distribution of D1, D2, and S2 receptors in the basal ganglia, specifically: highest D2 density dorsolaterally, S2 ventroposteriorally, and D1 receptors more uniformly distributed (Joyce et al., 1988; Pazos et al., 1987). This difference in regional receptor distribution can be utilized to study the mechanisms of action of neuroleptics. Standard neuroleptics are predicted to affect the dorsolateral areas, while clozapine is predicted to affect the ventromedial areas. We have found changes in glucose metabolic rate greater in putamen than caudate (Buchsbaum et al, 1987) as have others (Wik et al, 1989). The study further examines these regional differences.

METHODS

Twelve patients with schizophrenia (DSM-III-R criteria) received either clozapine (n=7) or thiothixene (n=5). Patients were scanned after 2-4 weeks drug-free and again after 4-6 weeks of medication. The FDG is taken up by the brain as a tracer of brain metabolic rate for a 30-minute period during which the subject does the Continuous Performance Test (CPT). An individually molded, thermoplastic headholder was made for each subject to minimize head movement and to allow the subject's accurate repositioning on the second scan. Nine planes were obtained parallel to the canthomeatal line at 10 mm increments. The caudate and putamen were measured using the stereotaxic coordinates derived from the neuroanatomical Matsui and Hirano, 1978 atlas. A four-way ANOVA with medication (clozapine, thiothixene), time (pre, post), hemisphere and structure (caudate, putamen) was used to assess regional effects.

RESULTS

A four-way interaction was observed (F=8.3, df 2,20, p=0.0026) demonstrating that clozapine and thiothixene have differential effects on FDG metabolism. The regional differences within the basal ganglia in metabolic effect of medication was relatively more uniform for clozapine than thiothixene. The clozapine group had higher metabolic rates than thiothixene across days, hemispheres, structures, and scan levels. A diagonal gradient was observed, with thiothixene effects greatest superiorly and anteriorly, and clozapine effects inferiorly and posteriorly.

DISCUSSION

These results demonstrate that clozapine differs significantly in its metabolic effects from a standard neuroleptic, thiothixene. A previous history of poor neuroleptic response was required to receive clozapine; therefore, patients in the two groups were not randomly assigned. This problem is being addressed in a new PET study comparing haloperidol with clozapine in the same patients. Errors from stereotaxic placement initially or during repositioning during the second PET scan need consideration. We have recently developed a computer algorithm which allows registration of MRI anatomically defined areas on to PET metabolic values to allow metabolic measurements of very precise structures. N-methylspiperone binding is similar in haloperidol responders and nonresponders suggesting that response to neuroleptics is more complicated than receptor number or occupancy (Wolkin et al, 1989). The FDG metabolic approach may be able to detect the net metabolic effects of neuroleptic drugs on the complex inhibitory and excitatory neural circuits that are important in understanding the mechanism of drug action.

1. Buchsbaum, M.S. et al.: Biological Psychiatry, 22(4):479-94, 1987.
2. Creese, I. et al.: Science, 192:481-483, 1976
3. Farde, L. et al.: Arch Gen Psychiatry, 45(1): 71-6, 1988.
4. Farde, L. et al.: Psychopharmacology, 99 suppl:S28-31, 1989.
5. Joyce, J.N. et al.: Synapse, 2(5):546-57, 1988.
6. O'Dell, S. et al.: Synapse, in press, 1990.
7. Pazos, A. et al.: Neuroscience 21:123-139, 1987.
8. Wik, G. et al.: Psychopharmacology Berlin, 97(3):309-18, 1989.
9. Wolkin, A. et al.: Am J Psychiatry, 146(7):905-8, 1989.

PET ANALYSIS OF GLUCOSE METABOLISM IN SCHIZOPHRENIC PATIENTS BEFORE AND DURING DRUG TREATMENT

F-A. WIESEL
Department of Psychiatry, Uppsala University, Uppsala, Sweden

Positron emission tomography (PET) enables the study of brain function in psychiatric patients. The condition so far most extensively studied is schizophrenia. The results are not unequivocal but suggest decreases in glucose metabolism both in frontal and posterior cortical areas (4). Subcortical structures are probably less changed. By studying the effects of neuroleptics on regional brain metabolism one may find out which regions that are of importance for the antipsychotic effect and in that way not only learn about the mechanisms of action of neuroleptics but also of the disease itself. These questions have been adressed in some PET-studies by investigating schizophrenic patients both before and during neuroleptic treatment.

ABSOLUTE RATES

In patients treated with different neuroleptics in various periods of time both increases and no changes in metabolism have been reported (cf. 4). A study by Wik et al (5) was specially designed to investigate effects of neuroleptics on regional glucose metabolism in patients with schizophrenia. Sulpiride, a selective D2-dopamine antagonist was found to increase glucose metabolism in the right lentiformis after 5 weeks treatment. Chlorpromazine did not demonstrate any effects on regional glucose metabolism. Another group has also reported an increase of neuroleptics on right basal ganglia metabolism (1). An increase in metabolism following neuroleptic treatment is in accordance with the finding that amphetamine decreases glucose metabolism (6). However, the more pronounced effect on right hemisphere metabolism is surprising considering that the number of D2-dopamine receptors are equally distributed between the right and the left nucleus (2). The finding of an asymmetric change in metabolism may indicate that the increase was not directly related to D2-dopamine receptor blockade but more related to changes in neuronal function as a consequence of the D2-dopamine blockade and the disease itself. In the study by Wik et al (5) the sulpiride treated patients were found to have a coupling between an increase in metabolism and a decrease in depressive symptoms. Chlorpromazine which is an unselective receptor antagonist did not demonstrate a similar relationship. The relationship for the sulpiride treated patients support the opinion of the necessity of D2-dopamine receptor blockade for therapeutic effects.

RELATIVE RATES

The calculation of relative rates means that the coupling between metabolism and neuronal activity is lost. However, relative rates may be useful to show minor changes in the pattern of metabolism induced by the drug. As for absolute rates Wik et al (5) and Buchsbaum et al (1) found increases also in relative rates in the right basal ganglia after neuroleptic treatment. Szechtman et al (3) have also reported increases of relative rates in the striatum.

DISCUSSION

Neuroleptic treatment seems to influence brain metabolism only to a low extent. There is no evidence that chronic neuroleptic treatment should influence brain metabolism differently from that of acute treatment (cf. 4). Receptor studies have shown that neuroleptic treatment results in a profound blockade of D2-dopamine receptors (cf. 4). This indicates that glucose metabolism is a too broad measure to study the mechanisms of action of neuroleptic treatment. Profound changes in neuronal circuits and function is probably induced by neuroleptic compounds but the net effect on the metabolism is very weak. In order to study mechanisms of action of neuroleptics in man glucose metabolism seems to be of limited value.

REFERENCES

1. Buchsbaum, M.S., Wu, J.C., DeLisi, L.E. et al. Positron emission tomography studies of basal ganglia and somatosensory cortex neuroleptic drug effects: Differences between normal controls and schizophrenic patients Biol. Psychiatry 22:479-494, 1987.
2. Farde, L., Pauli, S., Hall, H. et al. Stereoselective binding of ^{11}C-raclopride in living human brain - a search for extrastriatal central D2-dopamine receptors by PET. Psychopharmacol. 94:471-478, 1988.
3. Szechtman, H., Nahmais, G., Garnett, S. et al. Effect of neuroleptics on altered cerebral glucose metabolism in schizophrenia. Arch Gen Psychiatry 45:523-532, 1988.
4. Wiesel, F-A. Positron emission tomography in psychiatry. Psychiatric Developments 1:19-47, 1989.
5. Wik, G., Wiesel, F-A., Sjögren, I. et al. Effects of sulpiride and chlorpromazine on regional cerebral glucose metabolism in schizophrenic patients as determined by positron emission tomography. Psychopharmacol. 97:309-318, 1989.
6. Wolkin, A., Angrist, B., Wolf, A., et al. Effects of amphetamine on local cerebral metabolism in normal and schizophrenic subjects as determined by positron emission tomography. Psychopharmacol. 92:241-246, 1987.

DOPAMINE RECEPTOR ELEVATIONS IN DRUG NAIVE SCHIZOPHRENIA AND BIPOLAR AFFECTIVE ILLNESS MEASURED BY C-11 NMSP PET STUDIES: UPDATE AND METHODOLOGICAL CONSIDERATIONS.
DF Wong, L Tune, G Pearlson, T Young, E Shaya, C Ross, RF Dannals, AA Wilson, HT Ravert, J Links, HN Wagner, Jr, *A Gjedde. The Johns Hopkins Medical Institutions, Baltimore, Maryland, *Montreal Neuro Inst.

In 1986 we developed a quantitative procedure for measuring receptor density and affinity of D2 dopamine receptors in living human brain using 3-N-[C-11]-N-Methylspiperone (C-11-NMSP) (1)(2). We applied this procedure initially to 10 patients with drug naive schizophrenia (SCZ) and 5 who were drug free and found elevations in the mean receptor density (Bmax) compared to normal controls (3). Other methods employing C-11-raclopride (4) did not demonstrate such a difference. Recently Martinot (5) using a simpler method with Br-75 Bromospiperone did not demonstrate differences in overall populations although subtypes may have demonstrated differences. This finding was actually shown in 1985 by Wong et al (6) and has been suggested to be confounded by blood flow changes when receptor densities or affinities are high such as in young subjects (1).

We have continued to study drug naive schizophrenia with PET using C-11-NMSP to measure D2 dopamine receptor density Bmax and have more than doubled the number studied in 1986 (3). As a comparison group we have also studied patients with Bipolar Disorders (BIP). Both groups have been compared to normal controls.

Since a fall of D2 dopamine receptors with age has already been described for post mortem and PET data (7)(8) multiple regression model involving linear and polynomial terms of age vs Bmax was fitted to the combined normal and psychiatric subject data. Bmax of all groups fell linearly with age. SCZ and psychotic BIP revealed elevated Bmax in both groups compared with normal controls when regressed for age. Mean SCZ (33.07 ± 19.1 pmol/g, N=19) and mean Bmax of MDI ($28.7 \pm 12/4$ pmol/g, N=7) was higher and the intercept term of the regression model for psychotic MDI patients was significantly different from both non-psychotic MDI patients (16.9 ± 8.0, N=7) and normals (16.0 ± 8.1, N=19) but there was no difference between non-psychotic MDI and normals. When only the caudate/cerebellum ratio at 45 min. was employed for all measurements there was a significant fall with age for all groups but no significant difference in the means (as indicated by the y intercept) in the multiple regression analysis. This is consistent with previous studies (8) and Martinot's study (6). Hence the use of the model rather than simple tissue ratios provided the reported differences. Furthermore, there was a significant positive correlation between receptor density Bmax and the degree of psychosis as measured by the Present State Exam in the Bipolar subjects. These findings suggest that elevated Bmax may be important in disorders with prominent psychotic symptoms. Other important clinical variables and subsets including duration of illness effects of Bmax are under investigation (9).

We have continued to validate our D2 dopamine (DA) receptor Bmax PET quantification methods with C-11-NMSP. C-11 labeled metabolite corrections derived from our model were compared to direct HPLC measurements (up to 6 blood samples per PET study) in 21 normals or patients with SCZ, BIP, and other neuropsychiatric disorders. The mean of the differences between HPLC and modeled corrections were not significantly different from zero and no diagnostic group effect was evident employing a variable component model for intraclass correlation. Avg plasma protein binding of C-11-NMSP was 94.54% bound. No significant difference was noted between 32 patients and 6 controls nor between patient groups. Preliminary studies demonstrate robust resistance of [3H]-NMSP to competition with endogenous dopamine compared to [3H]-raclopride binding in rat striata.

In summary, we continue to find Bmax elevations in drug naive SCZ although clinical subtyping may effect some Bmax difference as previously alluded to at the 1987 Workshop (10) and may explain some of the discrepancies with the Farde data (4). However, pharmacology/ligand differences between C-11-NMSP and C-11-raclopride are likely to be very significant contributors to the discrepancy (11). The study of the same patient with both ligands is ongoing and will help elucidate this further. Acknowledgement: This work was supported in part by NIMH RO1MH42821.

1. Wong DF, Gjedde A, Wagner HN Jr. Quantification of neuroreceptors in the living human brain. Part I. Association rate of irreversibly bound ligands. J Cereb Blood Flow and Metab. 6:137-146, 1986a.
2. Wong DF, Gjedde A, Wagner HN Jr, et al. Quantification of neuroreceptors in the living human brain. Part II. Assessment of receptor density and affinity using inhibition studies. J Cereb Blood Flow and Metab. 6:147-153, 1986b.
3. Wong DF, Wagner HN Jr, Tune LE, et al. Positron emission tomography reveals elevated D2 dopamine receptors in drug-naive schizophrenics. Science. 234:1558-1563, 1986.
4. Farde L, Wiesel F-A, Stone-Elander S, Halldin C, Nordstrom A-L, Hall H, Sedvall G. D_2 dopamine receptors in neuroleptic-naive schizophrenic patients. Arch Gen Psychiatry. 47:213-219, 1990.
5. Martinot J-L, Peron-Magnan P, Huret J-D, Mazoyer B, et al. Striatal D2 dopaminergic receptors assessed with positron emission tomography and [76Br]bromospiperone in untreated schizophrenic patients. Amer Jnl of Psychiatry. 147(1):44-50, 1989.
6. Wong DF, Wagner HN Jr, Pearlson G, Dannals RF, et al. Dopamine receptor binding of C-11 3-N-methylspiperone in the caudate in schizophrenia and bipolar disorder: A preliminary report. Psychopharmacol Bull. 21(3):595-598, 1985.
7. Wong DF, Wagner HN Jr, Dannals RF, et al. Effects of age on dopamine and serotonin receptors measured by positron tomography in the living human brain. Science, 226:1393-1396, 1984.
8. Seeman P, Bzowej NH, Guan H-C, Bergeron C, Becker LE, et al. Human brain dopamine receptors in children and aging adults. Synapse. 1:399-404, 1987.
9. Tune LE, Wong DF, Pearlson GD, Young LT, et al. D2 dopamine receptors in drug naive schizophrenics: Update on 20 subjects. Schizophrenia Res. 2:114, 1989.
10. Andreasen N, Carson R, Diksic M, Evans AC, et al. Schizophrenia, positron tomography, and dopamine D2 receptors in the human enostriatum. Schizophrenia Bull. 14(3):471-484, 1987.
11. Seeman P, Guan H-C, Niznik HB. Endogenous dopamine lowers the dopamine D2 receptor density as measured by [3H]raclopride: Implications for positron emission tomography of the human brain. Synapse. 3:96-97, 1989.

COMPARISON OF METHODS USED WITH [11C]RACLOPRIDE AND
[11C]NMSP FOR THE PET-DETERMINATION OF CENTRAL D2-DOPAMINE
RECEPTORS.

L FARDE*, A-L NORDSTRÖM*, L ERIKSSON** C HALLDIN* and G SEDVALL
Department of Psychiatry and Psychology* and Departments of Neuroradiology
and Clinical Neurophysiology**, Karolinska Institutet, Stockholm, Sweden

The dopamine hypothesis states that the symptoms of schizophrenia are related to an increased dopaminergic neurotransmission. The hypothesis was supported when several groups reported increased densities of D2-dopamine receptors in brains of schizophrenic patients post mortem. However, the increased densities may have been caused by neuroleptic drug treatment during life-time.
We have used positron emission tomography (PET) and [11C]raclopride, a selective ligand for D2-dopamine receptors, to develop a quantitative method for the determination in vivo of central D2-dopamine receptor density in man (1, 2). We have examined [11C]raclopride binding in 20 healthy subjects and 18 newly admitted, young, neuroleptic-naive patients with schizophrenia (3). When the two groups were compared no significant difference in B_{max} or K_d-values were found in the putamen or in the caudate nucleus. These findings do not support the hypothesis that schizophrenia is related to a generally elevated D2-dopamine receptor density.
Our findings differ considerably from the findings of Wong and colleagues (4). They have used PET and [11C] NMSP, a ligand with a high affinity for both D2-dopamine and $5HT_2$-receptors, to examine D2-dopamine receptor densities in vivo in the caudate nucleus of 10 drug-naive schizophrenic patients. A two- to three-fold elevation in D2-dopamine receptor density was found in the patients (41.7 ± 4.6) compared to the healthy controls (16.6 ±2.5). This elevation is even higher than that found in post-mortem brains. This discrepancy between in vivo findings with PET calls for a critical examination of the methods and ligands used for the PET-determination of receptor binding.

SUBJECTS and METHODS
To compare the two methods for determination of D2-dopamine receptor density we have performed initial experiments both with [11C]raclopride and [11C]NMSP in the same healthy subjects. The healthy subjects were also controls in a study with [11C]NMSP on acutely ill neuroleptic-naive schizophrenic patients. The experimental procedure with [11C]NMSP and the strategy for calculations were based on information given in the litterature (4, 5). [11C]NMSP with a high specific activity was used in two separate experiments before and after oral administration of 7.5 mg haloperdiol. For the determination of D2-dopamine receptor density with [11C]raclopride two separate experiments were performed with a high and low specific activity, respectively (2,3)

RESULTS AND DISCUSSION

We have so far analysed data obtained from four healthy subjects and two neuroleptic-naive schizophrenic patients. The analysis was performed blindly, i.e. without knowing if a data set was obtained from a healthy subject or from a schizophrenic patient. In the healthy subjects the B_{max}-values obtained with [^{11}C]NMSP were higher than in the two schizophrenic subjects. (Table). These initial results do not confirm the findings of Wong et al (4).

Table. Central D2-dopamine receptor densities (pmol/ml)

	[^{11}C]NMSP	[^{11}C]raclopride
Healthy subjects	24	28
	64	35.2
	42	33
	75	-
Schizophrenic Patients	16	
	20	

The Bmax-values for the six subjects examined with [^{11}C]NMSP ranged from 16 to 75 pmol/ml. For a much larger sample of 38 subjects examined with [^{11}C]raclopride the range was smaller, 17 to 39 pmol/ml (3). One possible explanation for the high variation in densities obtained with [^{11}C]NMSP is that the rate constant k_3 (= k_{on} x (B_{max} - B)) was very small after administration of 7.5 mg haloperidol (0.02 ±0.01, mean±SD). The inverted value, $1/k_3$, is the value used for further calculations of B_{max}. Errors in a small k_3 are thus scaled to large variations in $1/k_3$. To further examine the effect of 7.5 mg haloperidol on k_3, [^{11}C]raclopride was used to examine the D2-dopamine receptor occupancy induced by 7.5 mg haloperidol. In two healthy subjects there was an 85 and 90% occupancy, respectively. This occupancy is higher than the occupancy of about 70 % induced by injection of [^{11}C]raclopride with a low specific activity (3).

Thus, the very high D2-dopamine receptor occupancy induced by 7.5 mg haloperidol reduces the potential for quantitative determinination of [^{11}C]NMSP binding with a high precision.

REFERENCES

1. Farde L et al, Quantitative analysis of D2-dopamine receptors in the living human brain. Science 231:258-261, 1986
2. Farde L et al, Kinetic analysis of central [11C]raclopride binding to D2-dopamine receptors studied by PET. JCBF 9:696-708, 1989
3. Farde L et al, D2-dopamine receptors in neuroleptic-naive schizophrenics. Arch Gen Psychiat 47:213-219, 1990
4. Wong D et al, PET reveals elevated D2 dopamine receptors in drug-naive schizophrenics. Science 234:1558-1563, 1986
5. Wong D et al, Quantification of neuroreceptors in the living human brain, JCBF 6:137-146, 1986

SUMMARY (FUNDAMENTAL BRAIN IMAGING 1: PET & SPECT)

T. YAMASAKI
Division of Clinical Research, National Institute of Radiological Sciences, Chiba, Japan

The recent development of imaging procedures such as X-ray CT, US and MRI is remarkable. However, these modalities are used mainly to detect morphological changes. On the contrary, nuclear medicine technics originated from the principle of tracer technic to study functional changes.
Among nuclear medicine technics, positron emission tomography (PET) is known as one of the best functional modality, and it provides more information than could be got by dissection or direct observation.
The special property of radioisotopes produced with a cyclotron and used in this tecnic , is as the short-life radionuclide and positron emitter. For example, O-15, N-13 and C-11 emit positrons and have half-life of about 2, 10, and 20 min, respectively. These short-life positron emitters are isotopes of the elements of the living body and have the advantage that their incorporation into biomolecules or drugs does not alter their metabolism.
To detect paired annihilation photons, resulting from the capture of emitted positrons, PET scanners are available. Initially, PET studies focused on the regional perfusion and energy metabolism. A lot of data have been reported in the brain research field. But the recent upsurge in interest in PET studies seems to be due to success in the noninvasive measurement of regional neuroreceptor density in the brain.
Using PET scanner and ligands labeled with positron emitters, many kinds of neuroreceptor such as dopamine D1, D2, serotonin 5-H2, opioid, benzodiazepine, muscarinic cholinergic receptors have been possible to measure.

For evaluating of receptor binding in the diseased brain by PET, it is necessary to know receptor binding in the healthy brain, especially age-related changes of receptor binding in healthy volunteers.
A couple of PET data using [C-11]N-methylspiperone(NMSP) and [C-11]SCH23390 will be shown here.
(1) Age-related decrease of in-vivo [C-11]NMSP binding in humans.
The association rate constant K_3 was calculated from the slope of radioactivity-ratio of striatum to cerebellum

versus the equivalent time in 11 healthy volunteers(22 to 72 years old).The equivalent time was calculated from the radioactivity of cerebellum as an input function. The exponential decrease of the K3 value with aging was observed. The K3 value of the youngest subject(22 years old,male)was 0.035/min,while that of the oldest one (72 years old,male)was found to be 0.020/min.
In addition ,[C-11]NMSP binding in frontal cortex was measured. The binding potential(BP) of receptors was estimated as the ratio of association rate constant K3 to dissociation rate constant K4 in the frontal cortex. The K3 and K4 value were calculated from nonlinear regression,given by a set of parameters that minimized the deviation between the measured kinetics and model prediction. The radioactivity in the cerebellum was used as an input function. A significant reduction in BP with age was obserbed. This decrease was found to be mainly due to the reduced K3 values whereas K4 values were not so much changed with age.
(2) Age-related changes in in-vivo dopamine D1 receptor binding with [C-11]SCH23390 in humans.
17 healthy male volunteers ranging in age from 20 to 72 years old participated. A two-compartment model was used to obtain quantitative estimates of rate constants of association(K3) and dissociation(K4). The value of K3 decreased 69% both in the striatum and in the frontal cortex, whereas the the value of K4 decreased 37% in the striatum and 69% in the frontal cortex over the age range(20to72). Details will be presented in other session by Suhara et al..
Since functional connection between D1 and D2 receptors has been indicated by numerous pharmacological experiments,combination use of [C-11]SCH23390 and [C-11]NMSP would have great value for PET studies on neurological and psychiatric disorders.

In addition to above mentioned data,some conventional and 3 dimensional images taken using a newly developed high resolution PET scanner will be shown. This PET scanner has five detector rings and can follow radioactivity in nine sections of the brain covering an 74 mm of the brain. The spatial resolution of the reconstructed images was 3.5 mm full width at half maximum.

Generally speaking, the center for the PET modality is not so common and the examination using this technic is very costly. On the contrary, Single Photon Emission Computed Tomography(SPECT) is an easier modality than PET. This technic is performed without any cyclotron in the campus. The success with PET now leads to the application of more easily available radiopharmaceuticals labeled with single photon emitters for perfusion and receptor studies.

NEUROENDOCRINE MARKERS OF SEROTONIN RESPONSIVITY IN DEPRESSION

STEPHEN M. STAHL, M.D., Ph.D.
Department of Psychiatry, University of California, San Diego and Veterans Administration Medical Center, San Diego, CA, U.S.A.

A number of new therapeutic agents including buspirone, gepirone, ipsapirone, and tandospirone bind to the $5HT_{1A}$ receptor as partial agonists. $5HT_{1A}$ receptors may play an important role in both anxiety disorders and in depressive disorders.

Study of $5HT_{1A}$ receptors in the human Central Nervous System (CNS) can be accomplished by utilizing neuroendocrine markers of human $5HT_{1A}$ receptors (1-3). Measurement of ACTH, cortisol, and prolactin after their release has been stimulated by a $5HT_{1A}$ agonist, may provide an index of CNS $5HT_{1A}$ receptor functioning in patients with various psychiatric disorders (3).

We have studied the effects of gepirone in untreated patients with major depressive disorder by determining gepirone-induced rises in cortisol compared to placebo-induced changes in cortisol. Our study also sought to determine whether gepirone-induced rises in plasma cortisol levels correlated with symptom severity in untreated patients with major depressive disorder. We also explored whether gepirone-stimulated plasma cortisol levels decreased (i.e., "down-regulated") after chronic administration of gepirone itself.

Single oral doses of 10 mg gepirone increased plasma cortisol levels significantly in unmedicated patients with major depressive disorder. Hamilton depression ratings correlated with serum cortisol levels after acute administration of gepirone. Thus, more severely depressed patients had greater plasma cortisol responses to a 10 mg oral gepirone challenge.

We also observed that gepirone-induced cortisol responses were significantly attenuated (i.e., "down-regulated") after 3-6 weeks of chronic gepirone administration. These findings lead us to hypothesize that gepirone increases plasma cortisol levels in depressed patients, in a manner correlated with severity of depression; this suggests a possible linkage of CNS $5HT_{1A}$ receptors to symptoms of depression. "Desensitization" of the gepirone-induced cortisol response was demonstrated in depressed patients whose symptoms improved after chronic gepirone treatment; this suggests that antidepressant effects of gepirone could be linked to $5HT_{1A}$ receptor desensitization.

Our study demonstrates the use of $5HT_{1A}$ agonist challenges, to increase secretion of neurohormones in man. We believe that this neuroendocrine strategy can also be employed to help clarify the potential relationship of $5HT_{1A}$ receptor "down-regulation" to the therapeutic actions of traditional and novel therapeutic agents in major depressive disorder.

REFERENCES

1. Gilbert, et al., (1988): Eur. J. Pharmacol., 147:431-39.
2. Lesch, K.P., Disselkamp-Tietze, J., and Schmidtke, A.: J. Neural. Trans., (in press).
3. Rausch, J.L., Stahl, S.M., and Hauger, R.L.: Biol. Psychiatry, (in press).

PHARMACOLOGY OF 5-HT$_{1A}$ AGONISTS

D.G. SPENCER, JR.*, J. DE VRY**, R. SCHREIBER**, and J. TRABER**
Central Project Management, Bayer AG, Wuppertal, FRG* and
Institute of Neurobiology, Troponwerke, Cologne, FRG**

The special link of the serotonin (5-HT) system with depression has become increasingly clear in the last decade. In particular, the idea that a serotonergic hypofunction may underlie depression is supported on the clinical level by the observation that reuptake-inhibiting drugs specific for 5-HT are fully effective anti-depressants. Furthermore, some evidence points to lower 5-hydroxy-indoleacetic acid (5-HIAA) in the cerebrospinal fluid of depressed patients (1), although this relation may be strongest in those depressed patients tending toward violent suicide (8,7). Blood platelets from depressed patients also appear to have a decreased 5-HT uptake as compared with normals, a finding that may indicate a parallel situation in the CNS (11). These findings are, however, very indirect and deal with 5-HT function averaged over the whole CNS or body. One can only conclude from this that 5-HT is involved in depression.

A more detailed appreciation of the 5-HT role can best be obtained through the more specific manipulation of functional subsets of the 5-HT system in the CNS. The 5-HT$_{1A}$ receptor is one of the many discrete 5-HT receptors in the CNS and is distributed presynaptically, on the 5-HT containing cells of the raphé nuclei, and postsynaptically, primarily in the limbic regions (i.e., hippocampus, septum, entorhinal/temporal cortex, amygdala; also: frontal cortex). 5-HT$_{1A}$ receptor partial agonists under clinical investigation include buspirone, ipsapirone, gepirone, and metanopirone (SM 3997), and exhibit varying degrees of affinity, intrinsic activity, and selectivity at or for this receptor. Thus, while buspirone is a partial agonist with low selectivity, ipsapirone has a similar intrinsic activity and high affinity and selectivity.

In the rat, partial 5-HT$_{1A}$ agonists appear to exert full agonistic intrinsic activity at the presynaptic somatodendritic receptor on the raphé cells (10), leading to an inhibition of their activity with a consequent reduction in brain 5-HT transmission. Conversely, at least some postsynaptic sites such as the hippo-campus, partial 5-HT$_{1A}$ agonists display an intermediate intrinsic activity, both with regard to adenylate cyclase second messenger (3) and electrophysiological responses (5). Other 5-HT$_{1A}$ postsynaptic sites exist which, even after 5,7-DHT lesions of the raphé cells, still mediate full stimulation of hypothermia and neuroendocrine hormones by these partial agonists, indicating a more full agonist profile. Thus, CNS 5-HT$_{1A}$ receptors are either themselves heterogenous or are heterogenously coupled to their effector systems. The importance of these findings for the therapeutic situation is emphasized by the fact that chronic administration of partial agonists like gepirone and ipsapirone results in a down-regulation of 5-HT$_{1A}$ receptors and a concurrent strong reduction in electrophysiological response to these drugs in the raphé but not in the hippocampus (6,2). Thus, in the first 1-2 weeks of administration, both raphé and hippocampus are affected; after 2 weeks, the hippocampal component must dominate.

In an attempt to determine what brain areas are most important in the putative antidepressant properties of these 5-HT$_{1A}$ partial agonists, we have examined the effects of central and systemic administration on immobility in the rat forced swimming test. Male Wistar rats were given a 20 min. trial swimming in a tank half-filled with water on day 1 and drugs were injected i.p. 23, 5, and 1 hour before the 5 min. swimming test on day 2 (group size = 6). Drug induced reductions in time spent immobile were expressed relative to vehicle control (immobility time: 150-180 sec). Ipsapirone (3-30 mg/kg), gepirone (10 mg/kg), as well as amitriptyline, nomifensine, and imipramine significantly reduced immobility; buspirone (0.3-30 mg/kg) did not. Both ipsapirone (30 ug/rat) and 8-OH-DPAT (10 ug/rat) also significantly reduced immobility when injected centrally into either the dorsal raphé or the lateral septum. In rats in which the raphé nuclei were lesioned due to a previous 5,7-DHT injection, the antidepressant effects of 8-OH-DPAT and ipsapirone were reduced but still present. Finally, ipsapirone (3 mg/kg) retained its antidepressant effect in this model after two weeks of chronic administration (3 mg/kg, given twice a day).

We interpret these data as indicating that both raphé as well as forebrain postsynaptic sites of 5-HT$_{1A}$ action are important for antidepressant efficacy. Furthermore, it may be possible that direct effects on the receptors in these regions may result in a rapidly-appearing antidepressant effect. Kennett et al. (4) noted that in a restraint stress model of depression, ipsapirone, but not desipramine or sertraline, reduced stress-induced behavioral deficits after acute as well as chronic administration. Similarly, in a study on the effects of ipsapirone in a collective of neurotic depressive in-patients, a rapid onset of clinical effect was noted, with significant differences noted against placebo at the first post-treatment time-point, 3 days (9).

REFERENCES
1. Asberg, M. et al. Acta Psychiatr. Scand. 69: 201-219, 1984.
2. Blier, P. and de Montigny, C. Synapse 1: 470-480, 1987.
3. Bockaert, J. et al. Naunyn-Schmiedeberg's Arch. Pharmacol. 335: 588-592, 1987.
4. Kennett, G.A., et al. Eur. J. Pharmacol. 134: 265-274, 1987.
5. Martin, K.F. and Mason, R. Eur. J. Pharmacol. 141: 479-483, 1987.
6. McMonagle-Strucko, K. and Fanelli, R.J. Soc. Neurosci. Abs. in press.
7. Montgomery, S.A. and Montgomery, D. J. Affect. Disorders 4: 291-298, 1982.
8. van Praag, H.M. J. Affect. Disorders 4: 275-290, 1982
9. Puechler, K. et al. VIII World Congress Psychiatry Athen 1989 638, 1989.
10. Sprouse, J.S. and Aghaijanian, G.K. Synapse 1: 3-9, 1987.
11. Tuomisto, J. and Tukianen, E. Nature 262: 596-598, 1976.

PRELIMINARY STUDIES OF 5HT$_{1A}$ AGONISTS IN DEPRESSION

N.M. KURTZ*, J. Keppel-Hesselink**, M. Beneke*** and A. H. Heller*
Miles Inc., Pharmaceutical Division*, West Haven, CT, U.S.A., Bayer AG**, Mijdrecht, Netherlands, Troponwerke***, Cologne, West Germany

There have been a number of reports in the preclinical and clinical literature indicating the potential effectiveness of 5HT$_{1A}$ partial agonists for the treatment of depression[1-4]. Ipsapirone, a potent and selective 5HT$_{1A}$ partial agonist is currently undergoing clinical development across a spectrum of depressive states.

SUBJECT AND METHOD

In Germany, a double-blind, parallel group placebo controlled trial was conducted in 34 inpatients who satisfied ICD-9 criteria for depressive neuroses[5]. Each patient was randomized to receive a 4-week treatment of either placebo (N=18) or ipsapirone (N=16). The dose of ipsapirone was fixed at 7.5mg TID. Throughout the study, each patient was rated for their response to therapy. The primary efficacy rating scale was the Hamilton Depression Scale (HAM-D). In addition, each patient was rated on global improvement and an assessment made of side effects. This information was used by the investigator to assess the risk/benefit ratio of the two treatments.

RESULTS

Hamilton Depression Scale: Change from Baseline
Intent-to-Treat, Last Observation Carried Forward

Values by Visit

Day	Ipsapirone N	Mean	S.D.	Placebo N	Mean	S.D.	p-Value
0	16	24.06	6.72	18	19.78	3.59	(Baseline)
4	16	-1.88	1.75	18	-0.22	1.70	0.0087
7	16	-4.88	3.48	18	-0.44	1.72	0.0001
11	16	-7.88	4.33	18	-1.28	1.93	0.0001
14	16	-10.25	5.34	18	-1.78	2.84	0.0001
18	16	-11.75	6.30	18	-2.06	3.70	0.0001
21	16	-12.75	6.04	18	-2.56	4.22	0.0001
25	16	-12.63	5.99	18	-2.72	5.64	0.0001
28	16	-13.13	6.05	18	-2.94	5.67	0.0001

Patients treated with ipsapirone exhibited a statistically significant decrease in the severity of their depressive signs and symptoms when compared to the group receiving placebo as measured by the change in the HAM-D score. The difference between the two groups was significant by Day 4 ($p<.009$) and grew in magnitude as study progressed [Day 28 ($p<.00018$)]. Ipsapirone treatment was safe and well tolerated. The overall risk/benefit as judged by the investigators was considered to be substantially in favor of ipsapirone ($p<.001$).

DISCUSSION

Data derived from this experiment is consistent with the finding from animal studies with ipsapirone and clinical trials with other $5HT_{1A}$ partial agonists. These compounds appear to offer significant therapeutic benefit to depressed patients. Further clinical trials will be necessary to determine whether this benefit exists across the full spectrum of depressive illness or will be ultimately confined to specific sub-groups. Future research will likely reveal that some of the $5HT_{1A}$ partial agonists will prove superior to others in the treatment of depression when the overall benefit to risk ratio is considered.

REFERENCES

1. Press, et al., (1989): Soc. Neurosci. ABS 15(1):225.

2. Goodwin, et al., (1987): Psychopharmacology 91:500-505.

3. Kennett, et al., (1987): Eur. J. Pharmacol. 138:53-60.

4. Kennett, et al., (1987): Eur. J. Pharmacol. 134, 265-274.

5. Heller, et al., (1990): Psychopharm. Bull. 26(2), (In Press).

POTENTIAL EFFECTIVENESS OF DRUGS WITH AN AFFINITY FOR 5-HT$_{1A}$ RECEPTORS IN OBSESSIVE COMPULSIVE DISORDER

S. A. MONTGOMERY, D. BALDWIN, N. FINEBERG, D. MONTGOMERY
Depart. Psychiatry, St Mary's Hospital Medical School, London UK

Obsessive compulsive disorder (OCD) coexists with depression in many cases. Reports that 5-HT uptake inhibitors such as clomipramine were effective were thought to merely reflect their antidepressant efficacy. Montgomery (1980) (3) demonstrated that clomipramine was effective compared with placebo in treating OCD in the absence of concomitant depression. This result had some unusual features. A low placebo response rate (5%) and a relatively high drug response rate (65%) measured on the CPRS obsessional scale (Montgomery & Montgomery 1980) (4) allowed efficacy to be demonstrated in small numbers.

In this study an early response to clomipramine compared with placebo was seen at weeks 1, 3 and 4. Deveaugh Geiss et al (1989) (1) in two large multicentre studies in non-depressed OCD patients reported almost identical findings with efficacy emerging at one to two weeks. In both of these studies the placebo response was low at 5% and the clomipramine response at 10 weeks 45% measured on the rather less sensitive YBOCS scale. Similar findings have been reported with fluvoxamine, a more selective 5-HT uptake inhibitor. These findings, together with the relative failure of conventional antidepressants without marked effects on serotonin, strongly suggest that OCD is a serotonin specific disorder. A single positive study with mianserin (2) which has 5-HT$_1$, 5-HT$_2$, and 5-HT$_3$ antagonist properties raises the question of whether a particular serotonin receptor sub-type is implicated in OCD.

mCPP, the metabolite of trazadone, was originally thought to be a selective 5-HT$_{1A}$ agonist and was used as a probe to determine serotonergic function. The initial studies were thought to show that an immediate worsening of obsessional symptoms was associated with effects at 5-HT$_{1A}$ receptors. However, mCPP has since been found to have effects on many other systems including 5-HT$_{1B}$, 5-HT$_{1C}$, and 5-HT$_2$ receptors, alpha$_2$ receptors, and to a lesser extent alpha$_1$, dopamine and muscarinic receptors. The effects of mCPP may have been non-specific anxiety provoking because it is so poorly tolerated. Similarly metergoline, a 5-HT$_{1A}$ and 5-HT$_2$ antagonist, has been reported to reverse the antiobsessional effects of clomipramine. This result is difficult to interpret in the light of a report that metergoline improves obsessional symptoms. The question as to whether a particular serotonin sub-type is directly implicated will not be resolved until properly conducted placebo controlled studies using more selective serotonin receptor subtype agonists or antagonists have been tested in the clinic.

REFERENCES

1. DeVeaugh Geiss J., Landau P., Katz R. Treatment of obsessive compulsive disorder with clomipramine. Psychiatric Annals 19:2, 1989

2. Jaskari M.O. Observations on mianserin in the treatment of obsessive neuroses. Curr. Med. Res. Opin. 6: Suppl.7 128-131, 1980

3. Montgomery S.A. Clomipramine in obsessional neurosis: a placebo-controlled trial. Pharmaceut. Med. 1: 189-192, 1980

4. Montgomery S.A. and Montgomery D.B. Measurement of change in psychiatric illness: new obsessional, schizophrenia and depression scales. Postgrad. Med. J. 56: Suppl1 50-52, 1980

5-HT REUPTAKE INHIBITION IN THE ELDERLY

I. KARLSSON
Dept. of Psychiatry and Neurochemistry, Gothenburg University, Gothenburg Sweden

In normal ageing brain the concentration of serotonin (5-HT) is reduced in parahippocampal cortex, caudate nucleus, putamen and hypothalamus (1). In an earlier study, no significant decrease age was found (2) while in the brain stem increased concentrations with age was found. The 5-HT in the brain reflects the concentration of 5-HT synapses. The data indicates a reduction with age of 5-HT containing nerve terminals in many, but probably not all, areas.

The end metabolite of 5-HT, 5-hydroxyindoleaceticacid (5-HIAA) has consistently been found not to decrease with age. The metabolite is supposed to reflect the turnover of the amine. The data thus in normal ageing the 5-HT activity is unchanged in spite of reduced amounts of 5-HT synapses.

5-HT disturbance in not demented elderly has yet not been associated with disease. However, state of depression as well as anxiety associated with organic changes is common in high age (3). If these changes are related to 5-HT disturbance have to be evaluated.

Several studies indicate that both 5-HT and 5-HIAA are reduced in the brains of Alzheimer's disease. The decreases are found in cortical areas as well as in basal ganglia and brain stem regions. Also in the hypothalamus, low concentrations of

The 5-HT sensitive Imipramine binding in brains from patients with Alzheimer's disease is reduced to about 50% of age-matched controls (4)

Also in vascular dementia, reduced levels of 5-HT and 5-HIAA have been reported in macroscopically normal brain tissue indicating a disturbed 5-HT function also in this form of dementia.

In a study of the effects of a selective serotonin uptake inhibitor, Citalopram, was given to 65 patients with Alzheimer's disease, mean age 77,2 years in a double blind study and a group of vascular dementia of 24 patients, mean age 78.5 years. Non of the patients had evidence of depressive disorder.

The effects were evaluated with the GBS-scale (5). After four weeks of treatment the Alzheimer group had evidence of improvements in emotional bluntness, confusion, irritability, anxiety, fear-panic and restlessness. There were no evidence of improvements in memory or other intellectual functions. No significant change was evident in the placebo group. The side effects were few.

The vascular dementia group did not show any significant changes.

A dexamethasone test was also done before and after 4 weeks of treatment. A great proportion of the patients had pathologic high response. In the treatment group the post-dexamethasone cortisol levels were significantly reduced. This indicates that the biochemical disturbance of the DST test was normalized by the 5-HT stimulation.

The results indicates that the 5-HT disturbance in dementia is related to emotional disturbances, at least in Alzheimer's disease. A stimulation of the 5-HT system by a selective serotonin uptake inhibitor seems to stabilize the emotional system.

1. Gottfries, C.G., Bartfai, T., Carlsson, A., Eckernäs, S.Å and Svennerholm, L. (1986) Progress in Neuropsychopharmacology and Biological Psychiatry, 10, 405-413.

2. Carlsson, A., Adolfsson, R., ASquilonius, S.M., Gottfries, C.G., Svennerholm, L. and Winblad, B. (1989) In Ergot compounds and brain function: neuroendocrine and neuropsychiatri aspects, (Goldstein M., Calne, D.B., Lieberman, A. and Thorner M.O eds.) pp. 295-304, Raven Press, New York

3. American Psychiatric Association. Diagnostic and Statistical manual of mental disorders (3rd ed. Revised) Washington DC: APA, 1987.

4. Marcusson, J., Alafusoff, I., Bäckström, I.T., Ericson, E., Gottfries, C.G. and Winblad, B. (1987). Brain Research, 425. 137-145.

5. Gottfries, C.G., Bråne, G., Gullberg, B. and Steen, G., (1982). Arch. Gerontol. Geriatr. 1, 311-330.

PHARMACO-VIGILANCE OF A 5-HT$_{1A}$ AGONISTS (BUSPIRONE)
J.J. López-Ibor Jr[a], J. Honorato[b], C. Ballús[c], V. Conde[d], J. Giner[e], J. Guimón[f] and A. Rodriguez[g].
(Departments of Psychiatry of Alcalá de Henares[a], Barcelona[c], Valladolid[d], Sevilla[e], Bilbao[f] and Santiago[g] and Department of Pharmacology Navarra[b], Spain)

Clinical trials with psychotropic drugs are based on a methodology which still has some drawbacks and pitfalls. Accordingly, it is quite normal, that after the marketing of a drug new aspects of it, both positive or negative, become manifest. The number of patients exposed to the drug is responsible for part of this phenomenon, but practicing habits might be even more important.

The introduction of a new type of agents such as 5HT$_{1A}$ agonists provide a good accession to study this phenomena. Drugs belonging to widely used pharmacological groups such as the Benzodiazepines, the Tricyclic Antidepressants or the Neuroleptics pose problems which are less relevant and very often the only new findings coming after the marketing of a drug relates to rare adverse reactions.

The prescription of 5HT$_{1A}$ agonists to treat anxiety disorders and other emotional symptoms relays on strategies to cope with several particularities which were unknown with the most widely used treatments for such disorders, specially with the Benzodiazepines. Long delay of action, the presence of initial side effects which are experienced by the patients as vegetative hyperfunction (and even as a worsening of their initial state) and the difficulty of changing from a Benzodiazepine to Buspirone are the most commonly mentioned of this phenomena.

A further aspect to be considered is that clinical trials are usually carried out in University or Research centers with selected groups of patients in conditions which are quite special and different from what is happening in normal clinical conditions. Such conditions are sometimes so extraordinary that the percentage of the placebo response in such clinical trials become very significant.

In order to investigate this aspects a multicenter study is being carried out in Spain. The study will include 7700 patients treated by 700 general practitioners. This general practitioners have been trained and are being monitored by 70 psychiatrists who have received a uniform training for this task under the direction of the authors of this paper. The main selection criteria of the patients is the presence of long standing anxiety but all the effort has been made to assure both a uniformity in the methodology and an approach as close as possible to everyday clinical practice. The presence of depressive symptoms does not exclude a patient from the study. Several scales used to measure modification in the symptoms of anxiety and depression are used for this propose and applied before and after the treatment period.

THE RELATION OF HYPNOTICS TO SLEEP AND WAKING FUNCTION

T. ROTH.
Henry Ford Hospital, 2799 West Grand Boulevard, Detroit 48202 MI U.S.A.

The rational and effective use of hypnotics in the symptomatic treatment of insomnia requires an understanding of the drug's effects on both sleep and waking behavior (1). Historically hypnotics were simply evaluated in terms of their effects on sleep duration and quality. More recently, it has become clear that effective hypnotics not only must improve sleep, but also need to be devoid of adverse effects on daytime functioning (2). Ideally, hypnotics should have a positive effect on an individuals ability to function during the day. Studies evaluating the effects of hypnotics on waking behavior have primarily focused on two issues : 1) how these drugs affect performance and alertness the day after the nocturnal administration of the drug, and 2) how they affect memory processes with special emphasis on anterograde amnesia.

The interest in waking function stems from the fact that individuals taking certain hypnotics reported decreased performance the day after drug ingestion. This occurs because hypnotics, by definition, produce sleepiness by reducing alertness, and thereby impairing performance efficiency. In fact, it has been demonstrated that hypnotic potency is directly related to the degree of performance decrement observed. The potency-decrement relation has been shown in studies using daytime drug administration in subjects remaining awake and nighttime administration in subjects awakened after some period of sleep (3). Hence, it is not surprising that one of the most frequent complaints of patients using hypnotics is a reduced ability to function in the morning following nighttime use. This side effect is essentially an extension of the drugs' nighttime use. This side effect is essentially an extension of the drugs' primary hypnotic effect.

A second reason for interest in hypnotics and performance relates to the potential benefits to be derived from hypnotic use. Sleep disorders clinicians generally agree that complaints of inadequate sleep cannot be considered insomnia without the accompanying complaint of some daytime consequence resulting from the presumed sleep disturbance. This distinction is necessary to difffferentiate an insomnia patient from an individual requiring less sleep than the norm, (i.e., short sleepers), as opposed to short sleepers who have tiredness or sleepiness following a poor night of sleep (5). Presumably, increased sleep time in the insomnia patient resulting from hypnotic use ought to lead to improved daytime functioning, although no study has demonstrated this.

Regardless of the mechanism, the probability of detecting a performance change in a given study depends on the nature of the drug under study (i.e., pharmacological factors) as well as the nature of subjects studied and performance measures utilized (i.e., non-pharmacological factors).

REFERENCES

1. Roth T, Zorick F, Wittig R and Roehrs T : Pharmacological and Medical Considerations in Hypnotic Use. Sleep 5(S1) : S46-S52, 1982.

2. Solomon F : Report of a Study : Sleeping Pills, Insomnia and Medical Practice. Institute of Medicine, Washington DC, 1979.

3. Nicholson AN : The Use of Short-and Long-Acting Hypnotics in Clinical Medicine. Brit J Clin Pharmacol 11 : 61S-69S, 1981.

4. Roth T, Hartse KM, Zorick FJ and Kaffeman ME : The Differential Effects of Short-and Long-Acting Benzodiazepines Upon Nocturnal Sleep and Daytime Performance. Drug Res 30(I) 5a : 891-894, 1980.

5. Association of Sleep Disorders Centers, Diagnostic Classification of Sleep and Arousal Disorders, 1st Ed. Prepared by the Sleep Disorders Classification Committee, Chairman HP Roffwarg. Sleep 2 : 1-137, 1979.

AMNESTIC PROPERTIES OF SEDATIVES/HYPNOTICS.

I. HINDMARCH, Robens Institute of Health & Safety, University of Surrey, Guildford, U.K.

Forgetfulness and disturbances of short term memory, as a sequelae to the nocturnal use of hypnotics, can severely compromise daytime functioning and performance of the cognitive tasks of everyday living. Many benzodiazepine hypnotics and sedatives produce amnesia, but some do not. Furthermore, other sedative agents, (e.g.) antihistamines have no proven memory disturbing properties, and it appears that sedation, per se does not necessarily lead to memory impairment. The cyclopyrrolone hypnotic, zopiclone is a potent sedative yet no residual amnestic activity has been measured during the day following nocturnal medication, in marked contrast to the impairment found with certain benzodiazepines, e.g. flunitrazepam. The lack of an amnestic "hangover" is an important consideration in the clinical management of sleep disturbance in the elderly where there is an established memory deficit and in other patients where the integrity of executive memory functions is essential for their daytime well being.

DAILY ACTIVITY AND PERSISTENT SLEEP-WAKE SCHEDULE DISORDERS

T. OHTA* and T. IWATA**
Department of Psychiatry* and Department of Clinical Laboratory**,
Nagoya University School of Medicine, Nagoya, Japan

Considerable numbers of patients with delayed sleep phase syndrome (DSPS) and non-24-hour sleep-wake syndrome (hypernychthemeral) have been reported in the last decade, but the definite method of treatment has not been established yet. We tried to treat DSPS and hypernychthemeral patients who had felt difficult to maintain their daily activity more than 6 months with non-pharmacotherapy and/or pharmacotherapy with or without hypnotics.

SUBJECT AND METHOD

(1) Eleven DSPS patients (8 adults and 3 adolescents) were selected with the diagnostic guidelines of Weitzman et al (3). They were treated with a combination of chronotherapy and pharmacotherapy under or after having their sleep-wake schedule reset. Three of the 11 patients were put on chronotherapy with the shift of phase advanced one hour weekly and the others with the shift of phase delayed 3 hours daily. Ten patients were polysomnographically recorded before and after chronotherapy and body temperature monitoring was also carried out.

(2) In two patients with hypernychthemeral syndrome (1 adult and 1 adolescent), the administration of Vitamin B12 (Methylcobalamin) was begun when each sleep-onset time was around 22:00-23:00. The blood concentration was monitored before and after administration.

All of our DSPS patients were shown in Table 1 and also hypernychthemeral patients were shown in Table 2.

TABLE 1. Patients with delayed sleep phase syndrome

Case No.	Age	Sex	Age of Onset	Chronotherapy	Pharmacotherapy
Adults:					
1	24	Female	18	Delay (L)	A, M
2	22	Male	18	Delay (L)	T, M
3	31	Male	18	Delay (L)	T, M
4	29	Male	20	Advance (H)	(-)
5	21	Male	20	Delay (H)	(-)
6	29	Female	23	Delay (L)	T, M
7	30	Male	27	Advance (L)	A
8	38	Male	37	Delay (L)	T
Adolescents:					
1	16	Female	14	Delay (L)	T, BAHS
2	17	Female	14	Delay (L)	(-)
3	17	Male	15	Advance (H)	(-)

Delay(Advance):chronotherapy by delayed (advanced) shift
(L):laboratory (H):home, T:triazolam, M:methylphenidate
BAHS:butoctamide hydrogen succinate A:antipsychotics(CP etc.)

TABLE 2. Patients with hypernychthemeral syndrome

Case No.	Age	Sex	Dose	Blood levels before	after
1	17	Male	3,000μg/day	590 pg/ml	2209 pg/ml
2	23	Male	3,000μg/day	510.0	970

RESULTS

(1) The delay of sleep phase of DSPS palient was attributable to a delay in REM sleep phase coupled with a delay in the body temperature cycle. According to the accumulation of the amplitudes of 0.5-2HZ delta-band EEG activities recorded before and after chronotherapy, the DSPS patient did not have any dysfunction of slow wave sleep as usually seen in the other types of insomniacs. The phase of body temperature advanced in relation to the phase of sleep. The mean value of the time interval between sleep onset and minimum rectal temperature of 4 cases was 166.3 minutes before chronotherapy, but was 299.3 minutes after chronotherapy. Resetting the circadian clock with chronotherapy was easy in all the DSPS patients, but it was not easy to maintain the reset rhythm without pharmacotherapy (triazolam etc.).

(2) Two hypernychthermal patients were successfully treated with the administration of vitamin B12 3mg/day. Effects of this drug on the entrainment to outside time-cues appeared soon after the administration and high blood levels were obtained. In one adolescent patient, his τ before administration of the drug was 24.6 hour and it was reset to 24.02 hour after treatment computed by a periodogram.

DISCUSSION

Chronotherapy made it possible to reset the circadian clocks of patients with DSPS, but maintaining the reset rhythm thereafter was not easy without additional therapy. Triazolam and some hypnotics seemed to be effective on the phase delay after chronotherapy but methylphenidate was not effective in advancing phases in most cases. All adlescent patients who had complained of not being able to attend school were able to return to their classes after treatment. Maintaining the reset rhythm in adolescent patients seemed to be easier than in adults. The treatment of two patients with Vitamin B12 was effective, nevertheless the mechanism of efficacy is still unknown. It shoud be done the study on the effects of methylcobalamin on sleep-wake rhythm of humans from two aspects of transmethylation and cholinergic metabolism of this agent.

REFERENCES

1. Kamgar-Parsi, B. et al. Successful treatment of human non-24-hour sleep-wake syndrome. Sleep 6:257-264, 1983.
2. Ohta, T. et al. On therapy of delayed sleep phase syndrome. Jpn J Psychiatr Neurol. 42:175-176, 1988.
3. Weitzman E.D. et al. Delayed sleep phase syndrome: A chronobiological disorder with sleep-onset insomnia. Arch Gen Psychiatry 38:737-746, 1981.

EFFECTS OF ZOPICLONE ON SUBJECTIVE EVALUATION OF DAY-TIME SLEEPINESS AND ON PSYCHOMOTOR AND PHYSICAL PERFORMANCES IN ATHLETES.

M. BILLIARD, M. TAFTI and A. BESSET.
Sleep and Wake Disorders Unit, Guy de Chauliac Hospital, Montpellier, France.

Prior to and during athletic competitions, increased incidence of sleep disruption, including longer sleep latency, shorter sleep duration, and more frequent awakenings is experienced by the athletes. Although many athletes are compelled to use hypnotic drugs in these conditions, the impact of this practice upon their performance is unknown.

The aim of this study was to evaluate the efffects of 7.5mg zopiclone on subjective (estimation, self-rating) and objective (psychomotor, physical) performances in athletes.

METHODS : A double blind cross over study was conducted with 8 athletes (National team of volley-ball), aged 22 to 29 years (median age 25 years). Two sessions of 2 nights with zopiclone or placebo administration were performed with 26 days of washout between the sessions. Residual effects on subsequent daytime functions were assessed at 0800, 1300 and 1800 by means of both psychomotor, physical and subjective self-assessment tests. These included choice reaction time (CRT) eye-hand coordination (EHC), critical flicker fusion (CFF), standing jump (SJ), running time (RT) and self-evaluations of sleep and daytime alertness.

RESULTS : All objective tests showed similar results in both conditions. Zopiclone slightly decreased EHC at 0800, and then rapidly increased performance to a level higher than that of placebo. Identical values were found for SJ in all scheduled tests with zopiclone and placebo while zopiclone slightly increased RT at 0800 and 1300. No significant differences were found in these objective tests.

Subjective assessments indicate that self-rated sleepiness (by means of the Stanford Sleepiness Scale) exhibited a significant improvement with zopiclone. In addition, subjects estimated their sleep to be significantly longer in duration with zopiclone . Sleep latency and the number of awakenings were not significantly modified. Finally, the subjects mentioned a better alertness, well-being and minimal fatigue under zopiclone.

CONCLUSION : The present study shows that psychomotor and physical performances are not modified with zopiclone. Moreover, the self-evaluation of sleep and daytime alertness point to some improvement with zopiclone.

HYPNOTIC-INDUCED DECREMENT AND ENHANCEMENT OF MEMORY

Wallace B. Mendelson
Department of Psychiatry, State University of New York,
Stony Brook, New York, USA

Increasingly more studies appear documenting cognitive deficits arising from the clinical use of hypnotics. The observation of retrograde enhancement of memory by a benzodiazepine (1) has led us to reassess a number of influences on the outcome of such drug studies. One major area of investigation has been examination of differential effects on various aspects of the process of registering, consolidating and retrieving memory traces. Other factors which need to be taken into account include:

1. The degree to which differing pharmacokinetics of various agents can explain their relative effects on memory processes. Our data suggests a close relationship between blood levels of benzodiazepines and duration of cognitive impairment (2), and other studies have emphasized the the contribution of kinetics to drug dynamics (3).

2. The presence of retrograde amnesia for the few minutes immediately before sleep onset, whether physiologic or drug-induced (4). This suggests that amnesic effects may often be secondary to the sleep induced by the drug, rather than by a more direct pharmacologic action on cognitive processes.

2. Alterations in learning secondary to impairment of vigilance and attention in awake subjects. Smirne et al. (5), for instance, found that decrements in immediate and short-term memory induced by flunitrazepam paralleled alterations in vigilance and attention.

3. Alterations in anxiety levels, which may influence learning. In principle, drugs which are more anxiolytic might enhance learning processes in subjects who are impaired by anxiety.

4. The possible influence of personality on drug effects. Friedman et al. (6), for instance, have reported that subjects characterized as introverted perform better on some tasks such as the Symbol Digit Modalities Test compared to those with higher scores for extroversion.

5. The brief phase of excitation or disinhibition from low doses of sedatives could conceivably enhance cognitive processes. This approach has been used to

explain retrograde enhancement of memory by low doses of alcohol (7). The challenge for this view comes from observations that potent hypnotics, which result in little or no evident excitatory phase, may retroactively enhance learning (1).

6. Genetic influences on memory effects of drugs. It has been speculated that one aspect of genetic influence might be mediated by the degree of drug-induced excitation (7), which may be partially under genetic control in animals.

In summary, the variability of results coming from studies of hypnotic effects on cognition reflects the many influences involved. Models of drug effect will have to include facilitation as well as decrements in cognitive processes.

REFERENCES

1. Mendelson, W.B. et al. Effects of two preparations of triazolam on cognition and performance in normal volunteers. Sleep Res. 18:63, 1989.
2. Mendelson, W.B. et al. Effects of benzodiazepine hypnotics on memory and EEG. Sleep Res. 16:107, 1987.
3. Greenblatt, D.J. et al. Pharmacokinetic determinants of dynamic differences among three benzodiazepine hypnotics. Arch. Gen. Psychiat. 46:326-332, 1989.
4. Roth, T. et al. Sleep and memory. In: Benzodiazepine receptor ligands, memory and information processing. (I. Hindmarch and H. Ott, eds.), Springer-Verlag, Heidelberg, 1988, pp. 140-145.
5. Smirne, S. et al. Effects of flunitrazepam on cognitive functions. Psychopharmacology 98:251-256, 1989.
6. Friedman, D.S. et al. Individual differences in the effects of triazolam on cognitive performance. Presentation at the American Psychological Assn. Annual meeting, New Orleans, Aug. 11-15, 1989.
7. Parker, E.S. et al. The alcohol facilitation effect on memory: a dose-response study. Psychopharmacology 74:88-92, 1981.

EFFECTS OF ZOPICLONE AND OTHER HYPNOTICS ON THE TRANSIENT CHANGE IN SLEEP-WAKE SCHEDULE

O. KANNO, H. WATANABE and H. KAZAMATSURI
Department of Psychiatry, Teikyo University school of Medicine, Tokyo, Japan

Recently, many kinds of hypnotic drugs are used for transient disorders of sleep-wake schedule(so called "Jet Lag" syndrome or "Work Shift" change). But, there have been no detailed reports on the effects of hypnotic drugs on these disorders.

SUBJECTS AND METHOD

Subjects were six healthy young volunteers, ranging in age from 21 to 28 years. After the two control nights with their usual sleep schedule, two experimental models were set up: one with subjects who were instructed to go to bed six hours earlier than their usual schedule (advanced shift, A-shift), and the other six hours later(delayed shift, D-shift). Then, the effects of four hypnotic drugs[Zopiclone 10mg(ZPC), Flunitrazepam 1mg(FNZ), Triazolam 0.25mg(TZM) and Levomepromazine 5mg(LPZ)], which had different chemical structures, elimination half-life and pharmacological properties, were compared with placebo. Polygraphic records and classification of sleep stages were made according to the methods and criteria of Rechtschaffen and Kales. The data were processed by the procedure of Williams et al. In view of "first night effect", the data on the first night were excluded from the study. The paired t-test was used to test for significant differences. Subjective evaluation of the drugs was also made.

RESULT

At A- and D-shift with placebo, total sleep time(TST) was shortened. At A-shift with placebo, sleep efficiency index(SEI) decreased, the percentage of stage REM(%SREM) decreased and non-REM/REM ratio increased. At D-shift with placebo, slow wave sleep latency(SWSL) was prolonged, percentage of stage 3 and 4(%S3+4) decreased, %SREM increased and non-REM/REM ratio decreased significantly. These changes supported the previous papers[1,2,3].

All drugs prolonged TST and increased SEI at A- and D-shift. At A-shift with TZM and LPZ, %SREM incresed and non-REM/REM ratio resumed to the control-night level. At D-shift with ZPC, FNZ and TZM, %SREM decreased and non-REM/REM ratio was recovered. SWSL was shortened to the control-night level by ZPC.

DISCUSSION

From the results of the polygraphic study, TZM and LPZ were effective

Fig.1: Advanced Shift(A-shift)

Fig.2: Delayed Shift(D-shift)

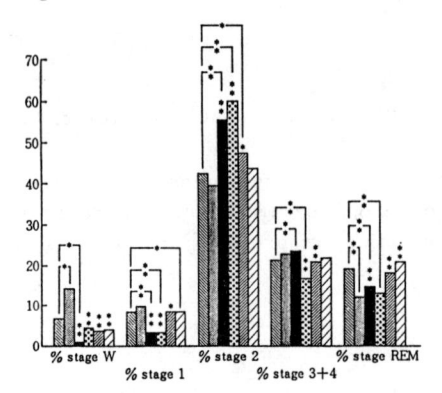

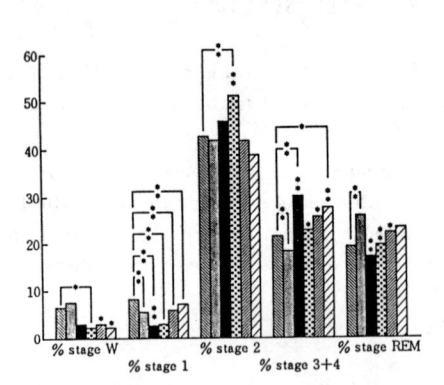

Fig.3: non-REM/REM ratio

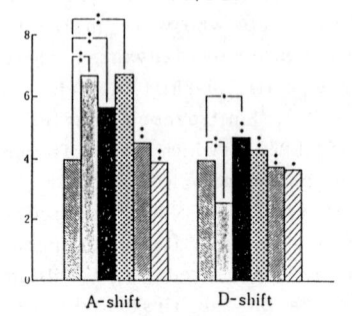

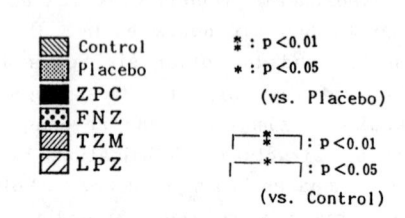

Control
Placebo
ZPC
FNZ
TZM
LPZ

**: $p<0.01$
*: $p<0.05$
(vs. Placebo)

$\lceil$**$\rceil$: $p<0.01$
$\lceil$*$\rceil$: $p<0.05$
(vs. Control)

in A-shift model. But LPZ showed hung-over effects in the subjective evaluation, so TZM could be recommended for the disorders like A-shift. In D-shift model, ZPC, FNZ and TZM were effective, and LPZ was slightly inferior to the other drugs. In some cases, TZM and LPZ had undesirable effects in mental and physical condition on the next day. ZPC was superior in increasing action in SWS(%S3+4) and in shortening action in SWSL, so ZPC had slightly better effect. But the effect of ZPC 10mg was a little too strong, therefore slightly smaller doses of ZPC could be recommended for this kind of disorders.

REFERENCE

1. Endo,S. et al: Persistence of the circadian rhythm of REM sleep; A variety of experimental manipulation of sleep-wake cycles. Sleep 4:319~328, 1981.
2. Taub,J.M. and Berger,R.J.:Sleep stage patterns associated with acute shifts in the sleep-wakefulness cycle. EEG Clin. Neurophysiol. 35:613~619, 1973.
3. Webb,W.B. and Agnew,H.W.Jr.: Sleep cycling within twenty-four-hour periods. J. Exp. Psycol. 74:158~160,1967.

GABA AND NORADRENERGIC MECHANISMS IN ANXIETY

D.J. NUTT, P. GLUE, C.W. LAWSON AND S. WILSON
Reckitt & Colman Psychopharmacology Unit, School of Medical Sciences, University of Bristol, Bristol, U.K.

The endogenous neurotransmitters that modulate anxiety have been the subject of much research although there is little in the way of definitive findings. Perhaps the two most relevant systems are noradrenaline (NA) and the GABA-A/benzodiazepine receptor complex, both of which may be abnormal, particularly in panic disorder. The present paper focuses on these and limits itself to the available human evidence.

NORADRENALINE
The evidence that NA dysfunction may predispose to anxiety is as follows:
1. Peripheral release\spillover\turnover of NA (6) and/or adrenaline (10) is often increased at baseline in anxious patients.
2. During episodes of anxiety, eg panic attacks (4) and alcohol withdrawal (8) such effects are increased.
3. This increase may reflect subfunctioning of central inhibitory α_2-adrenoceptors that control NA release (6,8).
4. There is evidence of downregulation of post-synaptic α_2-adrenoceptors eg those controlling growth hormone release and sedation (6,2), perhaps secondary to paroxysmal excessive NA release.
5. Drugs such as the tricyclic antidepressants (eg imipramine) which increase synaptic availability of NA are commonly anxiogenic in panic patients at the start of treatment (7).
6. Chronic administration of such antidepressants may act by reducing and\or stabilising a pathologically labile NA system (7).

However, there are some recent data that do not fully accord with this view, particulary the relative lack of anxiogenic action of the new selective α_2-adrenoceptor antagonists such as idazoxan. These compounds increase NA turnover in brain and should increase NA transmission. It is possible that this increase in central NA is not markedly anxiogenic because post-synaptic α_2-adrenoceptors are also blocked. The resolution of this paradox relies on the development of drugs selective for pre- and post-synaptic α_2-adrenoceptors, if such are possible.

GABA-A/BENZODIAZEPINE RECEPTOR COMPLEX
The obvious potency of benzodiazepines as rapidly-acting anxiolytics has produced at least three theories that incorporate dysfunction of this system into an explanation of anxiety. These are outlined in Table 1 and means of testing their predictions using the antagonist flumazenil in anxious patients are detailed. If an endogenous inverse agonist was to be released excessively in anxious patients then flumazenil would be anxiolytic and could be an effective therapy free from the risks of sedation and dependence which limit the current use of agonist benzodiazepines. Possible candidates for such compounds include Diazepam Binding Inhibitor (DBI,1) and derivatives (1), which are anxiogenic peptides, and Tribulin, an as yet unidentified substance whose excretion is increased in anxiety states (3). The second option is that there is an underproduction of endogenous anxiolytic benzodiazepine receptor ligands in the anxious. The recent discovery of desmethyldiazepam and other benzodiazepines in human brain (9) makes this a possibility. Thus flumazenil would oppose the tonic action of such compound and would be anxiogenic in volunteers as well as patients. The last hypothesis is that the "set-point" of the benzodiazepine receptor is altered in the brains of anxious people, so that GABA-inhibition is reduced. Such a shift of set-point has been suggested to occur in benzodiazepine withdrawal (5), a condition where anxiety can be marked. If this were the case then flumazenil would be

anxiogenic in patients but not in controls.

Our recently completed study of flumazenil (2 mg iv over 1 min) in 10 panic patients and 10 age and sex matched controls has revealed a profound anxiogenic action in patients but not in controls. Indeed, 80% of the patients but none of the controls experienced a clear panic attack. Ratings of anxiety before and at various time-points after the infusions are shown in fig 1. The lack of a significant anxiogenic response vehicle argues against a psychological explanation for this finding.

These data clearly refute both hypotheses that invoke the presence of an endogenous ligand. They are compatible with the altered "set-point" theory. Further evidence in support of this could be obtained by determining whether the actions of agonist benzodiazepines are also shifted in the inverse agonist direction (reduced agonism) in this population.

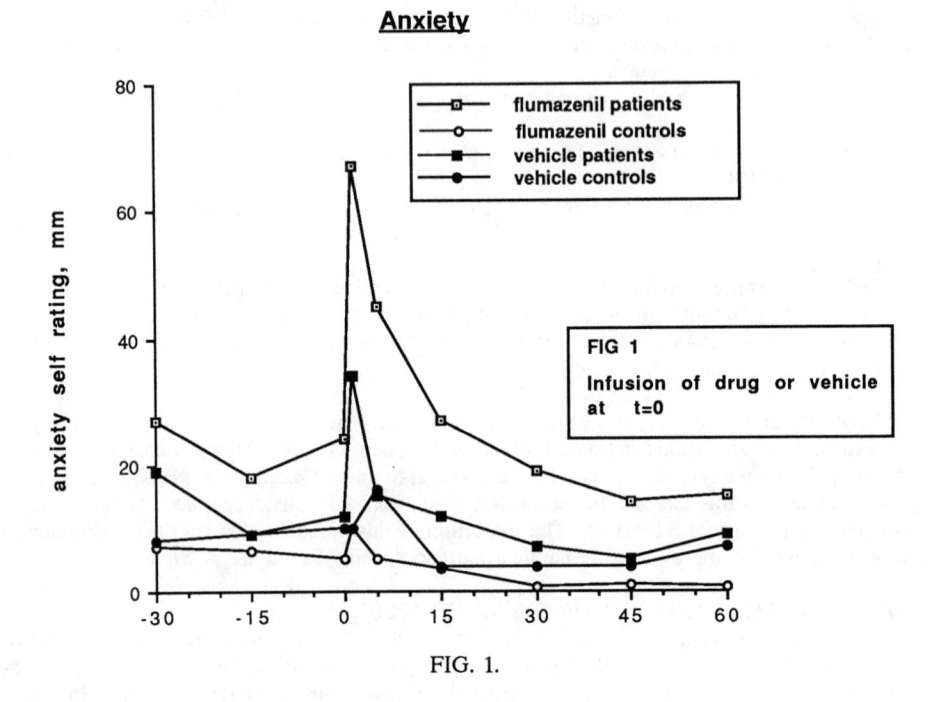

FIG. 1.

REFERENCES

1. Barbaccia, et al., (1986): Arch. Gen. Psychiat., 43:1143-1147.
2. Charney D.S. and Heninger G.R., (1986): Am. J. Psychiat., 43:1042-1054.
3. Clow, et al., (1988): Psychopharmacol., 95:378-380.
4. Ko, et al., (1983): Arch. Gen. Psychiat., 40:425-430.
5. Little H.J., Nutt D.J. and Taylor S.C., (1987): J. Psychopharmacol., 1:35-46.
6. Nutt D.J., (1989): Arch. Gen. Psychiat., 46:165-169.
7. Nutt D.J. and Glue P., (1989): Pharm. Ther., 44:309-334.
8. Nutt, et al., (1988): Alcohol:Clin. Exper. Res., 12:14-18.
9. Sangameswaran L., and De Blas A.L., (1985): Proc. Nat. Acad. Sci., 82:5560-5564.
10. Villacres, et al., (1987): Psychiat. Res., 21:313-321.

SEROTONERGIC MECHANISMS IN ANXIETY

ARLENE S. EISON and MICHAEL S. EISON
Preclinical CNS Research, Bristol-Myers Squibb Company, Wallingford, CT; U.S.A.

One approach to understanding the biological substrates of psychopathology is to infer from an understanding of the mechanism of action of drugs useful in treating psychiatric disorders what neurochemical aberrations may underlie these disorders. For many years the benzodiazepines (BZs) have been the mainstay of anxiolytic therapy, and it has been widely assumed that an appreciation for the neurochemical mediation of anxiety states would derive from an understanding of the dynamics of the BZ receptor complex. However, a new class of anxiolytic agent, the azapirones, has recently been described. These agents are clinically effective against generalized anxiety disorder (7,16) but do not interact with BZ receptors (4). Rather, these agents potently interact with brain serotonin (5HT) systems (4). The demonstrated efficacy of the azapirone anxiolytics has rekindled an interest in exploring the role of 5HT in anxiety.

Serotonin was first discovered in blood platelets (10). Changes in 5HT neurotransmission in brain, initially associated with depression, are now believed to be involved in multiple psychiatric disorders, including affective disorders, obsessive-compulsive, panic, and seasonal affective disorders (11). The complex pharmacology and anatomy of the 5HT system is appropriate to allow this transmitter substance to broadly affect behavior and mood (5). However, the complexity of central 5HT mechanisms and the potential for interactions between 5HT and other neurotransmitter systems has contributed to the generation of an often bewilderingly contradictory literature regarding the role of 5HT in anxiety disorders. This is particularly true of human studies. Despite relying upon often imperfect animal models, the types of experimental manipulations and independent measures available to animal researchers allows a more precise dissection of the 5HT effects of anxiolytic drugs. Consequently, this paper will summarize the preclinical evidence which supports the hypothesis that there is a clinically relevant serotonergic component to the expression of anxiety disorders.

Much of the early work which investigated the role of 5HT in anxiety employed so-called conflict tests, in which appetitive responding by animals is suppressed by punishment. Anxiolytic drugs release responding from punishment-induced suppression. It was observed that manipulations which result in diminished 5HT neurotransmission, such as PCPA-induced depletion of 5HT (15) or administration of 5HT antagonists (9) produced anxiolytic-like reduction of response suppression, while administration of 5HT precursors reversed depletion-induced release of suppression (15). In addition to punishment, conditions of novelty induce response suppression in rodents. Consistent with the notion that anxiolytic-like release from response suppression is associated with decreased 5HT function, it was observed that reduction of the activity of 5HT dorsal raphe cells produced by intracerebral administration of the inhibitory neurotransmitter (and important mediator of BZ effects) GABA, reduced novelty-induced neophobia in rats, while drugs that increased 5HT function exacerbated novelty-induced response suppression (14). Interestingly, BZs reduce 5HT turnover (2) and intraventricular administration of 5HT blocks BZ-induced (oxazepam) release from response suppression (19). Like BZs, the azapirone buspirone reduces firing of 5HT cells of the dorsal raphe in anesthetized preparations (18), and like the BZs (13), buspirone reduces 5HT cell firing in freely moving animals (17). The azapirones selectively interact with a particular subset of 5HT receptors, the 5HT-1A receptor (12,16). The azapirones may differ from each other by the extent to which they exhibit 5HT agonist effects at this site; buspirone and gepirone act as a partial agonists at postsynaptic 5HT-1A receptors (3,8) while ipsapirone appears to exert effects that are more like those of full 5HT agonists (8). Further support for the notion that anxiolytic effects are associated with reduced 5HT neurotransmission is provided by recent evidence that ritanserin, an antagonist of 5HT type 2 receptors, may also have anxiolytic potential (1). Results of animal studies, as well as clinical trials with non-BZ anxiolytics suggest that a functional excess in 5HT neurotransmission may underlie generalized anxiety disorder. It has been proposed that anxiety may reflect a state of hyperexcitability of 5HT receptors (10) or a plasticity disease of 5HT autoreceptors (6). Perhaps reduction of 5HT neurotransmission reflects a final common pathway for BZ and azapirone modulation of anxiety in man.

1. Ceulemans, et al., (1985): Pharmacopsychiatry, 18:303-305.
2. Corrodi, et al., (1971): Brain Res., 29:1-6.
3. Devivo, M. and Maayani, S. (1986): J. Pharmacol. Exp. Therap., 238:248-253.
4. Eison, et al., (1986): Pharmacol. Biochem. Behav., 24:701-707.
5. Eison, M.S. (1989): Psychopathology, 22(1):13-20.
6. Eison, M.S. (1990): J. Clin. Psychopharmacol., "In press".
7. Goldberg, H.L. and Finnerty, R.J. (1979): Am. J. Psychiat., 136:1184-1187.
8. Hamon, et al., (1988): J. Pharmacol. Exp. Therap., 246:745-752.
9. Iversen, S.D. (1984): Neuropharmacology, 23:1553-1560.
10. Kahn, et al., (1988): Biol. Psychiat., 23:189-208.
11. Lopez-Ibor, J.J. (1988): Br. J. Psychiat., 153(3):26-39.
12. Peroutka, S.J. 91985): Biol. Psychiat., 20:971-979
13. Preussler, et al., (1981): Soc. Neurosci. Abstr., 7:923
14. Soubrie, P. (1986): Behav. Brain Sci., 9:319-364.
15. Tenen, S.S. (1967): Psychopharmacologica, 10:204-219.
16. Traber, J. and Glaser, T. (1987): Trends in Pharmacol. Sci., 8:432-437.
17. Trulson, M.E. and Trulson, T.J. (1986): Neuropharmacology, 25:1263-1266.
18. VanderMaelen, et al., (1986): Eur. J. Pharmacol., 129:123-130.
19. Wise, et al., (1972): Science, 177:180-183.

TARGET RECEPTORS FOR ANXIOLYTIC DRUGS : THE RELEVANCE OF ANIMAL MODELS

D.J. Sanger, B. Zivkovic and S.Z. Langer.
Department of Biology, SYNTHELABO RECHERCHE (L.E.R.S), 58 rue de la Glacière, 75013 - Paris, France

The treatment of anxiety states has been dominated in recent years by the benzodiazepines. Although these drugs have many advantages they also have a number of undesirable side effects, and recent research has emphasized the search for new anxiolytics with novel chemical structures and original pharmacological profiles. As in many areas of contemporary psychopharmacology, the search for novel anxiolytics has involved an analysis of specific neurotransmitter systems with the hope of finding compounds with selectivity for different receptors. Systems currently of particular interest in this respect include ω receptors, 5HT receptor subtypes and glutamate receptors. In addition to the neurochemical studies necessary for this enterprise, behavioural models continue to play an important role in the screening and development of novel anxiolytics and in the analysis of their modes of action. Recent research have indicated, however, that the behavioural procedures previously found so effective for studying drugs such as benzodiazepines and barbiturates may not always be well-adapted to the analysis of newer putative anxiolytics.

One currently important research area involves the search for novel anxiolytics which, like benzodiazepines, bind to ω sites associated with the GABA receptor complex. A variety of compounds with chemical structures different from those of traditional benzodiazepine anxiolytics have now been shown to have this property. These include diazepines, triazolopyridazines, ß-carbolines, cyclopyrrolones, imidazopyridines and pyrazolopyridines. Although some of these compounds show pharmacological activity essentially similar to that of the benzodiazepines, some present interesting and important differences (Gardner, 1988).

In some cases these differences can be accounted for by partial agonist activity at the ω receptor sites. Bretazenil, for example, has anticonvulsant and antipunishment activity in some animal tests without sedative and muscle-relaxing effects, and will antagonise the depressant actions of benzodiazepines such as diazepam. This profile is most readily explained as indicating a low level of intrinsic activity at a single receptor site if it is assumed that the different pharmacological effects of benzodiazepines are all produced through this single receptor. However the profile of another anxiolytic drug, alpidem, which binds to ω receptors and shows anxioselective activity, is not explicable in this way. Alpidem has anticonvulsant activity and is active in some, but not all, punishment procedures. In addition, unlike bretazenil and many other ω receptor ligands it has discriminative stimulus properties in rats which differ from those of the benzodiazepines (Zivkovic et al, 1990). Although alpidem does have low intrinsic activity it has also been found to be selective for the ω_1 and ω_3 subtypes of receptors (Langer et al, 1990). However, as the ω_1 subtype has been associated with hypnotic effects (as with the imidazopyridine, zolpidem) and a functional role for the ω_3 site has not yet been defined, it is not clear to what extent this receptor selectivity is responsible for alpidem's pharmacological profile. At present, probably the most satisfactory explanation of the novel pharmacology of alpidem involves its combination of receptor selectivity and low intrinsic activity.

The recent discovery of a variety of subtypes of 5HT receptors has also had an important influence on anxiolytic drug research. It has been believed for some time that 5HT plays a significant role in anxiety and anxiolytic drug effects, and a variety of novel compounds acting at 5HT receptor subtypes ($5HT_1$, $5HT_2$, $5HT_3$) have been proposed as potential anxiolytics. Of particular importance has been the finding that the clinically active anxiolytic buspirone has affinity for $5HT_{1A}$ receptors. It has not yet been established with certainty that this mechanism mediates the clinical activity of buspirone. However, as a number of other compounds selective for $5HT_{1A}$ receptors are presently in clinical development, this problem may soon be resolved. The psychopharmacological profile of buspirone and related compounds in the laboratory differs substantially from that of benzodiazepine anxiolytics. Buspirone is active in some traditional behavioural tests but not in all. For example, it increases rates of punished responding in pigeons but has variable and less reliable effects in similar tests with rodents and primates. The discriminative stimulus properties of buspirone differ from those of benzodiazepines and barbiturates and it also shows some behavioural effects more usually associated with antidepressant or antipsychotic agents (eg. learned helplessness, conditioned avoidance).

These examples of recent research findings indicate that the experimental psychopharmacology of anxiolytics has entered a new era. A variety of novel anxiolytics are being developed with activity at different receptors. The animal models used traditionally for assessing anxiolytics may no longer be adequate to respond to the challenge presented by these new drugs. In the coming years it will certainly be necessary to re-evaluate laboratory tests in the light of clinical experience.

REFERENCES

1. Gardner C.R. Pharmacological profiles in vivo of benzodiazepine receptor ligands. Drug Dev Res 12: 1-28, 1988
2. Langer SZ, Arbilla S, Tan S, LLoyd KG, George P, Allen J, Wick A. Selectivity for omega receptor subtypes as a strategy for the development of anxiolytic drugs. Pharmacopsychiatry in press, 1990.
3. Zivkovic B., Morel E., Perrault Gh., Sanger D.J. and Lloyd K.G. Pharmacological and behavioural profile of alpidem as an anxiolytic. Pharmacopsychiatry in press, 1990

DRUG MODELS OF ANXIETY

T. W. Uhde
National Institute of Mental Health, Bethesda,
Maryland, U.S.A.

A historical overview of chemical and physiological models of anxiety, including the use of adrenergic agents (e.g. yohimbine, epinepheine, isoproterenol), lactate, carbon dioxide, metachlorophenylpiperazine, CCK, and inverse benzodiazepines agonists (e.g. FG 7142) to induce pathological anxiety states will be presented. The paper will present new data regarding the behavioral, physiological and biochemical effects of 1,3,7-trimethylxanthine (e.g. caffeine) in patients with primary anxiety disorders. Special attention will be given to possible mechanisms of caffeine-induced anxiety as they relate to noradrenergic, adenosinergic, dopaminergic and possible limbic and respiratory system dysfunction. Findings will be discussed within the context of the current DSM-III-R classification of the anxiety disorders.

FROM LABORATORY TO CLINIC

MALCOLM LADER
Department of Psychiatry, Institute of Psychiatry, University of London, U.K.

SYNDROMES OF ANXIETY

Clinicians, by and large, are much more concerned to have effective treatments for their patients than to be given elegant explicatory hypotheses for their patients' ills. Although, in a perfect world, the rational approach is preferable to the empirical one, most of psychiatry is too inchoate at present. Nevertheless, research must have some direction. To that end various models of anxiety have been proposed, usually on the basis of covert anthropomorphism, but occasionally on an ethological basis. Attempts are then made to validate those models using accepted human treatments as the criterion.

Anxiety is both a normal emotion and a pathological condition. Furthermore, anxiety of any type may result in the individual experiencing the emotion seeking medical or other professional advice. Abnormal or pathological anxiety is diagnosed when the intensity of the emotion felt and complained of (i.e. "state anxiety") seems quite disproportionate to the putative source of the anxiety (6).

However, the syndromes defined in nosological schemata such as that of the American Psychiatric Association (1) (DSM-IIIR) lay down rigid criteria such as unrealistic anxiety and worry about two or more life circumstances for six months or more. These requirements exclude from the category all but severe, chronic anxiety states.

In the 1960's and early 1970's, the benzodiazepines steadily replaced the barbiturates because they were perceived as much safer drugs. Indeed, in many countries, tranquillizer usage expanded appreciably as doctors prescribed them for more and more trivial conditions and patients demanded them to deaden normal responses to everyday stress. Inevitably, benzodiazepines became the yardstick against which animal models of anxiety were established. In all this, there was an assumption that the benzodiazepines were synonymous with tranquillisers - anxiety reduction without sedation - and it was widely believed that the key to understanding anxiety lay with unravelling the mode of action of these drugs (5).

The elucidation of the biochemical properties of the benzodiazepines has reinforced scepticism concerning selectivity of action. The benzodiazepines potentiate the effects of GABA at $GABA_A$ sites, modulating the opening of chloride ionophores. GABA is such an ubiquitous inhibitor neurotransmitter that selectivity of action seems unlikely unless clearly distinguishable subpopulations of benzodiazepine receptors exist (2). It is claimed that some newer compounds such as zuriclone and alpidem may have useful anxiolytic selectivity.

NEWER ANXIOLYTICS

A remarkable range of different compounds believed to act on one or other of the 5-HT_1, 5-HT_2 and 5-HT_3 systems have been synthesized recently and evaluated for therapeutic properties. The first of these drugs is buspirone, a 5-HT_{1A} partial agonist (3). It is as effective as benzodiazepines, (except in patients recently taking benzodiazepines), has few if any sedative properties, and its abuse and dependence potential seem limited or absent (4).

Another group of drugs acting on 5-HT mechanisms are the 5-HT_2 antagonists such as ritanserin and ICI 169,369. Compounds acting on 5-HT_3 pathways are also putative anxiolytics.

CONCLUSIONS

Several recognized methods exist for selecting behavioural and other animal models. One is the analysis of criterion behaviour. The second approach is through the analysis of criterion drugs. A third approach is to try to codify behaviour and then to seek compounds with different profiles of action. The limitations of these methods mean that many new anxiolytic drugs are still being discovered serendipitously.

Clinicians are the final arbiters of whether a drug will be a commercial success, and this is hopefully based on adequate clinical evidence concerning the risk/benefit ratio of the drug. Clinicians must assess quickly, accurately and dispassionately putative new anxiolytics and provide the feedback concerning efficacy which the behavioural psychopharmacologist needs. They can also provide new insights into anxiety. What they should avoid is ascribing spurious specificity to anxiolytic drugs.

REFERENCES

1. American Psychiatric Association. (1987). Diagnostic Criteria from DSM-III-R. Washington, DC: APA.
2. Braestrup, C., & Nielsen, M. (1980). Multiple benzodiazepine receptors. Trends in Neuroscience, 3, 301-3.
3. Eison, A.S. & Temple, D.L. (1986). Buspirone: Review of its pharmacology and current perspectives on its mechanism of action. American Journal of Medicine, 80 (3B, Suppl), 1-9.
4. Goa, K.L. & Ward, A. (1986). Buspirone: A preliminary review of its pharmacological properties and therapeutic efficacy as an anxiolytic. Drugs, 2, 114-29.
5. Insel, T.R., Ninan, P.T., Aloi, J., Jimerson, D.C., Skolnick, P. & Paul, S.M. (1984). A benzodiazepine receptor-mediated model of anxiety. Studies in non-human primates and clinical implications. Archives of General Psychiatry, 41, 741-50.
6. Lewis, A. (1967). Problems presented by the ambiguous word "anxiety" as used in psychopathology. Israel Annals of Psychiatry and Related Disciplines, 5, 105-21.

MOLECULAR CHARACTERIZATION OF THE RECEPTORS FOR DOPAMINE

Marc G. Caron, Allen Dearry, Jay A. Gingrich, Pierre Falardeau, Robert T. Fremeau, Jr., Michael D. Bates and Susan E. Senogles
Dept. of Cell Biology, Ophthalmology, Neurobiology and Medicine and Howard Hughes Medical Inst. Lab, Duke Univ. Med. Ctr., Durham, NC 27710 USA

The physiological effects of dopamine in the central nervous system and in the periphery are mediated by at least two receptors with distinct properties. D_1 dopamine receptors have been defined based on their ability to stimulate adenylyl cyclase (1) whereas D_2 dopamine receptors inhibit adenylyl cyclase but in addition, can stimulate K^+ channels through the intermediary of a G-protein (2). Over the past several years, a much better understanding of the properties of these receptors has been gained from studies of their biochemical characteristics and more recently from the cloning of the cDNAs and/or genes for these receptor proteins.

Early studies using specific affinity and photo-affinity probes indicated that both receptors represented distinct molecular entities, the D_2 receptor ligand binding site residing on a peptide of M_r = 90-120 kDa whereas the D_1 dopamine receptor was identified as a peptide of M_r = 72 kDa. Both receptors have been purified to apparent homogeneity: the D_2 receptor from bovine anterior pituitary and the D_1 receptor from rat striatum. The D_2 dopamine receptor was shown to interact selectively with the G_{i2} protein in a reconstituted system (3). A cDNA and gene for a D_2 dopamine receptor have been identified and isolated (4,5). The encoded protein possesses the 7 hydrophobic domains characteristic of other G-protein coupled receptors and shows significant homology to many other receptors of this class.

Based on the consideration that extensive homology exists between these receptors, we have used the molecular biology approach to elucidate the primary structure of a human D_1 dopamine receptor and its homologe from rat. A 72 base oligonucleotide probe based on the sequence of the rat brain cDNA for a D_2 dopamine receptor (aa 67-92) was used to screen a human retina cDNA library. A single clone encoding the partial sequence of the D_1 dopamine receptor was isolated. A fragment of this cDNA clone was used to screen a human genomic library from which a clone encoding the entire protein sequence was isolated. The single open reading frame encodes a protein of 446 aa suggesting that this receptor is intronless. The protein shows the typical 7 hydrophobic aa stretches presumed to be transmembrane domains (Fig. 1). Extensive homology, particularly within the transmembrane domains, is apparent with the D_2 dopamine

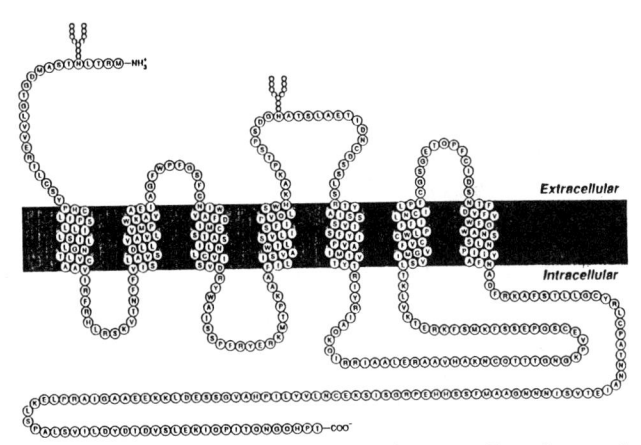

Fig. 1. Primary structure of a human D_1-dopamine receptor represented as it might exist within the plasma membrane.

receptor and other catecholamine receptors such as the various subtypes of α and β-adrenergic receptors. Two potential N-glycosylation sites are present, one in the amino terminus and another on the second extracellular loop. Expression of this DNA in COS-7 cells confers to these cells the ability to bind the specific ligands [^{3}H]SCH 23390 and [^{125}I]SCH 23982 with high affinity (K_D = 100 and 350 pM respectively) and typical D_1 dopaminergic pharmacology. In cells expressing the receptor, dopamine elevated cyclic AMP levels, suggesting that this clone represents the D_1 dopamine receptor coupled to stimulation of adenylyl cyclase. Northern analysis and in situ hybridization indicate that this receptor is predominantly expressed in the striatum. Availability of the gene encoding the D_1 dopamine receptor should facilitate studies of its relationship to the other dopamine receptor (D_2) and its potential implication in physiological and pathophysiological processes.

1) Kebabian, J.W. and Calne, D.B. Nature, 277:93-96 (1979).
2) Vallar, L. and Meldolesi, J. Trends Pharmacol. Sci. 10:74-77 (1989).
3) Senogles, S.E., Spiegel, A.M., Padrell, E., Iyengar, R. and Caron, M.G. J. Biol. Chem. 265:4507-4514 (1990).
4) Bunzow, J.R., Van Tol, H.M., Grandy, D.K., Albert, P., Salon, J., Christie, M., Machida, C.A., Neve, K.A. and Civelli, O. Nature 336:783-787 (1988).
5) Grandy, D.K., Marchionni, M.A., Makam, H., Stofko, R.E., Alfano, M., Frothingham, L., Fischer, J.B., Barke-Howie, K.J., Bunzow, J.R., Server, A.C. and Civelli, O. Proc. Natl. Acad. Sci. USA 86:9762-9766 (1989).

MULTIPLE D2 DOPAMINE RECEPTORS

Philip Seeman
Departments of Pharmacology and Psychiatry,
University of Toronto, Toronto, CANADA M5S 1A8

Although the antipsychotic action of neuroleptics may be explained by their common ability to block dopamine D2 receptors (1) in direct relation to their clinical potency (2), there is no such single explanation to account for the atypical lack of rigidity seen with the so-called atypical neuroleptics (3,4). In order to account for the low amount of rigidity caused by remoxipride and related benzamide antipsychotic drugs, it has been suggested (3) that there may be more than one type of D2 dopamine receptor which may have lower affinity for these benzamides and located in a brain region dominating the control of rigidity. Such different D2 receptors with different neuroleptic sensitivities, however, have not been found. For example, the in vitro neuroleptic sensitivities of D2 receptors in human limbic tissue are identical to those in human putamen (5,6). Although different forms of the D2 receptor have been cloned (7,8 and Refs. therein), their neuroleptic sensitivities appear to be similar. This brief report indicates that there are at least two classes of D2 receptors having different affinities to neuroleptics.

METHODS

The binding of [^{3}H]YM-09151-2 to D2 receptors in human caudate nucleus and in porcine anterior pituitary tissue was done as described earlier (9). The final concentration of [^{3}H]YM-09151-2 was 0.4 nM in a final incubation volume of 1.5 mL buffer (50 mM Tris·HCl, pH 7.4/1 mM EDTA/120 mM NaCl/5 mM KCl/1.5 mM CaCl$_2$/4 mM MgCl$_2$). The tube contents were filtered and rinsed with 7 ml of buffer through a 7034 filter, using a Skatron cell harvester.

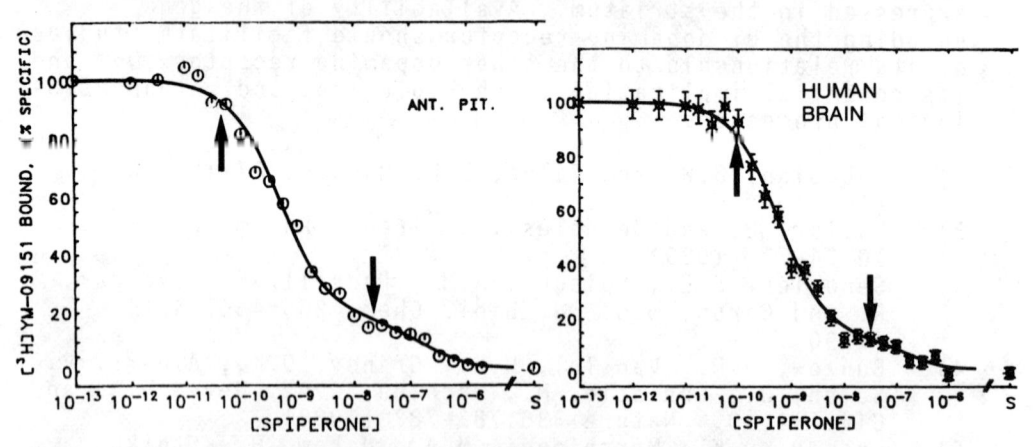

Fig. 1 Two D2 receptors for neuroleptic drugs can be detected by the competition of spiperone against [^{3}H]YM-09151-2 in porcine anterior pituitary or in human caudate nucleus (8 brains) homogenates. Specific binding defined by S (10 uM S-sulpiride). Arrows indicate the two dissociation constants for spiperone.

Nonspecific binding was defined as that occurring in the presence of 10 uM S-sulpiride (Ravizza).

RESULTS AND DISCUSSION

The binding of [^{3}H]YM-09151-2 was inhibited by spiperone in two phases, with dissociation constants of about 80 pM and about 20 nM, as indicated in Fig.1. Such data are similar to those obtained earlier (9), except that nonspecific binding was here defined as that in the presence of 10 uM S-sulpiride. In order to confirm that the site with low affinity for spiperone was dopaminergic, various agonists and antagonists were tested in the presence of 1 nM spiperone (to occlude the site having high affinity [80 pM] for spiperone); the rank order of potency was dopamine >> noradrenaline >> serotonin.

It is possible, therefore, that the extra D2 sites detected by [^{3}H]YM-09151-2, consistently amounting to about 30-40% more than those detected by [^{3}H]spiperone (Ref. 9), may have a different set of neuroleptic sensitivities (Fig. 1).

ACKNOWLEDGEMENTS

I thank Dr. H.-C. Guan for excellent assistance. Supported by the Medical Research Council of Canada, the Ontario Mental Health Foundation, and the Canadian Psychiatric Research Foundation.

1. Seeman, P., Wong, M., and Lee, T., (1974): Dopamine receptor block and nigral fiber impulse blockade by major tranquilizers. Fed. Proc., 33: 246.
2. Seeman, P., et al., (1975): Brain receptors for antipsychotic drugs and dopamine: direct binding assays. Proc. Nat. Acad. Sci., U.S.A., 72: 4376-4380.
3. Ogren, S.-O. and Hogberg, T., (1988): Novel dopamine D_2-antagonists for the treatment of schizophrenia. ISI Atlas of Sci., Pharmacol., 2: 141-147.
4. Seeman, P., (1990): Atypical neuroleptics: role of multiple receptors, endogenous dopamine, and receptor linkage. Acta Psychiatr. Scand. Suppl.: in press.
5. Reynolds, G.P., et al., (1982): Thioridazine is not specific for limbic dopamine receptors. Lancet 2: 499-500.
6. Seeman, P., and Ulpian, C., (1983): Neuroleptics have identical potencies in human brain limbic and putamen regions. Eur. J. Pharmacol. 94: 145-148.
7. Bunzow, J.R., et al., (1988): Cloning and expression of a rat D_2 dopamine receptor cDNA. Nature, 336: 783-787.
8. O'Dowd, B.F., et al., (1990): Cloning of two additional catecholamine receptors from rat brain. FEBS Letters.
9. Niznik, H.B., et al., (1985): Dopamine D_2 receptors selectively labeled by a benzamide neuroleptic: [^{3}H]YM-09151-2. Naunyn Schmiedeberg's Arch. Pharmacol. 329: 333-343.

INTRAMEMBRANE REGULATION OF DOPAMINE D2 RECEPTORS BY NEUROPEPTIDE RECEPTORS AND EXCITATORY AMINO ACID RECEPTORS. RELEVANCE FOR SCHIZOPHRENIA

K. FUXE[*], L.F. AGNATI[**], G. VON EULER[*], S. TANGANELLI[+], W. O'CONNOR[++], P. OSBORNE[++], T. ANTONELLI[+] and U. UNGERSTEDT[++]
Department of Histology and Neurobiology[*] and Department of Pharmacology[++], Karolinska Institute, Box 60400, 104 01 Stockholm, Sweden; Department of Human Physiology[**], University of Modena, Modena, Italy; Department of Pharmacology[+], University of Ferrara, Ferrara, Italy

During the eighties we introduced the concept of intra- and inter-synaptic intramembrane receptor-receptor interactions as a new computational mechanism in information handling in the brain (see 2,3) possibly mediated through allosteric interactions, G proteins or protein phosphorylation processes. In the present article we will review in vivo and in vitro evidence demonstrating that cholecystokinin (CCK) peptides, neurotensin (NT) and glutamate via activation of their respective receptors can reduce the sensitivity of neostriatal and subcortical limbic dopamine (DA) D2 receptors (see also 5).

Neurotensin/dopamine D2 receptor interactions

The available evidence demonstrates that NT in concentrations of 3-10 nM increases the K_D value of D2 agonist binding sites in membranes from subcortical limbic areas and from neostriatum of rat and postmortem human brain (see 1). The increase in the K_D value has been shown to be due to a preferential increase in the dissociation rate and appear to be microviscosity and G protein independent (1). The D1 receptors appear to be unaffected by these concentrations of NT.

Recent studies using in vivo intrastriatal microdialysis in freely moving rats also support this view. Local perfusion with NT (10 nM) enhanced the inhibitory effect of SKF38393 (D1 agonist) on extracellular DA levels, while it markedly reduced the inhibitory effect of pergolide (D2 agonist) on extracellular DA levels in the neostriatum (6,9). By favoring the D1 receptor population NT receptor activation has a potential therapeutic value in schizophrenia, since the ratio of D2/D1 receptors is increased in brains from schizophrenic patients (see 7).

CCK/DA D2 receptor interactions

A major action of CCK-4 and CCK-8 is to reduce the affinity of D2 agonist binding sites in striatal and subcortical limbic membranes in concentrations up to 10 nM (see 5). These results are supported by in vivo evidence demonstrating an involvement of CCK receptors in the control of striatal DA autoreceptors (10).

The available evidence indicates that D2 receptor sensitivity may be controlled by intramembrane feedback loops involving both NT and CCK receptors. It seems possible that the CCK receptors and NT receptors interact with the same transmembrane part of the DA D2 receptor to induce the increase of the K_D value (1).

In conclusion, also activation of CCK receptors in striatal and subcortical limbic regions may be helpful as a new principle for the treatment of schizophrenia in view of their ability to reduce D2 receptor sensitivity, thus favoring DA transmission via the D1 receptor population.

Glutamate/D2 receptor interactions

It is well known that phencyclidine, a blocker of ion channels linked to NMDA receptors produces schizophrenia-like syndromes (8). It is therefore of substantial interest that glutamate in membrane preparations reduces the affinity of D2 agonist binding sites of the neostriatum. This reduction of D2 receptor sensitivity may be related to a combined activation of several subtypes of excitatory aminoacid receptors (see 4). Furthermore, NMDA given in low concentrations into the ventricle of awake animals selectively reduces DA utilization within the anterior part of the nucleus accumbens and olfactory tubercle (see 5). On the basis of these observations it seems possible that deficiencies in the efferent cortico-limbic glutamate pathways innervating the nucleus accumbens and olfactory tubercle may contribute to the development of schizophrenia. Such a deficiency may lead to both an increase of DA release as well as to an increase of DA D2 receptor sensitivity.

In conclusion, the present results suggest that intramembrane receptor-receptor interactions involving NT, CCK and glutamate receptors may allow a selective reduction of D2 receptor sensitivity in the basal forebrain and the neostriatum opening up a new avenue for pharmacological treatment of schizophrenia.

REFERENCES

1. von Euler, G. (1989): Thesis: Interactions Between Neurotensin and Dopamine Receptors in the Brain, Repro Print, Stockholm.
2. Fuxe, K., and Agnati, L.F. (1985): Med. Res. Rev., 5:441-482.
3. Fuxe, K., and Agnati, L.F. (1987): Receptor-Receptor Interactions. A New Intramembrane Integrative Mechanism, MacMillan Press, London.
4. Fuxe, K., et al., (1984): Eur. J. Pharmacol., 100:127-130.
5. Fuxe, K., et al., (1989): In Neurochemical Pharmacology. A Tribute to B.B. Brodie, E. Costa, ed., pp. 211-227. Raven Press, New York.
6. Fuxe, K., et al., (1990): Science, in press.
7. Joyce, J., et al., (1988): Synapse, 2:546-557.
8. Quirion, R. (1986): In Neuromethods 4. Receptor Binding, A. Boulton, G. Baker, P. Hrdina, eds., pp. 499-542. Humana Press, Clifton, New Jersey.
9. Tanganelli, S., et al., (1989): Brain Res., 502:319-324.
10. Tanganelli, S., et al., (1990): Arch. Pharmacol., in press.

DOPAMINE RECEPTORS AND THEIR COUPLING TO ION CHANNELS

R.A. NORTH, M.G. LACEY, N. UCHIMURA and N. MERCURI
Vollum Institute, Oregon Health Sciences University, Portland OR97201, USA

Unclassified dopamine receptors

Potassium channel opening. A potassium conductance is increased by dopamine in *Aplysia* pleural (2,6) and abdominal ganglia (11); the conductance shows little voltage-dependence and a G protein is involved in coupling receptor to potassium channel. The same channels can be opened by agonists acting at distinct receptors (eg. histamine, muscarinic).

Calcium channel closing. A voltage-dependent calcium current is reduced by dopamine in neurons of the parietal ganglion of *Helix aspersa* (3). The effect is small (typically 30% inhibition), mimicked by guanosine-5'-O(3-thiotriphosphate)(GTP-γ-S), and blocked by pertussis toxin.

D_1 receptors

Activation of D_1 receptors in nucleus accumbens neurons of rat (15) and guinea pig (14) leads to a hyperpolarization resulting from a decrease in a membrane potassium conductance. This effect if mimicked by analogs of cyclic adenosine 3',5'-monophosphate (cAMP), consistent with the notion that elevation of cAMP is an intermediate step (14). Rat caudate nucleus neurons are also inhibited by agonists selective for D_1 receptors (1,10).

D_2 receptors

Potassium channel opening. Cell hyperpolarization resulting from potassium conductance increase by dopamine acting at D_2 receptors has been reported for rat substantia nigra neurons (7), human pituitary adenoma cells (5) and rat intermediate pituitary cells (8,13,16). The potassium conductance affected shows some inward rectification, and experiments with pertussis toxin (4) and GTP-γ-S (7) indicate the involvement of G_i or G_o in the coupling between receptor and channel. The same channels can be opened by agonists acting at γ-aminobutyric acid B (GABA$_B$) receptors (7).

Calcium channel closing. A reduction in the current flowing through voltage-dependent calcium currents is observed when dopamine is applied to melanotrophs of the pars intermedia of the pituitary gland (12,17). The effect is blocked by sulpiride and domperidone, and is mimicked by selective D_2 receptor agonists such as quinpirole. The maximum effect observed is about 40% inhibition. Pertussis toxin blocks the action of dopamine, whereas intracellular GTP-γ-S irreversibly depresses the calcium current.

Potassium channel closing. Dopamine (in presence of D_1 antagonists) and selective D_2 agonists depolarize neurons of guinea pig and rat nucleus accumbens by reducing a membrane potassium conductance (14,15). Depolarization and excitation of rat caudate nucleus neurons also involves the D_2 receptor (1,10). In nucleus accumbens, the same neurons are depolarized by 5-HT and by muscarine, acting respectively through 5-HT_2 and M_1 receptors, and by phorbol esters: this suggests the hypothesis that the D_2 receptors on these cells may stimulate phospholipase C.

Conclusions

Dopamine D_2 receptors on the dopamine-containing cells of the substantia nigra and on pituitary lactotrophs and melanotrophs, as well as an unclassified receptor on some invertebrate neurons, belong to the family of receptors which couple through a G-protein of the G_i/G_o type to inwardly-rectifying potassium channels and to high voltage-activated calcium channels (9). By contrast, activation of D_2 receptors on target cells of striatum leads to depolarization rather than hyperpolarization, through closure of a set of potassium channels: the mechanism of coupling D_2 receptor to channel in this case is unknown. The ionic mechanism whereby D_2 receptor agonists lead to inhibition of transmitter and hormone secretion is not understood: it may involve potassium conductance increase, calcium current decrease or some other mechanism. Agonists at D_1 receptors cause a hyperpolarization of striatal neurons, consistent with a pathway involving increased intracellular cAMP.

References

1. Akaike, A. et al. (1987): Brain Res. 418: 262-272.
2. Ascher, P. (1972): J. Physiol. 225: 173-209.
3. Harris-Warwick, R.M. et al. (1988): Neuron 1: 27-32.
4. Innis, R.B. and Aghajanian, G.K. (1987): Brain Res. 411: 139-143.
5. Israel, J.-M., Jaquet, P. and Vincent, J.-P. (1985): Endocrinology 117: 1448-1455.
6. Kehoe, J. (1972): J. Physiol. 225: 85-114.
7. Lacey, M.G., Mercuri, N.B. and North, R.A. (1987): J. Physiol.
8. MacVicar, B.A. and Pittman, Q.J. (1986): Neurosci. Lett. 64: 35-40.
9. North, R.A. (1989): Brit. J. Pharmacol. 98: 13-28.
10. Ohno, Y., Sasa, M. and Takaori, S. (1987): Life Sci. 40: 1937-1945.
11. Sasaki, K. and Sato, M. (1987): Nature 325: 259-262.
12. Stack, J. et al. (1990): Endocrinology (in press)
13. Stack, J., Surprenant, A. and Allen, R.G. (1987): Soc. Neurosci. Abstr. 13: 532.
14. Uchimura, N., Higashi, H. and Nishi, S. (1986): Brain Res. 375: 368-372.
15. Uchimura, N. and North, R.A. (1990): Brit. J. Pharmacol. 99: 736-740.
16. Williams, P.J., MacVicar, B.A. and Pittman, Q.J. (1989): Neuroscience 31: 673-681.
17. Williams, P.J., MacVicar, B.A. and Pittman, Q.J. (1990): J. Neurosci. 10: 757-763.

ROLE OF D-1 AND D-2 RECEPTORS IN BEHAVIOUR

S.O. ÖGREN
Astra Research Centre AB, CNS Research & Development, Södertälje, Sweden.

The purpose of this paper was to examine the degree to which the subtypes of DA receptors (D-1 or D-2), either alone or in combination, contribute to different behavioural responses in the rat. The effects of the D-2 antagonist raclopride (4) and the D-1 antagonist SCH 23390 (3) on different types of DA agonist-induced responses and on motor behaviours of presumed extrapyramidal origin (catalepsy) were studied.

SUBJECT AND METHOD

The ability to block apomorphine (1 mg/kg s.c.)-induced stereotypies and hyperactivity in the rat was examined as described previously. (4). The cataleptic effect was investigated in the bar test (4). In addition, the potencies to block the hypothermia induced by apomorphine (1 mg/kg s.c.), pergolide (0.1 mg/kg s.c.) and quinpirole (0.25 mg/kg s.c.) were studied (5). The compounds were injected i.p. (s.c.) 15/30 min (SCH 23390) or 60 min (raclopride) before the DA agonists.

RESULTS

The results are summarized in Table 1. Both raclopride and SCH 23390 blocked in a dose-dependent manner the hyperactivity and stereotypies induced by the D-1/D-2 agonist apomorphine. The combined treatment of SCH 23390 (0.1 mg/kg s.c.) and raclopride (1 μmol/kg i.p.) resulted in an enhanced potency to block the behavioural effects of apomorphine. SCH 23390 failed to attenuate the hypothermic effect of both apomorphine, pergolide (Fig 1) and quinpirole. In contrast, raclopride and haloperidol caused a dose-dependent blockade of the hypothermia effect of pergolide (Fig 1) and the other two DA agonists. When SCH 23390 (0.1 μmol/kg s.c.) was combined with raclopride (0.5 μmol/kg i.p.) it did not modulate the ability of raclopride to block the hypothermic effect of pergolide.

Fig 1. The effects of raclopride, SCH 23390 and haloperidol on the hypothermia caused by 0.1 mg/kg s.c. of pergolide. Results are means ± S.E.R. from at least six rats in each group.* p<0.05, **p<0.01, *** p<0.001

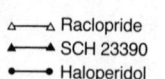

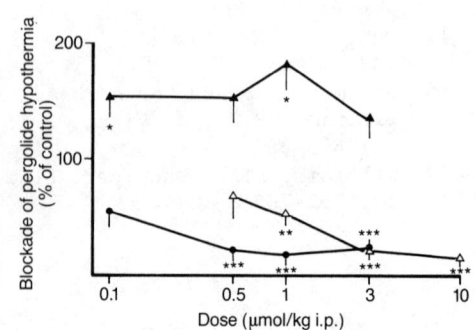

△——△ Raclopride
▲——▲ SCH 23390
●——● Haloperidol

TABLE 1: IN VIVO ACTIVITIES OF RACLOPRIDE AND SCH 23390 IN THE RAT (ED$_{50}$, µmol/kg i.p.)

Compound	Block of apomorphine-induced [a] stereo-typies	hyper-activity	hypo-thermia	Catalepsy, bar test [b]
Raclopride	1.80 (1.57-2.13)	0.13 (0.05-0.23)	0.20 [c]	11 (4.1)
SCH 23390	0.37 (0.28-0.52)	0.06 (0.02-0.09)	>1	0.99 (0.14)

a) The ED$_{50}$ values were calculated by regression analysis using Fieller's theorem for estimates of the 95 % confidence limits, b) ED$_{50}$ (SEM) was determined by probit analysis., c) 95 % confidence intervals not possible to determine

Both raclopride and SCH 23390 produced a dose-dependent induction of catalepsy in the bar test (Table 1). The combined treatment of raclopride (5 µmol/kg i.p.) and SCH 23390 (0.1 µmol/kg s.c.) resulted in an enhanced cataleptic response.

DISCUSSION

The present data are supportive of the notion that there is a reciprocal interaction between D-1 and D-2 receptors in DA agonist induced motor behaviours (see 1, 2, 6) and catalepsy. Dopamine agonist-induced hypothermia, on the other hand, appears to be mediated by activation of DA D-2 receptors.

REFERENCES

1. Arnt, J. Hyttel, J. and Perregaard. (1987): Europ. J. Pharmacol. 133:137-145,
2. Barone, P., Davis, T.A., Braun, A.R., et al. (1986): Europ. J. Pharmacol. 123:109-114.
3. Iorio, L.C., Barnett, A., Leitz, F.H., et al.(1983): J. Pharmacol. Exp. Ther. 226:462-468.
4. Ögren, S.O., Hall, H., Köhler, C., et al.(1986): Psychopharmacology 90:287-294.
5. Ögren, S.O. and Fuxe, K. (1988): Acta Physiol. Scand.. 133:91-95.
6. Ögren. S.O., Fuxe, K. and Köhler, C. (1988): In: Neurology and Neurobiology, M. Sandler, A. Dahlström, and R.H. Belmaker, eds. pp.27-31.

CLINICAL SIGNIFICANCE OF D1 AND D2 RECEPTORS

H. Beckmann
Department of Psychiatry, University of Würzburg, FRG

The blockade of dopamine receptors has been implicated in the clinical action of the available neuroleptics. This is suggested by various results from the laboratory, although overstimulated postsynaptic dopaminergic neurons have not been unequivocally identified in schizophrenic patients (2). Whereas the direct action on the receptors occurs within a short time, the clinical effects develop only after days or even weeks. Not all psychotic symptoms respond to neuroleptic treatment. Several attempts to define the symptoms which respond best have yielded unequivocal and unsatisfying results thus far. Experimental studies where remitted schizophrenic patients were challenged with dopamine agonists such as amphetamine or L-Dopa indicate that neuroleptic-free patients in whom those drugs produced transient symptom activation are more likely to relapse within a few weeks than patients in whom dopamimetics had little or no psychosis inducing effects. Traditional clinical subtypes as hebephrenic, catatonic, paranoid or undifferentiated schizophrenia have not been particularly helpful in predicting clinical response. Beside other attempts much attention has recently been focused on the positive and negative symptomatology, with the assumption that these two groups of symptoms may represent independent disease processes. However, clinical analyses of responses reveal that this view might be too simplistic, as several positive symptoms do not respond to even highest doses of neuroleptics whereas some negative symptoms do well ameliorate in acute as well as in chronic schizophrenia.
The first molecular action of the neuroleptics was found to be the inhibition of the dopamine-sensitive-adenylate-cyclase. However, not all clinically active substances showed this activity. In 1975 Seeman and Snyder using radioactively labelled haloperidol defined the D2 receptors showing a linear correlation between receptor affinity and clinical efficacy. The specific D1 receptor antagonist Sch 23390 has not been proven to be of clinical efficacy thus far. Discounting the effects of dopamine antagonists on other receptors as S2, α1, muscarinic and histamine receptors only haloperidol and the benzamides can be regarded as selective dopamine D2 receptor blockers both in vitro and

in vivo, whereas only Sch 23390 and SK and F 83566C can be regarded as dopamine D1 receptor selective compounds. The clinical significance of selective D1 versus D2 receptors is not well elaborated. In one double blind study by Kuny and Woggon (3) zuclopenthixol was compared to haloperidol in acute schizophrenia. The qualitative and quantitative antipsychotic effects were similar for both neuroleptics. Also, Heikkila et al. (1) comparing zuclopenthixol with haloperidol in a 12 week treatment design showed a nearly equal therapeutic effect, using the Brief Psychiatric Rating Scale as an evaluation system. The relative dose increase needed was significantly higher for haloperidol than for zuclopenthixol. It might be speculated that this was related to the selectivity of zuclopenthixol and haloperidol for dopamine D1 and D2 receptors. Wistedt et al. (4) compared flupentixol decanoate with fluphenazine decanoate treatment over 2 years. At the end flupentixol showed greater improvement than fluphenazine thus suggesting that the efficacy of fluphenazine decreased with time and showed a pharmacological tolerance phenomenon. One research group (Nordic Dyskinesia Group 1986) has determined the magnitude of aggravation of tardive dyskinesia after withdrawal from chlorprothixene, haloperidol and perphenazine. These researchers concluded that the thioxanthenes with its combined D1/D2 receptor blocking effect might have the lowest risk for developing tardive dyskinesia. New neuroleptics with a higher D1/D2 receptor blocking ratio may prove as advantageous for both therapeutic effects and lack of causing tardive dyskinesia.

1. Heikkila, L., Laitinen, J., and Vartiainen, H. (1981): Cis(Z)-clopenthixol and haloperidol in chronic schizophrenic patients - a double-blind clinical multicenter investigation. Acta Psychiatr Scand[Suppl 294] 64:30-38.
2. Hyttel, J., Arnt, J., and Van den Berghe, M. (1989): In Clinical pharmacology in psychiatry: from molecular studies to clinical reality, S.G. Dahl and L.F. Gram, eds., (Psychopharmacology series 7), pp 109-122. Springer Verlag, Berlin.
3. Kuny, S., and Woggon, B. (1984): In Proceedings of the symposium "Modern trends in the chemotherapy of schizophrenia". VII World Congress of Psychiatry, Vienna, P. Hall, ed., pp 13-24. Lundbeck A/S, Copenhagen.
4. Wistedt, B. (1984): In Proceedings of the symposium "Modern trends in the chemotherapy of schizophrenia". VII World Congress of Psychiatry, Vienna, P. Hall, ed., pp 44-59. Lundbeck A/S, Copenhagen.

PROSPECTIVE STUDIES OF TARDIVE DYSKINESIA DEVELOPMENT

J.M. KANE, M.D.[*], M. WOERNER, PH.D.[*], B. SALTZ, M.D.[*], J. LIEBERMAN, M.D.[*], K. BERGMANN, M.D.[*]
[*]Hillside Hospital, Long Island Jewish Medical Center, Glen Oaks, New York, U.S.A.

Tardive dyskinesia remains a major adverse effect associated with long-term neuroleptic therapy. Despite increasing attention and research in this area, no proven safe and effective treatments for tardive dyskinesia have emerged. At the same time no equally effective safer alternatives to neuroleptics have been developed, therefore, increased knowledge with regard to incidence and risk factors remains critical. We have been conducting prospective studies of tardive dyskinesia development in two distinct cohorts of patients. The first sample involves relatively young (mean age 28 SD 10) patients of whom 69% were diagnosed as either schizophrenic or schizoaffective. These patients had a median of 12 months of lifetime neuroleptic exposure at the point we began to follow them and had no evidence of abnormal involuntary movements. Among the first 616 neuroleptic treated patients, we found an incidence of approximately 4% per year of neuroleptic exposure for the first five years of treatment.

With regard to risk factors, older age, affective diagnosis and early occurrence of extrapyramidal side effects were significantly related to higher incidence.

In a second study we have focused on a substantially older population (mean age 77 SD 8.9) receiving neuroleptic drugs for the first time. Sixty-seven percent of this sample had an organic mental syndrome and 33% received a schizophrenic or affective disorder diagnosis. Results from the first 160 subjects who did not show dyskinesia at baseline and were neuroleptic-treated for at least 3 weeks after baseline, indicated that the cumulative incidence of new dyskinesia was 31% (95 to confidence $\pm$ 11%) after 43 weeks of cumulative neuroleptic exposure. The incidence in this group is strikingly higher than in the younger patients.

In terms of risk factors, patients who were given a "non organic" psychiatric diagnosis had a significantly higher incidence of TD as did patients with ratings of moderate or greater on any EPS measure during the first four weeks of treatment.

ANTECEDENTS OF VULNERABILITY TO TARDIVE DYSKINESIA AND CEREBRAL MRI IN SCHIZOPHRENIA

J.L.WADDINGTON*, E. O'CALLAGHAN**, C.LARKIN**, O.REDMOND***, J.STACK*** and J.T.ENNIS***
*Clinical Pharmacology, Royal College of Surgeons in Ireland, Dublin 2; **Cluain Mhuire Family Centre, Blackrock, Co. Dublin; ***Institute of Radiological Sciences, Mater Hospital, Dublin 7, Ireland.

In relation to the critical issue of vulnerability factors, there has been a long-standing debate as to whether more patients with pre-existing forms of organic brain dysfunction might be more likely to develop tardive dyskinesia if prescribed neuroleptics (1). There is now a considerable, but not entirely conclusive body of evidence suggesting that patients with tardive dyskinesia are more cognitively impaired than those who remain unaffected (2). If this relationship indicates more evident organic changes in those affected, what might be the antecedents of such an association? Obstetric complications are known to occur to excess in the early histories of schizophrenic patients. On the basis of the putative relationship of obstetric complications to aspects of structural brain pathology in schizophrenia, patients with a history of obstetric complications might be particularly vulnerable to tardive dyskinesia. However, we have recently reported that schizophrenic patients with tardive dyskinesia are less likely to have experienced obstetric complications, and more likely to have a family history of schizophrenia in a first degree relative, as well as being more cognitively impaired (3). To help to clarify these issues further, we give here a preliminary account of whether structural brain changes might be more evident in patients with tardive dyskinesia using magnetic resonance imaging (MRI).

SUBJECTS AND METHODS

Schizophrenic outpatients (DSM-III, N=47: 26M, 21F; mean age 35.3 ± 12.3 years; mean duration of illness 12.3 ± 9.3 years) and normal controls (N=25: 15M, 10F; mean age 34.4 ± 11.5) were examined by MRI, using a Siemens Magnetom 1.5T system. As previously described (4) images were obtained in three orthogonal planes, using T_1- and T_2-weighted spin echo and inversion recovery sequences to demonstrate tissue contrast behaviour and tissue pathology; resultant images were evaluated by a consultant MR neuroradiologist 'blind' to subject status, before proceeding to quantitative measures. Immediately prior to MRI, all patients were assessed using the Abnormal Involuntary Movement Scale.

RESULTS

Atrophy was evident in 12 of the 47 patients (qualified as 'age-related' in one case) and was absent in the 25 controls ($p<0.01$). Eighteen of the 47 patients (38%: 11M, 7F; age 37.1 ± 14.6) satisfied Schooler & Kane criteria for tardive dyskinesia, and orofacial movements were present in each case; the remaining 29 patients (15M, 14F; age

34.1±10.6) were unaffected. Atrophy was evident in 6(33%) of 18 patients with tardive dyskinesia and 6(21%) of 29 patients who appeared unaffected. Consideration of cerebral vs cerebellar atrophy, and of ventricular abnormalities or signal hyperintensities did not help to distinguish patients with and without tardive dyskinesia. However, the prevalence of cerebral cortical atrophy in patients with tardive dyskinesia (5/18) exceeded that in controls (p<0.02), while no significant excess was apparent in those patients without such movement disorder (5/29, NS).

DISCUSSION

We began these studies from the perspective of a substantial, though not conclusive body of studies which indicated that patients with tardive dyskinesia appear to be more cognitively impaired than otherwise indistinguishable patients without such movement disorder, and that this might support an association between tardive dyskinesia and organic brain dysfunction (1,2). In seeking potential antecedents of such an association, we found no evidence that obstetric complications, one putative cause of structural brain pathology in schizophrenia, were more common in the histories of patients who went on to develop tardive dyskinesia; however, such patients were more likely to have a family history of schizophrenia (3).

On examining more directly whether patients with tardive dyskinesia might show more evident structural brain pathology, a preliminary analysis of an extensive MRI study was inconclusive; though patients with tardive dyskinesia showed an excess of cerebral cortical atrophy in comparison with controls, while patients without such movements did not, no significant differences between patients with and without tardive dyskinesia were apparent. Several interpretations are possible: (i) our preliminary qualitative examination of MR images may be insensitive to more circumscribed structural changes; this would require the quantitative morphometric measures that are currently in progress. (ii) the inconsistent CT literature (2) suggests that any association between tardive dyskinesia and structural brain pathology may be more evident in older patients; to clarify this, it would be necessary to study prospectively our younger patient group, to determine if those currently showing atrophy but unaffected by tardive dyskinesia are more likely to develop such movement disorder subsequently. (iii) cognitive dysfunction as measured may not be a reliable marker for structural brain pathology in schizophrenia, and such pathology may be unrelated to vulnerability to tardive dyskinesia. However, the relationship between tardive dyskinesia and a family history of schizophrenia suggests that at least some feature(s) of the illness may be antecedents of such vulnerability.

This work was supported by the St. John of God Order.

REFERENCES

1. Edwards, H. (1970): Brit. J. Psychiat., 116: 271-275.
2. Waddington, J.L. (1989): Int. Rev. Neurobiol., 31: 297-353.
3. O'Callaghan, E. et al.: Brit. J. Psychiat. (in press).
4. O'Callaghan, E. et al.: (1988): Brit. J. Psychiat., 153: 394-396.

TRANSCULTURAL ASPECTS OF TARDIVE DYSKINESIA

H. KAZAMATSURI
Department of Psychiatry, Teikyo University School of Medicine, Tokyo, Japan

Tardive dyskinesia is a syndrome of abnormal involuntary hyperkinetic movements that occur in predisposed individuals during or following the cessation of long-term neuroleptic therapy. The increasing concern about this syndrome has led to a reconsideration of the proper indications for antipsychotic drugs. In addition, tardive dyskinesia has focussed substantial research into the mechanisms of current drug treatment and stimulated the pursuit of new antipsychotic agents that are free of late persistent side effects.
During past decades, many epidemiological studies on this syndrome were reported. However, the majority of investigations were conducted in western countries on Caucasian populations. In this presentation, recent studies on various cultural groups using identical rating of the symptoms are presented and discussed from a viewpoint of transcultural psychopharmacology.
The role of ethnicity in neuroleptic drug response, including tardive dyskinesia, is still controvertial.
Studies have reached conflicting conclusions about whether Asian patients are less or more likely to develop tardive dyskinesia. The reported prevalence of tardive dyskinesia among many ethnic groups gratly varies. Many risk factors which increase the frequency and severity of tardive dyskinesia have been proposed by

duration of neuroleptic treatment, type of neuroleptic drugs, trial period without neuroleptics, concomitant administration of anticholinergic drugs, psychiatric diagnosis and incidence of acute extrapyramidal symptoms. In addition to these risk factors, ethnic difference of sensitivity to provoke tardive dyskinesia is posturated.

In order to clarify the question whether there is some difference in the prevalence and risk factors of tardive dyskinesia among different ethnic groups, clinical studies were conducted in an ethnically homogeneous Japanese patient group in collaboration with foreign psychiatrist using Abnormal Involuntary Movements Scale (AIMS). In these studies, similar prevalence and risk factors of tardive dyskinesia were found in Japan and the West in spite of cross-cultural difference in psychiatric practice.

The fact that the results concerning prevalence and risk factors of tardive dyskinesia are similar to results from Western studies is remarkable considering differences in the practice of psychiatry among many countries.

PET STUDIES OF DOPAMINE RECEPTOR OCCUPANCY IN RELATION TO NEUROLEPTIC SIDE EFFECTS

A-L. NORDSTRÖM*, L. FARDE*, F-A. WIESEL** and G. SEDVALL*
*Department of Psychiatry and Psychology, Karolinska Institute, Stockholm, Sweden,
**Department of Psychiatry, Uppsala University, Sweden

It is widely accepted that the therapeutic effect of neuroleptic drugs is related to their ability to antagonize the action of dopamine by blockade of central dopamine receptors. This hypothesis was supported by the demonstration of a linear correlation between drug affinity for central D2-dopamine receptors in animals and antipsychotic potency in humans. Previously it has only been possible to test this hypothesis in animal models. The development of positron emission tomography (PET) has now made it feasible to study drug interaction with receptors in the living human brain. In this study the selective ligands 11C-SCH23390 and 11C-raclopride were used for PET-determination of central D1- and D2-dopamine receptor occupancy in schizophrenic patients treated with clinical doses of classical and atypical neuroleptics.

Methods

11C-SCH23390 or 11C-raclopride with a high specific activity (mass <1µg) was injected intravenously. Regional brain radioactivity was measured using a Scanditronix PC-384-7B PET-scanner. Specific binding to D1- or D2-dopamine receptors in the putamen (B) was defined as the difference between total radioactivity in putamen and the cerebellum. Radioactivity in the cerebellum was used as an estimate of the free radioligand concentration in the brain (F). Dopamine receptor occupancy was defined as the per cent reduction of the ratio B/F in relation to the expected value in the neuroleptic-free state. The expected value for D2-dopamine receptor binding was obtained from experiments in 20 drug-naive schizophrenic patients (mean 3.55; SD=0.63). The expected value B/F for D1-dopamine receptor binding was based on experiments in seven healthy subjects (mean 2.9; SD 0.37). A presupposition for this method is that the ratio B/F is reliable which has been investigated in a separate test-retest study.

D1- and D2-dopamine receptor occupancy in neuroleptic treated patients

Treatment with conventional doses of ten chemically distinct classical neuroleptics resulted in a 70-89% occupancy of D2-dopamine receptors. This finding represents strong support for the hypothesis that the mechanism of action of classical antipsychotic drugs is related to a substantial degree of D2-dopamine receptor occupancy. In three patients treated with conventional doses of the atypical neuroleptic clozapine, the D2-dopamine receptor occupancy was 38-63%, the lowest values so far obtained. Clozapine seems to be different from classical neuroleptics also regarding D1-dopamine receptor binding. In the patients treated with clozapine the D1-dopamine receptor occupancy was high (42%) as compared to patients treated with classical neuroleptics (0-40%).

D1- and D2-dopamine receptor occupancy in patients with EPS

In some patients treated with classical neuroleptics, akathisia or parkinsonism was recorded in connection with the PET experiment. These patients with extrapyramidal side effects (EPS) tended to have higher D2-dopamine receptor occupancy as compared to patients with no EPS. Worth noting is that treatment with clozapine results in a low D2-dopamine receptor occupancy and is associated with a low frequency of extrapyramidal side effects. An explanation may be that treatment with clozapine does not induce the high D2-dopamine receptor occupancy found in patients with EPS during treatment with classical neuroleptics.

Table 1: D2-DOPAMINE RECEPTOR OCCUPANCY IN PATIENTS TREATED WITH ANTIPSYCHOTIC DRUGS

CLASSICAL NEUROLEPTICS

Drug	Dose	D2-occupancy	D1-occupancy	
Chlorpromazine	100x2	78		
Flupentixol	3x2	70	40	
Flupentixol	5x2	70		
Flupentixol dec	40/weekly	81	36	eps
Haloperidol	4x2	82		
Haloperidol	6x2	84		eps
Haloperidol	3x2	89		eps
Haloperidol dec	50/3 week	85		eps
Haloperidol	3x2	84		eps
Haloperidol	2x2	75		eps
Haloperidol	2x2	84		eps
Melperone	100x3	70		
Melperone	100+150	71		
Pimozide	4x2	79		eps
Perphenazine	4x2	76	0	
Perphenazine	30x2	84		eps
Sulpiride	400x2	78	-7	
Thioridazine	150x2	74		
Thioridazine	100x2	81	29	
Trifluoperazine	5x2	75		
Zuclopent. dec	200/2week	81	11	

ATYPICAL NEUROLEPTICS

Clozapine	300x2	63		
Clozapine	150x2	40	42	
Clozapine	250x2	38	42	

eps= extrapyramidal side effects

<u>Dynamics of D2-dopamine receptor occupancy after single oral doses of haloperidol</u>

Central D2-dopamine receptor occupancy was followed by repeated PET-scans after administration of a single oral dose of a neuroleptic drug. 7.5 mg haloperidol was given to a healthy male volunteer. D2-dopamine receptor occupancy was determined 3, 6 and 27 hours after haloperidol administration. Adverse events were recorded hourly. After 3 hours the subject reported discomfort (inner restlessness), the feeling reached its maximum after 4-6 hours but did not completely disappear until 24 hours later. The D2-dopamine receptor occupancy in the putamen was 92 % after 3 hours, 89 % after 6 hours and 76 % after 27 hours. Another healthy volunteer was also given a single oral dose of 7.5 mg haloperidol. D2-dopamine receptor occupancy determined in PET-experiments was 83% after 3 hours and 84% after 6 hours. The subject reported moderate akathisia during both PET-experiments. A high D2-dopamine receptor occupancy was accordingly established 3 hours after administration of 7.5 mg haloperidol. Of particular interest is that reported and observed side effects were most severe when D2-dopamine receptor occupancy was very high.

Discussion

An important potential with positron emission tomography is to examine relationships between central dopamine receptor occupancy and drug effects during neuroleptic treatment. Such relationships may be useful for optimal clinical monitoring of neuroleptic drugs.

References
Farde, L., Wiesel, F-A.,Nordström, A-L., Sedvall, G.: D1- and D2-dopamine receptor occupancy during treatment with conventional and atypical neuroleptics. <u>Psychopharmacology</u>(1989) 99:S28-S31

NEUROLEPTIC-INDUCED PARKINSONISM IN SCHIZOPHRENIA

W.F. HOFFMAN, L. C. BALLARD, G. A. KEEPERS, T.E. HANSEN, AND D.E.CASEY
Psychiatry Service, VA Medical Center and Department of Psychiatry, Oregon Health Sciences University, Portland, OR, USA

Neuroleptic drug-induced parkinsonism (DIP) and tardive dyskinesia (TD) occur more in the aged. DIP results from striatal dopaminergic (DA) blockade by neuroleptics. The etiology of TD is less well understood, but up-regulation of DA receptors due to chemical denervation is a popular hypothesis. According to this model, the severity of TD and DIP would be negatively correlated. However, the syndromes frequently coexist and their prevalence may even be positively associated (6). Prospective examination of parallel changes in these syndromes during neuroleptic withdrawal should provide information about the extent of their coupling. DIP usually resolves if neuroleptic drugs are withdrawn, while TD frequently (albeit often transiently) worsens (1,2), but simultaneous change in the disorders has not been extensively studied.

Subjects and Methods

Twenty-seven stable outpatients over age 40 with a DSM-III-R diagnosis of schizophrenia were randomly assigned, in a double-blind fashion, to neuroleptic withdrawal (n=13) or control (n=14) groups. Eight of the patients were also being treated with anticholinergic agents. Neuroleptic and anticholinergic doses were expressed in chlorpromazine (CPZE) and benztropine (BNZE) equivalents, respectively. In the withdrawal group, neuroleptics were tapered by 10% per day starting on day 3 of the study. After withdrawal was complete, subjexts were maintained on no neuroleptics for 21 days. Anticholinergic drugs were also withdrawn in 4 patients (2 in each group). Patients received TD and DIP ratings three times weekly throughout the course of the study. TD was assessed with the Abnormal Involuntary Movement Scale (AIMS, 4) and DIP with the Sct. Hans Scale for Extrapyramidal Symptoms (3). Diagnoses of probable TD and probable DIP were made according to the criteria of Schooler and Kane (7) and Hoffman et al. (5), respectively. Four patients did not complete the study: two were withdrawn because of psychotic relapse and two withdrew for personal reasons. Only data on patients who completed the protocol were entered into further analysis.

Table 1. Comparison of Control and Withdrawal Groups

	Control (N = 13) Initial	Control (N = 13) Final	Withdrawal (N = 10) Initial	Withdrawal (N = 10) Final
Age	48.9 ± 8.2	-	66.5 ± 7.6[c]	-
Neuroleptic (CPZE)	386 ± 294	386 ± 294	400 ± 575	0
Anticholinergic (BNZE)	2.3 ± .86	0.43 ± 0.82[c]	1.5 ± .71	0.30 ± 0.68[c]
Total AIMS	3.7 ± 2.0	3.5 ± 3.0	6.1 ± 4.2	11.7 ± 5.1[a]
%TD	61.5	30.8	80.0	90.0
Mean Change in AIMS	-	-0.8 ± 1.5[b]	-	5.4 ± 4.3[b,d]
Total Sct. Hans	7.5 ± 8.0	6.1 ± 5.9	12.3 ± 5.1	9.4 ± 5.8
%DIP	30.1	30.8	50.0	40.0
Mean Change in Sct. Hans	-	-0.2 ± 2.0[b]	-	-2.9 ± 3.0[b,e]

[a]Final different from initial $p < .001$. [b]Change scores calculated from regression equations for each subject. [c]Final different from initial $p < .05$. [d]Withdrawal differs from control $p < .001$. [e]Withdrawal differs from control $p < .05$

Results

In the overall sample (N = 27), 4 patients (15%) had DIP only, 11 (41%) had TD only, 8 (29%) had both and 4 (15%) had neither. The 23 study completers did not differ from the total sample on any of the variables examined. Summary statistics for the completers are given in Table 1. The age of the withdrawal group was higher than that of the control group (p < .001) and subsequent analyses were controlled (where appropriate) for age. Comparisons of the groups initially and on study day 33 are given in Table 1. Repeated measures analysis revealed significant time by group interactions for both total AIMS (p < .01) and total Sct. Hans (p < .05) scores. AIMS increased and Sct. Hans decreased in the experimental group but remained constant in the control group (FIG. 1). Changes in total AIMS and Sct. Hans were negatively correlated (r = -0.60, p < .05) in the withdrawal group and unrelated (r = .02, p = .9) in the controls (FIG. 1). There was no relationship between magnitude of TD or DIP change and size of neuroleptic dose.

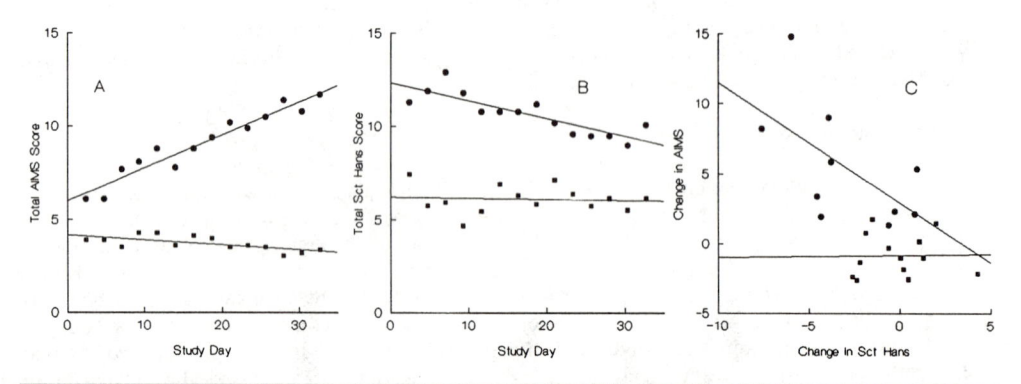

FIG. 1. Circles and squares indicate the neuroleptic withdrawal group the control group, respectively. Changes in mean daily total AIMS and Sct. Hans scores as a function of time are shown in graphs A and B. Graph C illustrates the relationship between changes in AIMS and Sct. Hans. Lines represent least squares regressions.

Discussion

Symptoms of DIP decreased on withdrawal of neuroleptics, while symptoms of TD increased in concert. The latter increase is best understood as withdrawal dyskinesia, secondary to stimulation of unmasked up-regulated striatal dopamine receptors, and is expected to diminish somewhat with time (2,7). The negative correlation of changes in TD and DIP partially supports the simple dopaminergic model of the TD/DIP relationship. Interestingly, however, the absolute value of the rate of change in parkinsonism was substantially less than the rate of change in hyperkinesia. Cerebral structures synaptically downstream of the corpus striatum (pallidum, thalamus, and cortex), which are necessary for the expression of symptoms, may be differentially responsive to dopaminergic stimulation.

References

1. Crane, G.E., (1978): Am. J. Psychiatry 135:619-620.
2. Gardos, G. et al., (1985): Arch. Gen. Psychiatry 41:1030-1035.
3. Gerlach, J., (1979): Dan. Med. Bull. 26:209-244.
4. Guy, W., (1976) ECDEU Assessment Manual for Psychopharmacology (Revised). US Government Printing Office, Washington, D.C.
5. Hoffman, W.F. et al., (1987): Biological Psychiatry 22:427-439.
6. Richardson, M.A. and Craig, T.J., (1982): Am. J. Psychiatry 139:341-343.
7. Schooler, N.R. and Kane, J.M., (1982): Arch. Gen. Psychiatry 39:486-487.

NEUROLEPTIC MALIGNANT SYNDROME

G.M. SIMPSON* and S. GRATZ*
*Department of Psychiatry, Medical College of Pennsylvania/EPPI, Philadelphia, PA, U.S.A.

Laborit (2) introduced neuroleptics into medical practice in his work with hibernation anesthesia. Thus, by giving a mixture of drugs, he showed that you could lower the temperature of individuals about to undergo surgery. The drug that essentially satisfied his criterion was chlorpromazine. His observations on this led him to recommend it for use in psychiatry. Some two years later, the world knew that a unique pharmacological agent was now available which, in addition to its effect on temperature control, for the first time produced an amelioration of psychotic symptoms and, at the same time, extrapyramidal side effects (EPS) indistinguishable from idiopathic parkinsonism. All of the above pharmacological properties are important in our understanding of the "neuroleptic malignant syndrome" (NMS). This ill-defined syndrome has been associated with both neuroleptics and non-neuroleptics and certainly, has not always been malignant. It is uncertain whether the hyperthermic syndromes associated with non-neuroleptics are part of a more generalized syndrome that may occur in some predisposed individuals. Nonetheless, changes in thermoregulation associated with rigidity, autonomic disturbances and altered mental status does occur in patients undergoing neuroleptic treatment and, on occasion, can be fatal. The treatment is equally ill-defined but in nearly all cases, consists of controlling the temperature, withdrawing the neuroleptic, maintaining hydration, watching for concomitant physical illnesses and treating the rigidity present. This syndrome seems to appear at any time throughout treatment, but in our experience is mainly seen early in treatment or occasionally associated with dosage changes. We suggest that high potency neuroleptics in acutely excited patients, particularly if given parenterally, may be a factor in producing this disorder. We have stated elsewhere that we consider the designation "NMS" undesirable in that it may potentially foster misinterpretation and confusion, thereby resulting in treatment delays and have, therefore, suggested alternatively "extrapyramidal side effects with fever," which at the very least, is a better description of what is going on and if so, then methods for prevention and treatment become more logical. Thus, if EPS are a necessary part of this disorder, then we should monitor carefully at all times for the presence of EPS and as far as possible avoid them (this is not always easy in acute treatment situations). When present, neuroleptics should be reduced and/or antiparkinson agents utilized. Lower dose strategies for treating schizophrenia have a long history but have only recently begun to impact in practice in psychiatry. The use of low dose strategies which, in our opinion, do not interfere with efficacy should cut down on the amount of neuroleptic malignant syndrome, and at the very least, is testable. This would seem to be so in our own hospital where we have seen very little of this disorder and where we teach about the undesirability of akathisia, and rigidity and have tended to use low dosages of drugs. Moreover, the diagnosis of NMS suggests a unique illness with unknown treatments and perhaps diminishes the focus of what we believe is the cardinal feature, the EPS. If EPS are present long enough, particularly if akathisia and agitation are present, then dopaminergic and cholinergic mechanisms can begin to interfere with the heat control system and all the consequences of NMS can arise. On the other hand, if EPS are avoided, neuroleptics are used in low dosages, and benzodiazepines used concomitantly in agitation, then we should see little or none of it. Our suggested treatment strategy for patients with severe EPS emphasized vigorous and aggressive initial usage of anticholinergic agents to reverse the neuroleptic-induced rigidity. We suggest, however, that these agents be avoided or employed with caution in patients with a fever of 101°F or greater (1). In our clinical practice, nevertheless, we have frequently encountered cases where aggressive efforts to treat the drug-induced muscle rigidity is either never attempted or even delayed for several days. Since the discovery of the antipsychotic agents over 30 years ago and the determination of their utility in the treatment of mental disorders, the signs of EPS have led to claims that such sequelae are an essential feature of these agents. Controversy still exists as to the therapeutic significance of these extrapyramidal disturbances. Hopefully, these reflections on this relatively-rare phenomenon - NMS - and our emphasis on early treatment and management will clarify some of the more relevant and important issues regarding the management of this condition.

REFERENCES

1. Gratz, S., Levinson, D.F. and Simpson G.M. (in press): In Adverse Effect of Psychotropic Drugs, J.M. Kane and J. Lieberman, eds., Guilford Press, New York.

2. Laborit, H. and Huygenard, P. (1954): Practique. Del'hibernotherpaie in Chirurgie et en Medecine, Paris, Massin.,

ADVANCES IN THE TREATMENT OF DEPRESSION

P. KIELHOLZ
Badweg 1
Seengen, AG, Switzerland

Essential for the success of treatment is always a combination of pharmacotherapy, psychotherapy, and sociotherapy. The type of basic treatment indicated can be inferred from the nosological classification of the depressive disorder, and the choice of an appropriate antidepressant can be decided upon the light of the phenomenology of the clinical picture. Biological research has revealed new aspects relating to the mechanisms of action of antidepressants. Reference is also made to newly developed Antidepressants which to some extent display specific effects, as well as to Type A MAO inhibitors. In cases of severe depression involving suidical tendencies or showing resistance to treatment, it is recommended that antidepressants be administered by intravenous drip infusion or employed in combination with lithium and carbamazepine or a neuroleptic agent.

REFERENCES

1. Freyhan, F.A.: How long should prophylactics be continued in affective disorders? Pharmakopsychiat. 9, 137, 1976
2. Kielholz, P. (Ed.): Die larvierte Depression, Verlag Hans Huber, Bern, Stuttgart, Wien, 1973
3. Kielholz, P., Adams, C.: Pharmakotherapie der larvierten Depression. Dtsch. med. Wschr. 104, 375, 1989
4. Kielholz, P., Adams, C.: Die larvierte Depression. Der informierte Arzt (Schweizer Ausgabe) 1, 14, 1980
5. Okuma, T.: Therapeutic and prophylactic efficacy of carbamazepine in manic-depressive psychosis. In: Emrich, H.M., Okuma, T., Muller, A.A. (Eds.): Anticonvulsance in affective disorders. Experta Medica 76-87, Amsterdam 1984
6. Okuma, T., Yamashita, I., Takahashi, R. et al.: Double-blind control studies on the therapeutic efficacy of carbamazepine in affective and schiophrenic patients. Psychopharmacology 96, 1988
7. Sartorius, N., Davidian, G., Ernberg, F.R. et al.: Depressive disorders in different cultures. Report on the WHO Collaborative Study on Standardized Assessment. World Health Organization, Geneva 1983.

CURRENT PROBLEMS OF PSYCHONEUROIMMUNOLOGY

M.E.VARTANIAN, G.I.KOLYASKINA
National Mental Health Research Centre,
Moscow, USSR

Neurvous tissue was widely considered to be "immunologically privileged". But it is clear that this longstanding idea is not absolute: both immune and autoimmune responses can accur there. Recent works have deepened our understanding of the mechanisms controlling the immune response to neuronal antigens, and how that response may be manipulated.

Ther are several shared antigens both in the immune and nervous systems: Thy-1, T4, T8, GFAP. There are some neuroendocrine peptides produced by the immune system: ACTH, enkephalins, somatostatin, oxitocin, neurophysin and others. The neuroendocrine effects of lymphokines and monokines (α- and β- interferons, interleukin-1, interleukin-2, thymosin-α1, thymosin-β4) and immunoregulatory effects of neuroendocrine peptides (ACTH, α- and β-endorphins, Leu- and Met-enkephalins, substance P, somatostatin and others) have been described. At last immune and nerve cells have the same receptors: ACTH, β-endorphin, enkephalins, substance P, insulin. Therefore, any alteration in these substances or receptors of immune system might result in disturbed functions of immune system as well as neuronal transmission mechanisms and vice versa. The data suggest that abnormalities of immune system may be of major significance in pathogenesis of neurological and psychiatric diseases. In fact many different peculiarities of the immune system have been described in multiple sclerosis, myastenia gravis, schizophrenia and others. Moreover there are some data that immunomodulators were successfully used in treatment of patients with different neurological and psychiatric diseases.

The development of immunological research in psychiatry has run parallel to that of immunology, reflecting the methodological and theoretical advances made in the latter field. The 1970s and 1980s have seen a resurgence of activity in this area and the appearance of new centers in which impairment of immunity in endogenous psychoses is being examined. These matters are being studied at present by experts from Yugoslavia, the United States, France, the Soviet Union, Finland, Canada and many other countries. It should be emphasized that the active development of immunological research in psychiatry was largely promoted by the Division of Mental Health of WHO which, since 1978, has organized one or two symposia as part of the World Congress of Biological Psychiatry, at which the results of research in that field are discussed. In recent years, three conferences devoted entirely to "Viruses, Immunity and Mental Disorders" were organized with the help of WHO (Louvain, Belgium, 1983; Montreal, Canada, 1984; Mont-Gabriel, Canada, 1988), and the results have been published in two monpgraphs (25, 30).

ADVANCES IN MEMBRANE RESEARCH
LEONID PRILIPKO
Division of Mental Health, World Health Organization, Geneva

The brain has a high oxygen consumption and is rich in oxidizable substrates, mainly catcholamines and unsaturated lipids. The membranes of the central nervous system are therefore at a high risk from the destructive biochemical processes associated with free radical mediated lipid peroxidation (LPO). Therefore, the interests of some groups of practitioners in biological psychiatry have been directed to investigations of the role of LPO in the pathogenesis of mental and neurological disorders.

A collaborative study on schizophrenic patients in three research centres in Ireland, Scotland and England has been carried out and as a result it has been shown that in all three groups the n-6 essential fatty acid levels (EFA) were significantly reduced in both plasma and red cell phospholipids whereas n-3 EFA levels were elevated in plasma but reduced in red cells. The linoleic acid and arachidonic acid, two of the most unsaturated phospholipids compounds, were significantly reduced also.[1]

Another research group[2] has discovered a strong negative correlation between glutathione peroxidase (one of the most important enzymes responsible for the degradation of the reactive by-products of oxidative metabolism) in both isolated platelets and erythrocytes and CT scan measures of brain atrophy and ventricle-brain ratios in schizophrenics, but not in the control population. Moreover, the direct measurements of LPO products in the blood of schizophrenic patients demonstrate their significant elevation correlated with the clinical status of patients[3]. Similar results have been found in patients with manic depressive psychosis in depressive phase.[4]

It is also worthwhile to mention here the well-known fact concerning the accumulation of granules of lipofuscin (one of the products of LPO) in the neurons of patients with schizophrenia, Alzheimer disease, Parkinson's disease and some other neurological disorders. Moreover, in postmortem material from patients with Parkinson's disease it has been found that polyunsaturated fatty acid levels (an index of the amount of substrate available for lipid peroxidation) were reduced in substantia nigra compared to other brain regions and to control tissue. However, basal malondialdehyde (MDA) (an intermediate in the lipid peroxidation process) levels were increased in parkinsonian nigra compared to other parkinsonian brain regions and control tissue[5].

These results are in harmony with another group of successful studies aimed to improve the clinical state of psychiatric patients with tardive dyskinesia with antioxidant therapy or treatment with essential fatty acids.[6,7]

Preliminary results are also available showing a significant improvement in therapy-resistent depressive patients when treated by alpha-tocopherol in addition to the standard antidepressants.

Taking into account the briefly-mentioned results of this recent research, it is clear that the study of the phospholipid matrix and its components indicate a promising new avenue in biological psychiatry, which can increase our knowledge about some of the real causes of mental disorders and consequently improve future treatment prospects.

References
1. Horrobin, D.I., et al, (1989) Essential fatty acids in plasma phospholipids in schizophrenics. Biol. Psych. 25: 562-568
2. Buckman, T.D., et al, (1987) Glutatione peroxidase and CT scan abnormalities in schizophrenia, Biol. Psych. 22: 1349-1356
3. Prilipko, L., Liedeman, R. (1982) Lipid peroxidation as a causative factor in membrane-bound protein modification in nervous cells of schizophrenic patients. Vestnik Akad. Med. Nank SSSR (USSR) 1, 33-36
4. Kovaleva, E., et al, (1988) The lipid peroxidative process in patients with manic depressive psychosis. J. Neuropathol. & psych. 4: 69-71
5. Dexter, D., et al Increased lipid peroxidation in substantia nigra in Parkinson's Disease. J. Neurochem, (in press)
6. Lohr, J., et al (1987) Alpha-tocopherol in tardive dyskinesia. The Lancet, 1987, 18: 913-914
7. Vaddadi, K., et al (1989) A double-blind trial of essential fatty avid supplementation in patients with tardive dyskinesia Psychiatry Research, 1989, 27: 313-323

ADVANCES IN GENETIC RESEARCH IN PSYCHIATRY
J. MENDLEWICZ
University clinics of Brussels, Erasme Hospital - Free University of Brussels - Department of Psychiatry - route de Lennik 808 - 1070 Brussels, Belgium

Linkage studies have provided evidence of the presence of a single gene located on the X chromosme, in manic-depression (1,2) however this type of inheritance has not been observed in all families (1). In recent DNA recombinant studies a close linkage has been demonstrated between manic depression and Factor 9 (Hemophylia B) on the distal end of the long arm of chromosome X (3). Conversely, the localisation of a gene situated on chromosome 11 has also been reported (4), but this chromosomal linkage has not yet been confirmed in other pedigrees (5-7). Furthermore, a recent reevaluation of the Amish family (8) showed lod scores to be considerably weakened. Furthermore, genetic probes on the long arm of the X-chromosome are suggesting the presence of a major locus for manic-depression between ST 14 and factor IX genes. Thus the new chromosomal linkage findings reveal the existence of several distinct genetic forms of bipolar illness. Other pedigrees of bipolars have been reported not to show linkage with the above genetic markers (1). These results provide strong support for the hypothesis of molecular heterogeneity in the genetic etiology of bipolar manic-depressive illness. Most twin and family studies as well as adoption studies have indicated that Schizophrenia seems to have a polygenic mode of transmission, but the involvment of a major gene locus with variable penetrance can not be excluded. Indeed, there has been a recent report mapping a major gene for schizophrenia in the q11-q13 region of chromosome 5 (9), but these findings could not be confirmed (10-12). It is therefore essential to collect further large multiplex kindreds of both schizophrenic and affectively ill probands in different laboratories in order to confirm previously reported linkages and assess the other chromosomal regions of the human genome with new polymorphic DNA markers. Cytogenetic studies have also shown a trisomy 5q11-q13 in two schizophrenics in a family of Chinese origin (13). The discovery of linkage in mental disorders will also utlimately lead to the isolation, sequencing and cloning of the mutant genes and thus help providing some rational for etiological and preventive therapeutic approaches. Ethical issues and guidelines are essential to develop on a cross national basis for further advancement of molecular genetic research in mental disorders.

REFERENCES

1. J. Mendlewicz. Population and family studies in depression and mania. British Journal of Psychiatry, 153 (suppl. 3) 16-25, 1988.
2. J. Mendlewicz. X-linked transmission of affective illness : current status and new evidence. Biological Psychiatry. Eds. C. Shagass, R. Josiassen, W. Bridger, K. Weiss, D. Stoff, G. Simpson, Elsevier, vol. 7, 46-48, 1986.
3. J. Mendlewicz, P. Simon, F. Charon, H. Brocas, S. Legros, G. Vassart. A polymorphic DNA marker on X chromosome and manic-depression. The Lancet, 1230-1232, 1987.
4. J.A. Egeland, D.S. Gerhard, D.L. Pauls, J.S. Sussex, K.K. Kidd, C.R. Allen, A.M. Hostetter, D.E. Housman. Bipolar affective disorders linked to DNA markers on chromosome 11. Nature, 325, 783-787, 1987.
5. S.D. Detera-Wadleigh, W.H. Berretini, L.R. Goldin, D. Boorman, S.B. Anderson, E.S. Gershon. Close linkage of C-Harvey-ras-1 and the insulin gene to affective disorder is ruled out in three North American pedigrees. Nature, 325, 806-808, 1987.
6. S. Hodgkinson, R. Sherrington, H. Gurling, R. Marchbanks, S. Reeders, J. Mallet, M. McInnes, H. Petursson, J. Brynjolfson. Molecular genetic evidence of heterogeneity in manic-depression. Nature, 325, 805-806, 1987.
7. G. Michael, P. McKeon, P. Humphries. Linkage analysis of manic depression in an Irish family using H-ras 1 and INS DNA markers. Journal of Medical Genetics, 25, 634-637, 1988
8. J.R. Kelsoe, E.I. Gings, J.A. Egeland, D.S. Egeland, A.M. Golstien, S.J Bale, D.L. Pauls, R.T. Long, K.K. Kidd, G. Conte, D.E. Housman, S.M. Paul. Reevaluation of the linkage relationship between chromosome 11 p loci and the gene for bipolar affective disorder in the old order Amish. Nature, vol 342, 238-243 1983.
9. R. Sherrington, J. Brynjolfsson, H. Petursson, M. Potter, K. Dudleston, B. Barraclough, J. Wasmuth, M. Dobbs, H. Gurling. Localization of a susceptibility locus for schizophrenia on chromosme 5. Nature, vol 336, 164-167, 1988.
10. J.L. Kenedy, L.A. Guiffrat, H.W Moises, L.L. Cavalli-sforza, A.J. Pakistis, L. Wetterberg, J.R. Kidd . Evidence against linkage of schizophrenia to markers on chromosme 5 in a northern Swedich pedigree. Nature, vol 336, 167-170, 1988.
11. D. St. Clair, D. Blackwood, W. Muir, D. Baillie, A. Hubbard, A. Wright, H.J. Evans. No linkage of chromosome q11-q13 markers on schizophrenia in Scottish families. Nature, vol 339, 305-309, 1989.
12 S.D. Detera-Wadleigh, L.R. Goldin, R. Sherrington, I. Encio, C. de Miguel, W. Berettini, H. Gurling, E.S. Gershon. Exclusion of linkage to 5q11-13 in families with schizophrenia and other psychiatric disorders. Nature, vol 340, 391-393, 1989.
13. A.S. Basset, B.C. McGillivray, B.D. Jones, J Tapio Pantzar. Partial trisomy on chromosome 5 cosegregating with schizophrenia. The Lancet, 799-800, 1988.

BIOLOGICAL MARKERS: PAST AND FUTURE

I.YAMASHITA and T.KOYAMA
Department of Psychiatry, Hokkaido University School of Medicine, Sapporo, Japan

Drug therapy and biological studies of affective disorders have produced a number of hypotheses, and many markers or marker-candidates related to these hypotheses. For instance, reduced MHPG in urine or 5-HIAA in CSF, decreased plasma free tryptophan, blunted GH response to clonidine, phase advance of daily rhythm, etc. However, there are only three markers that have attracted world-wide attention and provoked a great number of studies in the present decade. They are 1)non-suppression by dexamethasone (DST), 2) reduced imipramine binding of platelets, and 3) sleep EEG abnormalities in depression. These 3 markers were also extensively investigated by the group of WHO Collaborative Centers in Biological Psychiatry and Psychopharmacology.

Epsom (Coppen) and 12 centers worked on DST, Paris (Langer) and Copenhagen (Mellerup) and 8 centers on platelet imipramine binding, and Brussels (Mendlewicz) and 7 centers on sleep EEG. These studies were unique in that a large number of patients from various ethnic populations were investigated, using the same protocols and standardized laboratory methods, in order to obtain conclusive findings for conflicting reports, and to detect possible ethnic differences by the world-wide multi-center collaboration.

The results of these studies were briefly as follows: (1) An abnormal DST response was confirmed to be the steady biological characteristic of depression, and indicated a certain difference between Europeans and Japanese. (2) Sleep EEG showed abnormalities specfic to depression, including shortened REM latency and increased REM density. (3) Platelet imipramine binding failed to show any difference in membrane binding sites between depressed and normal subjects, partly due to complicated methodological problems.

It must be admitted however that, at the present time, there is no marker of affective disorders which is as useful as markers of cancers, which are routinely utilized for screening, diagnosis and therapeutic evaluation. So, what about the future of markers of affective disorders?
I believe that there must be two prospects in the future. One is the further development of research techniques and the other is a more appropriate clinical categorization.

Recently, our colleague Mori found that the increase of inositol-1-phosphate of platelets by epinephrine stimulation through α-2 receptor was more pronounced in depressives (151.5±5.5%) than in controls (129.0±4.2%) ($P<.005$). Sugano in Fukushima reported increased Bmax of α-2 receptor binding at platelet membrane using UK14304, which is more specific to α-2 receptor than clonidine. Our colleague Kusumi is estimating 5-HT2 receptor-mediated intracellular Ca^{++} increase in platelets induced by 5-HT stimulation. There is a possibility that rapid progress of experimental techniques in neuroscience, including molecular biology and brain imaging, may provide more reliable markers of affective disorders in the future.

It should also be stressed that affective disorder is not a uniform illness. It is possible that it may consist of a variety of disease entities with different biological pathology. It has been well recognized that abnormal DST is more frequent in endogenous than non-endogenous depression. Progress of clinical nosology is also a prerequisite for the further investigation of markers.

There will be a long way to go for the establishment of useful markers of affective and other psychiatric disorders. However, biological markers have long been the dream of psychiatrists and it is eagerly hoped that this dream will sometime be fulfilled. But, even when it becomes possible to diagnose depression by test tube, thoughtful interviews with patients for diagnosis will not cease, as these will always be the task and responsibility of psychiatrists.

1. A World Health Organization Collaborative Study; The dexamethasone suppression test in depression. Brit.J. Psychiat. 150:459-462,1987

PHARMACOLOGICAL MODIFICATION OF POST-ISCHEMIC BRAIN CELL INJURY

KYUYA KOGURE and HIROYUKI KATO
Department of Neurology, Institute of Brain Diseases, Tohoku University School of Medicine, Sendai, Japan

Recent experimental evidence has led us to hypothesize that selective vulnerability of neurons to ischemia is initiated by glutamate receptor activation which causes a loss of calcium homeostasis and an alteration of intracellular signal-transduction system such as increased protein kinase C activities, leading to disruption of functional and structural integrity of membrane and cytoskeleton, and finally to neuronal death (1).

According to this hypothesis, ischemic neuronal damage can be prevented by pharmacological modification of the chain of reactions leading to neuronal death. This includes 1). blockade of glutamate receptor activation, 2). enhancement of activities of inhibitory neurotransmitters, such as GABA and adenosine, 3). blockade of intracellular calcium influx, 4). inhibition of increased protein kinase C activities, and 5). protection of membrane damage by encouraging repair process or by free radical scavengers.

To test the working hypothesis, various pharmacological intervention was made to examine whether hippocampal neuronal damage induced by cerebral ischemia is prevented. The experimental animal models which we employed are 1). 5-min bilateral carotid artery occlusion in the Mongolian gerbils, 2). three 2-min bilateral carotid artery occlusions at 1-hr intervals in the Mongolian gerbils("R" in Table), and 3). 10 or 20 min of 4-vessel occlusion in the rat. Neuronal density of the hippocampal CA1 subfield was determined using traditionally stained sections after long-term survival, usually seven days.

Pharmacological agents used in this systematized experimental series are as follows: NC-1200(glutamate blocker), MK-801(NMDA antagonist), Mg^{2+}(receptor-operated calcium channel blocker), pentobarbital(GABA-A receptor-effector), vinpocetine, vinconate and propentofylline(inhibitory neuromodulators), methoxamine(a1-adrenoceptor agonist), naftidrofuryl (serotonine S2 antagonist), NC-1100, KB-2796 and flunarizine (calcium antagonists), staurosporine and K-252a(protein kinase C inhibitors), S-adenosyl methionine(SAM) and CDP-choline(cofactors of phosphatidylcholine synthesis), and a-tocopherol and KB-5666(free radical scavengers). The results are summarised in Table. The neuronal density of the hippocampal CA1 subfield (% control) in vehicle-treated and drug-treated animals are tabulated.

Table

drug/dose/route	animal	vehicle	drug	
1). blockade of glutamate receptor				
NC-1200/40mg/kg/ip/post	gerbil	5%	69%	$p<0.01$
MK-801/3mg/kg/ip/pre	gerbil(R)	6%	50%	$p<0.05$
Mg2+/50mM/topical/pre	rat	15%	45%	$p<0.01$
2). inhibitory neuromodulation				
pentobarbital/40mg/kg/ip/pre	gerbil	19%	56%	$p<0.01$
pentobarbital/40mg/kg/ip/post	gerbil	13%	52%	$p<0.01$
pentobarbital/40mg/kg/ip/pre	gerbil(R)	6%	51%	$p<0.01$
vinpocetine/50mg/kg/ip/pre	gerbil	19%	50%	$p<0.05$
vinconate/100mg/kg/ip/pre	gerbil	2%	49%	$p<0.01$
propentofylline/20mg/kg/ip/pre	gerbil	14%	72%	$p<0.05$
methoxamine/10mg/kg/ip/post	gerbil	3%	75%	$p<0.01$
naftidrofuryl/50mg/kg/ip/pre	gerbil	15%	87%	$p<0.01$
3). calcium antagonists				
NC-1100/30mg/kg/ip/post	gerbil	11%	71%	$p<0.01$
KB-2796/10mg/kg/ip/post	gerbil	13%	47%	$p<0.01$
flunarizine/30mg/kg/ip/pre	gerbil	19%	7%	ns
flunarizine/30mg/kg/ip/pre	gerbil(R)	6%	6%	ns
4). protein kinase C inhibitors				
staurosporine/10ng/topical/pre	gerbil	33%	82%	$p<0.01$
K-252a/10ng/topical/pre	gerbil	20%	57%	$p<0.05$
5). protection of membrane damage				
SAM/120mg/kg/iv/post	rat	18%	81%	$p<0.01$
CDP-choline/150mg/kg/iv/post	rat	18%	12%	ns
a-tocopherol/50mg/kg/iv/post	gerbil	20%	56%	$p<0.05$
KB-5666/10mg/kg/ip/post	gerbil	13%	50%	$p<0.01$

As the results indicate, pharmocological modification of post-ischemic events at at least five aspects presented above can effectively prevent ischemic neuronal damage in the hippocampus. These agents which were experimentally proved to be effective can be the candidates for cerebral protective drugs for cerebrovascular diseases in man.

Reference
1. Kogure K, Tanaka J, Araki T; The mechanism of ischemia-induced brain cell injury. The membrane theory. Neurochem Pathol 9:145-170,1988

COMPONENTS OF HYPOXIC NEURONAL INJURY IN HIPPOCAMPAL SLICES WHICH ARE INDEPENDENT OF CALCIUM INFLUX

J.E. PARSONS, R.A. WALLIS and C.G. WASTERLAIN
Epilepsy Research Laboratory, VAMC Sepulveda, Department of Neurology and Brain Research Institute, UCLA School of Medicine, Los Angeles, CA, USA.

Recent studies have emphasized the role of calcium influx through NMDA-operated channels and voltage-dependent channels in hypoxic-ischemic neuronal injury. We studied hypoxic injury to CA1 neurons of hippocampal slices in medium containing zero calcium, 0.1-1 mM EGTA, so that calcium influx is minimal and other components of hypoxic injury can be identified. Stimulation of the alveus produced an antidromic (A) population spike (PS), and stimulation of the Schaffer collaterals produced an orthodromic PS (O) in CA1 cells. The measure of cell injury was the ratio of PS after perfusion with nitrogenated medium and 60 minutes recovery to prehypoxic PS. Perfusion with 0 Ca^{2+}, 0.1 mM EGTA medium during hypoxia provided only 27% protection, suggesting that a large component of hypoxic injury was independent of calcium influx. Low Cl- and Low Na+ media offered no protection from hypoxic injury, but total removal of Na+ from the medium proved too toxic to be testable during hypoxia. In the absence of extracellular calcium, 10 mM Mg and MK-801 (10 mg/l) were highly protective (88% and 81% respectively), suggesting that these blockers of NMDA-associated channels reduce hypoxic injury even in the absence of calcium influx implying either that their protective action is separate from their ability to block NMDA-associated ionic channels, or that in the absence of extracellular calcium another cation enters through NMDA channels and mediates the injury. In calcium-free medium, tetrodotoxin (1 μM) reduced hypoxic injury by 53%, suggesting that calcium-independent hypoxic injury is in part mediated by sodium influx. Finally, in complete artificial cerebrospinal fluid (ACSF) dantrolene (20 μM) reduced hypoxic injury by 88%, presumably by blocking release of intracellular calcium stores.

These data suggest that while calcium influx through voltage-dependent and NMDA receptor-operated channels may in part mediate hypoxic injury in CA1 neurons, other mechanisms of injury in CA1 are independent of calcium influx. Significant components of hypoxic CA1 injury in the hippocampal slice involve the release of intracellular calcium stores, the influx of sodium through sodium channels, and possibly the influx of sodium through NMDA receptor-operated ionic channels.

FIGURE 1.

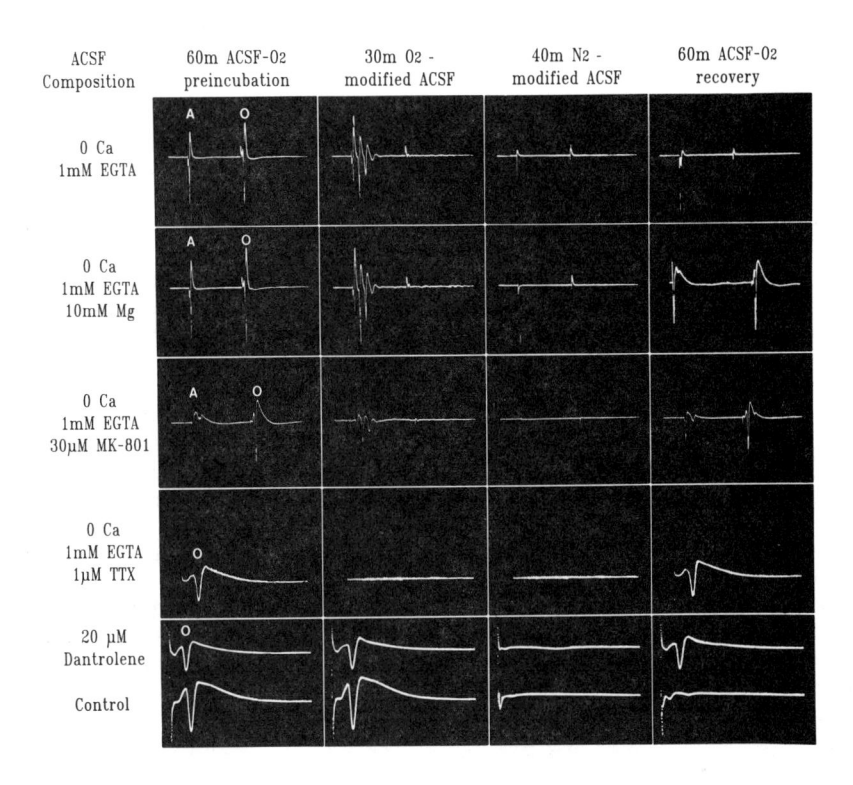

ACSF Composition	60m ACSF-O2 preincubation	30m O2 - modified ACSF	40m N2 - modified ACSF	60m ACSF-O2 recovery
0 Ca 1mM EGTA				
0 Ca 1mM EGTA 10mM Mg				
0 Ca 1mM EGTA 30µM MK-801				
0 Ca 1mM EGTA 1µM TTX				
20 µM Dantrolene / Control				

Legend: Representative samples of PS evoked in CA1 cells by antidromic (A) or orthodromic (O) stimulation. O2 refers to perfusion with ACSF equilibrated with 95% O2-5% CO2, and N2 to perfusion with ACSF equilibrated with 95% N2-5% CO2. Note that during perfusion with low calcium ACSF, the antidromic PS becomes multiphasic, and the orthodromic PS disappears since transmitter release is blocked. Tetrodotoxin (TTX) experiments included a recovery period of 90 minutes since washout was not completed in 60 minutes. In dantrolene experiments, the slice treated with drug (top tracing) was paired with a slice from the same hippocampus exposed to the same hypoxic treatment without dantrolene (bottom tracing). Both slices were perfused with nitrogenated ACSF until 5 minutes past the disappearances of the hypoxic injury potential in the control slice, then reoxygenated together. The dantrolene treated slices recovered a greater porportion of their evoked potentials than the control slices.

Supported by Research Service of the VA, by Grant NS13515 from NINDS, and by the American Epilepsy Society.

MECHANISMS OF DRUG ACTIONS AGAINST NEURONAL DAMAGE CAUSED BY ISCHEMIA

J. KRIEGLSTEIN, C. BACKHAUß, C. KARKOUTLY, J. PREHN and M. SEIF EL NASR
Institut für Pharmakologie und Toxikologie, Philipps-Universität,
Ketzerbach 63, D-3550 Marburg (F.R.G.)

Ischemia leads to biochemical, morphological, and functional disturbances of the brain. Any drug that could protect brain tissue against ischemic damage would be of therapeutic interest. Various in vivo and in vitro models have been developed to test anti-ischemic or anti-hypoxic drug effects. In the present study we induced focal ischemia by permanent occlusion of the middle cerebral artery (MCA) in mice and a transient forebrain ischemia in rats. Using these models we tested possible neuroprotective effects of calcium antagonists, NMDA antagonists, 5-HT$_{1A}$ agonists and radical scavengers.

METHODS

Focal ischemia was performed with male NMRI mice by electrocoagulation of MCA. Two days after MCA occlusion, brains were perfused with carbon black and fixed with formaldehyde phosphate buffer solution (pH 7.4). The infarct surface was determined planimetrically by means of an image analyzing system (IBAS 2000, Kontron, Eching, F.R.G.).

Forebrain ischemia was induced for 10 min by clamping both carotid arteries and lowering the mean arterial blood pressure to 40 mm Hg in male Wistar rats. After 7 days of recovery, neuronal damage in the hippocampal subfields was determined as the percentage of cells stainable with acidic fuchsin.

RESULTS

Focal ischemia of the mouse seems to be a useful screening model to test neuroprotective effects of drugs. Calcium antagonists of the dihydropyridine type (nimodipine, CRE 319), NMDA antagonists (phencyclidine, memantine), 5-HT$_{1A}$ agonists (urapidil, CM 57493), and scavengers of free oxygen radicals (dimethylthiourea, dihydrolipoic acid) proved to be capable of reducing the infarct area of the mouse brain (Table 1).

These results were confirmed by the experiments with the rat forebrain ischemia model. In untreated rats a high percentage of damaged neurons was found in the hippocampal CA1 subfield after ischemia. Pre- or postischemically administered drugs protected the neurons against ischemic damage.

DISCUSSION

Ischemia of brain tissue disturbs the very sensitive regulation of the cytosolic Ca^{2+} concentration ($[Ca^{2+}]_i$) fundamentally. Voltage-

TABLE 1: NEUROPROTECTIVE DRUG EFFECTS AGAINST BRAIN DAMAGE CAUSED BY FOCAL ISCHEMIA IN THE MOUSE

Drug	Control	Drug-treated
Calcium antagonist CRE 319 (0.3 mg/kg, s.c.)	24.2 + 3.6 (n = 10)	18.7 + 5.0** (n = 11)
NMDA antagonist Memantine (20 mg/kg, i.p.)	20.5 + 4.9 (n = 10)	15.0 + 3.7* (n = 13)
5-HT$_{1A}$ agonist CM 57493 (5 mg/kg, i.p.)	26.1 + 2.9 (n = 13)	21.5 + 3.6** (n = 11)
Radical scavenger Dihydrolipoic acid (100 mg/kg, i.p.)	26.5 + 3.6 (n = 11)	21.3 + 3.6** (n = 9)

Values are given as means + S.D. in mm .
Drugs were administered 1 h (CRE 319, dihydrolipoic acid), or 30 min (memantine, CM 57493) prior to ischemia. * $p < 0.05$, ** $p < 0.01$

---

sensitive and receptor-operated ion-channels allow Ca^{2+} to enter neurons. $[Ca^{2+}]_i$ may increase tremendously and causes neuronal damage by inhibition of mitochondrial function and energy production as well as stimulation of lipases, proteases and endonucleases leading to membrane destruction during postischemic recirculation of the tissue (for ref. see 1). Calcium and NMDA antagonists can inhibit Ca^{2+} entry and, therefore, protect neurons against ischemic damage (Table 1).

Reintroduction of oxygen to ischemic brain tissue produces a burst of oxygen free radicals resulting in extensive cellular destruction and disturbed calcium homeostasis (1). Drugs such as dihydrolipoic acid capable of scavenging free radicals obviously reduce ischemic brain lesions (Table 1).

5-HT$_{1A}$ receptors in brain tissue are linked to adenylate cyclase and in rat hippocampus they are coupled directly to neuronal K^+ channels (2). Whether 5-HT$_{1A}$ agonists could also influence calcium homeostasis and protect neurons during postischemia by these mechanisms remains to be shown.

REFERENCES

1. Krieglstein, J. (1989): Pharmacology of cerebral ischemia 1988. Wissenschaftliche Verlagsgesellschaft and CRC, Stuttgart and Boca Raton.
2. Fozard, J.R. (1987) TIPS 8: 501-506

THE PHARMACOLOGY OF NMDA RECEPTORS IN RELATION TO NEURONAL DEGENERATION

A.C. FOSTER, C.L. WILLIS, M.H.M. BAKKER AND R. TRIDGETT
Merck Sharp and Dohme Research Laboratories, Neuroscience Research Centre, Terlings Park, Eastwick Road, Harlow, Essex, CM20 2QR, UK.

The N-methyl-D-aspartate (NMDA) sub-type of receptors for the excitatory amino acid neurotransmitters glutamate and aspartate is believed to play an important role in neurodegenerative phenomena. In animal models of cerebral ischaemia, NMDA receptor antagonists reduce the degeneration of neurones resulting from the large elevations of extracellular glutamate and aspartate levels which occur in the vicinity of vulnerable neurones. One way to mimic this situation is by direct injection of an NMDA receptor agonist into the brain. We have used this model to investigate the neuroprotective effects of antagonists which act at different sites within the NMDA receptor complex, and to explore the mechanisms involved in this type of neurodegeneration.

MK-801 (dizocilpine) is the most potent of a group of drugs which block the ion channel of the NMDA receptor (6). The degeneration of rat striatal or hippocampal neurones caused by direct injection of NMDA or the endogenous NMDA receptor agonist quinolinate, is prevented by pretreatment of animals with MK-801 (2,3). Unexpectedly, a single dose of MK-801 (ip) was found to prevent degeneration of rat striatal neurones when administered up to 5h after quinolinate or NMDA injection (3), and revealed a differential time course of degeneration of neuronal populations. Thus, pretreatment with MK-801 protected all hippocampal neuronal types from the neurodegenerative effects of quinolinate, whereas CA1 and CA3 pyramidal cells required administration of the drug by 1 or 2h after the excitotoxin, and dentate granule cells and GABAergic interneurons were still protected by delaying MK-801 administration to 3h. These results suggest that NMDA receptors on vulnerable neurones are activated for several hours after excitotoxin injection to produce a delayed degeneration. This is supported by measurement of the CSF concentrations of MK-801 required for neuroprotection when the drug was administered as a continous i.v. infusion from 0.5 to 4.5h after quinolinate injection into the rat striatum. A range of MK-801 concentrations from 25-91nM were required, close to the known affinity of MK-801 for the NMDA receptor (8).

Delayed administration of the competitive NMDA receptor antagonist 3-[(±)-2-carboxypiperazin-4-yl]propyl-1-phosphonate (CPP) also prevented quinolinate induced neurodegeneration in the rat striatum with an ED_{50} of approximately 30mg/kg (ip), 1h after quinolinate. Other pharmacological agents, such as haloperidol (0.5mg/kg, ip) and diazepam (10mg/kg, ip) were inactive, as was ifenprodil (50mg/kg, ip), which has been suggested to exert its neuroprotective effects through NMDA receptor antagonism (1).

Antagonists at the glycine site on the NMDA receptor (5) are neuroprotective in this model when injected directly into the brain (4). The full antagonist 7-chlorokynurenate (7-Cl KYNA) showed a similar timecourse of neuroprotective effects to MK-801, being effective when injected up to 5h after quinolinate in the striatum, and producing complete protection after a delay of 1h in the hippocampus. The neuroprotective effects were reversed by the selective glycine site agonist D-serine. The partial agonist HA-966 showed similar characteristics, although the degree of neuroprotection was less. Recently, the separate enantiomers of HA-966 have been prepared, and affinity for the glycine site found to reside in (+)HA-966, whereas (-)HA-966 produced potent sedative effects by a distinct mechanism (7). As shown in Table 1, this stereoselectivity is also apparent in the neuroprotective effects of HA-966 when tested by measuring the marker enzymes choline acetyltransferase (CAT) and glutamate decarboxylase (GAD) in the rat striatum.

Table 1 Neuroprotective effects of HA-966 enantiomers in the rat striatum

	CAT	GAD	(n)
Vehicle Control	74.1 ± 3.9	79.4 ± 2.7	(8)
(±)HA-966 500nmol	32.4 ± 7.2*	52.2 ± 10.1*	(5)
(+)HA-966 500nmol	20.0 ± 5.6*	40.9 ± 5.8*	(8)
(-)HA-966 500nmol	78.1 ± 5.3	81.8 ± 4.1	(8)

HA-966 was injected into the striatum 1h after 200nmol quinolinate. Values are the percent reduction of enzyme activity in the injected vs contralateral striatum and are the mean ± SEM of n animals. * $P<0.01$ significance of difference from control, Duncan's Test.

Similar effects were noted in the rat hippocampus where protection by (+)HA-966 was almost complete.

In conclusion, NMDA receptor antagonists which block the ion channel or compete at the glutamate or glycine recognition sites can prevent delayed neuronal degeneration caused by NMDA receptor agonists. This NMDA receptor-dependent process may be similar to the delayed degeneration which occurs following cerebral ischaemia and further studies may shed light on the neurochemical mechanisms involved.

1. Carter, et al., (1988): J. Pharmac. Exp. Therap. 247: 1222-1232.
2. Foster, et al., (1987): Neurosci. Lett. 76: 307-311.
3. Foster, A.C., Gill, R. and Woodruff, G.N., (1988): J. Neurosci. 8: 4745-4754.
4. Foster, A.C., Willis, C.L., and Tridgett, R., (1990): Eur. J. Neurosci. 2: 270-277.
5. Johnson, J.W., and Ascher, P., (1987): Nature 325: 529-531.
6. Kemp, J.A., Foster, A.C., and Wong, E.H.F., (1987): Trends Neurosci. 10: 294-298.
7. Singh, et al., (1990): Proc. Natl. Acad. Sci. (USA). 87: 347-351.
8. Willis, C.L., Brazell, C., and Foster, A.C., (1990): Br. J. Pharmac. Proc. Suppl. (in press).

NON-NMDA ANTAGONISTS PROTECT AGAINST DELAYED NEURONAL CELL DEATH INDUCED BY CEREBRAL ISCHEMIA

T. HONORÉ*, M.J. SHEARDOWN*, A.J. HANSEN*, K. ESKESEN* and N. DIEMER**
Novo Nordisk CNS Division* and Institute of Neuropathology, Univ. of Copenhagen**, Soeborg and Copenhagen, Denmark.

The massive release of glutamate during cerebral ischemia in rat hippocampus (1) may be the most important trigger of the cascade reaction leading to neuronal cell death. The glutamate released is supposed to interact with postsynaptic glutamate receptors.

The glutamate receptors comprise a group of receptor subtypes which are named NMDA, kainate and AMPA-receptors, after the most selective agonists (2). Besides the classical ionchannel coupled receptors, recently described subtypes exist (3).

Compounds interacting with the NMDA receptor complex, such as MK-801, have been reported to protect against delayed neuronal cell death especially when administered before initiation of the cerebral ischemia (4). Contradictionary results have however been obtained when MK-801 is administered after reperfusion (5). Here we report that NBQX (2,3-dihydroxy-6-nitro-7-sulfamoyl-benzo(F)quinoxaline), a selective antagonist for non NMDA-receptors protect against delayed neuronal death following cerebral ischemia.

METHODS

Mongolian gerbils and Wistar rats underwent bilateral carotide and four-vessel occlusion, respectively for 5 and 10 min. NBQX was in both groups administered i.p. (90 mg/kg over a period of 25 min) immediately or a number of hours (1-4) after the ischemic challenge. Hippocampal CA_1 damage was quantitated in frontal sections 4-7 days after ischemia.

RESULTS

The table summarizes the result obtained with NBQX. Significant ($P < 0.01$) protection of delayed neuronal cell death induced by cerebral ischemia was obtained at all time points tested.

DISCUSSION

Since NBQX is a highly selective AMPA antagonist, the result suggests that delayed neuronal cell death after a period of global ischemia is mediated not only by NMDA receptors as previously suggested (4), but also by a mechanism involving non-NMDA receptors.

Furthermore, the fact that NBQX inhibits Schaffer collateral CA_1 transmission (data not shown) suggests the importance of glutamate mediated synaptic transmission for the development of ischemic damage in the CA_1 region. This conclusion is in agreement with earlier studies in which Schafferectomi produced protection of ischemic damage in the CA_1 region (6).

Treatment	Mongolian gerbils % undamaged CA_1 pyramidal cells	Wistar rats mean % CA_1 pyramidal cell loss
Control	9	81
NBQX 90 mg/kg i.p. immediately after recirculation	71	11
1 hour after recirculation	93	15
4 hours after recirculation	45	nt

REFERENCES

1. Benveniste, H., Drejer, J. and Schousboe, A.: Elevation of the extracellular concentrations of glutamate and aspartate in rat hippocampus during transient cerebral ischemia monitored by intracerebral microdialysis. J. Neurochem. 43:1359-1374, 1984.
2. Watkins, J.C., Krogsgaard-Larsen, P. and Honoré, T.: Structure-activity relationships in the development of excitatory amino acid receptor agonists and competitive antagonists. TIPS 11:25-33, 1990.
3. Sugiyama, H., Ito, I. and Hirono, C.: A new type of glutamate receptor linked to inositol phospholipid metabolism. Nature 325:531-533, 1987.
4. Woodruff, G.N., Foster, A.C., Gill, R., et al. The interaction between MK-801 and receptors for N-methyl-D-aspartate: Functional consequences. Neuropharmacol. 26:903-909, 1987.
5. Perkins, W.J., Lanier, W.L., Karlsson, B.R., et al. The effect of the excitatory amino acid receptor antagonist dizocilipine maleate (MK-801) on hemispheric cerebral blood flow and metabolism in dogs: Modification by prior complete cerebral ischemia. Brain Res. 498:34-44, 1989.
6. Benveniste, H., Jorgensen, M.B., Sandberg, M., et al. Ischemic damage in hippocampal CA_1 is dependent on glutamate release and intact innervation from CA_3. J. Cereb. Blood Flow Metab. 9:629-639, 1989.

MORPHOMETRIC STUDIES OF BRAIN ANATOMY WITH MRI IN NORMAL MONOZYGOTIC TWINS AND MONOZYGOTIC TWINS DISCORDANT FOR SCHIZOPHRENIA

D.R. Weinberger, R. Suddath, M. Casanova, G.W. Christison, E.F. Torrey
Clinical Brain Disorders Branch, NIMH Neuroscience Center at St. Elizabeths, Washington, D.C. USA

The application of MRI to the study of brain morphology in patients with schizophrenia (Sz) has made it possible to identify subtle anatomical deviations in such patients during life and thus to confirm findings from postmortem studies which are inherently more problematic. We (1) and other groups (2,3) have reported that patients with schizophrenia evidence slight reductions in size of medial temporal grey matter structure as compared with normal controls. The results have been based on group mean comparisons and have not clarified whether such structural deviations characterize most or only a small subgroup of patients with this disorder. In an effort to address this question by comparing each patient to an ideal individualized control, we have studied monozygotic (MZ) twins discordant for schizophrenia. The results of these studies have been published in detail elsewhere (4,5).

SUBJECTS AND METHODS

Fifteen sets of MZ twins discordant for Sz by DSM III R criteria (8 male, 7 female, mean age 32 ± 5.3, range 25-44) and 7 sets of normal MZ twins (mean age 30.6, range 19-44) underwent a spin echo T1 weighted MRI scan (contiguous 5mm thick coronal sections) for determination of size of frontal and temporal lobes, amygdala and hippocampus, and ventricles and a midline T1 weighted sagittal scan for determination of corpus collosal (CC) dimensions. The scans were digitized, coded and transferred to a computerized image analysis station for morphometric analyses.

RESULTS

The table shows the results for structures measured in the first two slices through the amygdala-pes hippocampal region. It illustrates that at this location in the brain the affected twin with few exceptions has larger ventricles and smaller hippocampi than the unaffected twin. On visual inspection of the scans, the affected twin could be correctly identified in 12 of the pairs simply by choosing the scan that showed the larger CSF filled spaces. Measurements of the thickness and length of the CC did not discriminate between twins. However, the affected twin had a significantly more "bowed" CC, as determined by an angle of curvature measurement, consistent with the finding of ventriculomegaly in the affected twin. None of these differences were observed in the normal twin pairs.

Table: Area Measurements (cm^2) in MRI slices Through the Temporal Lobe in Monozygotic Twins Discordant for Schizophrenia

Structure	Unaffected Twin	Affected Twin	Percent Difference	p Value	Predictive Accuracy
Right lateral ventricle					
Slice 1	1.09 ± 0.60	1.33 ± 0.55	21	0.005	13
Slice 2	0.96 ± 0.63	1.20 ± 0.59	25	0.001	13
Left lateral ventricle					
Slice 1	1.10 ± 0.61	1.27 ± 0.64	16	0.005	14
Slice 2	1.01 ± 0.65	1.19 ± 0.65	18	0.003	14
Third ventricle					
Slice 1	0.33 ± 0.12	0.37 ± 0.10	12	0.04	11
Slice 2	0.34 ± 0.12	0.42 ± 0.13	23	0.001	13
Right hippocampus					
Slice 2	1.50 ± 0.26	1.35 ± 0.25	10	0.02	12
Slice 3	1.21 ± 0.28	1.09 ± 0.20	10	0.001	13
Left hippocampus					
Slice 2	1.50 ± 0.19	1.23 ± 0.25	19	0.001	14
Slice 3	1.18 ± 0.25	1.07 ± 0.26	9	0.06	13

DISCUSSION

The results of this study indicate that, at least in this twin population, signs of subtle neuroanatomical deviations are consistently associated with schizophrenia. Since the identical anatomical findings have been described in nontwin patients, it is likely that the results of this study are applicable to general clinical populations. Thus, it is reasonable to assume that if an ideal anatomical baseline were available for each individual patient with schizophrenia, evidence of subtle anatomical changes would be found in most patients. Finally, since similar anatomical deviations have been reported in patients at the time of their initial hospitalization (3), the findings do not appear to be the result of chronicity or of psychiatric treatment.

REFERENCES

1. Suddath, R.L., Casanova, M., Goldberg, T., et al.: Temporal lobe pathology in schizophrenia: A quantitative MRI study. Am. J. Psychiat. 146:464-472, 1989.
2. DeLisi, L.E., et al.: Perinatal complications and reduced size of brain limbic structures in familial schizophrenia. Schizophr Bull, 14(2):185-192, 1988.
3. Bogerts, B., Ashtari, M., Degreet, G., et al.: Reduced temporal limbic structure volumes on magnetic resonance images in first episode schizophrenia. Psychiatry Res. (in press).
4. Suddath, R.L., Christison, G.W., Torrey, E.F., Casanova, M., and Weinberger, D.R.: Anatomical abnormalities in the brains of monozygotic twins discordant for schizophrenia. N. Engl. J. Med. 322:789-794, 1990.
5. Casanova, M.F., Sanders, R.D., Goldberg, T.E., et al.: Morphometry of the corpus callosum in monozygotic twins discordant for schizophrenia: A magnetic resonance imaging study. J. Neurol. Neurosurg. Psychiat. (in press).

EEG MAPPING IN DIAGNOSIS AND TREATMENT OF DEMENTIA: ON RELATIONS TO COMPUTED TOMOGRAPHY AND PSYCHOMETRY

B. SALETU*, E. PAULUS*, P. ANDERER*, P.K. FISCHHOF**, L. WICKE***
Department of Psychiatry, School of Medicine, University of Vienna*
Psychiatric Hospital, Vienna**
Institute for Diagnostic Imaging, Rudolfinerhaus, Vienna, Austria***

Topographic brain mapping of the electroencephalogram (EEG) has become an important method in the field of neuropsychiatry and specifically in geriatric medicine. In this latter field the possibility arises to relate functional EEG brain mapping to other imaging techniques such as computed tomography (CT) showing structural morphological changes as well as to clinical psychopathological and psychometric data obtained at the behavioral level. The aim of the present study was to investigate psychopathology, mental performance, brain function and brain morphology in dementia of the Alzheimer type (SDAT) and multi-infarct dementia (MID) before and after nootropic drug treatment as well as to study the interrelation between the respective measures.

SUBJECT AND METHOD

In 111 demented hospitalized patients (77 females, 34 males) aged between 58 and 98 (mean 82) years, clinical and psychometric studies as well as morphological CT and functional EEG imaging were carried out, with the patients being off psychopharmaceutical agents for at least 14 days. They were diagnosed according to the DSM III criteria and sub-diagnosed according to the Hachinski score ($\leq$ = SDAT; ≥ 7 = MID) and CT in 54 SDAT and 57 MID patients. The groups did not differ in regard to sex nor in the SCAG score (1). Evaluations were carried out before as well as 8 weeks after treatment. Patients were randomly allocated to treatment with either 3 x 1 g xantinolnicotinate or placebo (3 x 1 tablet).

CT measures included 10 CSF space variables according to Meese at al.: A/greatest (gr.) distance between the anterior horns; B/distance between the caudate nuclei; C/width of third ventricle; D/distance between the choroid plexuses; E/gr. distance between the lateral ventricles at the level of the cella media; F/gr. ext. diameter of the frontal bone; G/gr. internal diameter between the temporal bones; H/gr. external diameter between the temporal bones; F/A: frontal horn index; A/G: Evans index; D/A: ventricular index; H/E: cella media index; A/B: Huckman number. In addition, cortical density was measured in 1,7 mm^3 cubes under 17 EEG electrodes (Hounsfield units).

EEG brain mapping was based on 3-minutes V-EEG recorded by a Nihon Kohden 4317 as well as on off-line-spectral analysis and subsequent mapping utilizing Hewlett Packard Vectra-Computers (1).

Clinical and psychometric evaluations included the Sandoz Clinical Assessment Geriatric (SCAG) scale, the Clinical Global Impression (CGI) scale, the Digit Symbol Substitution Test (DSST), the Trail Making Test (ZVT) and the Digit Span Forward test.

Statistical analysis included the Wilcoxon test, the Mann-Whitney U-test, the Manova, Hottelling's T^2 test, the t-test as well as the Spearman rank correlation.

RESTULTS

Untreated SDAT patients demonstrated, as compared with normals, an increased delta/theta activity, decreased beta activity and slowing of dominant frequency and centroid of the total activity specifically over the parietal and temporal regions. MID patients showed these differences, as compared with normals, over all brain regions. These neurophysiological findings indicate a deterioration in vigilance. Differences between SDAT- and MID-patients were found mostly in specific measures concerning differences between max-min power and left/right power asymmetry. Concerning the three reference conventions, differences appeared slightly more marked based on common average reference (AV) and source derivation (SDV) than averaged mastoid reference (A1/2) (1). Based on SDV. 66,7 % of the patients could be correctly classified into SDAT and MID types of dementia.

Correlation maps regarding the relationship between 11 CT, 9 clinical and 36 quantitative EEG variables demonstrated: The less the cortical density and the wider the CSF spaces measured in the CT, the higher was the relative power in the delta/theta and the less in the alpha and beta frequency range and the slower the centroid of the total activity. Furthermore: The more pronounced the slowing of the brain function as determined by means of quantitative EEG variables, the worse was the psychopathology as evaluated by the clinician utilizing the SCAG score as well as SCAG factors. Finally, significant correlations were obtained between EEG brain mapping and psychometric variables; the slower the brain activity, the worse was the performance in regard to recognition and memory of the patients as evaluated by means of the psychometric test battery.

From the therapeutic aspect, a significant improvement was observed both in SDAT and MID patients treated with 3 g xantinolnicotinate while placebo-treated patients showed either no or only minimal changes. The active medication was significantly superior to placebo. EEG brain maps demonstrated in xantinolnicotinate-treated SDAT patients as compared with placebo-treated ones mostly a increase of slow alpha activity, while in MID patients an attenuation of delta/theta and increase of beta-activity was observed as compared with placebo-treated patients. MANOVA suggested that drug-induced changes could be seen best by SDV evaluations. They were located in SDAT patients mostly over the frontal regions, in MID patients mostly over the fronto-temporal regions.

REFERENCES

1. Saletu, B. et al. (1985). EEG brain mapping in SDAT and MID patients before and during placebo and xantinolnicotinate therapy: Reference considerations. In: Statistics and Topography in Quantitative EEG, D. Samson-Dollfus ed., pp. 251-275. Elsevier, Paris.

EFFECTS OF TYPICAL AND ATYPICAL NEUROLEPTICS ON IN VIVO BRAIN GLUCOSE METABOLISM EVALUATED BY PET

DAVID PICKAR[1], WILLIAM E. SEMPLE[2], PAUL ANDREASON[2], RICHARD R. OWEN[1], P. ERIC KONICKI[1], THOMAS NORDAHL[3] and ROBERT M. COHEN[2]
[1]Section on Clinical Studies, Clinical Neuroscience Branch and [2]Section on Clinical Brain Imagining, Laboratory of Cerebral Metabolism, National Institute of Mental Health, Bethesda, MD 20892; [3]Department of Psychiatry, University of California (Davis), Sacramento, CA 95817

The effectiveness of the atypical neuroleptic, clozapine, in treating otherwise treatment resistant patients with schizophrenia (1) represents a significant contribution to the field of neuropharmacology. Clozapine, a prototype atypical neuroleptic, shares some, but not all pharmacologic properties with typical neuroleptic drugs. The delineation of differences in mode of action between typial and atypical neuroleptic drugs may provide important information for both understanding the pathophysiology of schizophrenia as well as mechanisms of drug response. We have initiated studies of brain glucose metabolism using PET in schizophrenic patients during typical and atypical neuroleptic treatment in order to pursue these questions.

SUBJECTS AND METHODS

Subjects who met RDC criteria for schizophrenia granted informed consent to participate in this procedure and participated when drug free (>15 days), when treated with fluphenazine and cogentin (> 4 weeks) and clozapine (>4 weeks). The subjects, with eyes patched, began an auditory discrimination task several minutes prior to the injection of 3-5 mCi of [^{18}F]FDG and completed the task 35 minutes after injection. Arterial blood samples were taken from the left arm for quantification of [^{18}F]FDG uptake. Following the 35 minute uptake period subjects were placed in the scanner. Slices were parallel to the canthal meatal (CM) line and the interslice interval was 13 mm. Raw pixel values were converted to glucose metabolic rate and the extraction of regional glucose metabolic rate were performed as previously described (2). Data was analyzed after normalization to whole brain glucose metabolism.

RESULTS

In paired data analysis (n=9), fluphenazine significantly increased glucose metabolism in the putamen ($p < 0.01$), caudate ($p < 0.05$) and hippocampus ($P < .05$). Clozapine also increased glucose metabolism in the putamen ($p < 0.1$) and caudate ($p < 0.05$), although these effects were significantly less than those of fluphenazine ($p < .05$). The two brain regions which best discriminated between typical and atypical neuroleptic were the hippocampus and the cingulate cortex. Fluphenazine, but not clozapine, increased glucose metabolism in the hippocampus (p<.05 for drug comparison) whereas clozapine, but not fluphenazine increased metabolism in the cingulate cortex (P<.05 for drug comparison). Further analysis of these and additional data, including their correlation with clinical response are in progress.

COMMENT

The marked (approximately 25%) fluphenazine-induced increase in glucose metabolism in the caudate and putamen is consistent with some previous findings (3) and is thought to be related to reductions in the inhibitory properties of CNS dopamine systems. The localization of the most marked neuroleptic effects to the striatum is consistent with their putative mechanism of action involving acute dopamine post-synaptic receptor blockade followed by adaptational reductions in presynaptic function in the striatum and limbic structures (4). The atypical neuroleptic, clozapine, produced more modest increases in subcortical metabolism than fluphenazine, presumably because of its less pronounced effects on nigrostriatal neurons. This difference in basal ganglia metabolic activity was unlikely due to anticholinergic properties of clozapine since fluphenazine treated patients were also receiving the anticholinergic agent, cogentin, to treat drug-induced EPS. Thus, differences in the propensity of typical and atypical neuroleptics to produce extrapyramidal side effects may be manifest by their differences in glucose metabolism in the basal ganglia.

The differences between fluphenazine and clozapine on hippocampal and cingulate cortex metabolism have not been previously reported and may relate to differences in pharmacologic mechanisms other than differential dopamine receptor binding in the striatum. For example, clozapine, but not fluphenazine, exerts significant α_2 antagonist effects resulting in enhanced noradrenergic function, an effect which may alter metabolism in cortical brain regions. Other distinct properties of clozapine such as its prominent anti-serotoninergic effects are thought to be related to its unique therapeutic properties and may also contribute to differences from typical neuroleptics effects on brain metabolism.

REFERENCES

1. Cohen RM et al. (1988): From syndrome to illness: delineating the pathophysiology of schizophrenia with PET. Schizophr Bull 14(2):169-76.
2. DeLisi LE et al. (1985): Positron emission tomography in schizophrenic patients with and without neuroleptic medication. J Cereb Blood Flow Metab 5(2):201-6.
3. Kane J et al. (1988): Clozapine for the treatment-resistant schizophrenic: a double-blind comparison with chlorpromazine. Arch Gen Psychiatry 45:789-96.
4. Pickar D (1988): Perspectives on a time-dependent model of neuroleptic action. Schizophr Bull 14:255-68.

MRI-SPECT AND PET-EEG FINDINGS ON BRAIN DYSFUNCTION IN SCHIZOPHRENIA

W. GUENTHER

Psychiatric University Hospital links der Isar, Munich, F.R.G.

In our studies on brain dysfunction in schizophrenia, we investigated initially 30 neuroleptic-treated schizophrenic patients (DSM-III 295.1,2,3), using a psychomotor activation paradigm and 16-channel EEG Mapping. We obtained in **resting conditions** increased power values in slow frequency bands delta and theta, predominant in frontal areas, as reported by other groups (1,5). Additionally, in **motor activation conditions**, we found signs of reduced left hemisphere activation and increased right hemisphere involvement (3).

For further evaluation we used a multimodal approach involving MRI/SPECT and PET/EEG measurements and drug-naive, wash-out and neuroleptic treated patients. Psychopathology was studied especially using the "positive-negative" dimension.

MRI/SPECT FINDINGS

31 schizophrenic patients and 31 control persons were investigated using magnetic resonance imaging (MRI) and single photon emission computerized tomography (SPECT). MRI was used to obtain midsagittal planes for planimetry of the area of Corpus Callosum. SPECT yielded measurements of regional cerebral blood flow (rCBF) in the same persons during resting condition and simple motor activity of the dominant right hand (details in 4).

As in our previous SPECT study (2), we found a "diffuse" (i.e. cortical and subcortical) bihemispherical hyperactivation on motor stimulation in patients with little negative symptomatology (SANS below 15). In contrast, "negative" schizophrenics (SANS above 35) showed a complete non-reactivity (although they performed the task!). For normals a 25% rise in contralateral sensorimotor area exclusively was found, as known from the literature (2).

Callosal area in the "positive" schizophrenics was significantly greater than in "negative" patients. However, when both schizophrenic subgroups were taken together, the callosal area was equal to that found in normal persons (however with a threefold SD!).

PET/EEG MAPPING FINDINGS

Simultanous measurements of cerebral glucose uptake (11-2-Deoxy-Glucose as tracer, PETT VI, Bartlett et al. in press) and 21-channel EEG mapping (Cadwell, Brain Research Laboratories, NYU Medical Center) was performed in 9 neuroleptic-treated chronic schizophrenic patients (DSM III-R 295.1,3,9). Non-reactivity on complex motor stimulation was found in these patients, concordant with our previous SPECT findings, and PET findings on other types of cerebral activation (5).

Interestingly, PET/EEG correlation coefficents in 16 regions of interest differed to those in normals, as reported by Buchsbaum et al. (1). As shown in fig. 1, differences are maximal in left frontotemporal areas.

References

Buchsbaum MS et al. (1984): In Pfurtscheller et al. (eds) Brain Ischaemia, pp. 263-269. Elsevier, Amsterdam (1)

Guenther W et al., (1986): Biol. Psychiatry 21:889-899 (2)

Guenther W et al., (1988): Biol. Psychiatry 23:295-311 (3)

Guenther W et al., (1989): Psychiatry Res. 29:453-455 (4)

Guich SM et al., (1989): Schiz.Res. 2:439-448 (5)

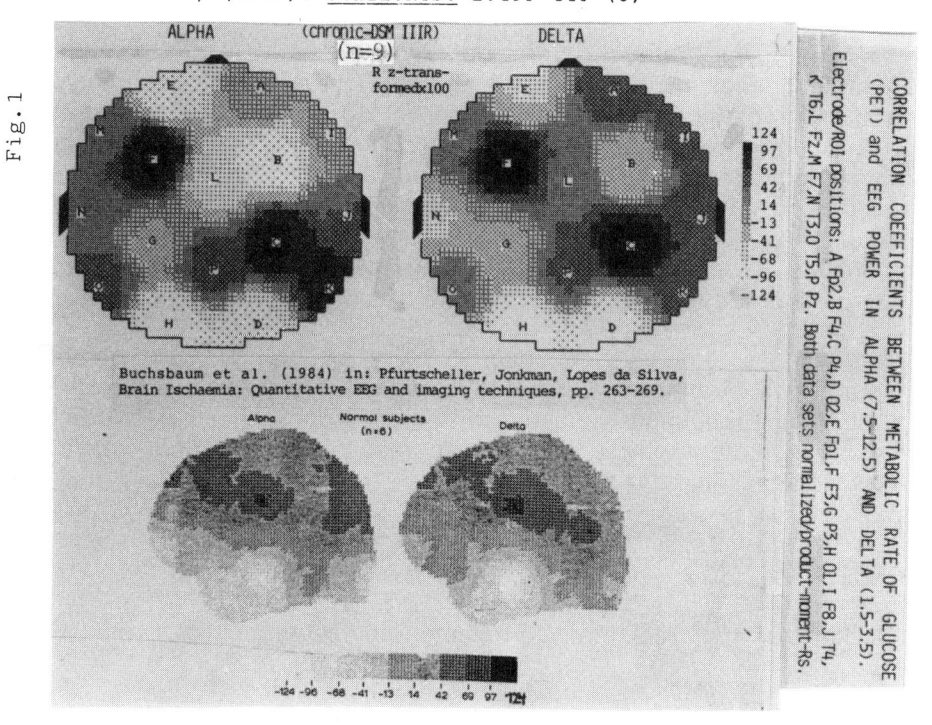

Fig. 1

QUANTITATIVE RECEPTOR MAPPING IN POSTMORTEM BRAIN HUMAN AS IT RELATES TO IN VIVO NEUROIMAGING

J. E. KLEINMAN
NIMH Neuroscience Center at St. Elizabeths; Washington, D.C., U.S.A.

Neuropathological research has experienced a renaissance as the result of advances in in vivo neuroimaging and neurochemistry. The latter has led to numerous postmortem studies in neuropsychiatry in the last 25 years. The vast majority of these studies have involved neurochemical analyses of dissected brain regions. There has been no shortage of findings, but unfortunately few replications. One possible explanation for the latter could be difficulties in standardizing brain dissections.

One of the more replicable finding in the postmortem neurochemical literature involves increased dopamine receptors in the basal ganglia of schizophrenics (1) Not surprisingly, basal ganglia structures (caudate, putamen and nucleus accumbens) are relatively easy to identify and dissect. This is not the case with structures that are very small, i.e., locus coeruleus and ventral tegmentum, or very large, i.e., cerebral cortex. A review of the literature in these areas reveals few replicable findings (1).

An alternative strategy for elucidating neurochemical abnormalities in postmortem studies involves autoradiography. This approach has been used by a number of investigators over the last 10 years to study the locus coeruleus (2), the basal ganglia (3) and the cortex (4). Although a pathognomonic lesion for neuropsychiatric disorder has proved elusive, this approach has the advantage of reducing the variability of dissection while allowing for large areas to be screened. In addition it allows comparisons between quantitative in vivo neuroimaging approaches and their counterparts with autoradiography.

A comparison of in vivo iodinated QNB single photon emission computed tomography will be made with tritiated iodinated QNB using autoradiography on postmortem specimens. Results with these approaches are surprisingly similar. Autoradiography is a useful approach for confirming the validity of in vivo imaging studies.

REFERENCES

1. Jaskiw G and Kleinman: Postmortem neurochemistry studies in

schizphrenia. In: Schulz SC and Tamminga CA (eds.): Schizophrenia: Scientific Progress. New York, Oxford University pp. 246-255, 1988.

2. Ko GN, Unnerstall JR, Kuhar MJ and Kleinman JE: Alpha-2 agonist binding in schizophrenic brains. Psychopharmacology Bull 22:1011-1016, 1986.

3. Joyce JN, et al: Organization of dopamine D1 and D2 receptors in human striatum: receptors autoradiographic studies in Huntington's disease and schizophrenia. Synapse 2:746-557, 1988.

4. Lang W and Henke H: Cholinergic receptor binding and autoradiography in brains of non-neurological and senile dementia of Alzheimers-type patients. Brain Research 267:271-280, 1983.

L-DOPA IN VERY IMPAIRED SCHIZOPHRENIC PATIENTS

D.G.C. OWENS*, P.E. HARRISON-READ** AND E.C. JOHNSTONE*
*Department of Psychiatry, Northwick Park Hospital, Harrow, U.K.
**Department of Psychiatry, St. Mary's Hospital, London., U.K.

In the last 15 years there has been considerable investigation of dopamine (DA) mechanisms in schizophrenia, particularly relating to the effectiveness of DA blockade in the control of 'positive' features. There has in addition also been interest in the effects of DA agonists in both 'positive' and 'negative' states. Controlled, long-term studies are few and results difficult to interpret. We present results of a long-term, double blind study assessing the efficacy of L-Dopa (as SINEMET 110) added to standard chlorpromazine (CPZ) regimes, in severely disabled chronic schizophrenic in-patients.

SUBJECTS AND METHODS

The subjects were 8 Feighner positive, highly dependent schizophrenic men (age range 41-64 years) who continued to show a marked degree of 'positive' and 'negative' symptomatology despite being maintained long-term on oral CPZ. The study was a double-blind, cross-over design consisting of 2 experimental and 2 control conditions (Table 1) each of 8 weeks duration.

Group 1 (n=4)	Exp. 1	Control	Exp. 2	Control
Group 2 (n=4)	Control	Exp. 1	Control	Exp. 2

Experimental condition 1 = full-strength CPZ + active L-Dopa

Experimental condition 2 = half-strength CPZ + placebo L-Dopa

Control condition = full-strength CPZ + placebo L-Dopa

Experimental condition 2 was included to examine the possibility that adding L-Dopa is merely equivalent to reducing neuroleptic doses. Sinemet or placebo was increased to a maximum of 7.5 tabs per day (active L-Dopa equivalent 4gms) by week 5 of each period. Ratings performed by nurses were, Venables Activity/Withdrawal Scale (daily) and NOSIE (bi-weekly). Medical ratings performed at mid and end points of each period included mental state (Krawiecka Scale) and neurological status (AIMS and TAKE) and in addition videotaped interviews were evaluated subsequently using Videotask, a computerised technique for measuring affect-related behaviour.

RESULTS

All patients completed the study. Neither experimental condition affected Krawiecka ratings of negative symptoms. Venables scores at mid period were increased by L-Dopa but not by halving CPZ. Krawiecka ratings of positive features tended to be reduced by L-Dopa and NOSIE ratings of 'manifest psychosis' significantly reduced.

Some Videotask items correlated significantly with negative feature scores on Krawiecka and of these items eyebrow movements significantly increased on L-Dopa. AIMS scores significantly increased on half-strength CPZ but not L-Dopa.

DISCUSSION

These results indicated that L-Dopa has significant effects on both positive and negative features of severe and otherwise treatment-resistent schizophrenia. The Videotask technique may provide a sensitive measure of negative features.

EFFECTS OF MIANSERIN ON NEGATIVE SYMPTOMS IN SCHIZOPHRENIA

Y. MIZUKI
Department of Neuropsychiatry, Yamaguchi University School of Medicine, 1144 Kogushi, Ube 755, Japan

Crow (1) presented the hypothesis that schizophrenic symptoms can be divided into positive and negative categories, and that exaggerated DA function may underlie the positive symptom dimension, while structural impairment may underlie the negative symptom dimension in schizophrenia. Despite an increase of reports on the remission of negative symptoms by medication, there are at present no convincing data that any medication is more effective in negative symptoms. In the present study, the possible efficacy of mianserin as a supplement in treating chronic schizophrenia was tested by monitoring the BPRS as well as the concentrations of monoamine metabolites (HVA, MHPG and 5-HIAA) in plasma.

METHODS

The subjects were 20 inpatients who were diagnosed as schizophrenic by DSM-III criteria, with an illness of more than 5 years' duration. The patients continued to receive their regular maintenance doses of neuroleptics throughout the study. Initial BPRS and blood testing were performed before mianserin administration. Fixed doses of 60 mg/day of mianserin for the first 2 weeks, flexible doses of 60 or 90 mg/day for the second 2 weeks, and flexible doses of 60, 90 and 120 mg/day for the third 2 weeks were given orally in an open study for 6 consecutive weeks. A period of no mianserin treatment followed for the next 1 week. BPRS scoring was carried out once weekly throughout the study, and blood samples were obtained after mianserin treatment.

RESULTS

The total BPRS scores decreased over the entire study period. There were significant reductions in the scores for somatic concern, anxiety, emotional withdrawal, tension, depressive mood, motor retardation and blunted affect, respectively. In order to identify those responses which accompany mianserin treatment, the patients were divided into two groups, i.e., a responding group who showed more than a 3-point decrease in total BPRS scores after medication (n=11) and a nonresponding group who showed less than a 2-point decrease or no change in the values of total BPRS scores (n=9). As shown in Table 1, plasma 5-HIAA concentrations were increased after medication in both responding patients and nonresponding patients. However, the 5-HIAA values of responders were lower than those of nonresponders. Plasma HVA levels were slightly increased by mianserin in the responders. There were no significant changes in MHPG levels.

TABLE 1: EFFECTS OF MIANSERIN ON PLASMA MONOAMINE METABOLITES

		Before treatment	After treatment
5-HIAA	Responder	5.6 ± 2.1	6.7 ± 1.7B
	Nonresponder	7.2 ± 2.2	9.8 ** ± 2.1C
	All patients	6.4 ± 2.3	8.1 ± 2.5C
HVA	Responder	9.4 ± 3.0	11.6 ± 3.9A
	Nonresponder	12.6 ± 9.0	11.5 ± 3.8
	All patients	10.9 ± 6.4	11.6 ± 3.8
MHPG	Responder	3.5 ± 1.3	3.6 ± 1.2
	Nonresponder	4.2 ± 1.2	4.0 ± 1.3
	All patients	3.8 ± 1.3	3.7 ± 1.2

A: $p<0.10$; B: $p<0.05$; C: $p<0.001$; **: $p<0.01$.

DISCUSSION

Mianserin is a tetracyclic antidepressant, and its pharmacological profile is characterized by potent antagonism of presynaptic α2 receptors and postsynaptic 5-HT2 receptors, and weak antagonism of D2 receptors (3). Furthermore, mianserin also antagonizes heterotypical α2 receptors (2) and 5-HT3 receptors (4). Considering the results of the studies up to this point, chronic mianserin treatment combined with neuroleptics in schizophrenia may cause an increase of HVA but a decrease of MHPG and 5-HIAA concentrations. Therefore, the present results suggest that mianserin does not affect NA turnover in chronic schizophrenics, and that it potentiates DA turnover and inhibits activation of 5-HT turnover in the responding patients. The reason for this may be that α2 receptors are damaged in chronic schizophrenics, and that D2 and 5-HT2 receptors are still functional in only some patients (responding patients), however, they are damaged in the remaining patients with severely negative symptoms (nonresponding patients).

REFERENCES

1. Crow, T.J. (1980): Molecular pathology of schizophrenia: more than one disease process? Brit. Med. J., 280: 66-68.
2. Maura, G. et al. (1985): α2-adrenoceptors in rat hypothalamus and cerebral cortex: functional evidence for pharmacologically distinct subpopulations. Eur. J. Pharmacol., 116: 335-339.
3. Pinder, R.M. (1985): Adrenoreceptor interactions of the enantiomers and metabolites of mianserin: are they responsible for the antidepressant effect? Acta Psychiat. Scand., 72 (Suppl. 320): 1-9.
4. Schmidt, A.W. and Peroutka, S.J. (1989): Antidepressant interactions with 5-hydroxytryptamine3 receptor binding sites. Eur. J. Pharmacol., 163: 397-398.

DOPAMINE AUTORECEPTOR AGONISTS IN THE TREATMENT OF POSITIVE AND NEGATIVE SCHIZOPHRENIA

O. BENKERT, H. WETZEL and K. WIEDEMANN
Department of Psychiatry, University of Mainz, D-6500 Mainz, FRG

In dopaminergic neurons, dopamine synthesis and release as well as the firing rate of dopaminergic neurons is controlled by stimulation of autoreceptors via a negative feedback regulation. In relation to the dichotomization of schizophrenic syndromes in a positive subtype associated with increased mesolimbic dopaminergic function and a negative subtype possibly related to structural brain abnormalities, we conducted open clinical trials with the dopamine autoreceptor agonists B-HT 920 (1) and roxindole (EMD 49990) (2) in patients with positive or negative schizophrenic symptomatology free of neuroleptic pretreatment for at least 3 months. B-HT 920 may also exert some weak agonistic effects on postsynaptic dopamine receptors (3) and stimulate α_2-adrenergic receptors in higher dosages. Roxindole has also 5-HT uptake inhibiting and 5-HT_{1A} agonistic actions.

1. B-HT 920 in positive schizophrenia

Ten patients suffering from a paranoid schizophrenia according to DSM-III were given B-HT 920 in doses from 0.3 to 1.2 mg/day for up to 28 days. In 3 patients, B-HT 920 medication was discontinued after 21 days. Fig. 1 shows the time course of mean total BPRS scores under B-HT 920. Endpoint analysis demonstrated a non-significant decrease of mean total BPRS scores from 49.3 ± 10.7 at day 0 to 39.0 ± 19.6 at day 28. In 4 patients however, a substantial psychopathological improvement (reduction of initial BPRS scores by more than 50 %) could be observed. Seven patients showed a marked psychomotor activation (4).

2. Roxindole in positive schizophrenia

Roxindole was administered for 28 days to 7 patients suffering from a paranoid or undifferentiated type of schizophrenia (DSM-III-R) in increasing dosages from 0.3 up to 30 mg/day. Three patients were drop-outs because of deterioration of symptoms after 3, 23 and 27 days of treatment, respectively. The time course of mean total BPRS scores under roxindole treatment is demonstrated in Fig. 1. The initial mean total BPRS score (day 0) was 59.9 ± 7.8, and endpoint analysis of data revealed a mean total BPRS score of 56.7 ± 18.9 at day 28. Only 2 patients showed a sufficient treatment response. Profound dose-dependant psychomotor activation was observed in 3 patients and prompted premature termination of the trial in all cases.

3. Roxindole in negative schizophrenia

In contrast to positive schizophrenia, a dopamine deficiency rather than an excess has been suggested in negative symptoms (5, 6). Since neither B-HT 920 nor roxindole demonstrated a satisfying antipsychotic efficacy with regard to positive schizophrenic symptoms, and because of the psychomotor activating and possibly anti-anergic effects of both drugs, we conducted an additional open trial with roxindole in 10 neuroleptic-free patients with primary

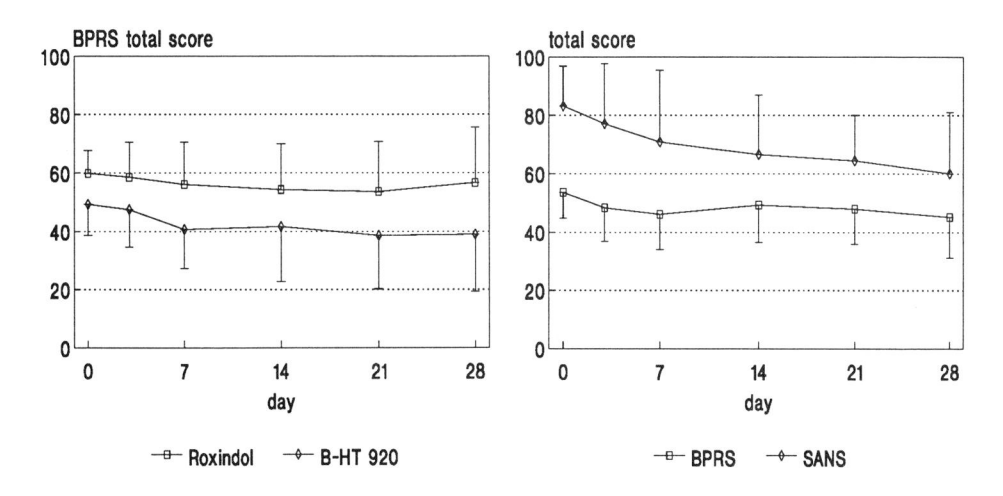

Fig. 1. Time course of mean total BPRS scores in patients with positive schizophrenia treated with B-HT 920 or roxindole.

Fig. 2. Time course of mean BPRS and SANS scores in patients with negative schizophrenia treated with roxindole.

negative symptoms suffering from a disorganized or residual type of schizophrenia. Roxindole dosages extended from 0.3 mg/day in the beginning up to 30 mg per day. As shown in Fig. 2, mean total BPRS scores demonstrated only a minor reduction from 53.6 ± 8.8 at day 0 to 45.2 ± 14.0 at day 28 while in the SANS a moderate 25 % decrease from 83.2 ± 13.7 (day 0) to 60.1 ± 21.0 (day 28) was observed. Two patients showed a significant amelioration of negative symptomatology, and another 2 patients were rated as partial responders. Beneficial effects were mostly observed in symptoms like reduced energy, apathy, anhedonia and depressive mood. However, 2 patients had to be withdrawn from the study because they developed positive symptoms after 14 days under roxindole dosages of 1.2 and 15 mg/day, respectively.

As to side effects, roxindole as well as B-HT 920 were well tolerated and did not cause any untoward extrapyramidal symptoms.

In <u>conclusion</u>, our data do not support the hypothesis that dopamine autoreceptor stimulating drugs might have antipsychotic effects on positive symptoms. With regard to negative symptomatology, our findings of beneficial effects in some patients do not yet allow a reliable judgment and remain to be clarified by double-blind placebo-controlled studies.

REFERENCES

1. ANDEN, N.E., et al., (1982): Naunyn-Schmiedeberg's Arch.Pharmacol. 321:100-104
2. SEYFRIED, C.A., et al., (1989): Eur.J.Pharmacol 160:31-41
3. SCHMIDT, C.J., et al., (1986): Naunyn-Schmiedeberg's Arch.Pharmcacol. 334:377-382
4. WIEDEMANN, K., et al., (1990): Pharmacopsychiat. 23:50-55
5. MACKAY, A.V.P. (1980): Br.J.Psychiatry 137:379-383
6. WEINBERGER, D.R. (1987): Arch.Gen.Psychiatry 44:660-669

TREATMENT OF A NEW BENZAMIDE DERIVATIVE EMONAPRIDE(YM-09151) FOR SCHIZOPHRENIA

Y.Kudo
Institute of Clinical Pharmacology, Aino Hospital, Ibaraki, Osaka, Japan

Emonapride(YM-09151) is a benzamide derivative which has been newly developed in Japan(1)-(3). It has been shown that emonapride has a broad spectrum of antipsychotic effect on schizophrenia. A double-blind comparative study using sulpiride as control drug was conducted in schizophrenia to assess the effectiveness and safety of emonapride objectively.

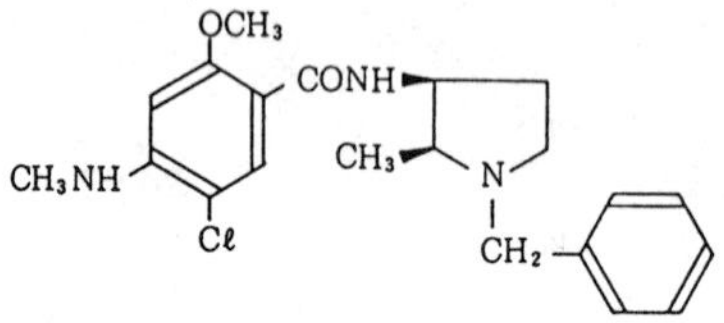

FIGURE 1. CHEMICAL STRUCTURE OF EMONAPRIDE(YM-09151)

SUBJECT AND METHOD

A total of 186 schizophrenic patients, including 92 cases in the emonapride group and 94 cases in the sulpiride group, were subjected to analysis. Three mg tablets of emonapride and 100 mg tablets of sulpiride were used. The initial daily dosage was 9 or 18 mg with emonapride and 300 or 600 mg with sulpiride, and thereafter adjusted depending on the symptoms of the patients and the responsiveness to drugs, with the maximum daily dosage up to 36 mg with emonapride and 1200 mg with sulpiride. The administration period was determined to be 8 weeks. The psychiatric symptoms were evaluated by using BPRS and SANS.

RESULTS

In the final global improvement, moderate and marked improvement numbered 22(24%) in emonapride and 19(20%) in sulpiride, slight to marked improvement numbered 47(51%) and 48(51%), and slight aggravation and worse numbered 21(23%) and 11(12%). No significant difference was observed between the two groups with the final global improvement. In overall safety, no significant difference was observed between the two groups. However, number of extrapyramidal symptoms was slightly greater in emonapride group. No significant difference was observed between the two groups in usefulness.

TABLE 1: OVERALL EVALUATION OF EMONAPRIDE AND SULPIRIDE

FINAL GLOBAL IMPROVEMENT	EMONAPRIDE (N=92) N (%)	SULPIRIDE (N=94) N (%)
MARKED IMPROVEMENT	4 (4)	1 (1)
MODERATE IMPROVEMENT	18(20)	18(19)
SLIGHT IMPROVEMENT	25(27)	29(31)
NO CHANGE	22	32
SLIGHT AGGRAVATION	11(12)	3 (3)
MODERATE AGGRAVATION	8 (9)	5 (5)
MARKED AGGRAVATION	2 (2)	3 (3)
INDETERMINABLE	2	3

DISCUSSION

Emonapride showed not only antihallucinatory and antidelusional actions, but high improvement percentages in several negative symptoms and several items representing anxiety and tension. The results of this study indicate that emonapride has a good efficacy and safety and is fit for practical use as an antipsychotic.

REFERENCES

1. Terai, M., Usuda, S., Maeno, H., et al.: Selective binding of YM-09151-2, a new potent neuroleptic, to D_2-dopaminergic receptors. Japan J. Pharmacol., 33: 749-755, 1983.
2. Usuda, S., Nishikori, K., Noshiro, O., et al.: Neuroleptic properties of cis N-(1-benzyl-2-methyl-pyrrolidin-3-yl)-5-chloro-2-methoxy-4-methylamino-benzamide(YM-09151-2) with selective antidopaminergic activity. Psychopharmacol., 73: 103-109, 1981.
3. Yamamoto, M., Usuda, S., Tachikawa, S., et al.: Pharmacological studies on a new benzamide derivative, YM-09151-2, with potential neuroleptic properties. Neuropharamacol., 21: 945-951, 1982.

SEROTONIN 5-HT$_2$ RECEPTOR BLOCKERS IN SCHIZOPHRENIA

Y.G. Gelders, S.L.E. Heylen, G. Vanden Bussche, A.J.M. Reyntjens and P.A.J. Janssen
Janssen Research Foundation, B-2340 Beerse, Belgium

Notwithstanding the important therapeutic activities of the selective dopamine D$_2$ antagonist haloperidol in psychotic disorders, clinical experience with pipamperone gave an early indication of the advantages of mixed serotonin 5-HT$_2$ and dopamine D$_2$ antagonism in the treatment of schizophrenia.These benefits include anti-autistic effects, regulation of disturbed sleep-wakefulness rhythms and low EPS-inducing liability. Such efficacity is consistent with the suspected role of the serotonergic system in schizophrenia, which has been recently reviewed by Bleich et al. (1).

More recently, following the discovery of the selective and potent serotonin antagonist ritanserin (5), an important role for selective 5-HT$_2$ receptor blockade in the treatment of negative symptoms and disturbed sleep in schizophrenic patients has been suggested (7). Moreover, EPS due to the basic neuroleptic treatment were found to be attenuated during treatment with ritanserin.

Although the use of ritanserin offers these advantages in the treatment of schizophrenia, especially when combined with oral or depot neuroleptic maintenance treatments, the need for an acceptable monotherapy remains undeniable. Subsequent chemical and pharmacological research has therefore focussed on the search for new substances with combined central serotonin 5-HT$_2$ and dopamine D$_2$ antagonism.

Major progress was made with the synthesis of risperidone in 1984. Characterized by potent 5-HT$_2$ and catecholamine antagonism (mainly dopamine D$_2$ and alpha$_1$ adrenergic receptor blockade) (4), risperidone has proven to be a novel type of antipsychotic medication. Whilst controlling hallucinations and delusions during the maintenance therapy of chronic schizophrenia, risperidone as well has important effects on the negative symptomatology, with negligible EPS (2,3). The treatment with risperidone is well tolerated and may thus considerably enhance patient compliance. As of early 1990, over 1700 patients have been treated with risperidone and long-term follow-up data are available for over 100 patients. International multicentre studies for which 2200 patients are envisaged, featuring a fixed-dose parallel-group design are in progress.

Next, with the synthesis of R 79 598 in 1988, a new compound with very potent dopamine antagonism and nearly equipotent serotonin antagonism became available, providing new perspectives on the treatment of psychotic patients (6). This pharmacological activity predicts neuroleptic efficacy with reduced EPS liability as compared with haloperidol. The first pilot clinical study performed in Belgium demonstrates that therapy-resistant schizophrenic patients with acute psychotic symptoms can be efficaciously treated with R 79 598 , whilst only mild EPS were observed in only part of the patients.

It can thus be concluded that with the advent of the new centrally active serotonin and dopamine mixed antagonists, substantial progress in the treatment of psychotic disorders can be expected.

REFERENCES:

1. Bleich, A., Brown, S.L., Kahn, R. and van Praag, H. (1988): The role of serotonin in schizophrenia. Schizophrenia Bulletin **14**: 297-315
2. Castelao, F., Ferreira, L., Gelders, Y.G., Heylen, S.L.E. (1989). The efficacy of the D2 and 5-HT$_2$ antagonist risperidone (R 64 766) in the treatment of chronic psychosis: an open dose-finding study. Schizophrenia Research, **2**, 411-415.
3. Gelders, Y.G. (1989) Thymosthenic agents, a novel approach in the treatment of schizophrenia. Br. J. Psych., **155**, suppl. 5, 33-336.
4. Janssen, P.A.J., Niemegeers, C.J.E., Awouters, F., Schellekens, K.H.L., Megens, A.A.H.P., Meert, T.F. (1988). Pharmacology of risperidone (R 64 766), a new antipsychotic with serotonin-S$_2$ and dopamine-D$_2$ antagonistic properties. J. Pharmacol. Exp. Ther., **244**, 685-693.
5. Leysen, J.E., Gommeren, W., Van Gompel, P., Wynants, J., Janssen, P.F.M. and Laduron, P.M. (1985). Receptor-binding properties *in vitro* and *in vivo* of Ritanserin. A potent and long-acting serotonin-S$_2$ antagonist. Mol. Pharmacol., **27**, 600-611.
6. Megens, A. A. H. P., Lenaerts, F.M., Awouters, F.H.L., Meert, T. F., Van Gorp, W., Schellekens, K.H.L., Niemegeers, C.J.E. (1989) *In vivo* pharmacological comparison of the new potent neuroleptic R 79 598 with risperidone, haloperidol and ritanserin in rats and dogs. Janssen Research Products Information, Preclinical Research Report R 79 598/7.
7. Reyntjens, A., Gelders, Y.G., Hoppenbrouwers, M.-L.J.A. and Vanden Bussche, G. (1986). Thymosthenic effects of ritanserin (R 55 667), a centrally acting serotonin-S$_2$ receptor blocker. Drug Dev. Res., **8**, 205-211.

DEPRESSION AND SUICIDE IN LATE LIFE

M.Shimizu. Dept. of Psychiat. Jikei Univ., School of Medicine,
3-25-8, Nishi-Shinbasi, Minato-ku, Tokyo 105, JAPAN

INTRODUCTION
Among those over 65 years of age, suicide ranks rather low as a cause of death in Japan in recent years (7th at 65〜69 and 8th at 70〜75 in 1987). The ranking keeps going down as age goes up. However, we should not depreciate the significance of suicide in late life, when death caused by various physical diseases increases conspicuously.

SUICIDE RATE IN LATE LIFE
If one compare suicide curve of 1982 to that of 1957, several differences can be noted. One is the general decrease in suicide rate. Another is disappearance of the unique peak of suicide rate among youth and the emergence of a elevation of suicide rate among middle aged males in 1982. The last but not least feature is steep upward curve of suicide rate in late life for both sexes and pose a grave problem for our society.

Fig.1 illustrates suicide rate of male population for each age group in various countries. Denmark has the highest suicide rate for most age groups with unique curve pattern. France, West-Germany, Japan, and U.S. exhibit similar pattern of steep rising in populations of 65 years and older. While in Engeland and in Sweden, rising in 65 years and older is less steep.

Fig.2 illusturates suicide rate of female population. The most conspicuous finding is prominent uprise for Japanese and Hong Kongese suicide rate curves for 65 years and older, showing highest suicide rate in various countries. This peculiar pattern has been noted for these 3 decades in Japan, since the end of the IInd World War. In other developed countries however, no prominent rising of elderly female suicide rate is noted.

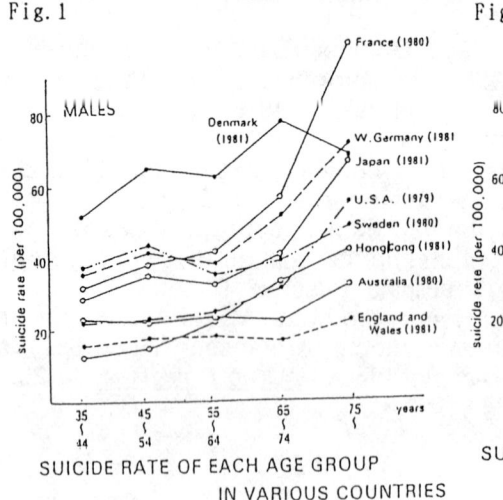

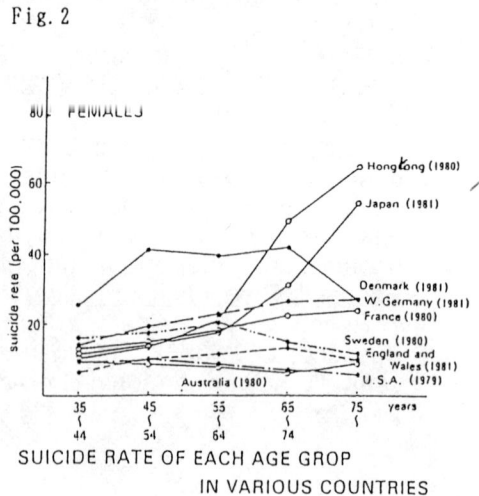

Fig.1

SUICIDE RATE OF EACH AGE GROUP
IN VARIOUS COUNTRIES

Fig.2

SUICIDE RATE OF EACH AGE GROP
IN VARIOUS COUNTRIES

Speculatively, this unique phenomenon may have something to do with innovation of our family system in the past few decades, diminishing trend of extended families in Japan. It is likely that they are vulnerable to depressive syndrome in solitary situation, particularly following their husbands death. The similar speculation may be applicable to Hong Kongnese elderly female. The present speculation would be testifed if the prominent uprise of elderly female suicides diminishes in the future, when our aged population addapted to the cultural innovation.

FACTERS CONTRIBUTING TO SUICIDE IN LATE LIFE

Preparatory state of suicide can be provoked by various factors. Several investigaters have unanimously pointed out the importance of depression or depressive syndrome in terms of suicide in late life. Some of the results are summarized in the tabele.

Table. SUICIDE IN LATE LIFE AND PSYCHIATRIC DIAGNOSIS

	Number	Diagnosis of Psychosis
Batschelor, IRC (1953)	?	82% : depression and organic dementia
O'neal, P (1956)	N=19	89% : depression (58%), dementia, acute confusional state, alcoholism
Ohara, K (1961)	N=11	91% : psychotic depression (64%), depressive state (27%)
Barraclough, BM (1971)	N=30	87% : psychotic depression (63%) depressive state (23%) with physical illness, delirium, alcoholism

There is no doubt that suicide in elderly population is closely related to depressive syndrome. On the other hand, its relationship with socio-economical factors should not be overlooked. The probable example is the transient uprise of suicide rate curve among Japanese elderly population around 1973 when we experienced socio-economical crisis by sudden rise in petroleum price, so-called "oil shock".

METHOD OF SUICIDE AND SUICIDE NOTE

Method of suicide may reveal the attitude toward death of those who commit suicide. The more fatal method one uses, the more determined one's will toward death. The ratio of fatal suicidal methods, such as hunging and strangulation, increases with advancing age. Similar fatal suicidal methods are used by psychiatic patients, suggesting close relationship between the two suicidal groups. Less elderly suicides leave note than young suilcides do. Ohara(1) indicated 90% of elderly suicide notes are brief and self-reproachful which presumably written in depressive state.

REFERENCES
1. Ohara K, Shimizu M.(1975) In:Kuromaru S, Shinfuku N, Hosaki, H(eds) Geriatric Psychiatry. Nakayama Shyoten, Tokyo, pp 363-396

NEUROENDOCRINEIMMUNE REGULATION OF AGING

JOSEPH MEITES
Department of Physiology, Michigan State University, East Lansing, MI 48824, U.S.A.

Aging can be defined as a decline in body structure and function with time, associated with a decrease in ability to maintain homeostasis. Many of these decrements in body functions begin relatively early in life in animals and man. In man it has been demonstrated that there is a progressive reduction from 30 to 90 years of age in metabolic rate, cardiovascular function, nerve conduction velocity, renal function, vital capacity, etc. (Shock, 1977). Although it is generally agreed that the genome determines the length of the lifespan among different species, the role of the genome in regulating the rate of aging in body tissues is not clear. I believe that the genome and environment determine the rate of aging mainly via the major integrative mechanisms of the body, namely the central nervous system (CNS), endocrine system, and immune systems, or what is termed collectively the "neuroendocrineimmune system." These three components of the neuroendocrineimmune system constantly interact with each other throughout life to regulate or influence development, growth, and function of every tissue in the body. Any major dysfunction that develops in one component may affect operations of the other components and thereby alter the rate of aging in body tissues.

Studies reported during the past 25 years, primarily in rats, have demonstrated that dysfunctions appear in all components of the neuroendocrineimmune system with time. Deficiencies develop in hypothalamic, pituitary, target gland, and immune function, as well as in the tissues they regulate. However, the major defect appears to be the decline in hypothalamic function due to the decrease in secretion of catecholamines (CAs), particularly dopamine (DA) and norepinephrine (NE). The decrease in NE leads to reduced release from the hypothalamus of gonadotropin releasing hormone (GnRH), leading to lower secretion of pituitary gonadotropins, reduced ovarian and testicular function and cessation of estrous cycles. The decline in DA and particularly NE leads to a fall in release of growth hormone releasing hormone (GHRH) and to decreased GH and somatomedin (IGF-1) secretion, resulting in decreased protein synthesis. Since hypothalamic DA is the major inhibitor of prolactin (PRL) secretion, its decline in aging rats leads to a marked increase in PRL secretion and development of numerous mammary and pituitary tumors. The gonadotropins, GH and PRL, as well as other hormones influence functions of the thymus, the chief component of the immune system. The reduction in GH secretion is believed to contribute to decreased immune function with age. These observations have been reviewed previously (Meites et al., 1987, 1988).

Correction of the deficiency of CAs in the hypothalamus of old rats by administration of L-dopa (CA precursor) or other dopaminergic drugs, results in restoration of estrous cycles in females and elevation of testosterone secretion in males, a rise in GH and somatomedin secretion and increased protein synthesis, and reduced PRL secretion and regression of mammary and pituitary tumors. Increased GH levels in old rats were reported to elevate thymus size and function. Administration of L-dopa also was reported to prolong the lifespan of a short-lived strain of mice (Cotzias et al., 1974), and L-deprenyl (a specific MAO-B inhibitor which retards DA catabolism) prolonged reproductive activity and the lifespan of old male rats (Knoll et al., 1989). The causes for the decrease in hypothalamic secretion of CAs with time are not entirely known at present, but it has been shown that the chronic action of some hormones, particularly estrogens, can damage neurons in the hypothalamus, including dopaminergic neurons (Sakar et al., 1982). Also, "free radicals" are produced by the catabolism of CAs, and exposure to toxins such as quinones or other deleterious agents may damage neurons.

The relevance of the changes reported here in the neuroendocrineimmune system in aging rats to those that appear in aging men and women is not entirely clear at present. Relatively few studies have yet been reported on neuroendocrineimmune function in elderly as compared to that in young or middle-aged individuals. The closest parallel to aging rats in elderly human subjects is the similar decline in GH and somatomedin secretion (Florini et al, 1985). There is also evidence that CAs are decreased in the hypothalamus (Hornickiewicz, 1987), and CAs can promote GH secretion in man (Martin and Reichlin, 1987), but it has not been determined whether the decrease in CAs is responsible for the reduction in GH and somatomedin secretion or whether it influences other endocrine functions in aging man.

REFERENCES
1. Cotzias, G., Miller, S., Nicholson, A., Matson, W., Tang. L. Levo-dopa, fertility, and longevity. Proc. Natl Acad. Sci. USA 71:2466-2469, 1974.
2. Florini, J.R., Prinz, P.N., Vitiels, M., Hintz, R.L. Somatomedin-C levels in healthy young and old men: relation to peak and 24-hour integrated levels of growth hormone. J. Gerontology 40:2-7, 1985.
3. Horniekiewicz, O. Neurotransmitter changes in human brain during aging. In: Govoni, S., Buttaini, F., eds. Modification of Cell to Cell Signals During Normal and Pathological Aging. Springer-Verlag, pp. 169-182, 1987.
4. Knoll, J., Dallo, J., Yen, T.T. Striatal dopamine, sexual activity and lifespan. Life Sciences 45:525-531, 1989.
5. Martin, J.B., Reichlin, S. Clinical Neuroendocrinology, 2nd Ed., F.A. Davis Co., Philadelphia, 1987.
6. Meites, J., Goya, R., Takahashi, S. Why the neuroendocrine system is important in aging processes. Exper. Gerontol. 22:1-15, 1987.
7. Meites, J. Neuroendocrine basis of aging in the rat. In: Everitt, A.V., Walton, G.R., eds. Regulation of Neuroendocrine Aging. Karger, Basel, 37-50, 1988.
8. Sarkar, D.K., Gottschall, P.E., Meites, J. Damage to hypothalamic dopaminergic neurons is associated with development of prolactin-secreting pituitary tumors. Science 218:684-686, 1982.
9. Shock, N. Systemic integration. In: Finch, C.E., Hayflick, L., eds. Handbook of the Biology of Aging. Van Nostrand Reinhold, New York, pp. 639-665, 1977.

LIMBIC HYPOTHALAMIC PITUITARY ADRENAL-AXIS DYSFUNCTION IN ELDERLY DEPRESSED PATIENTS

I.J. HEUSER*, H.-J. WARK, D. BORCHARDT and L. HERMLE
Department of Psychiatry, University of Freiburg, Freiburg, F.R.G.
*now at: Max-Planck-Institute for Psychiatry, Munich, F.R.G.

Patients with depression frequently have a central alteration of corticotropin-releasing hormone (CRH) regulation. Furthermore, data from animal studies suggest that repeated episodes of glucocorticoid (GC) excess - e.g. depressive illness - might facilitate degenerative cell loss in the hippocampus, consequently weakening its GC-feedback capacity and thus possibly propelling forward the aging process (1). The present, ongoing study addresses neuroendocrine, cognitive and psychopathological concomitants of depressive illness in later life.

SUBJECTS AND METHODS

17, otherwise healthy, inpatients (1 male, 16 females) with a major depressive episode (DSM-III-R) completed the study. Mean age was 70.6 ± 7 (SD), ranging from 60 to 82 years. Overall duration of illness varied from 0 to 46 years, mean 21 ± 15 years, duration of the index episode averaged 5 ± 3 weeks, 1 to 12 weeks. Mean number of episodes was 7 ± 6, 1 to 20. Degree of severity of depression ranged from moderate to severe (Hamilton depression rating (HDR) scores: 26 ± 6, 18 to 41). At admission, any previous medication was tapered. Thereafter, patients received placebo for 7 days. During this baseline interval (BL) psychopathological and cognitive studies were performed as well as a combined dexamethasone-corticotropin-releasing hormone challenge (DEX/CRH) test to probe limbic-hypothalamic-pituitary-adrenal(LHPA)-axis function(2). Following BL evaluation, all patients received a slow release preparation of 75 mg amitriptyline orally at bedtime for 42 days. Psychopathological, cognitive and neuroendocrine studies were repeated after weeks 1, 3 and 5 of active treatment.

RESULTS

86% of the pratients showed mild to moderate cognitive impairment during baseline (mean 28 ± 11, 96 to 139, Mattis dementia rating scale (DRS); normal: $\geq$ 140), which improved steadily during treatment to normal values in 58% of the patients. Another 10% of all patients clearly regained cognitive capacity, but fell short to reach DRS scores > 140, whereas 27% showed unchanged cognitive performance and 5% decreasing cognitive capacity during course of treatment. No significant relationship between severity of depression and degree of cognitive impairment was found.
Comparing DEX/CRH-test results of 6 depressed patients with 6 strictly age-matched controls revealed significantly higher basal plasma cortisol levels after dexamethasone (DEX) administration (61 ± 48 vs. 8 ± 6 ng/ml; $p < 0.02$) in patients, but undistinguishable CRH-stimulated cortisol release (net area: 9017 ± 5668 vs. 11965 ± 10235 ng x min/ml x 10^3). DEX-pretreated basal ACTH levels were almost double in depressives as compared to controls (21.2 ± 9 vs. 12.9 ± 3 pg/ml; $p < 0.05$), but CRH-stimulated ACTH release was similar in both groups. In the entire group of depressed patients, DEX-CRH-test results normalized during treatment (net area: 6100 ± 6000 at BL vs. 1275 ± 3000 ng x min/ml x 10^3 cortisol after 42 days of treatment; $p < 0.003$). 53% of the patients were considered responders (RES) and 47% non-responders (N-RES) to treatment. RES and N-RES did not differ in age (69 ± 7 vs. 74 ± 5 years), severity of depression 24 ± 4 vs. 26 ± 4 HDS-score) or cognitive impairment (127 ± 13 vs. 128 ± 15 DRS-score) at BL. However, DEX-pretreated basal cortisol levels (7.7 ± 4 vs. 36 ± 33 ng/ml; $p < 0.01$) and cortisol response

to CRH (net area: 3103 ± 4000 vs. 10000 ± 7150 ng x min/ml x 10^3; $p \leq 0.02$) were significantly higher in N-RES as compared to RES during BL. Among patients, multiple stepwise regression analysis revealed a significant impact of overall duration of illness upon CRH-induced cortisol and ACTH secretion, whereas age, severity of depression or degree of dementia had only minor effects upon DEX-CRH test results. In contrast, age and CRH-induced cortisol release correlated positively among the normal controls.

CONCLUSIONS

From these data we conclude that normal aging is associated with heightened LHPA-axis activity, probably reflecting cumulative effects of experienced stressful life events as they inevitably occur during one's life. Interestingly, in depressed patients, overall duration of depressive illness seems to override age effects on LHPA-axis function, suggesting that depression-prone individuals might have persistent yet subtle and may-be progressing LHPA-axis dysregulation even during psychopathological "remission". Although a high percentage of the studied patients had cognitive deficits, no statistically significant association between degree of dementia and LHPA-axis disturbances were found. Interestingly, neither severity of depression, degree of dementia nor age predicted beneficial effects of short-term antidepressive treatment, whereas degree of LHPA-axis disturbances did.

REFERENCES

1. Sapolsky, R.M., Krey, L.C., McEwen, B.S.: The neuroendocrinology of stress and aging: the glucocorticoid cascade hypothesis. Endocr. Rev. 7:284-301, 1986.
2. von Bardeleben, U., Holsboer, F.: Cortisol response to a combined dexamethasone-human corticotropin-releasing hormone challenge in patients with depression. J. Neuroendocrinol. 1:485-488, 1989.

PHARMACOKINETIC ASPECTS OF ANTIDEPRESSANT TREATMENT IN LATE LIFE

T.R. NORMAN and G.D. BURROWS
Department of Psychiatry, University of Melbourne Austin Hospital, Heidelberg, Victoria, AUSTRALIA.

Depression is a relatively common disorder in late life and is frequently treated with antidepressants. Both the tricyclic antidepressants and the newer agents have been evaluated in elderly populations in controlled studies. In general these medications are as effective in older patients as they are in younger subjects, but usually at lower dose ranges. Altered pharmacokinetics in the elderly is usually offered as the explanation for the lower dose requirements. While differences in antidepressant kinetics in the elderly have been demonstrated, changes in receptor sensitivity with ageing may also account for dose alterations. Testing of the pharmacodynamic hypothesis 'in vivo' is difficult and few studies have convincingly demonstrated changes in drug sensitivity with age [3].

PHYSIOLOGICAL CHANGES AFFECTING PHARMACOKINETICS

Changes in body composition and physiology with age potentially may alter drug pharmacokinetics. Although a number of alterations of gastrointestinal physiology occur with age, it has not been demonstrated that the absorption of drugs is impaired. Drug distribution may be affected by the ageing process. Lean body mass and total body water decrease with age but body fat increases [2]. Depending on the lipid or aqueous solubility of a drug the volume of distribution may be increased for highly lipid soluble compounds e.g., diazepam or decreased for water soluble substances e.g., paracetamol. Distribution of extensively protein bound drugs may also be influenced by the age-related decline in albumin concentrations. The activity of liver microsomal enzymes is reduced with age and some studies indicate an increase in plasma drug half-life [6]. Oxidative drug metabolism (i.e., demethylation and hydroxylation) are often impaired but glucuronide-conjugation is least affected [3]. The glomerular filtration rate declines with age. Drugs excreted by the kidneys without prior metabolism e.g., lithium persist at higher concentrations, for longer periods in the elderly.

ANTIDEPRESSANT PLASMA LEVELS AND AGE

Age as a factor influencing both single dose pharmacokinetic studies and steady-state concentrations of antidepressant drugs has been studied in recent years. Nies et al. [5] reported older patients treated with amitriptyline or imipramine developed higher steady state levels than younger patients. This was associated with decreased rates of elimination for imipramine treated subjects. Braithwaite et al [1] showed that amitriptyline and nortriptyline steady-state plasma concentrations were correlated with age. Single dose studies with these drugs showed decreased clearance and increased plasma half-life. More significantly there was much greater variability in the elderly than in younger subjects. Although the greater susceptibility of the elderly to the side effects of antidepressants is generally attributed to pharmacokinetic alterations this is not always apparent in clinical studies. Nelson et al [4] for example showed that major adverse reactions to desipramine treatment were higher in patients over 60 years old but plasma concentrations were not different from those under 60. The presence of concurrent medical illness may be more likely to predispose patients to side effects. Other studies also find no evidence of an association between age, elevated plasma concentrations and side effects. Nevertheless single dose studies in healthy elderly volunteers for both tricyclic antidepressants and the newer agents show decreased clearance and increased plasma elimination half-life.

Pharmacokinetics and steady-state plasma levels of antidepressants are likely to show much more variability in elderly than in younger patients. Factors such as race, sex, smoking status, the presence of somatic illnesses, co-administered prescription and non-prescription drugs are likely to contribute more to the observed variability than does age. Due to the large inter-individual variability in plasma levels, therapeutic drug monitoring can be useful in the elderly to avoid sub-therapeutic concentrations or toxic levels.

REFERENCES

1. Braithwaite, R.A., Montgomery, S.A. and Dawling, S. (1979) In Drugs and the Elderly, J. Crooks I.H. Stevenson, eds, pp 133-144, Macmillan Press, London.

2. Bruce, A. et al. (1980) Scand. J. Clin. Lab. Invest. 40:461-473.

3. Greenblatt, D.J., Sellers, E.M. and Shader, R.I. (1982) New Engl. J. Med. 306:1081-1088.

4. Nelson, J.C. et al. (1982) Arch. Gen. Psychiat. 39:1055-1061.

5. Nies, A. et al. (1977) Am. J. Psychiat. 134: 790-793.

6. Norman, T.R. et al. (1979) Med. J. Aust. 1:273-274.

MAO INHIBITORS, OLD AND NEW : SIMILARITIES AND DIFFERENCES

B.A. CALLINGHAM
Department of Pharmacology, University of Cambridge, Tennis Court Road, Cambridge, CB2 1QJ, U.K.

It is now more than thirty years since inhibitors of monoamine oxidase (MAO; EC 1.4.3.4) were first employed in the treatment of depression. Since that time these agents have had a chequered history. From the beginning there was concern about their safety. First, there was the toxicity of hydrazine-based agents and second, there were reports of hypertensive crises, which proved fatal in some patients, following the ingestion of food or drink containing sympathomimetic amines. Called the "cheese effect" as a result of tyramine-containing cheese being high on the list of culprit foods (1), this reaction acquired such a sinister reputation that patients and physicians alike lost confidence and turned towards alternative medication. While it is likely that these MAO inhibitors (MAOI) gained their unenviable reputation through the highly emotive impact of their bizarre toxicity, with proper dietary restrictions and care they could be very successful in the treatment of certain forms of depression (2). This coupled with the comparative lack of other side effects of these drugs has proved to be a powerful stimulus to the search for safe MAOI as antidepressants that do not need tiresome attention to what can, or cannot, be eaten or drunk. At first sight however, such a quest seems ill advised. MAO-A, which appears to be the target for the antidepressant action (3) is also found in the sympathetic nerve endings and in the gastrointestinal tract where it provides a defence against a wide range of endogenous and exogenous amines, many of which, including tyramine, possess substantial sympathomimetic activity (4). Thus any significant inhibition of MAO-A at these sites, in parallel with the therapeutic inhibition of the enzyme in the brain, ought, inevitably, to lead to the cheese effect.

IRREVERSIBLE (OLD) MAO INHIBITORS

Until recently, nearly all available MAOI, for clinical use as antidepressants, were suicide (mechanism-based or k_{cat}) inhibitors (5) leading to irreversible inhibition of both MAO-A and MAO-B, which would then require synthesis of new enzyme for recovery of catalytic activity. The oral administration of such inhibitors leads inevitably to the irreversible inhibition of the protective MAO of the gastrointestinal tract. This allows access of amines such as tyramine into the hepatic portal system and beyond, since any protection afforded by the liver would be dissipated as well. Thus, the poor esteem in which these MAOI are held, is due less to their shortcomings as antidepressants but more to fear of cardiovascular catastrophe. Pharmacologically, it could be reasoned that to combine an MAOI with a tricyclic antidepressant, which inhibits, *inter alia,* neuronal uptake of sympathomimetic amines, both directly, and indirectly-acting, would prevent or limit the cheese effect and enable use of the compounds with confidence. While this turns out largely to be the case, fear of drug interactions, real and imagined, has prevailed. Not all is bad news for irreversible inhibitors. The discovery that treatment of patients suffering from Parkinson's disease with *L*-dopa combined with selegiline (*l*-deprenyl; an irreversible inhibitor of MAO-B) improved the condition and prolonged life-span more than with *L*-

dopa alone (6), is most important since the cheese effect is absent as MAO is virtually unaffected.

REVERSIBLE (NEW) MAO INHIBITORS

For use as antidepressants however, a new strategy is required if MAOI are to have any future at all. This appears to have been realised through the development of competitive inhibitors of MAO. Although concurrent inhibition of MAO-B by a non-selective MAOI would not appear to be disadvantageous, most compounds that have been examined are selective for MAO-A. The effects of these compounds are concentration dependent and would be opposed by an ingested amine such as tyramine, greatly reducing the risk of any cheese reaction. Studies with the short acting MAO-A inhibitor, brofaromine (7), clearly demonstrate a close correlation between concentration of inhibitor and pressor response to administered amine. But, provided the concentration of reversible MAOI does not exceed $3 \times K_i$, any rise in blood pressure can be kept within acceptable limits (8). The short-acting and reversible MAOI, moclobemide, has been studied in great detail by Da Prada and his colleagues (9). While some potentiation of pressor responses to orally administered tyramine was seen in rats, it was much less than that seen with the irreversible MAOI, clorgyline. Moclobemide appears to increase in potency with time both *in vivo* and *in vitro*, which may be important in sparing the MAO of the gut even more than would be the case with a conventional competitive agent. A further advantage of this compound is the lack of antimuscarinic activity, which represents a substantial advantage over the extensively used tricyclic antidepressants. Indeed, it is suggested that a combination of moclobemide and a tricyclic could be efficacious (9). In short, moclobemide offers a promising new start in the life of MAOI.

REFERENCES

1. Da Prada, M. et al. (1988): On tyramine, food, beverages and the reversible MAO inhibitor moclobemide. J. Neural Transm. [Suppl] 26: 31-56.
2. Dowson, J.H. (1987): MAO inhibitors in mental disease: their current status. J. Neural Transm. [Suppl] 23:121-138.
3. Lipper, S. et al.(1979): Comparative behavioural effects of clorgyline and pargyline in man: a preliminary evaluation. Psychopharmacology, 62: 123-128.
4. Callingham, B.A. (1986): Some aspects of monoamine oxidase pharmacology. Cell Biochem. Function, 4: 99-108.
5. Da Prada, M., Kettler, R. and Cesura, A.M. (1988): Reversible enzyme-activated monoamine oxidase inhibitors: new advances. Pharmacol. Res. Commun. 20 (Suppl. IV): 212-33.
6. Riederer, P., Jellinger, K. and Seemann, D. (1984): Monoamine oxidase and parkinsonism: In Monoamine oxidase and disease. Prospects for therapy with reversible inhibitors, K.F. Tipton, P. Dostert and M. Strolin Benedetti, eds., pp. 403-415. Academic Press, London.
7. Bieck, P. et al. (1984): Tyramine pressor effects of CGP 11305A in comparison to tranylcypromine after prolonged treatment of human volunteers: In Monoamine oxidase and disease. Prospects for therapy with reversible inhibitors, K.F. Tipton, P. Dostert and M. Strolin Benedetti, eds, pp. 505-513. Academic Press, London.
8. Strolin Benedetti, M. et al. (1983): Intestinal metabolism of tyramine by both forms of monoamine oxidase in the rat. Biochem. Pharmacol, 32: 47-52.
9. Da Prada, M. et al. (1989): Pharmacological profile of moclobemide, a short-acting and reversible inhibitor of monoamine oxidase type A. J. Pharmacol. Exp. Ther., 248: 391-399.

PRECLINICAL PROFILE OF MOCLOBEMIDE

M. Da Prada
Pharmaceutical Research Department, F. Hoffmann-La Roche Ltd, CH-4002 Basel, Switzerland

Depressive disorders, for which new therapeutic agents with improved efficacy and with negligible side effects are needed, pose a challenge to pharmaceutical research. The new generation of reversible monoamine oxidase (MAO) inhibitors, which includes moclobemide (p-chloro-N-[2-morpholinoethyl]-benzamide, Ro 11-1163, Aurorix®), is an attempt to meet this challenge (2-5).

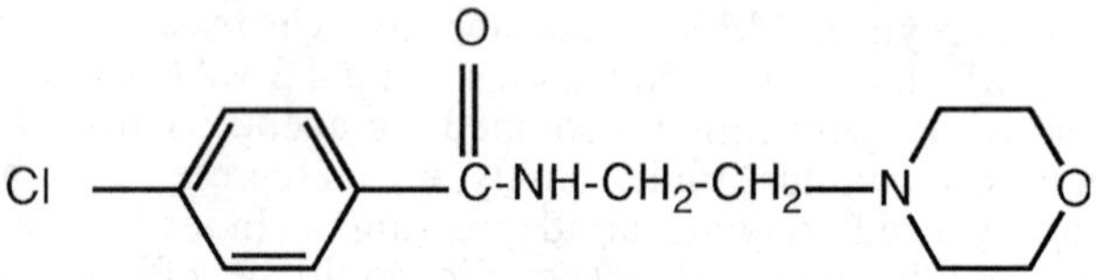

Fig. 1. Chemical structure of moclobemide

MAO exists in two functional enzymic forms, i.e. MAO-A and MAO-B, which as recently shown have different primary structures (1).The MAO-A isoenzyme preferentially deaminates 5-hydroxytryptamine (5-HT) and noradrenaline (NA) whereas the MAO-B isoenzyme prefers phenylethylamine (PEA) as substrate. This discovery stimulated the search for novel, reversible and selective MAO-A inhibitors, in an attempt to find new antidepressant compounds with much greater safety than the clinically available irreversible and non-selective inhibitors.

The characterization of moclobemide as a MAO A inhibitor is a classic example of serendipitous drug discovery. Moclobemide, initially synthesized as a potential lipid lowering agent, was then investigated because of its benzamide structure as a potential neuroleptic, to be finally identified as a reversible MAO-A inhibitor.

Moclobemide, a benzamide carrying a morpholine ring, bears no chemical relation to irreversible MAO inhibitors such as hydrazine derivatives (iproniazid, isocarboxazid, phenelzine), propargylamine derivatives (pargyline) or amino-cyclopropyl derivatives (tranylcypromine). Rat experiments show that moclobemide, in contrast to the irreversible MAO inhibitors phenelzine and tranylcypromine which produce long-lasting effects, increased the level of brain biogenic amines and decreased that of their main metabolites merely for 8-16 h (6). This indicates that moclobemide is short-acting. *In vitro* moclobemide seems to behave as a time-dependent (slow-binding) inhibitor since in tissue homogenates its inhibitory activity increases in parallel with the time of incubation. MAO-A inhibition induced by moclobemide in the rat brain *in vivo* is reversed by dialysis as well as by simple incubation at 37°C of the brain homogenates, indicating a relatively rapid dissociation of the inhibitor from the enzyme at physiological temperature. This prompt reversibility is a unique feature of moclobemide as compared to other short-acting or irreversible MAO inhibitors. In contrast to irreversible MAO inhibitors which are much more potent *in vitro* than *in vivo*, moclobemide is virtually equipotent in both conditions. Moclobemide does not inhibit other enzymes involved in the synthesis or in the catabolism of the biogenic amines (tyrosine hydroxylase and aromatic L-amino acid decarboxylase) and does not affect the uptake or the release of endogenous biogenic amines (2,3,5,6). In man, moclobemide acts as a selective MAO-A inhibitor and only affects to a minor extent platelet MAO-B activity (5). In the rat, a metabolite of moclobemide is formed which blocks MAO-B (4). It is important to stress that MAO inhibition is not synonymous with hepatotoxicity. Thus, moclobemide, due to its chemical structure, is not converted into isopropyl-hydrazine, the hepatotoxin which is suspected to induce liver necrosis after iproniazid, and in fact, experiments in rats show that moclobemide is completely devoid of hepatotoxic effects (7). In contrast to the clinically available irreversible inhibitors (e.g. tranylcypromine) moclobemide very weakly potentiates the pressor effects of orally administered tyramine (8).

In conclusion the reversible MAO-A inhibitor moclobemide, due to its neurochemical characteristics, belong to the so-called RIMA (**r**eversible **i**nhibitors of **m**onoamine oxidase type **A**) antidepressants (4). Moclobemide due to its well documented safety characteristics, to its lack of anticholinergic effects and to its good tolerability will provide an innovative tool for clarifying the role of MAO-A inhibitors in the treatment of endogenous as well as non-endogenous depressive states.

REFERENCES

1. Bach, A.W.J., Lan, N.C., Johnson, D.L. et al., (1988): Proc. Natl. Acad. Sci. USA, 85:4934-4938.
2. Burkard, W.P., Bonetti, E.P., Da Prada, M. et al., (1989): J. Pharmacol. Exp. Ther., 248:391-399.
3. Burrow, G.D., and Da Prada, M., (eds) (1989): Reversible MAO-A inhibitors as antidepressants. Basic advances and clinical perspectives. J. Neural Transm., [Suppl. 28].
4. Da Prada, M., Kettler, R., Burkard, W.P. et al., (1990): Acta Psych. Scand. Suplementum (in press).
5. Da Prada, M., Kettler, R., Keller, H.H. et al., (1989): J. Pharmacol. Exp. Ther., 248:400-414.
6. Priest R.G., (ed) (1989): Brit. J. Psych., 155, Supplementum 6.
7. Schläppi, B., (1985): Drug. Res., 35:800-803.
8. Youdim, M.B.H., Da Prada, M., and Amrein, R. (eds) (1988): J. Neural Transm. [Suppl. 26].

NEWER ASPECTS OF THE SELECTIVE, REVERSIBLE INHIBITOR OF MAO-A, BROFAROMINE

P.C. WALDMEIER, J. KRAETZ and L. MAITRE
Research Department, Pharmaceuticals Division, CIBA-GEIGY Ltd., CH-4002 BASLE, Switzerland

This contribution deals with two aspects of the new, reversible and selective inhibitor of monoamine oxidase A (MAO-A), brofaromine: the role of its serotonin (5-HT) uptake inhibiting properties [4] in its therapeutic effect, and with a safety issue, i.e. the interaction with sympathomimetic amines used in OTC medications [1].

There are not many alternatives to investigate 5-HT uptake inhibiting effects of drugs in humans. The most common consists in measuring 5-HT uptake or levels in thrombocytes ex vivo. However, this may yield misleading results because of an elevation of circulating 5-HT even in the case of a specific MAO-A inhibitor, even though thrombocytes themselves only contain MAO-B. This might be circumvented by studying the interaction with the binding of the 5-HT uptake inhibitor, ^{3}H-paroxetine [2,3], to human platelets under ex vivo conditions. As a feasibility study, we have therefore investigated the interaction of brofaromine with ^{3}H-paroxetine binding in human thrombocytes in vitro.

Interactions of MAO inhibitors have been reported with a number of drugs. While case reports of pharmacodynamic interactions with the sympathomimetic amines DL-phenylpropanolamine (PPA) and (+)-pseudoephedrine (PE) are relatively rare, the matter deserves attention because these agents are commonly used in OTC medications, e.g. as nasal decongestants[1]. We have therefore compared pressor and heart-rate responses to PPA and PE after brofaromine and phenelzine pretreatment in rats.

MATERIALS AND METHODS

^{3}H-Paroxetine binding in platelets: 50 µl ^{3}H-paroxetine (28.8 Ci/mmol, NEN, Boston, Mass.) in Tris-HCl buffer 0.15 M pH 7.5, 50 µl Tris-HCl buffer containing graded concentrations of brofaromine and imipramine, and 100 µl Tris-HCl buffer containing or not 10^{-4} M fluvoxamine to define specific binding, were added to 800 µl platelet—rich plasma (PRP) or a partly purified platelet preparation (PPPP). The latter was prepared by centrifugation of PRP at 1200 x g for 10 min and resuspension of the platelets in a buffer consisting of 0.05 M Tris-HCl buffer pH 7.5, 0.12 M NaCl and 0.005 M KCl. The final concentrations of ^{3}H-paroxetine were 1 nM with PRP and 0.5 nM with PPPP. The samples were incubated for 2 h at room temperature with occasional shaking and then centrifuged at 1200 x g for 10 min. The pellet was rinsed with 0.2 ml ice-cold Tris-HCl buffer and subsequently dissolved in 500 µl 0.1 M HCl, of which 400 µl were counted.

Pressor interactions with PPA and PE: Male Tif:RAIf(SPF) rats weighing 310 - 450 g were treated once daily for 4 days with 3 or 10 mg/kg p.o. brofaromine HCl (these doses correspond to 3 and 10 times the ED_{50} to inhibit rat brain MAO-A) or 5 or 15 mg/kg p.o. phenelzine sulphate (1 and 3 times the ED_{50}; with the higher dose, 4/9 rats died after surgery for haemodynamic experiments and with 50 mg/kg p.o., i.e. 10 times the ED_{50}, all rats died in the course of the treatment). Controls received solvent (H_2O). One h after the last treatment, rats were anesthetized with 90 mg/kg i.p. thiopentone sodium. The trachea was cannulated and the right carotid artery and the left jugular vein were catheterized for the measurement of arterial blood pressure and injection of PPA (cumulative doses of 0.01 - 1 mg/kg at 10 min intervals) and PE (single doses of 0.5 and 5 mg/kg, because of occurrence of tachyphylaxis). The injections were started about 30 - 45 min after completion of surgery, and pulsatile and mean arterial blood pressure (MAP), and heart rate (HR) were from the pulse-wave recorded on a Hellige recorder.

RESULTS AND DISCUSSION

^{3}H-Paroxetine binding in platelets: ^{3}H-paroxetine bound with an apparent K_D of 1.3 nM to human thrombocytes in PRP. In resuspended platelets (PPPP), the apparent K_D dropped to 0.23 nM.

In PRP, imipramine showed an IC_{50} of about 40 nM, which was not changed when incubation was with PPPP. On the other hand, brofaromine in PRP was completely ineffective up to 1 µM in PRP, but showed an IC_{50} of about 300 nM in PPPP. This difference seems to be due to a strong binding of this compound to plasma proteins (about 98 %), and in turn suggests that the 5-HT uptake inhibiting properties of brofaromine in humans cannot be investigated using this or any other technique related to blood platelets.

Pressor interactions with PPA and PE: Neither brofaromine at both doses nor phenelzine at 5 mg/kg daily affected basal MAP or HR. In the rats surviving 15 mg/kg daily, phenelzine lowered basal MAP (-34 mm Hg vs. controls), but not HR; this dose was therefore not included in the comparison. Pretreatment with brofaromine (3 and 10 mg/kg/day) and phenelzine (5 mg/kg/day) had no influence on the pressor and tachycardic responses to PPA (0.01 - 1 mg/kg i.v.; data not shown). On the other hand, pressor responses to 0.5 and 5 mg/kg i.v. PE were increased by both MAOI, more so by 10 mg/kg brofaromine than by its lower dose and by 5 mg/kg phenelzine (table 1). However, when compared in relation to the ED_{50} with respect to brain MAO-A inhibition, phenelzine was more potent to increase

Table 1 Effect of 4 once-daily treatments with brofaromine or phenelzine on the effects of single doses of PE on MAP and HR in anesthetized rats

	ΔMAP (mm Hg)		ΔHR (beats/min)	
	PE 0.5 mg/kg	PE 5 mg/kg	PE 0.5 mg/kg	PE 5 mg/kg
controls	10 ± 2 (4)	17 ± 1 (6)	36 ± 8 (4)	71 ± 2 (6)
brofaromine 4 x 3 mg/kg p.o.	15 ± 1 (3)	31 ± 7 (4)	45 ± 2 (3)	104 ± 8 (4)
brofaromine 4 x 10 mg/kg p.o.	21 ± 2 (4)	46 ± 7 (4)	56 ± 3 (4)	99 ± 17 (4)
phenelzine 4 x 5 mg/kg p.o.	22 ± 4 (4)	29 ± 5 (4)	66 ± 4 (4)	90 ± 7 (4)

Rats were subjected to surgery 1 h after the last MAOI treatment. PE was injected 30 - 45 min after completion of surgery. Data are means ± SEM. Numbers or animals are given in brackets.

the pressor effects of PE: its effects at 1 x ED_{50} were similar or greater than those of 3 x ED_{50} of brofaromine. The PE-induced tachycardia was increased to a similar extent by both MAOI (table 1).

Therefore, the risk of hypertensive reactions in response to treatment with medications containing PE is likely to be greater in patients treated with phenelzine than in those receiving brofaromine. Preparations containing PPA are less apt to interact with MAOI, probably because the pressor effects of this amine results from a direct stimulation of smooth-muscle α-adrenoceptors. PE, in contrast, acts through stimulation of catecholamine release.

REFERENCES

1. Decongestant, cough, and cold preparations (1986). In: AMA Drug Evaluations, K.F. Lampe, S. McVeigh, B.J. Rodgers (eds.). Am. Med. Assoc., Chicago, p. 372.
2. D'Haenen, H., De Waele, M. and Leysen, J.E. (1988): Psychiatry Res., 26: 11-17.
3. Mellerup, E.T., Plenge, P. and Engelstoft, M. (1983): Eur. J. Pharmacol., 96: 303-309.
4. Waldmeier, P.C. and Stöcklin, K. (1989): Eur. J. Pharmacol., 169: 197-204.

MOCLOBEMIDE: DRUG AND ALCOHOL INTERACTIONS
A.J. PUECH and I. BERLIN
Dpt of Clinical Pharmacology, Hôpital Pitié-Salpêtrière, Paris, France

Because of the apparition of selective and reversible monoamine oxidase inhibitors (MAOIs) the interactions of MAOIs with other drugs need to be reevaluated. The interactions of these new compounds with other drugs should be discussed in the light of present knowledge about irreversible and non-selective MAOIs-drug interactions in order to evaluate whether new MAOIs represent an advantage over classical MAOIs.

Interactions of moclobemide
Interaction with tyramine

Tyramine interaction of moclobemide and brofaromine has extensively been studied. We dispose published results with regard tyramine sensitivity after administration of oral tyramine in healthy subjects. The interaction of brofaromine with tyramine has been evaluated in two studies (1, 2), in the first one the reference drug was TCP, in the second one phenelzine. Tyramine sensitivity on moclobemide has been compared in a controlled study with TCP (3). Since in all three studies the measure of tyramine sensitivity was the tyramine threshold dose required to increase systolic BP by 30 mmHg, the results can be compared. Tyramine sensitivity was increased 56fold by TCP after an overnight fast or 38fold after meal (3). Brofaromine increased tyramine sensitivity only by a factor of 7-8.5 and moclobemide by a factor of 5. Phenelzine 30 mg/d had the same effect than moclobemide (600 mg/d), phenelzine 45/d as brofaromine (150 mg/d). The relative order of tyramine sensitivity seems to be moclobemide ^{2} brofaromine ^{2} phenelzine ^{2} TCP.

Interaction with sympathomimetics
The possible potentiating effect of moclobemide on phenylephrine induced BP increase was investigated in two open cross over studies. Single dose of 100 mg and repeated doses of 3x100 mg/d for a week moclobemide did not change phenylephrine induced BP increase. In contrast, a slight potentiation (1.6fold) of the phenylephrine pressor effect was observed at the end of a 21 days' treatment period with 3x200 mg/d moclobemide.

Interaction with alcohol
The interaction of alcohol-clomipramine and alcohol-moclobemide was compared in a double blind study in 24 young healthy subjects. With a blood alcohol concentration of 0.6 g/l no clear cut differences were observed between clomipramine (50 mg/d) and moclobemide (600 mg/d). In interaction with alcohol, clomipramine increased body sway and choice reaction time more than did moclobemide but it diminished alcohol induced memory impairment. The most important difference occured in adverse effects: subjects taking clomipramine had more adverse effects after alcohol ingestion than did subjects taking moclobemide.
In another study the possible interaction between alcohol and moclobemide (600 mg/d) were compared to that of alcohol-trazodone in

older subjects (mean age 66 yr). The effect of alcohol on psychometric performance and body sway were potentiated by trazodone but not by moclobemide.

Interaction with TCAs
The possible interaction of moclobemide with amitryptyline was investigated in an open study in 21 depressive patients. In this study moclobemide could be substituted by amitryptyline without a therapy free interval; the addition of amitryptyline to moclobemide and the combined moclobemide-amitryptyline therapy were well tolerated.

In another study in healthy volunteers, desipramine decreased tyramine sensitivity which was not modified by moclobemide co-administration.

Further evidences suggest that the switch from moclobemide to maprotiline, doxepin and mianserine and the long-term moclobemide-TCAs co-administration is safe and well tolerated.

Interaction with other psychotropic drugs
To our knowledge no prospective studies were conducted to assess the interaction of moclobemide with other psychotropic drugs although these will most probably be co-administered with moclobemide. Data originating from studies with moclobemide in which different psychotropic drugs were co-administered show that combined moclobemide-neuroleptic and moclobemide-lithium treatments may be safely given and that lithium did not interfere with moclobemide in terms of efficacy.

The co-administration of antiparkinsonian drugs with moclobemide is insufficiently documented. The safety/tolerability of BZD co-administration shows no specific adverse events but the therapeutical interest and efficacy were, to this time, not evaluated.

From these observations it cannot be concluded that there is no interaction between moclobemide and psychotropic drugs. Specific studies and larger observation period are needed to assess the presence or absence of potential interactions between moclobemide and other psychotropic drugs.

Interaction studies with non-psychotropic drugs
Specific studies were conducted to evaluate a possible interaction between moclobemide and phenprocoumon, digoxin, oral contraceptives, metoprolol, nifedipine, hydrochlorothiazide, glibenclamide and cimetidine. Positive results concerne metoprolol and cimetidine. On combined treatment of metoprolol and moclobemide BP was lower than on metoprolol alone, a similar potentiation of the BP reduction was not seen in the groups treated with nifedipine or hydrochlorothiazide. A clear pharmacokinetic interaction was found between cimetidine and moclobemide. Cimetidine prolonged elimination half-life of moclobemide, increased its maximal plasma concentration and AUC of about 100 %. Therefore, it is recommended if moclobemide is initiated in patients treated by cimetidine, to start with a low moclobemide dose and adapt it to clinical needs.

References:
1. Bieck PR et al.:J Clin Psychopharmacol 1988;8:237-45
2. Biek PR et al.:Clin Pharmacol Ther 1989; 45:260-9
3. Berlin I et al: Clin Pharmacol Ther 1989; 46:344-51

OVERVIEW OF CLINICAL INVESTIGATIONS WITH BROFAROMINE

J.A. SNAITH
Research & Development, Ciba-Geigy Ltd., Basle, Switzerland

Classical monoamine oxidase inhibitors (MAOI) are effective antidepressants, however, their usefulness is limited because of their irreversibility and lack of selectivity. Interaction with dietary tyramine or sympathomimatic drugs can produce rare but serious increases in blood pressure.

Brofaromine is a reversible, selective, inhibitor of MAO-A and is less liable to potentiate pressor responses to tyramine in man compared to classical MAOI (1). Initial dose finding trials indicated antidepressant effects in the dose range 100-150 mg/d (2). The efficacy and safety of brofaromine has been further evaluated in four separate, comparative trials versus imipramine (2 studies), tranylcypromine, and phenelzine.

PATIENTS AND METHODS

Patients were selected according to standardised criteria for all trials and were in-patients, (except in one trial versus imipramine) of either sex, aged 18-65 years, with a primary diagnosis of major affective disorders, according to DSM-III criteria. At two successive examinations, at least 3 days apart, patients scored at least 18 on the Hamilton Rating Scale for Depression (HRSD). Major exclusion criteria were: psychosis, rapid cycling bipolar disorder, obvious suicide risk, hypertenison and clinically relevant cerebrovascular, cardiovascular, hepatic or renal abnormalities.

Eligible patients were randomised double-blind to brofaromine 100-150 mg/d or comparator at the following dosages: imipramine, 100-150 mg/d; tranylcypromine, 20-30 mg/d; phenelzine, 45 mg/d.

Normally, treatment duration was for 6-8 weeks. No other psychotropic medication was allowed except of chloral hydrate or benzodiazepines for night-time sedation. The trials versus imipramine were performed without dietary restrictions.

Patients were evaluated every one or two weeks using HRSD and Zung or Van Zerssen self rating scales for depression. Volunteered adverse events, blood pressure, pulse and body weight were recorded at each visit. Routine laboratory measurements were performed at baseline and on at least one other occasion during the study.

RESULTS

More than 700 patients were randomised to treatment in the 4 studies. At the time of preparation of this abstract only the results of the first trial versus imipramine have been analysed and reported.

In this study, involving 241 patients, there were no significant differences in total reduction of HRSD between treatments, however, the number of patients achieving a reduction in HRSD of $\geq$ 50% was higher in the brofaromine group (61% vs 51% [p = 0.06]).

Overall 5% of patients in both treatment groups were withdrawn because of adverse events (AEs). Most commonly recorded AEs were
- brofaromine: dry mouth, 13%; sleep disturbance, 12%; nausea, 6%;
- imipramine: dry mouth, 24%; hyperhydrosis, 12%; sleep disturbance, 7%.

There were no significant effects on blood pressure, pulse, body weight or laboratory parameters during treatment with brofaromine

In conclusion, brofaromine was at least as effective as imipramine with fewer anticholinergic side effects. There were no hypertensive episodes sociated with its use in patients receiving unrestricted diet. The results of this and the other 3 studies will be presented in detail and discussed.

REFERENCES

1. Bieck, P.R. and Antonin, K.H., (1989):
   J. Neural. Transm. (Suppl.), 28:21-31.

2. Schiwy, W. et al., (1989):
   J. Neural. Trans. (Suppl.), 28:33-44.

CLINICAL OVERVIEW ON MOCLOBEMIDE

J.W.G. TILLER
Dept. of Psychiatry, University of Melbourne, Melbourne,
The Royal Melbourne Hospital, Victoria, 3050, Australia.

INTRODUCTION

Moclobemide is the first of the new class of reversible inhibitors of monoamine oxidase A (RIMAs) generally available for clinical use.

DOSAGE AND METABOLISM

Moclobemide is an effective antidepressant in doses of 300-600mg/day. It is rapidly and completely absorbed and rapidly metabolised in the liver (half-life 2-4 hours) with little change in metabolism after the first week of treatment. Excretion is 90% renal. Dosage and metabolism in the elderly is no different to that for younger adults.

PLACEBO CONTROLLED STUDIES

In four major double blind placebo controlled studies moclobemide reduced the Hamilton Depression Rating Scale (HDRS) by more than 50% in 62% of patients with endogenous depression (n=151) and 43% with non-endogenous depression (n=197) compared with 24% and 27% respectively for placebo.

COMPARISONS WITH TRICYCLICS AND OTHER ANTIDEPRESSANTS

In double blind comparisons with tricyclic antidepressants in 1070 patients there were no significant differences in effectiveness between moclobemide and the comparator drugs imipramine, desipramine, clomipramine and amitriptyline. Similar clinical efficacy was found for moclobemide and the irreversible non-selective MAOI tranylcypromine. However, moclobemide was better tolerated than tranylcypromine and relieves endogenous as well as non-endogenous depressions, unlike older MAOIs. Moclobemide had similar efficacy to the second generation antidepressants maprotiline, mianserin and nomifensine. In the elderly (>60 years) moclobemide is also effective in approximately 60% of depressions.

DIET AND TYRAMINE PRESSOR EFFECTS

In clinical use, there is no need for dietary restrictions with moclobemide for patients eating a normal balanced diet who take their moclobemide after meals. Most meals contain less than 50mg tyramine and its absorption is slowed by food. Nevertheless, patients should be advised to avoid large quantities of tyramine rich food (>100mg tyramine) while on moclobemide. Moclobemide increases the pressor effects of oral tyramine, on average, about 4.4 times (range 2.8-10) more than no treatment. This is only 0.13 times the enhancement caused by the traditional MAOIs like tranylcypromine, resulting in a greater safety margin.

DRUG INTERACTIONS

Because of its short duration of action, moclobemide is unlikely to significantly interfere with medicines used in emergencies. Tricyclic antidepressants can be substituted with no drug free interval between treatments. Of drugs likely to be taken concomitantly, there were no major interactions with alcohol, digoxin, phenprocoumon, hydrochlororthiazide, nifedipine or oral contraceptives. Metoprolol's antihypertensive actions were enhanced, and moclobemide clearance was reduced to 25% by cimetidine suggesting the need to, at least, halve moclobemide doses when co-administering cimetidine. Phenylephrine reactivity was unchanged at low doses of moclobemide but increased up to 1.8 times at 200mg tid of moclobemide. Phenylephrine is unlikely to reach significant pressor effect concentrations with recommended use as a nasal decongestant or mydriatic.

TOLERABILITY AND SAFETY

Moclobemide is well tolerated, with clinician ratings of very good/good given to 90% on moclobemide compared with 93% on placebo. It lacks anticholinergic effects, is better tolerated and has fewer effects on sleep than other antidepressants. Adverse effects were few and most occurred with similar frequencies to placebo. Those occurring more frequently with moclobemide included nausea (4.7%), insomnia (2.6%), increased anxiety (2.4%), dry mouth (2.3%), diarrhoea (2.1%) and constipation (2.0%). It has been taken in single doses up to 2000mg, in overdose, without fatality. In long term treatment, 358 patients completed a mean of 184 days treatment, with 107 patients treated for 10 months or longer. Tolerability was very good/good for 89% and no new adverse effects were reported which were not present in the initial treatment phase. Efficacy continued, with initial mean HDRS scores of 25.1 falling to 9.0 at six weeks and to between 5.0 and 6.5 after 5 months or longer.

SUMMARY

Overall, moclobemide appears to be a novel, safe, effective and well tolerated antidepressant providing a useful alternative to available treatments for depression.

REVERSIBLE MAO INHIBITORS IN COMPARISON TO ESTABLISHED ANTIDEPRESSANTS
R.L. Borison. Department of Psychiatry, Augusta VA Medical Center
and Medical College of Georgia, Augusta, Georgia, 30910, USA.

The reversible monamine oxidase inhibitors (MAOI), such as moclobemide, promise a new generation of therapeutic and safer agents in the treatment of depression. In clinical trials versus standard tricyclic antidepressants, moclobemide reduced the Hamilton Depression Rating Scale score by approximately 50%, which was equivalent to the therapeutic action of imipramine. Similarly, moclobemide was therapeutically equivalent to the irreversible MAOI tranylcypromine. In contrast, moclobemide demonstrates a side-effect profile which is superior to that of the tricyclic antidepressants. Anticholinergic side-effects, such as dry mouth, blurred vision, and constipation occur significantly more frequently with tricyclic antidepressant therapy. Furthermore, dizziness, sweating, and tremor were significantly less common side-effect with moclobemide treatment. Sedation was also a more common problem in the tricyclic treated group. In comparison with standard MAOI, moclobemide produces less hypotension, and does not produce the cheese reaction. It therefore appears that the reversible MAOI produce an antidepressant action on par with standard antidepressant treatments, but with significantly fewer side-effects.

SEROTONERGIC AND DOPAMINERGIC NEURONAL CHANGE, INCLUDING RECEPTOR CHANGES, AFTER CHRONIC LITHIUM

T.KOYAMA, Y.ODAGAKI, A.MURAKI and I.YAMASHITA
Department of Psychiatry, Hokkaido University School of Medicine, Sapporo, Japan

Lithium (Li) is currently well established as the most specific agent for the acute management and prophylaxis of affective disorders. However, despite nearly 40 years of widespread clinical use, the action mechanisms whereby Li exerts its psychotropic effects remain unclear. This presentation will summarize our recent research on the effects of Li treatment on serotonergic and dopaminergic neurones.

EFFECT OF LITHIUM TREATMENT ON SEROTONERGIC SYSTEM

In the terminal regions of various serotonergic neurones, maintenance of rats on a diet containing Li carbonate (0.23%) for 3,7 or 21 days resulted in a significant increase in the concentrations of tryptophan and 5-hydroxyindoleacetic acid (5-HIAA). When loaded with l-tryptophan (25mg/kg and 50mg/kg,i.p.), the concentrations of tryptophan and 5-HIAA in these brain regions were increased significantly by the Li treatment for 21 days. There was also a significant increase in the accumulation of 5-hydroxytryptophan (5-HTP) after the inhibition of the activity of aromatic l-amino acid decarboxylase with 3-hydroxybenzylhydrazine (NSD 1015, 100mg/kg), suggesting a possible enhancement of the serotonin (5-HT) synthesis and release due to an increase in the active uptake of tryptophan into the brain.

The inclusion of Li in the diet for 21 days led to a significant decrease in $5-HT_1$ receptor binding in the hippocampus, with no changes noted in $5-HT_1$ or $5-HT_2$ receptor binding in the cerebral cortex. It was confirmed that this reduction of Bmax value of the $5-HT_1$ receptor in the hippocampus was accompanied by no significant changes in both the adenylate cyclase activity and 8-hydroxy-2-(di-n-propylamine) tetralin (8-OH-DPAT)-induced hypothermic reaction, which coupled with $5-HT_{1A}$ receptor. The inhibition of forskoline-stimulated adenylate cyclase activity by 5-HT, which may be coupled with $5-HT_{1A}$ receptor, was not also changed by the long-term Li treatment for 21 days. Chronic lithium consumption resulted in a significant enhancement of the 5-HTP, quipazine or 5-Methoxy-N.N-Dimethyltryptamine (5-MeODMT)-

induced increase in the corticosterone secretion, which may be mediated by 5-HT$_2$ receptors. These results suggest that lithium treatment enhances the pre-and postsynaptic serotonergic activity, especially 5-HT$_2$ receptor mediated-biological function.

EFFECT OF LITHIUM TREATMENT ON DOPAMINERGIC SYSTEM

In the terminal regions of various dopaminergic neurones, dietary Li treatment for 3,7 or 21 days resulted in a significant increase in the in vivo accumulation of dihydroxyphenylalanine (DOPA) during 30 min after the injection of NSD 1015. There was also a significant increase in the concentrations of dopamine metabolites ; dihydroxyphenylacetic acid (DOPAC), homovanillic acid (HVA) and 3-methoxytyramine (3-MT), in these brain regions of rats given Li for 21 days when compared to control rats, suggesting a possible enhancement in the dopamine (DA) systhesis and release.

Futhermore, we investigated the effects of co-administration of Li and haloperidol or SCH 23390 on dopaminergic receptor-adenylate cyclase system in rat striatum. Long-term treatment of rats with haloperidol resulted in a siginificant increase in dopaminergic D$_2$ receptor binding. There was also a significant increase in dopaminergic D$_1$ receptor binding in the rats injected with SCH 23390 for 21 days. This up-regulation of dopaminergic D$_1$ or D$_2$ receptor was accompanied by the supersensitivity of DA-sensitive adenylate cylase system. Rats treated concurrently with Li and haloperidol or SCH 23390 faild to develop both the up-regulation and the supersensitization of dopaminergic D$_1$ or D$_2$ receptor. These results may be related, in part, to our finding that chronic Li treatment enhances the DA systhesis and release in the various brain regions including striatum ; i.e., the increase in the synaptic content of DA might counteract the receptor blockade by haloperidol or SCH 23390.

These results are suggestive that Li treatment enhances the presynaptic dopaminergic activity. Previously Koyama et al. (1) reported the Li-induced reduction of prolactin concentrations in serum and anterior pituitary glands, and the suppressed secretion of prolactin in vitro from anterior pituitary tissue. An icreased release of DA from tuberoinfundibular dopaminergic neurone may account for these findings.

REFERENCE

1. Koyama,T. et al. Lithium treatment enhances the activity of tuberoinfundibular and tuberohypophyseal dopaminergic neurons. Soc.Neurosci. Abstr. 11:658, 1985.

GABA RECEPTOR ALTERATIONS AFTER CHRONIC LITHIUM--IN COMPARISON WITH CARBAMAZEPINE AND SODIUM VALPROATE--

N. MOTOHASHI
Department of Neuropsychiatry, Yamanashi Medical College, Tamaho, Yamanashi, Japan

Gamma-aminobutyric acid (GABA) is one of the major inhibitory neurotransmitters in the mammalian central nervous system. The GABA hypothesis of affective disordes has been proposed for several reasons (3). Lithium has been widely used for the acute and prophylactic treatment of affective disorders. Recently, carbamazepine and sodium valproate have been reported to have potential therapeutic action in affective disorders. These three drugs are classified as mood stabilizers. Although they act on the cerebral GABAergic system, effects of these agens on GABA receptors have rarely been examined. I have now reported the influence of lithium, carbamazepine and sodium valproate on $GABA_A$ and $GABA_B$ receptors in rat brain.

MATERIALS AND METHOD

Male Wistar-Kyoto rats weighing between 200 and 250 g were used. [^{3}H]Muscimol (MUS) and [^{3}H](-)baclofen (BAC) were used to label $GABA_A$ and $GABA_B$ receptors, respectively. Lithium chloride (1.5 mEq/kg), carbamazepine (50 mg/kg) and sodium valproate (150 mg/kg) were injected i.p. once daily for 14 days. The rats were decapitated 24 h after the last injection and brain regions rapidly removed, frozen on dry ice and stored at -80°C up to the time of binding assays. Synaptic membranes were prepared according to Herschel and Baldessarini (2). [^{3}H]MUS binding to $GABA_A$ receptors and [^{3}H]BAC binding to $GABA_B$ receptors were performed by the methods of Herschel and Baldessarini (2) and Motohashi et al. (4), respectively. The final concentration of [^{3}H]MUS was 4 nM and that of [^{3}H]BAC, 10 nM.

RESULTS

Single treatment with lithium, carbamazepine or sodium valproate did not induce any change in $GABA_A$ and $GABA_B$ receptors in the frontal cortex, hippocampus and thalamus (data not shown). $GABA_B$ receptors were increased in the hippocampus following chronic treatment with either of these three drugs (Table 1). In the frontal cortex, thalamus and striatum, $GABA_B$ receptors did not change significantly (Table 1). Moreover, $GABA_A$ receptors were unchanged in any

Table 1: Effects of chronic lithium, carbamazepine and valproate on $GABA_A$ and $GABA_B$ receptors in rat brain. Results are expressed as mean±SEM (fmol/mg rotein) for 6-8 rats.

	Frontal cortex	Hippocampus	Thalamus	Striatum
$GABA_A$				
Control 1	487±12	239±20	971±45	310±24
Lithium	506±27	265±7	1080±64	328±15
Carbamazepine	503±14	258±9	1057±53	359±24
Control 2	490±19	256±9	1120±33	342±20
Valproate	558±31	282±17	1081±63	369±12
$GABA_B$				
Control 1	219±12	28±3	101±5	29±4
Lithium	201±10	40±3**	115±9	28±5
Carbamazepine	227±10	43±4**	104±2	28±2
Control 2	232±11	27±2	110±5	27±2
Valproate	277±19	37±3*	122±7	32±2

**: $p<0.01$ as compared to Control 1.
*: $p<0.05$ as compared to Control 2.

of the regions examined (Table 1).

DISCUSSION

The present findings demonstrate that chronic treatment with lithium, carbamazepine or sodium valproate increased hippocampal $GABA_B$ receptors. The results are in agreement with the previous report that all of these drugs decreased the turnover rate of GABA in mouse brain (1). One common mechanism of action of these mood stabilzers may be mediated by $GABA_B$ receptors in the hippocampus. Moreover, the results further support the view that GABA is involved in the pathophysiology of affecive disorders.

REFERENCES

1. Bernasconi, R. (1982): In Basic Mechanisms in the Action of Lithium, H.M. Emrich, J.B. Aidenhoff and H.D. Lux, eds., pp. 183-192. Excepta Medica, Amsterdam-Oxford-Princeton.
2. Herschel, M. and Baldessarini, R.J. (1979): Life Sci.,24: 1849-1854.
3. Motohashi, N. (1988): Jpn. J. Psychiat. Neurol., 42:869-870.
4. Motohashi, N., et al. (1989): Eur. J. Pharmacol., 166:95-99.

MECHANISMS OF LITHIUM IN MODULATION OF AMINERGIC RECEPTOR FUNCTIONS

Arne Geisler and Arne Mørk

Department of Pharmacology, University of Copenhagen, 20, Juliane Maries Vej, 2100 Copenhagen Ø, Denmark.

Very many clinical investigations, supported by the widespread therapeutic use of lithium, have demonstrated its effeciency as an antimanic drug and as a prophylatic agent against recurrent mood disorders, especially manic-depressive psychosis or bipolar mood disorders. Despite numerous experimental studies, trying to elucidate different cerebral processes, the mode of action of lithium is still unknown.

My colleagues and I have aimed to study the influence of lithium on the enzyme adenylate cyclase. The reason for this approach is that in some early studies we showed that chronic lithium treatment inhibits vasopressin-stimulated renal adenylate cyclase both ex vivo and in vivo. This effect may be the cause of lithium-induced polyuria.

Extensive research has revealed that the structure of the adenylate cyclase is complex. Thus, the adenylate cyclase system consists of three subunits. A stimulatory or inhibitory receptor at the outside of the cell membrane, a catalytic unit at its inner side; this part of the enzyme forms cyclic AMP from ATP. In between a so-called G-protein is localized, which transmits the neurotransmitter-receptor signal to the catalytic unit. There are both a stimulatory G-protein, termed Gs, and an inhibitory protein-Gi. The activity of the adenylate cyclase is regulated by GTP, magnesium and calcium-calmodulin. We - and other researchers - have demonstrated that lithium in vivo and ex vivo, i.e. after chronic treatment inhibits stimulated activities of the enzyme in various brain regions, for example the cortex, the striatum, and the limbic system. We assume that lithium may have two effects on the adenylate cyclase system. The first effect may be an "in situ" effect, i.e. the effect of lithium in the brain during treatment, which may be similar to the in vitro effect of lithium, and a second effect caused by the chronic influence of lithium on the enzyme itself or proteins or other enzymes by which it may indirectly be modulated - e.g. the phosphoinositide system.

It is possible to activate the single subunits of adenylate cyclase. Studies of the influence of lithium in vivo have shown that lithium inhibits norepinephrine-stimulated cyclic AMP formation in various brain regions, including cerebral cortex and the dopamine-stimulated adenylate cyclase in the striatum - both in the rat and in the human brain. Further, lithium in vivo inhibits GTP and Gpp (NH)p as well as fluoride-stimulated cyclic AMP formation. Finally lithium in vivo inhibits forskolin, Ca^{2+}-CaM and Mn^{2+}-CaM activities by an influence on the catalytic subunit. It is likely that the effect of lithium in vivo or in situ is an antagonizing influence on the stimulation of magnesium.

The effect of lithium ex vivo, i.e. after chronic lithium treatment giving serum levels about 0.7 mM Li^+ is an inhibition of norepinephrine cyclic AMP formation, while serotonin-stimulated cyclic AMP synthesis is increased. Lithium ex vivo inhibits stimulation via the G-protein and the catalytic subunit.

However, it should be emphazised that the mode of action of lithium is still unknown, but studies on the mechanism by which lithium influences neurotransmitter effects may be of significance in the search for the basis of the therapeutic effect of lithium and thereby the neurobiological dysfunction underlying abnormal mood swings.

INTRACEREBROVENTRICULAR INOSITOL DOES NOT REVERSE HIGH DOSE LITHIUM TOXICITY IN RATS.

O. KOFMAN* & R.H. BELMAKER
Beer-Sheva Mental Health Center, Ben-Gurion University,
P.O.B. 4600, Beer-Sheva, Israel.

Lithium is a therapeutic mainstay of bipolar affective disorder, yet the pharmacological basis of its therapeutic and prophylactic action is unclear. Lithium has a narrow therapeutic index, and at high doses may cause a variety of central and peripheral toxic effects. Several mechanisms of action have been suggested for the therapeutic effect of lithium. Lithium inhibits the increase in noradrenergic agonist-stimulation of cyclic AMP accumulation in the brain (4), an effect which may be explained by its inhibition of G-protein binding stimulated by muscarinic and adrenergic agonists (2). Lithium also reduces brain levels of myo-inositol in rats by inhibiting the dephosphorylation of two inositol lipids: inositol monophosphate and Ins (1,4) P_2, thereby reducing the pool of myo-inositol available for resynthesis of the critical inositol lipids (1, 7, 8). In rats, 10 meq/kg LiCl reduced cortical myo-inositol levels by 30-35% and increased inositol monophosphate levels 20 fold after 6 hr and 40 fold after 24 hr (1, 7).

In vitro, inositol (10 mM) reversed lithium inhibition of agonist-stimulated insulin release in pancreas islet cells (9), and lithium-induced accumulation of CMP-phosphatidate in rat cortical slices following stimulation by carbachol (5). Myo-, but not epi-inositol attenuated the teratogenic effects of lithium in frog embryos (3).

Kaplan et al. (6) unsuccessfully attempted to reverse the toxic effects of lithium (35 meq/kg) by intraperitoneal injection of myo-inositol or forskolin. Mice were injected with either one or multiple doses of forskolin (6 or 12 mg/kg) or myoinositol (0.5, 1.0, 1.5, or 2 gm/mouse) intraperitoneally. Neither drug attenuated the toxic effects of lithium.

Since inositol crosses the blood brain barrier poorly, the following study examined the effect of intracerebroventricular (icv) injections of myo-inositol (INOSITOL) on hypoactivity induced by a high doses (10meq/kg) of lithium chloride (LiCl).

Male Charles-River rats (250-350 gm) were anesthetized and implanted with guide cannulae into the dorsal part of the third ventricle using standard stereotaxic procedures. To examine the effects of inositol on LiCl-induced suppression of motor activity, rats were divided into four groups: NaCl-VEHICLE (n=5), LiCl-VEHICLE (n=6), NaCl-INOSITOL (n=4), or LiCl-INOSITOL (n=4). Rats were injected with either 10 meq/kg LiCl or 10 meq/kg NaCl in a volume of 10 cc/300 gm body weight. Twenty four hours later, rats were injected icv with vehicle (artificial CSF) or 10 mg inositol in vehicle, and 15 minutes later placed in a photocell activity monitor (Columbus Opto-varimax). Rearing, ambulatory and total activity were automatically monitored for a period of 30 min. Cannula placement was confirmed by injecting the rats intracranially with cell dye, perfusing them intra-cardially with 10% formalin and examining the site of the cannula tip and spread of the dye throughout the ventricular system.

LiCl significantly reduced all measures of activity in rats treated with vehicle or inositol (Table I). Inositol significantly reduced rearing activity, but did not significantly affect ambulatory or total activity. Separate one-way analyses of variance were performed between the groups that received icv injections of vehicle or inositol for NaCl- and LiCl- treated animals. Inositol significantly reduced rearing in the NaCl ($F(1,7)= 7.949$, $p=.025$), but not in the LiCl rats. There were no significant interactions on any of the activity measures, indicating that inositol does not mitigate or reverse LiCl-induced hypoactivity. These results contrast with the ability of inositol to reverse depression of rearing induced by a lower dose of lithium (5 meq/kg) (Kofman et al., unpublished) and could suggest a different mechanism of action for high dose LiCl toxicity than for behavioural effects of low doses.

Table I. Effects of icv inositol on activity following systemic NaCl or LiCl. (Mean+ S.D.)

	ICV/ip	CSF	INOSITOL
Total Activity	NaCl	4590 ± 725	3652.25 ± 1036
	LiCl	3013 ± 1294	2538.5 ± 470.2
	Lithium main effect: $F(1,15) = 7.015$, $p=.017$		
Ambulatory Activity	NaCl	2909.2 ± 637	2265 ± 734
	LiCl	1970 ± 965	1532 ± 500.8
	Lithium main effect: $F(1,15) = 4.44$, $p=.05$		
Vertical Activity	NaCl	751.4 ± 137.4	386.5 ± 203
	LiCl	270 ± 187.6	235 ± 84
	Lithium main effect: $F(1,15)=13.857$, $p=.002$		
	Inositol main effect: $F(1,15)=5.532$, $p=.031$		

1. Allison et al., (1976) Biochem. Biophys. Res. Comm. 71:664-670.
2. Avissar et al., (1988) Nature 331:440-442.
3. Busa and Gimlich (1989) Developmental Biol. 132:315-324.
4. Ebstein et al., (1980) J. Pharm. Exp. Ther. 213:161-167.
5. Godfrey, P.P. (1989) Biochem. J. 258:621-624.
6. Kaplan et al., (1988) J. Neural Transm. 72:167-170.
7. Sherman et al.,(1981) J. Neurochem. 36:1947-1951.
8. Sherman et al.,(1985) J. Neurochem. 44:798-807.
9. Zawalich et al., (1989) Biochem. J. 262:557-561.

*Supported by the Israel Institute for Psychobiology Grant 31-89.

AUGMENTATION OF 5-HT NEUROTRANSMISSION BY LITHIUM

C. de Montigny and P. Blier
Neurobiological Psychiatry Unit, Department of Psychiatry, McGill University, Montréal, Québec, CANADA H3A 1A1

Using a behavioral paradigm in the rat, Grahame-Smith and Green had concluded that lithium, at "therapeutic" plasma levels, enhanced the function of 5-HT neurons (7). We devised an electrophysiological in vivo paradigm whereby the efficacy of the 5-HT synapse can be assessed in the rat. It consists of electrically stimulating the ascending 5-HT pathway while recording from postsynaptic neurons in the dorsal hippocampus. In this paradigm, it was found that short-term lithium, resulting in plasma levels of 0.4-1.1 mEq/L, enhanced the efficacy of the stimulation of the ascending 5-HT pathway (1). The 5-HT nature of this effect was ascertained by showing that prior lesionning of 5-HT neurons with the neurotoxin 5,7-dihydroxytryptamine virtually abolished the effect of the stimulation and that lithium had no effect in these rats. That the enhancement of the efficacy of the stimulation by lithium was indeed attributable to a presynaptic effect of lithium was suggested by the observation that the responsiveness of the same neurons to the microiontophoretic application of 5-HT and of the selective 5-HT$_{1A}$ agonist 8-OH-DPAT was not modified (1). Furthermore, the mean firing activity of dorsal raphe 5-HT neurons was unchanged in lithium-treated rats, as previously observed by Sheard and Aghajanian (11). Hence, it was concluded that short-term lithium treatment results in a net enhancement of 5-HT neurotransmission. This effect of lithium appeared not to be attributable to a desensitization of terminal 5-HT autoreceptors, as the function of these autoreceptors, assessed electrophysiologically, was unaltered in lithium-treated rats. Rather, it might be attributable to an increased synthesis of 5-HT (4,9) and/or to an increase of the releasable pool of 5-HT (12).

In a more recent series of experiments, we have documented a sensitization of a sub-set of 5-HT$_{1A}$ postsynaptic receptors by short-term lithium (2). This conclusion was reached from the observation that the efficacy of systemic injection of 8-OH-DPAT in depressing the firing activity of dorsal raphe 5-HT neurons was enhanced by a short-term lithium treatment. That this was not due to an increased sensitivity of somatodendritic 5-HT$_{1A}$ receptors was ascertained by showing that the responsiveness of dorsal raphe 5-HT neurons to microiontophoretically-applied 5-HT, LSD and 8-OH-DPAT, and also to the systemic injection of LSD was not modified. Hence, consistent with the finding that the effect of intravenous 8-OH-DPAT on the firing activity of dorsal raphe 5-HT neurons was not modified in the presence of a desensitization of the somatodendritic 5-HT$_{1A}$ receptor of these neurons following long-term administration of a 5-HT$_{1A}$ agonist (3), it is proposed that the effect of systemic 8-OH-DPAT on dorsal raphe 5-HT neuron firing activity is mediated by a sub-set of postsynaptic 5-HT$_{1A}$ receptors presumably located on neurons which are part of a transneuronal negative feedback loop controlling the firing activity of these neurons.

Hence, it would appear that lithium exerts an enhancing effect both on 5-HT neurons themselves and on some postsynaptic 5-HT$_{1A}$ receptors. Whether only one of these effects or both underlie the efficacy of lithium addition in treatment-refractory depression (5,6,8,10) remains to be determined.

REFERENCES

1. Blier, P. and de Montigny, C.: Short-term lithium administration enhances serotonergic neurotransmission: Electrophysiological evidence in the rat CNS. Eur. J. Pharmacol. 113:69-77, 1985.
2. Blier, P. and de Montigny, C.: Short-term lithium treatment enhances responsiveness of postsynaptic 5-HT$_{1A}$ receptors without altering 5-HT autoreceptor sensitivity. Synapse 1:225-232, 1987.
3. Blier, P. and de Montigny, C.: Modification of 5-HT neuron properties by sustained administration of the 5-HT$_{1A}$ agonist gepirone: electrophysiological studies in the rat brain. Synapse 1:470-480, 1987.
4. Broderick, P. and Lynch, V.: Behavioral and biochemical changes induced by lithium and L-tryptophan in muricidal rats. Neuropharmacology 21:671-679. 1982.
5. de Montigny, C., Cournoyer, G., Morissette, R. et al.: Lithium carbonate addition in tricyclic antidepressant-resistant unipolar depression. Arch. Gen. Psychiat. 40:1327-1334, 1983.
6. de Montigny, C., Grunberg, F., Mayer, A. et al.: Lithium induces rapid relief of depression in tricyclic antidepressant drug non-responders. Br. J. Psychiat. 138:252-256 1981.
7. Grahame-Smith, D.G. and Green, A.R.: The role of brain 5-hydroxytryptamine in the hyperactivity produced in rats by lithium and monoamine oxidase inhibition. Br. J. Pharmacol. 52:19-26, 1974.
8. Heninger, G.R., Charney, D.S. and Sternberg, D.E.: Lithium carbonate augmentation of antidepressant treatment. Arch. Gen. Psychiat. 40:1335-1342, 1983.
9. Knapp, S. and Mandell, A.J.: Effects of lithium chloride on parameters of biosynthetic capacity for 5-hydroxytryptamine in rat brain. J. Pharmacol. Exp. Ther. 193: 812-823, 1975.
10. Nelson, J.C. and Byck, R.: Rapid response to lithium in phenelzine nonresponders. Br. J. Psychiat. 141:85-86, 1982.
11. Sheard, M.H. and Aghajanian, G.K.: Neuronally activated metabolism of brain serotonin: effect of lithium. Life Sci. 9:285-290, 1970.
12. Treiser, S.L., Cascio, C.S., O'Donohue, T.L. et al.: Lithium increases serotonin release and decreases serotonin receptors in the hippocampus. Science 213: 1529-1531, 1981.

POTENTIAL TARGETS FOR THE ACTION OF LITHIUM IN THE BRAIN:
MUSCARINIC RECEPTOR REGULATION

R.H. LENOX and J. ELLIS
Neuroscience Research Unit, Department of Psychiatry, University of
Vermont, College of Medicine, Burlington, Vermont 05405

INTRODUCTION

Accumulating evidence from our laboratory and others suggests that muscarinic receptor regulation in the hippocampus may be a site for the action of chronic lithium in the brain. Clinical as well as basic studies have indicated a role for changes in the relative activity of the central muscarinic system in the evolution of affective illness (3). Muscarinic receptors in the hippocampus are coupled to the generation of phosphoinositide - derived second messengers, i.e. inositol 1,4,5-trisphosphate (IP_3) and diacylglycerol; and data from our laboratory have demonstrated that this response will desensitize in hippocampal slices preexposed to carbachol (4). Lithium effectively blocks the breakdown of IP_3 by inhibiting the conversion of inositol monophosphate (IP) to inositol, which may significantly affect the regeneration of critical pools of phosphoinositide 4,5-bisphosphate required for the elaboration of the second messengers (2). It is also of note that the accumulation of IP in the brain following lithium administration can be blocked by the presence of the muscarinic antagonist, atropine (1). These data suggest that the muscarinic receptor in the hippocampus might be predisposed to an interaction with lithium, and our investigations have focussed upon the effects of chronic lithium on the dynamic regulation of receptors and their coupling to the second messenger response.

RESULTS and DISCUSSION

Groups of rats were exposed to chronic lithium per diet for a period of 3 weeks during which time the concentration of lithium in their brain was approximately 0.72 meq/kg tissue. During the third week groups of animals received either atropine (10 mg/kg/day) or saline subcutaneously via implanted osmotic minipumps. Twenty-four hours after removal of the pumps, preparations of hippocampal slices and membranes were prepared for determination of muscarinic receptor binding studies and carbachol stimulated IP response. Up regulation of muscarinic receptor binding sites occurred in the hippocampus following chronic atropine in both control and lithium treated animals (Table 1). Chronic atropine did not alter the proportion of muscarinic receptor subtypes. While the control animals demonstrated an associated increase in the carbachol stimulated IP response in hippocampal slices, the chronic lithium animals showed no evidence for an atropine induced supersensitivity. These data suggest that chronic lithium did not alter the appearance of new receptor binding sites but in some way altered the coupling of these muscarinic sites to the IP second messenger response.

TABLE 1: MUSCARINIC RECEPTOR BINDING AND RESPONSE IN HIPPOCAMPUS

Specific Binding of $[^3H]QNB$ (1nM) (% of Control)   Carbachol (1mM) Stimulated IP Response (% of Control)

	Hippocampus	Hippocampus
Lithium	105 ± 5.7	114 ± 15
Atropine	125 ± 5.4*	131 ± 8*
Lithium & Atropine	120 ± 6.0*	101 ± 10

* significantly different than Control p<.01

Since muscarinic receptors have been shown to be coupled to the IP response through a guanine nucleotide binding (G) protein, we examined the possibility that lithium might alter the activity of the receptor-G protein complex. Membranes were prepared from control and lithium treated animals, and the effect of GTP analogs to alter the binding of agonist to the receptor site was examined. Conversely, other studies were carried out to examine the effect of lithium on agonist induced release of GTP$\gamma[^{35}S]$ from G proteins. These studies were carried out with membranes from several tissues, including: brain, heart, platelet and cell lines. We did not observe any effect of lithium, either in vitro or by chronic administration in vivo, on these receptor-G protein interactions. It appears likely that the effect of lithium in preventing sensitization of the muscarinic PI response is a result of more complex interactions, possibly through indirect changes in the regulation of protein kinase C mediated phosphorylation of protein substrates.

REFERENCES

1. Allison, J.H., Blisner, M.E.: Inhibition of the effect of lithium on brain inositol by atropine and scopolamine. Biochem. Biophys. Res. Commun. 68:1332-1338, 1976.
2. Berridge, M.J., Downes, P.C. and Hanley, M.R.: Neural and Developmental Actions of Lithium: a unifying hypothesis. Cell. 59:411-419, 1989.
3. Dilsaver, S.C. and Coffman, J.A.: Cholinergic hypothesis of depression: a reappraisal. J. Clin. Psychopharmacol. 9:173-179, 1989.
4. Lenox, R.H., Hendley, D. and Ellis, J. Desensitization of muscarinic receptor coupled phosphoinositide hydrolysis in rat hippocampus: comparisons with the alpha 1 adrenergic response. J. Neurochem. 50:558-564. 1988.

ORGANIZATION AND PLASTICITY OF EXCITATORY AMINO ACID RECEPTORS IN THE RODENT AND HUMAN BRAIN

C. W. COTMAN*, J.W. GEDDES**, and J. ULAS*
Department of Psychobiology* and Division of Neurosurgery**, University of California, Irvine, CA, U.S.A.

Recent evidence indicates that an excitatory amino acid (EAA) is the major neurotransmitter in the CNS. EAAs interact with at least five specific membrane receptors to elicit two types of responses: One response involves the operation of ion channels directly linked to the EAA receptor. The other response is linked to the generation of second messengers via the breakdown of phosphatidylinositol biphosphate (PI). The ionophore-activating receptors separate into different subtypes based on the relative specificities of agonists in electrophysiological experiments. The three main subtypes are known as N-methyl-D-aspartate (NMDA), kainic acid (KA), and α-amino-3-hydroxy-5-methylisooxazole-4-propionic acid (AMPA). The AMPA receptor has also been called the quisqualic acid (QA) receptor. However, as QA has the ability to act at other receptors (KA, NMDA, and the PI-linked receptor), the receptor is more appropriately called the AMPA receptor. A fourth receptor has also been identified by the action of 2-amino-4-phosphonobutyric acid (AP4) and appears to represent an inhibitory autoreceptor.

The PI-linked receptor can be distinguished pharmacologically from the ionotropic receptors. Various glutamate agonists function as agonists for this receptor, with the most potent agonists being trans-aminocyclopentane dicarboxylic acid (ACPD), ibotenic acid (IBO), and QA. The most specific agonist is ACPD, with IBO and QA having affinity for the ionotropic receptors NMDA, KA, and AMPA. This receptor linked to PI metabolism that is stimulated by QA does not correspond to the ionotropic receptor. In addition to various receptors there are various transport systems that remove glutamate. A key question concerns the organizational, functional role and the plasticity of these systems.

RESULTS AND DISCUSSION

NMDA-displaceable [^{3}H]L-glutamate binding sites are found throughout the brain but predominantly within the telencephalon. The highest levels in the entire brain are found in strata oriens and radiatum of the hippocampal area CA1. Most of area CA3 and dentate gyrus have moderate levels, where as the mossy fiber termination zone (stratum lucidum) is quite low in NMDA receptors. The human hippocampus has a similar distribution of NMDA sites; the CA1 region, Sommer's sector, contains the highest density of sites.

It is significant that the highest levels of binding are found in CA1 fields, because long-term potentiation (LTP) in this region has been shown to involve NMDA receptors. In contrast to area CA1, LTP in the mossy fiber system is insensitive to NMDA antagonists, as might be predicted by the low density of NMDA sites observed by autoradiography. Thus, receptor patterns appear to predict function.

Brain regions that are sensitive to excitotoxicity exhibit particularly high densities of NMDA receptors. Furthermore, this vulnerability should also be dependent on the amount of glutamate present, the level of which is regulated, in part, by glutamate transport.

Autoradiographic studies of glutamate uptake sites indicated heterogeneity and differential distributions, both of which should affect excitotoxic vulnerability. Area CA1 of the hippocampus, for example, which is particularly sensitive to excitotoxic injury, exhibits a high density of receptors but a low density of transport sites. In contrast, the molecular layer of the dentate gyrus, which is less sensitive to excitotoxicity, has high densities of both receptors and transport sites. Thus, each component of the excitatory transmission systems, including ligand, regulatory, and transport sites, must be analyzed mutually to properly evaluate excitotoxic vulnerability.

The response of NMDA and kainate receptors to deafferentation and subsequent reinnervation following unilateral entorhinal cortex lesions was studied in the rat hippocampus using quantitative *in vitro* autoradiography. The first changes in KA receptor distribution were observed 21 days postlesion when the dense band of KA receptors occupying the inner one-third of the molecular layer expanded into the denervated outer two-thirds of the ipsilateral molecular layer. The spreading of the KA receptor field into previously unoccupied zones continued 30 and 60 days postlesion. At these time points, the zone enriched in [^{3}H]KA binding sites became significantly (on average 50%) wider than in unoperated controls. No changes were observed in either the distribution or binding levels in other hippocampal areas or in the contralateral hippocampus at any studied time point. The pattern of KA receptor distribution was similar to the well-characterized pattern of sprouting of commissural/associational systems from the inner one-third into the outer two-thirds of the molecular layer after entorhinal lesions.

The pattern of changes in hippocampal KA receptors following the loss of the entorhinal input differs from the time course of responses reported for NMDA and quisqualate receptors in the same experimental model. The distinct responses of the various EAA receptors are evident especially during the early postlesion days: At this time point, the binding levels of KA receptors in the deafferented molecular layer on the operated side remain unchanged, whereas binding levels of quisqualate (and to a lesser degree, NMDA) receptors are diminished. Thirty to 60 days postlesion, the KA, NMDA, and quisqualate receptors respond in a more uniform pattern. Elevated KA receptor levels in the ipsilateral molecular layer are similar to those found for NMDA receptors in the outer two-thirds of the ipsilateral dentate gyrus molecular layer; increases in the binding to quisqualate receptors are of smaller magnitude. NMDA and quisqualate receptors change bilaterally at long post-lesion times. Changes in KA receptor binding are found only in the ipsilateral molecular layer. This implies that although related to the same neurotransmitter(s), the EAA receptors in the molecular layer of the hippocampus are differentially regulated in response to the loss of the entorhinal projection and to the subsequent circuit reorganization.

REFERENCES

1. Anderson, K.J., et al. Autoradiographic characterization of putative excitatory amino acid transport sites. Neuroscience, (in press).

2. Cotman, C.W., et al. The role of the NMDA receptor in central nervous system plasticity and pathology. J. NIH Res., 1: 65-74, 1989.

3. Ulas, J., Monaghan, D., Cotman, C. Plastic response of hippocampal excitatory amino acid receptors to deafferentation and reinnervation. Neuroscience, 34: 9-17, 1990.

4. Ulas, J., Monaghan, D.T., and Cotman, C.W. Kainate receptors in the rat hippocampus: A distribution and time course of changes in response to unilateral lesions of the entorhinal cortex. J. Neurosci., (in press).

THE GLUTAMATE RECEPTOR GENE FAMILY

Heinemann, S., Bettler, B., Boulter,J., Deneris, E., Duvoisin,R., Gasic, G., Hartley, M., Hermans-Borgmeyer, I., Hollmann, M., Johnson,D., O' Shea-Greenfield, A., Papke, R. and Rogers, S. Molecular Neurobiology Laboratory, The Salk Institute P.O. Box 85800 San Diego, California 92138.

The glutamate receptor system is thought to be involved in the first steps of learning and memory acquisition and is perhaps the most important excitatory receptor system in the mammalian brain. We have used an expression cloning approach to identify a family of glutamate receptor genes. One gene that we have called GluR K1 codes for a functional glutamate receptor of the kainate subtype. The primary structure and the physiology of the GluR K1 glutamate receptor indicates that it is a member of the ligand-gated channel family, Hollmann,M., O' Shea-Greenfield, A., Rogers, S.W. and Heinemann, S., Nature **342** 643-648 (1989). Four additional genes that code for proteins with sequence homology to the GluR K1 glutamate receptor have been identified. Two of these genes code for functional glutamate receptors. In situ hybridization data suggest that the genes code for different glutamate receptors that are expressed in specific brain regions.

The GluR K1 glutamate receptor protein has been expressed in bacteria and the protein used to immunize rabbits. Antisera from rabbits immunized with the GluR K1 glutamate receptor protein recognize brain proteins of about 107 kd. This is close to the predicted size of the protein encoded by the GluR K1 cDNA. The antisera detects the 107 kd protein at high levels in the hippocampus and at moderate levels in the cortex, midbrain and cerebellum. No detectable antigen was seen in either the brainstem or liver. The 107 kd protein is shown to be present in the post-synaptic membrane and it is a glycoprotein.

The Rat-2 cell line has been engineered by transfection to express the GluR K1 glutamate receptor and as expected these cells produce the 107 kd antigen. The transfected Rat-2 cell lines are being used to study the effects of glutamate on cytotoxicity.

GLUTAMATE CHANNEL KINETICS UNDERLIE THE SLOW EPSC IN HIPPOCAMPAL NEURONS.

G.L. Westbrook, R.A.J. Lester, J.D. Clements and C.E Jahr
Vollum Institute, Oregon Health Sciences University, Portland, OR, U.S.A.

Recent studies of central excitatory synapses in vertebrates have revealed a number of important differences from the classical model of excitatory neurotransmission, the neuromuscular junction. These differences reflect the great potential for modulation of synaptic efficacy at excitatory amino acid-mediated pathways in the CNS. Synaptic release of L-glutamate generates an excitatory postsynaptic current (epsc) in many central neurons resulting from activation of non-NMDA and NMDA receptors which appear to be colocalized on the postsynaptic membrane.The channels linked to non-NMDA receptors generate a brief conductance increase lasting approximately 1 millisecond. In contrast the NMDA receptor mediated component has a duration of up to 500 ms. The mechanism responsible for the long duration of the NMDA-mediated synaptic potential is unclear, as the mean open time of NMDA channels in single channel recordings is only 5-10 msec (for review, see Ref. 2).

RESULTS

To determine whether the long duration of the NMDA-receptor mediated synaptic current is due to residual transmitter in the synaptic cleft, or to long openings (e.g. bursts or clusters) of the NMDA channel, we have used two complementary experimental approaches. In the first, monosynaptic epscs were evoked between pairs of cultured hippocampal neurons using whole cell patch recording. Rapid applications of magnesium (Mg) or a competitive NMDA antagonist were delivered to the synapse either immediately before, or at progressive intervals after, synaptic activation. As expected, Mg (100 μM) blocked the slow epsc with an onset time constant of 20 ms; this was used to definedthe approximate time constant of drug delivery. However the competitive NMDA antagonist 2-amino-5-phosphonovalerate (AP5, 100 μM) had no effect on the NMDA receptor mediated slow epsc when delivered following synaptic activation. AP5 delivered 20 msec before stimulation of the presynaptic neuron completely blocked the slow epsc. This conclusively demonstrates that rebinding of free transmitter in the synaptic cleft does not contribute to the slow epsc, but rather suggests that transmitter molecules can be continuously bound to NMDA receptors for periods of 500 msec or longer (1).

To examine the channel kinetics directly, brief pulses (2-10 ms) of L-glutamate were delivered to outside-out membrane patches taken from cultured hippocampal neurons. The extracellular solution contained 0 Mg, 10 μM glycine, and 2 μM CNQX (6-cyano-7-nitroquinoxaline-2,3-dione) to block non-NMDA receptors. L-glutamate was applied and removed by pushing a 2-barreled flowpipe with a piezoelectric translator, so that the patch pipette tip rapidly crossed the solution interface; open pipette controls using two concentrations of NaCl showed a solution exchange time constant of <500 μs. Clusters of bursts of NMDA channel openings lasting hundreds of milliseconds were observed following complete removal of agonist. Channel openings to a single 10 ms pulse of 10 mM L-glutamate are shown in Figure 1. The decay of the ensemble current generated by averaging repeated glutamate pulses was fitted with two exponentials ($\tau_1 \approx 100$ ms, $\tau_2 \approx 1000$ ms). These values were virtually identical to the decay of the slow epsc. Decays following longer applications of L-glutamate (500-2000 ms) consisted primarily of the slow time constant (τ_2), perhaps suggesting that an increasing proportion of the channels entered a desensitized state during prolonged transmitter exposure.

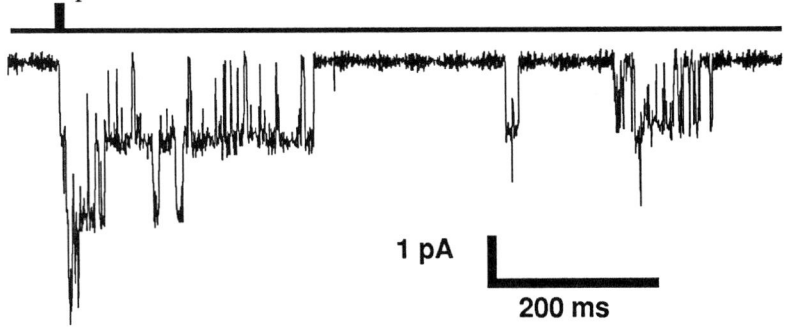

FIGURE 1. Brief applications of L-glutamate result in prolonged channel openings. Excised outside-out patch from a cultured hippocampal neuron held at -70 mV. Patch pipette contained cesium-based electrolyte solution with pCa buffered to ≈ 8.

DISCUSSION

The prolonged NMDA channel activity following brief exposure of excised patches to L-glutamate suggests a kinetic model in which τ_1 represents clusters of channel bursts and τ_2 represents escape from an inactivated or desensitized state. This behavior of the NMDA channel make it likely that channel kinetics play an important and previously unrecognized role in shaping the NMDA receptor-mediated component of synaptic transmission. For example, asynchronous opening of NMDA channels by spontaneous release of transmitter could appear as 'tonic' activation of the voltage-dependent NMDA conductance. Our data also predicts that lower affinity ligands such as L-aspartate or homocysteate, if released at synapses, should result in synaptic currents with shorter durations than seen with L-glutamate.

ACKNOWLEDGEMENTS

This work was supported by grants from the Public Health Service (NIH and ADAMHA) and the McKnight Foundation to GLW and CEJ.

REFERENCES

1. RAJ Lester, JD Clements, GL Westbrook and CE Jahr (1990). The time course of synaptically activated NMDA receptors depends on channel kinetics. submitted.

2. GL Westbrook & CE Jahr (1989). Glutamate receptors in excitatory neurotransmission. Sem. Neurosci., 1:103-114.

ACTIVITY AND EXCITATORY AMINO ACID RECEPTORS IN THE DEVELOPING AND REGENERATING VISUAL SYSTEM

Ronald L. Meyer
Developmental and Cell Biology, University of California, Irvine, CA 92717, U.S.A.

Activity is a critical process for the formation of visual circuits. In carnivores and primates including humans, abnormal visual experience during early life can produce permanent abnormalities of the electrophysiological response properties of neurons in striate cortex. These alterations can be quite specific. For example, optical misalignment of the two eyes leads to a loss of electrophysiologically measured binocular responses while leaving other response features unaltered (1). The cellular basis of these altered electrophysiological responses, however, has, in most cases, been obscured by the complexity of the underlying circuitry.

A simpler model is obtained in the retinotectal projection of lower vertebrates where activity dependent changes are expressed in the anatomical distribution of optic fibers. When the optic nerve of a goldfish is cut, optic fibers will regrow to reform their original retinotopic projection onto the contralateral tectum in the course of about 2 months. During the first month, fibers form a roughly ordered projection in which quadrant level retinotopy is restored. The projection becomes more refined in the ensuing month to generate retinotopic order that can be indistinguishable from normal (4). This latter refinement but not the initial rough order is absolutely dependent on activity. If activity is eliminated by periodic injections of tetrodotoxin into the eye, refinement is blocked but can continue upon resumption of activity (5). The critical feature of activity is thought to be the correlated activity of neighboring retinal ganglion cells which optic fibers decode in tectum according to the rule: fibers that fire together, terminate together.

Excitatory amino acids (EAA) are thought to play a critical role in mediating these activity dependent changes in both mammals and lower vertebrates. One reason is that EAA are the candidate neurotransmitter used by optic fibers and geniculocortical neurons. In goldfish, there are two lines of evidence indicating that optic fibers use EAA neurotransmission. One is immunohistochemistry using a double affinity purified antibody against gluteraldehyde conjugated glutamate made by Wenthold at NIH. In this study (3), strong immunoreactivity was localized to retinal ganglion cells and optic fibers. Densely reactivity was associated with the main optic innervation layer, the SFGS, and this was greatly reduced 2 days after enucleation. At the ultrastructural level, putative optic terminals in tectum were found to be densely reactive.

The other evidence for EEA transmission is pharmacologic (6) using a newly developed *in vitro* preparation in which the entire tectum together with the entire optic nerve is placed in a slice type recording chamber. This preparation permits efficient and selective stimulation of the nerve while permitting infusion of various pharmacologic probes. Various kainate and quisqualate receptor antagonists such as DNQX were highly effective in blocking the field potential. In addition, a slight decrement which included the earliest components of the potential was also seen with NMDA antagonist like APV and MK-801. Contrary to previous *in vivo* studies, nicotinic cholinergic antagonists had no inhibitory effect.

A critical test for the hypothesis that EAA mediate activity dependent changes comes from *in vivo* pharmacologic inhibition studies. Since the NMDA receptor has been implicated in neuroplasticity such LTP and the development of visual cortex and tectum (see 1), we asked whether NMDA might be involved in activity mediated ordering during nerve regeneration. Although previous studies had used direct infusion of APV with minipump or slow release matrices, there were several reasons for not using this method. Specific antagonism of NMDA receptors with APV is concentration dependent. Infusion techniques usually produce a higher than optimal concentration at the infusion site and slow release matrices show an initial spurt followed by progressive decline. APV can also have cytotoxic effects. To avoid these problems, we used MK801 which is a highly potent NMDA antagonist that crosses the blood brain barrier. When fish were injected intraperitoneally with MK801 beginning at 30 days, the late retinotopic refinement were prevented at 2-3 months.

The latter result not only indicates that EAA transmission may be required for activity dependent refinement but additionally suggests a particular role for NMDA receptors which normally generate a comparatively small amount of the postsynaptic current. The NMDA receptor may represent a synaptic "plasticity" receptor.

REFERENCES

1. Constantine-Paton, M., et al., (1990): *Annu. Rev. Neurosci.*, 13:129-54.
2. Hubel, D.H. and Weisel, T.N. (1965): *J. Neurophysiol.*, 28:1041-59.
3. Kageyama, G.H. and Meyer, R.L. (1989): *Brain Res.*, 503:118-27.
4. Meyer, R.L. (1980): *J. Comp. Neurol.*, 189:273-89.
5. Meyer, R.L. (1983): *Brain Res.*, 6:293-98.
6. VanDeusen, E.B. and Meyer, R.L. (1990): *Brain Res.*, in press.

LINKS BETWEEN SYNAPTIC PLASTICITY AND BEHAVIOR

C. A. BARNES, C. A. ERICKSON, and B.L. MCNAUGHTON
Center for Neural Systems, Memory and Aging, Department of Psychology, University of Arizona, Tucson, AZ, 85721, U.S.A.

It has been proposed that the long-lasting changes in synaptic transmission that can be induced at certain hippocampal synapses, called either long-term potentiation (LTP; for review see 2) or long-term enhancement (LTE; 5), may be used by the nervous system to store information. The evidence that supports this idea comes from experiments, for example, that have found correlations between the persistence of LTE and memory (1), the disruption of memory by saturating the LTE process (3,6) or by blocking NMDA receptors which appear to regulate the induction of LTE (7). It must, however, be emphasized that no experiment has demonstrated the occurrence of LTE as a consequence of the neuronal activity that naturally accompanies learning. Sharp et al. (8) have recently reported conditions under which there are robust increases in perforant path-granule cell synaptic responses in hippocampus that occur as a result of exploratory behavior. Although it is premature to conclude that this process represents synaptic changes involved in information storage, a number of possible alternative interpretations have been ruled out. These include the observations that the exploration-induced synaptic response increases are not due to changes in the distribution of current sources and sinks along the granule cell dendrites or to the number of perforant path fibers activated; the effect is independent of hippocampal theta rhythm and is not a direct results of the motor activity accompanying exploration; and finally the medial septum need not be functional for the synaptic increase to occur (4). Whether this behaviorally-induced synaptic change involves the same pharmacological receptors as electrically-induced LTE is the subject of this report.

METHODS

Rats were prepared for chronic recording of granule cell evoked field potentials elicited by stimulation of the perforant path. Responses were recorded over a baseline period of 90 minutes while rats were alert but still in their home cages, then for 20 minutes while they were encouraged to explore on an open platform in the same room, and again for 90 minutes after they were returned to their home cages. One hour before the exploratory period saline or doses of 0.30 mg/kg or 0.08 mg/kg of the NMDA receptor blocker MK-801 were administered by i.p. injection.

RESULTS

In control (saline) sessions, exploratory activity produced a gradual but robust growth in the field EPSP that persisted long after the rat was returned to its home cage (see Figure 1A). This growth was significantly reduced (F(2,6) = 15.98, p < 0.001) in a dose-dependent fashion during MK-801 sessions (see Figure 1B).

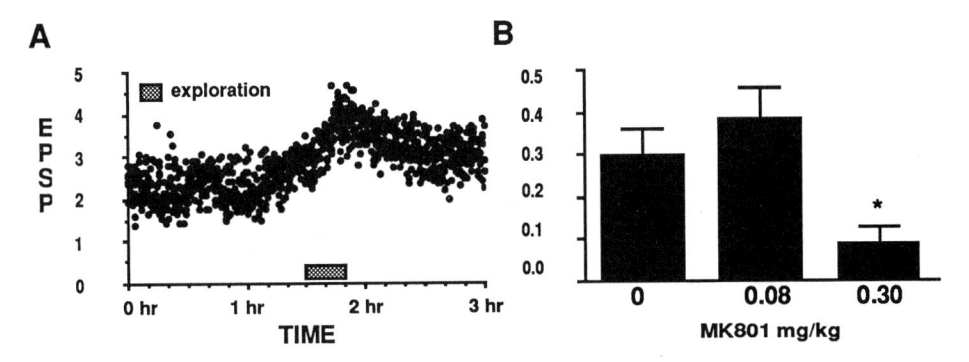

FIGURE 1. A: Amplitude (mV) of field EPSP measured over a 3 hour recording session in a chronically-prepared rat. At the bar, the rat continuously moved about on a triangular platform. Note that the synaptic increase outlasted this exploratory behavior. B: Fractional change in the EPSP between baseline and exploration periods following i.p. injections of saline, 0.08 mg/kg or 0.30 mg/kg MK-801. The environmental exploration effect was blocked by the high dose of MK-801 (0.30 mg/kg) but not by the low dose.

DISCUSSION

These data provide preliminary evidence that exploration-induced synaptic enhancement involves activation of NMDA receptors in a manner similar to that which regulates the induction of high-frequency stimulation induced LTE/LTP. In addition, blockade of NMDA receptors appears to disrupt the same type of spatial memory tasks as does saturation of LTE (3,6,7). It is possible, therefore, that exploration-induced increases in synaptic efficacy, artificially-induced LTE, and certain forms of memory may share common underlying mechanisms. However, it remains possible that MK-801 disrupts the neural activity patterns that are necessary for the induction of the exploration effect, rather than acting directly on the synapses in question. Further studies are required in which MK-801 or other NMDA antagonists are applied in a restricted fashion to the site of perforant path termination in the hippocampus before this question can be resolved.

This work was supported by an NSF grant to BLM, and AG03376 to CAB. The MK-801 was kindly provided by Merck, Sharp, and Dohme.

REFERENCES

1. Barnes, C. A. (1979): J. Comp. Physiol. Psychol., 93:74-104.
2. Bliss, T. V. P., and Lynch, M. A. (1988): In Long-term potentiation: From biophysics to behavior, P. W. Landfield and S. A. Deadwyler, Eds., pp. 3-72. Alan R. Liss, New York.
3. Castro, C.A., Silbert, L.H., McNaughton, B.L., and Barnes, C.A. (1989): Nature 342:545-548.
4. Green, E. J., McNaughton, B. L., and Barnes, C. A. (1990): J. Neurosci., (in press).
5. McNaughton, B. L. (1982): J. Physiol., 324:249-262.
6. McNaughton, B.L., Barnes, C.A., Rao, G., Baldwin, J., and Rasmussen, M. (1986): J. Neurosci., 6:563-571.
7. Morris, R. G. M. (1989): J. Neurosci. 9:3040-3057.
8. Sharp, P. E., McNaughton, B. L., and Barnes, C. A. (1989): Psychobiol., 17:257-269.

SEROTONIN RECEPTORS

M.B. TYERS
Department of Neuropharmacology, Glaxo Group Research Ltd, Park Road, Ware, Hertfordshire SG12 0DP

Serotonin (5-HT) is widely distributed in the body, primarily in platelets, enterochromaffin cells in the GI tract and in neurones. Serotonin has many varied actions when injected, some of which are apparently opposing. For example serotonin can both contract and relax smooth muscle and can depolarise as well as hyperpolarise neurones in the CNS. To account for these many actions the receptors for serotonin have now been classified into three or possibly four categories: $5-HT_1$, $5-HT_2$, and $5-HT_3$ (and possibly $5-HT_4$, although this subtype has not yet been fully characterised). The $5-HT_1$ receptor is now known to comprise several sub-types: $5-HT_{1A}$, $5-HT_{1B}$, $5-HT_{1C}$ and $5-HT_{1D}$. There are some additional serotonin receptors which fit best into this group but also have not been fully characterised; these are referred to as $5-HT_1$-like receptors. $5-HT_2$ receptors are probably homogenous but some recent evidence from binding studies suggest that there may be two sub-types. The $5-HT_3$ receptors can only be sub-divided between species. Evidence for species variants of this receptor is considerable but within a single species there is no evidence for $5-HT_3$ subtypes.

In the CNS, $5-HT_1$ receptors are generally inhibitory on neuronal activity. $5-HT_{1A}$ receptors are present on serotonin cell bodies in the raphé nuclei and inhibit serotonin release. The $5-HT_{1B}$ (rodents) and $5-HT_{1D}$ (non-rodents) receptors appear to function as terminal inhibitory autoreceptors on serotonin neurones. The only current clinical applications for drugs acting on $5-HT_1$ receptors are $5-HT_{1A}$ agonists (e.g. buspirone) which have anxiolytic and antidepressant activity. In addition, evidence emerging from clinical studies suggest that $5-HT_1$-like agonists (e.g. sumatriptan) are effective in treating migraine.

$5-HT_2$ receptors generally stimulate central neurones. Antagonists for this receptor (e.g. ritanserin) are generally silent in behavioural models in animals but are being evaluated in anxiety and schizophrenia.

$5-HT_3$ receptors are located on neurones in both the peripheral and central nervous systems. Antagonists for this receptor (e.g. ondansetron) have several important effects on behaviour. These drugs inhibit mesolimbic dopaminergic activity and may therefore be effective in treating schizophrenia and/or drug abuse states. $5-HT_3$

antagonists also release suppressed behaviour in animals exposed to a novel and aversive stimulus suggesting a possible use in anxiety. And finally, evidence from neurochemical and behavioural studies suggest a role in enhancing cognitive deficiencies.

Clinical trials are in progress with drugs which are selective for each of these classes of receptor. Data from these trials will have important implications not only in the treatment of psychiatric disorders but also in the design of psychopharmacological studies in animals.

Clinical Effects of 5HT-1A Partial Agonists, Buspirone and Gepirone, in the Treatment of Depression.

D.S. Robinson, R.E. Gammans, R.C. Shrotriya, S.W. Jenkins, J.J. Andary, D.R. Alms, M.E. Messina
Bristol-Myers Squibb, CNS Clinical Research
Wallingford, CT, U.S.A.

Many clinically effective antidepressants modulate serotonergic neurotransmission, most indirectly by altering serotonin disposition. Both tricyclics and monoamine oxidase inhibitors enhance synaptic serotonin and norepinephrine inducing adaptive changes in receptors on those neurons. Recently, selective serotonin uptake inhibitors, also acting indirectly to alter serotonin receptors by decreasing synaptic serotonin clearance, have established that selectively modulating serotonergic neurotransmission is sufficient for antidepressant efficacy.

We have investigated the antidepressant effects of buspirone and gepirone, partial agonists that act selectively at 5HT-1A receptors. Both compounds are active in animal behavioral models predictive of antidepressant activity and induce adaptive changes in serotonin neurotransmission like those produced by indirectly acting antidepressants. We report here results of placebo-controlled studies that indicate clinical antidepressant activity for both buspirone and gepirone These data confirm results of predictive animal models and suggest that direct, selective modulation of 5HT-1A receptors can produce clinically important therapeutic effects.

TABLE 1: IMPROVEMENT SCORES ON CLINICAL OUTCOME MEASURES FOLLOWING BUSPIRONE OR GEPIRONE TREATMENT OF DEPRESSED PATIENTS

OUTCOME MEASURE	BUSPIRONE STUDIES Buspirone (n=183)	Placebo (n=199)	GEPIRONE STUDIES Gepirone (n=80)	Placebo (n=38)
HAM-A IMPROVEMENT	-9.2*	-5.6	-7.9	-6.6
HAM-D (17 item) IMPROVEMENT	-8.4*	-5.3	-8.4*	-5.1
HAM-D RETARDATION FACTOR IMPROVEMENT	-2.6*	-1.6	-	-
RESPONDERS (CGI)	101 (55%)*	63 (32%)	48 (59%)*	15 (39%)

* drug placebo difference $p<0.05$

METHODS

The buspirone data are from studies employing a common protocol conducted at 5 sites throughout the U.S. After granting informed consent 382 patients who met DSM-III-R criteria for Major Depression with at least 18 on the HAM-A and HAM-D were randomized to receive buspirone (up to 90 mg/day) or placebo. Response was evaluated weekly.

The gepirone data are from a similar study conducted at one of the same clinics. After granting informed consent 118 outpatients meeting DSM-III-R criteria for Major Depression and HAM-D scores of at least 18 were randomized to one of two dose ranges of gepirone (5-30 mg/day or 10-60 mg/day) or placebo, and response was evaluated weekly.

Data were evaluated by ANOVA (HAM-A, HAM-D) or Cochran Mantzel Hanzel (CGI) procedures using the last efficacy observation for each patient on treatment.

RESULTS

Buspirone and gepirone produced significant improvement in depressive symptoms on all three major outcome measures. The mean dose of buspirone responders was approximately 45 mg/day while the most effective dose range for gepirone was 5-30 mg/day.

DISCUSSION

Selective 5HT-1A partial agonists have been shown in animal models to produce behavioral and neurochemical changes similar to other antidepressants that interact nonspecifically with the serotonergic system. The clinical data presented confirm that buspirone has antidepressant effects and give preliminary indication that gepirone is also a useful antidepressant. These findings support the hypothesis based on pharmacologic evidence that selective 5HT-1A partial agonists modulate serotonergic systems leading to antidepressant activity.

THE 5-HT₂ RECEPTORS: WHAT DO THEY DO? POSSIBLE ROLES IN AFFECTIVE DISORDERS.

J.E. LEYSEN
Department of Biochemical Pharmacology, Janssen Research Foundation, B-2340 Beerse, Belgium.

The role of 5-HT₂ receptors has to be considered from three points of view: 1. their role, amply demonstrated, in pharmacological tests; 2. the role in normal physiological conditions, about which new ideas were recently put forward based on receptor regulation studies; 3. the role in clinical pathologies which can be surmised from clinical studies with 5-HT₂ antagonists.

1. 5-HT₂ receptors play a role in various pharmacological effects elicited by exogenous serotonin agonists. In rodents they mediate behavioural excitation (head twitches, forepaw treading, coarse body tremors) and discriminative stimulus effects. In the periphery 5-HT₂ receptors mediate serotonin-induced platelet aggregation and vascular, tracheal and ileal smooth muscle contraction (1). Biochemical and molecular biological studies have demonstrated that 5-HT₂ receptors belong to the family of G-protein coupled receptors: they activate the phosphatidyl inositol turn-over system for signal transduction and the receptor is a protein monomer with seven putative transmembrane domains (1,2,3). The drug binding properties of 5-HT₂ receptors are well documented: recently we reported on forty-eight antagonists, belonging to twenty different chemical classes, with nanomolar affinity for 5-HT₂ receptors (4). Known agonists with various chemical structures display micromolar affinity. Analysis of the receptor binding profile of the compounds revealed that only two antagonists fulfilled the criteria of 5-HT₂ receptor selectivity, namely of: pipamperone and cinanserin. They display at least 50 times higher binding affinity for 5-HT₂ receptors than for any other known 5-HT receptor subtype or for various other neurotransmitter or peptide receptors, ligand gated ion channels or neurotransmitter transporters (4). All the various 5-HT₂ antagonists block the various pharmacological effects elicited by agonist activation of 5-HT₂ receptors. However, in mammals, 5-HT₂ antagonists by themselves cause only mild effects in physiological conditions: in man and laboratory animals they significantly increase slow wave sleep and in rats they abolish behavioural inhibition induced by natural aversive stimuli. But, 5-HT₂ antagonists do not disrupt or stimulate autonomic, motor and intellectual functions.

2. In view of the rather weak effects of 5-HT₂ antagonist the question has been raised to what extent 5-HT₂ receptors are activated under normal physiological conditions. Direct experimental information on this problem is hard to obtain; we have approached the issue by analysing 5-HT₂ receptor regulatory responses. It has been amply demonstrated that 5-HT₂ receptors do not up-regulate following serotonergic denervation or chronic receptor blockade. Chronic treatment with high dosages of various non-selective antidepressants and 5-HT₂ antagonists caused an anomalous 5-HT₂ receptor down-regulation. In contrast, chronic treatment with specific 5-HT uptake inhibitors did not affect 5-HT₂ receptor numbers (2). We recently found that 5-HT₂ receptors very rapidly desensitize and down-regulate by repeated agonist stimulation [complete abolishment of

behavioural response and 50 % reduction in frontal cortical 5-HT$_2$ receptor numbers following 4 administrations in 24 h of DOM (2.5 mg/kg, s.c.) to rats]. Based on these observations we suggested that 5-HT$_2$ receptors probably receive little stimulation under normal physiological conditions. They may only function in emergencies or during short periods of the day-night cycle, e.g. to interrupt slow wave sleep. Thus, the receptors may normally exist in a supersensitive state. Acute blockade does not disrupt the normal situation, which explains the minor apparent effects of 5-HT$_2$ antagonists. Nor will denervation or chronic blockade cause development of supersensitivity or receptor up-regulation. Specific inhibition of serotonin re-uptake will not affect 5-HT$_2$ receptor numbers since normally there will be little or no free serotonin in the receptor vicinity. However, acute stimulation of 5-HT$_2$ receptors by exogenous agonists causes marked and detrimental effects, and repeated stimulation promptly induces desensitization, which probably is a defensive reaction of the system against noxious receptor activity.

3. Whereas 5-HT$_2$ receptors should normally be silent they may receive too much activation in pathological conditions and, in view of the above, it could be speculated that the down-regulatory response could be deficient. Observed therapeutic effects with 5-HT$_2$ antagonists provide indications of the involvement of 5-HT$_2$ receptors in pathologies. In vascular pathologies, the 5-HT$_2$ antagonist ketanserin was found to improve impaired microcirculation, probably owing to its antiplatelet aggregation and antivasoconstrictive action. In psychiatric applications, ritanserin, a very potent and long-acting centrally active 5-HT$_2$ antagonist, revealed thymostenic effects. Therapeutic activity was observed in dysthymia, generalized anxiety, neurotic depression and on negative symptoms in schizophrenia (5). The studies with ritanserin confirm early observations with pipamperone, which was introduced as a neuroleptic twenty years ago, but which now appears to be the most selective known 5-HT$_2$ antagonist according to drug receptor binding profiles. Pipamperone has long been noted for its unique capacity to regulate disturbed sleep rhythms in psychiatric patients and to improve social contact in withdrawn patients. It can be concluded that enhanced 5-HT$_2$ receptor stimulation may be a cause of mood disorders; it can also be speculated that the ability of the 5-HT$_2$ antagonists to improve the quality of sleep adds to their therapeutic action.

REFERENCES

1. Leysen, et al. (1984) Neuropharmacology, 23: 1493-1501.
2. Conn, P.F., and Sanders-Busch (1987) Psychopharmacology 92: 267-277.
3. Pritchett, et al. (1988) EMBO Journal 7: 4135-4140.
4. Leysen, J.E. (1990) Neuropsychopharmacology, in press.
5. Reyntjens, et al. (1986) Drug. Dev. Res. 8: 205-211.

SEROTONIN AND COGNITION

J.M. BARNES, N.M. BARNES, B. COSTALL, A.M. DOMENEY, M.E. KELLY and R.J. NAYLOR
Postgraduate Studies in Pharmacology, The School of Pharmacy, University of Bradford, Bradford BD7 1DP, UK.

Disturbances in cognitive performance have long been associated with deficits in cerebral acetylcholine but attempts to find ameliorative therapy which directly influences cholinergic function has met with limited success. Recently, it has been discovered that cerebral cholinergic function is modulated via serotonin, specifically via the $5-HT_3$ receptor subtype. This has lead to a completely novel approach to the enhancement of cognitive performance, and selective $5-HT_3$ receptor antagonists are now in clinical trial as potential cognitive enhancers. Here we report on the preclinical work which lead to the clinical appraisal of the $5-HT_3$ receptor antagonists as cognitive enhancers.

METHODS

The techniques employed mice, rats and marmosets. A habituation test assessed time taken for a mouse to learn to move from an aversive white compartment into a preferred dark compartment (3). Rat studies used an alternation task in an elevated T-maze where rats were required to learn to move in alternate directions, initially dictated by a barrier, to gain food rewards when starved to 85% of body weight. Rats were also subject to a water maze task in which they learned to swim from different island quadrants to locate a submerged island in opaque liquid, using spatial cues (3). Impairments in performance were induced by scopolamine, lesions of the nucleus basalis, ischaemic intrusion and by old age (3).

The primate test of cognition utilised a Wisconsin General Test Apparatus and determined performance in an object discrimination reversal task. Trained marmosets were required to select to criterion between two junk objects to obtain a food reward. The positive stimulus changed from one object to the other in one test session (4).

The questions posed were whether the $5-HT_3$ receptor antagonists could improve basal cognitive performance and/or influence deficits caused by scopolamine, nucleus basalis lesions, ischaemic insult or by the ageing process.

Neurochemical correlates for the influence of the selected $5-HT_3$ receptor antagonists, ondansetron, zacopride, granisetron and ICS 205-930, were also established using standard radioligand binding techniques (^{3}H.zacopride, rodent and human tissue) (2) and influence on K^+ stimulated ^{3}H.acetylcholine release from rodent entorhinal cortex (1).

RESULTS

Mouse basal habituation performance was improved by low doses of the 5-HT$_3$ receptor antagonists (e.g. 10 ng/kg i.p. b.d. ondansetron) such that the latency of movement from the aversive white compartment was reduced (from 10-12 to 1-2 sec on day 2). Impairments in habituation induced by scopolamine, nucleus basalis lesions and old age were also significantly improved by agents such as ondansetron and zacopride. Similarly, in low µg/kg doses, ondansetron or zacopride could inhibit the disturbed performance of scopolamine treated or aged rats in the T-maze task, or the disturbance associated with scopolamine or ischaemic damage in the water maze task. Primate performance in the WGTA was also dramatically improved, with ng/kg and low µg/kg doses of the 5-HT$_3$ receptor antagonists improving poor performance on the initial task and the more flawed performance of the reversal task. For example, in one assessment the number of trials to criterion on the reversal task was reduced from 20-35 to 2-15. Animals made less errors and worked more efficiently to make more correct decisions.

5-HT$_3$ recognition sites were located in areas relevant to cognitive performance, including the entorhinal cortex, hippocampus and amygdala. Using slices of entorhinal cortex loaded with ^{3}H.choline, 5-HT$_3$ receptor antagonists were shown to prevent an inhibitory 5-hydroxytryptaminergic action.

DISCUSSION

The 5-HT$_3$ receptor antagonists have been shown to improve cognitive performance of mice, rats and primates in situations where (a) basal performance is poor and (b) performance is impaired by loss of cortical and limbic cholinergic function, whether this be by scopolamine or a surgical intervention. Performance of aged animals is also improved. It is proposed that these novel compounds, including ondansetron and zacopride, act in limbic and cortical areas to improve cholinergic function and, as a consequence, cognitive performance. This awaits confirmation in man.

REFERENCES

1. Barnes, J.M. et al. 5-HT$_3$ receptors mediate inhibition of acetylcholine release in cortical tissue. Nature 338 (6218):762-763, 1989.
2. Barnes, N.M. et al. Identification of 5-HT$_3$ recognition sites in human brain tissue using ^{3}H.zacopride. J. Pharm. Pharmac. 40(9): 668, 1988.
3. Costall, B. et al. The effects of ACE inhibitors captopril and SQ29,852 in rodent tests of cognition. Pharmacol. Biochem. Behav. 33(3):573-579, 1989.
4. Costall, B. et al. Effects of GR38032F on performance of marmosets (Callithrix jacchus) in an object discrimination reversal task. Br. J. Pharmac. 98:637P, 1989.

ROLE OF 5-HT RECEPTORS IN ADDICTIVE DISORDERS

E.M. Sellers, M.B. Sobell, G.A. Higgins
Departments of Medicine and Pharmacology, University of Toronto, and Addiction Research Foundation, Toronto, Ontario, Canada

Addictive behaviour is characterized by the repeated non-therapeutic self-administration of a psychoactive drug which is harmful to an individual or society. For some individuals stopping such use is very difficult, hence discovery of medications for prevention or treatment is important. The focus of this presentation will be on serotonin receptor selective strategies for developing drugs as medications to treat addictive disorders. Mechanisms whereby medications could modify drug taking include: antagonize the reinforcing properties; serve as a primary substitute for the reinforcing properties; decrease the urge or desire to initiate use; improve learning of new behaviours; produce a conditioned or unconditioned aversive reaction; suppress primary or secondary withdrawal symptoms; provide a non-specific internal stimulus substitution; treat a primary or secondary mental disorder; improve mood or affect; increase ability to control or cope with stress; alter the metabolic/kinetic features of the abused drug; prevent, reduce or treat drug toxicity. Current data suggest at least 3 classes of serotonergic drug may have efficacy by some of these mechanisms.

$5-HT_3$ RECEPTOR ANTAGONISTS

Increasing evidence highlights the importance of the dopaminergic mesolimbic system in drug self-administration, discrimination and dependence for opiates, nicotine, alcohol and stimulants (e.g. amphetamine, cocaine). Thus, nicotine and morphine (and possibly ethanol) increase the firing rate of DA neurons in the VTA resulting in elevated DA turnover in the N. accumbens. Recently, $5-HT_3$ antagonists (e.g. ICS205-930) have been shown to inhibit both the increased VTA neuronal firing induced by morphine and the elevated accumbens DA turnover produced by morphine, nicotine and ethanol (3). Furthermore, both nicotine and morphine reinforcement as measured by place preference may be attenuated by ICS205-930 and MDL72222 (2). In the marmoset the $5-HT_3$ antagonist ondansetron (GR38032F) and other $5-HT_3$ antagonists decreased post-drug dependent anxiety behaviour in animals pre-treated for 7 days with alcohol, nicotine, diazepam or cocaine (5, Oustall et al, unpublished). In non-dependent ethanol-preferring rats similar but smaller effects on self-administration have been reported (7). Interestingly, conflicting findings have been observed with respect to antagonism of amphetamine-induced place preference by these drugs. This may be due to a direct effect of amphetamine on terminal DA release. Thus, $5-HT_3$ antagonists may find greatest utility against treatments whose primary based reinforcement is dependent upon enhanced mesolimbic activity mediated at the level of the VTA.

$5-HT_{1A}$ RECEPTOR COMPOUNDS

The pharmacology and function of compounds acting at $5-HT_{1A}$ sites is complex because of their pre- and post-synaptic actions which may be conflicting and critically dependent on dose selection. Chronic administration of the $5-HT_{1A}$ partial agonist (gepirone) produces a desensitization of $5-HT_{1A}$ somatodendritic receptors resulting in an increase in central 5-HT tone (1). Such an increase could be associated with effects on alcohol consumption and possibly other drugs of abuse, since presumably 5-HT uptake blockers similarly raise serotonin function.

However, several 5-HT$_{1A}$ partial agonists (e.g. buspirone, WY-47846) acutely decrease ethanol self-administration in rats (Sellers EM, unpublished observation) and monkey (3) and in man uncontrolled clinical observations suggest buspirone may have such an effect.

SEROTONIN UPTAKE INHIBITORS (SUI)

A number of studies have shown that selective specific SUI (e.g. sertraline) decrease ethanol self-administration by rats and monkeys (see references in 5). Similarly, SUI also decrease food but not water intake. This hypophagia may be medicated via increased activation of 5-HT$_{1B}$ (rat) or 5-HT$_{1C}$ receptors (8). Further studies are required to identify the subtype(s) involved on ethanol consumption by these drugs. We have studied the effects of sertraline on ethanol consumption in the rat. Acute sertraline administration (3, 10 mg/kg) selectively decreases bout number and slows the rate of E consumption, suggesting an important role of serotonin in regulating these phenomena. Interestingly, the size of each drinking bout was unaffected. In clinical trials, citalopram, viqualine, zimelidine and fluoxetine decrease mean drinking by 10-18% in low dependent drinkers (mean standard drinks/day at baseline 6.5-8.0 [88-109 g ethanol/d]) (5). Citalopram in another short-term ethanol treatment study decreased ethanol drinking and desire to drink (Naranjo et al, personal communication). These data therefore support the pre-clinical findings suggesting an effect on drinking initiation.

CONCLUSIONS

5-HT$_3$ and 5-HT$_{1A}$ receptor selective drugs and SUI may be important leads to treat substance abuse and dependence. In addition, their potential efficacy in anxiety, depression, cognitive impairment and impulse disorders, suggest further ways in which such compounds could be useful in addictive disorders. However, a far more systematic study of the effects of such drugs on self-administration, drug discrimination, drug withdrawal and dependence-behaviour are needed. Because of the anticipated pattern of clinical use, chronic administration pre-clinical studies are important. In addition, clinical trials must be designed in such a way that the putative therapeutic mechanism is consistent with the drug's pharmacologic mechanisms of action. Since human addictive behaviour is a chronic disorder based upon the complex interaction of drug, patient and context, medications must be combined with non-pharmacologic treatment.

REFERENCES

1. Blier, P. and DeMontigny, C. Modification of 5-HT neuron properties by sustained administration of the 5-HT$_{1A}$ agonist gepirone: Electrophysiological studies in the rat brain. Synapse 1: 470-480, 1987.
2. Carboni, E., et al. 5-HT$_3$ receptor antagonists block morphine- and nicotine-induced place-preference conditioning. Eur. J. Pharmacol. 151: 159-160, 1988.
3. Carboni, E., et al. Differential inhibitory effects of a 5-HT$_3$ antagonist on drug-induced stimulation of dopamine release. Eur. J. Pharmacol. 164: 515-519, 1989.
4. Collins, D.M. and Myers, R.D. Buspirone attenuates volitional alcohol intake in the chronically drinking monkey. Alcohol 4: 49-56, 1987.
5. Naranjo, C.A., et al. Fluoxetine differentially alters alcohol intake and other consummatory behaviours in problem drinks. Clin. Pharmacol. Ther., 1990 (in press).
6. Oakley, N.R., et al. The effect of GR38032F on alcohol consumption in the marmoset. Br. J. Pharmacol. 95: 870P, 1988.
7. Sellers, E.M. et al. The 5-HT$_3$ antagonist GR38032F decreases alcohol consumption in rats. Abst. 18th Ann. Mtg. Soc. Neurosci. 14 (Part I): 41, 1988.
8. Wilkinson, L.O. and Dourish, C.T. Serotonin and animal behaviour. In: Sertonin Receptor Subtypes: Basic and Clinical Aspects. S.J. Peroutka, ed. Alan R. Liss, 1990 (in press).

CLINICAL IMPORTANCE OF MULTIPLE SEROTONIN RECEPTORS:
SUMMARY AND FUTURE DIRECTIONS

Edmund G. Anderson
Department Pharmacology, University of Illinois Col.
Medicine Chicago, IL, U.S.A.

The proliferation of 5-HT receptor subtypes belies the history of the dopamine receptor, in that experience is expanding more than merging receptor subtypes. This is resulting in many new sites for pharmacological attack, and new drug entities in clinical trial. What lies ahead?

A clearer definition of receptor subtype pharmacology and function is much needed. More specific agonists and antagonists would accelerate the growing understanding of the functional roles of these receptors, and help rationalize new drug design.

The 5-HT1A receptor system is emerging as an important inhibitory system. Though 8-OH-DPAT is a selective high-affinity ligand for the 1A receptor, functional studies report confusing results, because its' low efficacy results in mixed agonist-antagonist properties. Buspirone possesses similar limitations with lower potency. However, its' effectiveness in anxiety and depression suggests therapeutic potential for drugs that are full 1A agonists. The confused category of 5-HT1-like receptors needs better nomenclature and sharpened pharmacological definition. Despite this confusion, some of these agents (GR-43175 and AH-25086, which selectively contract cerebral vessels) reportedly terminate migraine headache. The complex smooth muscle effects of this receptor group suggests significant potential for new drugs with selective actions.

The 5-HT2 receptors have been implicated in the actions of hallucinogens, antidepressants and in drug dependance, but their exact role remains unclear. 5-HT2 receptor down-regulation is thought important to the action of some antidepressants. The future holds potential for better therapy through understanding 5-HT2 receptor regulation.

Functional characterization of the more recently discovered 5-HT3 receptor system is occurring rapidly, because highly selective antagonists are available. Early trials indicate that these antagonists are highly effective antiemetic agents in cancer chemotherapy. These antagonists also block 5-HT evoked release of dopamine, and modulate dopaminergic behaviors leading to potential applications as antipsychotics with reduced side effects as well as treatment of drug dependance. The 5-HT4 receptor system is just emerging, but its prominence in the hippocampus and other brain structures suggest new opportunities for serotonergic drug development.

5-HT-1A RECEPTOR-MEDIATED EFFECTS OF ANTIDEPRESSANTS: RELATION TO G PROTEIN FUNCTION

M.E. NEWMAN AND B. LERER
Yaacov Herzog Centre for Brain and Psychiatry Research, and Dept. of Psychiatry, Hebrew University, P.O.B. 140, Jerusalem, Israel.

Serotonergic mechanisms have been proposed to be involved both in the pathogenesis of depression and in the mechanism of action of antidepressant drugs. Recently, attention has been focussed on the 5-HT-1A receptor as a possible site of antidepressant action. In mice, a reduction in the hypothermia induced by the 5-HT-1A agonist 8-OH-DPAT was shown after administration of a variety of antidepressant treatments including electroconvulsive shock (ECS), and also after administration of lithium (Li). In rats short-term Li enhanced the 8-OH-DPAT behavioural syndrome but had no effect on the concomitant hypothermia. We have demonstrated a biochemical correlate of these findings by showing that chronic desimipramine (DMI), ECS and Li each reduced the degree of inhibition of forskolin-stimulated adenylate cyclase by 5-HT in rat hippocampal membranes (1,2). These studies have now been extended to other antidepressants. Chronic administration of fluoxetine or zimelidine (each at 15 mg/kg i.p. for 3 wk) were each found to reduce the 5-HT-1A response, while administration of iprindole or mianserin had no effect. Similarly, it has been shown that chronic administration of MAO A but not MAO B inhibitors reduces the degree of inhibition of forskolin-stimulated cyclase by 8-OH-DPAT (3). These studies point to the 5-HT-1A receptor as an important putative locus of antidepressant action, and indeed 5-HT-1A receptor agonists are now being evaluated for antidepressant efficacy.

In human platelets, 5-HT induces both stimulation of basal adenylate cyclase activity and inhibition of forskolin-stimulated activity, as has indeed been reported for the 5-HT-1A receptor in hippocampus. Evaluation of the pharmacological characteristics of the enzyme in human platelet membranes is under way. Maximal inhibition in platelet membranes from 6 control subjects was 37.6 $\pm$ 3.3% and the EC50 for 5-HT, 35.5 $\pm$ 29.4 nM. This finding provides a tool for examining whether 5-HT-1A function is altered in depressed patients as compared to normal subjects, and also for evaluating the effects of antidepressant treatments. A recent report showed that the hypothermic response to the 5-HT-1A specific ligand ipsapirone was attenuated in depressed patients and further reduced by chronic treatment with amitryptyline (4), but no further data on the effects of other antidepressants on this system is as yet available.

We have investigated whether the actions of Li and antidepressants on inhibition of adenylate cyclase are confined to the effect mediated by 5-HT-1A receptors, by studying the degree of inhibition of forskolin-stimulated cyclase by carbachol in rat hippocampal membranes. Carbachol induced inhibition was reduced after both chronic ECS and DMI (1), and a similar effect was obtained after long- or short-term Li administration. These results suggest that the primary action of the antidepressants may occur at the G protein distal to the receptor. Work on binding of labelled GTP to rat cortical membranes has suggested that this is the case for Li (5).

In order to obtain more evidence for an action at this site, we have also studied the effects of Li on neurotransmitter-stimulated inositol monophosphate (IP) formation in rat cortical and hippocampal slices. Administration of Li for either 10 days or 3 weeks significantly reduced the degree of stimulation of IP formation in cortical slices by either noradrenaline or 5-HT, but had no effect on carbachol-induced IP formation. Since alpha-1 adrenoceptor number is generally thought to be unaffected by Li administration, these results imply that the noradrenaline and carbachol responses are mediated by different G proteins.

In hippocampal slices, Li also reduced the noradrenaline-stimulated IP response but had no effect on the responses to carbachol or 5-HT. When carbachol and 5-HT were present simultaneously, 5-HT reduced the degree of carbachol stimulation of IP formation by 28 ± 6%. This effect, which has been shown to be mediated by 5-HT-1A receptors (6), was completely abolished after Li administration. The 5-HT-1A site thus seems to be of particular importance for Li action since both second messsenger reactions mediated by this receptor are reduced after Li administration. Further experiments are required to show whether all the effects of Li and antidepressants on second messenger systems can be explained by a single action at the G protein level, or whether a specific effect at the 5-HT-1A receptor occurs.

1. Newman, M.E. and Lerer, B. Eur. J. Pharmacol. 148: 257-260, 1988.
2. Newman, M.E., Drummer, D., Lerer, B. J. Pharmacol. Exp.Ther. , in press, 1990.
3. Sleight, A.J., Marsden, C.A., Palfreyman, M.G., Mir, A.K. and Lovenberg, W. Eur. J. Pharmacol. 154: 255-261, 1988.
4. Lesch, K.P., Disselkampe-Tietze, J., Schmidtke, A. J. Neural Transm. 80: 157-161, 1990.
5. Avissar, S., Schreiber, G., Danon, A., Belmaker, R.H. Nature 331: 440-442, 1988.
6. Claustre, Y., Benavides, J., Scatton, B. Eur. J. Pharmacol. 149: 149-153, 1988.

(Supported in part by NIMH Grant # 43873)

PROTEIN PHOSPHORYLATION AFTER ACUTE AND CHRONIC ANTIDEPRESSANT TREATMENT

N. BRUNELLO, J. PEREZ, D. TINELLI, E. BIANCHI and G. RACAGNI

Center of Neuropharmacology, Institute of Pharmacological Sciences, University of Milan, Italy.

Neurochemical, electrophysiological, behavioral and clinical studies have been conducted in an attempt to better understand the relationship among antidepressant drug action, brain function and neurochemistry. Substantial data exist to support a link between the symptoms of affective illness and alterations in monoaminergic transmission. Noradrenergic as well as serotonergic receptor system seem to be particularly vulnerable to change by antidepressant drugs. Receptor binding studies have indicated that chronic, but not acute, treatment with clinically effective antidepressants induces a decrease in beta-adrenergic and $5HT_2$ receptor binding in rat brain cortex (3). Although receptor binding studies are useful as an initial screening device to understand drug mechanisms, they are quite limited in revealing functional changes. Therefore more recent studies have been focussed on neuronal signal transduction processes beyond the receptor level as potential target sites for the action of antidepressant drugs. The most commonly described effective mechanism for second messengers depends on protein phosphorylation mediated by activation of specific protein kinases (1). It is now well established that cAMP dependent protein kinase type II (PK II) is mainly associated with microtubules, indicating that cell surface receptors linked to cAMP could regulate microtubule function (4). We have recently demonstrated that repeated treatment with desmethylimipramine (DMI) modified the cAMP dependent phosphorylation system (2). It was therefore of interest to study whether PK II associated with microtubules could be an intracellular target for the action of different antidepressant drugs. We have thus measured the photoaffinity labelling with $8-N_3-{}^{32}P$-cAMP of the regulatory subunit of PK II in the microtubule fraction of rat cerebral cortex after prolonged treatment with DMI and with other antidepressant drugs, such as fluoxetine, a specific 5HT uptake blocker and (+) oxaprotiline, an inhibitor of NE reuptake. Fig. 1 shows that chronic treatment with DMI, fluoxetine and with (+) oxaprotiline induced an increase in the photoactivated incorporation of $8-N_3-{}^{32}P$-cAMP into a protein band with apparent molecular weight of 52 KDa which could be the regulatory subunit of PK II. The band labelled were shown to be specific since their labelling was prevented by the presence of excess unlabelled cyclic AMP. Acute administration or in vitro addition of any of the above drugs did not induce any modification in the covalent

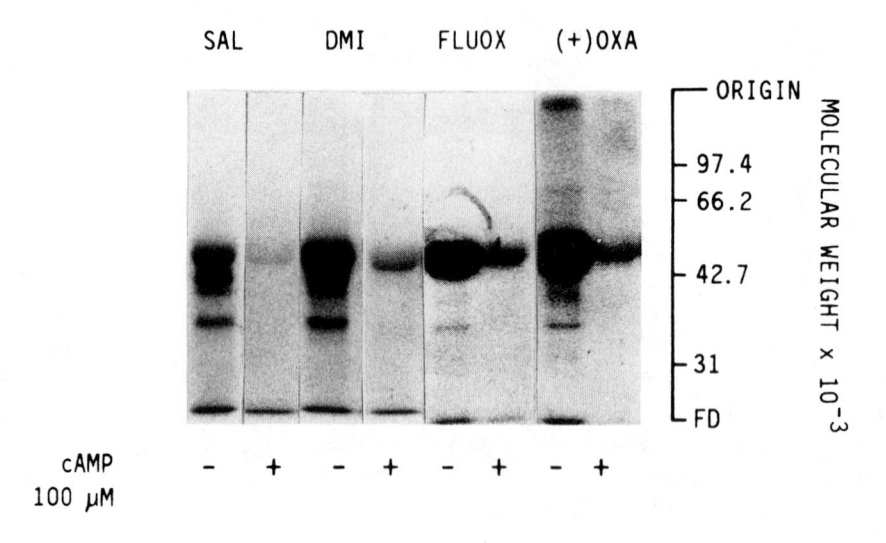

Fig. 1: Autoradiography of the photoaffinity labelling with 8-N$_3$-^{32}P-cAMP of rat cerebrocortical microtubule fraction after 10 days of treatment with saline (SAL), desmethylimipramine (DMI), fluoxetine (FLUOX) and (+) oxaprotiline (+OXA).

binding of 8-N$_3$-^{32}P-cAMP to 52 KDa protein band. These results indicate that chronic treatment with antidepressant drugs might affect the regulatory subunit of PK II associated to the microtubule fraction. In conclusion we can suggest that, besides the modifications elicited at the receptor level, antidepressants might modulate signal transduction mechanisms beyond the receptor and that cAMP dependent phosphorylation system associated with microtubules could be a target in the mechanism of action of antidepressant drugs.

REFERENCES

1. Edelman A.M., Blumenthal D.K. and Krebs E.G. (1987): Annu. Rev. Biochem., 56: 567-613
2. Perez J. et al. (1989): Eur. J. Pharmacol. Mol. Pharmacol. Sec., 172: 305-316
3. Racagni G. and Brunello N. (1984): Trends Pharmacol. Sci., 5: 527-531
4. Theurkauf W.E. and Vallee R.B. (1982): J.Biol.Chem., 257: 3284-3290

ELECTROPHYSIOLOGICAL STUDIES WITH ANTIDEPRESSANT DRUGS IN HIPPOCAMPAL SLICES FROM THE RAT

Helmut L. HAAS and Susanne BIRNSTIEL
Department of Physiology, Johannes Gutenberg-University
Saarstr. 21, D-6500 Mainz, FRG

Acute exposure of nervous tissue to antidepressant drugs is known to interfere with amine transmitter receptors and uptake (1). Recent investigations indicate also an inhibitory role of antidepressant drugs at the N-methyl-D-aspartate (NMDA) receptor complex which is involved in synaptic plasticity (2,3). We have therefore studied the interactions of several antidepressants with a number of paradigms relevant to neuronal excitability, amine transmitter effects and synaptic plasticity in hippocampal slices in vitro.

METHODS

Transverse slices of 500 μm thickness were chopped from the hippocampi of young rats and completely submerged in a recording chamber, where they were allowed to equilibrate for one hour before recording started in oxygenated artificial cerebrospinal fluid. Stimulation was on the Schaffer collate-ral/commissural pathway, and recording in the CA 1 stratum radiatum (for synaptic dendritic responses) or pyramidale (for synaptically driven population spikes and intracellular recording from cell bodies).

RESULTS AND CONCLUSION

Extracellularly registered field potentials: Amitryptiline, imipramine, desipramine, (+)- and (-)-oxaprotiline (the latter, levoprotilene, is devoid of uptake inhibiting properties) had negligible effects on the dendritically recorded excitatory postsynaptic potential at 10 μM perfused for 10 min periods. With longer exposure times and higher concentrations depressant effects became apparent. The population spike (the summed action potential of CA 1 pyramidal cells in response to afferent, synaptic, stimulation) was al-so decreased upon longer lasting applications but could be enhanced transiently or with brief applications. Double shocks at distances of 20-40 ms were delivered in another series of experiments. The paired pulse pattern (facilitation or inhibition of the second pulse) which would have changed if transmitter release or interneurone (GABA) inhibition had been affected, was not different from control.
In Mg^{2+}-free medium we recorded the multiple population discharge in response to stratum radiatum stimulation, which is sensitive to NMDA antagonists. The first and the third population spike were chosen for evaluation. Imipramine at

10 µmol/l slightly increased population spikes. This effect became significant at 50µmol/l. After 20 min of perfusion, however, the spikes began to decline. The transient excitation could be caused by an initial stronger effect on interneurons which fire high frequency bursts.

Long term potentiation (LTP): Stimulation was adjusted to give 50% or 67% of the maximal population spike. LTP, a cellular learning phenomenon, was elicited by tanic stimulation (4 trains of 100 Hz, spaced by 10 s) at test intensity. All responses were registered as averages of 8 sweeps. Posttetanic potentiation (PTP) was defined as the average obtained during the first 90 s after tetanus, LTP was defined as the one recorded 22 min after tetanus. Imipramine, oxaprotiline and levoprotiline were added to the perfusion medium 11 min before the tetanus and were present until the end of the experiment: At 67% of maximum stimulation, imi-pramine and levoprotiline slightly decreased PTP and LTP. For (+)-oxaprotiline a significant decrease in LTP was found. At 50% of maximum stimulation, all antidepressants tested enhanced PTP and LTP. LTP could be obtained even after 30 min perfusion with a high concentration of imipramine (50 µmol/l).

In low Ca2+-medium in the absence of synaptic transmission (4), imipramine caused a dose-dependent decrease of spontaneous firing at all concentrations tested (10, 20 and 50 µmol/l). At 10 µmol/l, (+)-oxaprotiline and levoprotiline caused an initial decrease in firing rate that was followed by an increase after 25-30 min of perfusion. The higher concentrations 20 and 50 µmol/l caused dose-dependent decreases of firing rate.

Intracellular recording: (+) and (-)-oxaprotilin (10 µM) caused a small depolarisation on 15 CA 1 pyramidal neurones tested (+3.5 ± 1.6 mV). The following parameters were not significantly changed: input resistance and inward rectification, "Q-sag" (as measured by hyperpolarizing current injection), the long lasting afterhyperpolarization, the accommodation of firing.

Thus antidepressant drugs do not block induction of LTP their mechanisms of action are not likely to include interference with NMDA-receptors. All measured effects were subtle and probably not specific for the antidepressant properties. A study with these paradigms including amine transmit-ter effects in slices from chronically treated rats is underway.

REFERENCES
1. Costa, E. and Racagni, G. Typical and atypical antidepressants. Raven Press, New York 1982
2. Sernagor, E. et al. Open channel block of NMDA receptor responses evoked by tricyclic antidepressants. Neuron 2:1221-1227, 1989.
3. Reynolds, I.J. and Miller R.J. Tricyclic antidepressants block NMDA receptors: similarities to the action of zinc Br.J.Pharmacol. 95:95-102
4. Haas, H.L. et al. (1984) Modulation of low calcium induced field bursts in the hippocampus by monoamines and cholinomimetics. Pflügers Arch. 400: 28-33

MONOAMINE HYPOTHESES OF DEPRESSION: IS LEVOPROTILINE THE STUMBLING-BLOCK?

P.C. WALDMEIER and L. MAITRE
Research Department, Pharmaceuticals Division, CIBA-GEIGY Ltd., CH-4002 BASLE, Switzerland

Levoprotiline, the (-)-enantiomer of oxaprotiline which in contrast to the (+)-enantiomer does not inhibit noradrenaline (NA) uptake [5], exhibits antidepressant properties, contrary to the prediction by the catecholamine hypothesis [8]. It enhances the functional responsiveness towards 5-hydroxytryptophan (5-HTP) and dopamine (DA) agonists [1,2,3] and reduces 5-HT synthesis in several rat brain areas, more strongly after two consecutive than after a single treatment, and even more so after repeated administration [6]. In the present study, we have extended these investigations to a number of antidepressants devoid of 5-HT uptake or MAO inhibiting properties, known to cause inhibition of 5-HT synthesis. Thus, the effects of the (+)-enantiomer of levoprotiline, CGP 12104, desmethylimipramine (DMI) and trimipramine were studied at various intervals after a single administration of high doses, and the effects of graded doses were checked after two consecutive administrations. Moreover, since levoprotiline was also reported to enhance the functional activity of the dopaminergic system, preliminary studies of its effects and those of CGP 12104 and DMI on DA synthesis were also made.

MATERIALS AND METHODS

Levoprotiline, CGP 12104 and DMI (hydrochlorides) and trimipramine maleate were administered i.p. to female Tif:RAIF (SPF) rats (Tierfarm Sisseln, Switzerland) weighing 160-200 g once at various intervals before or twice, 18 and 2 h before 100 mg/kg i.p. NSD 1015 (m-hydroxybenzylhydrazine x 2HCl). The accumulation of 5-HTP in the cortex or of DOPA in the striatum within 30 min after was determined by HPLC with coulometric detection essentially as described previously [4,7].

RESULTS

Levoprotiline caused a markedly and significantly reduced 5-HT synthesis in the rat cortex for nearly 24 h. CGP 12104 had a similar, though shorter effect, and DMI caused a slightly more marked reduction which lasted even longer; trimipramine did not exhibit a significant effect (Fig. 1 upper panel). These drugs were used at a lower dose (50 mg/kg i.p.) than levoprotiline (100 mg/kg i.p.) for tolerability reasons. Levoprotiline and CGP 12104 showed a similar dose-response relationship after two consecutive administrations, both reaching a reduction of 5-HT synthesis of 20 - 30 % at 30 mg/kg i.p. DMI seemed to be somewhat more potent, and trimipramine was inactive (Fig.2). The effects of each of the four drugs were very similar in hippocampus and striatum (not shown). Also, a long-lasting decrease of the synthesis of DA was induced by levoprotiline (100 mg/kg i.p.); CGP 12104 and DMI at 50 mg/kg i.p. had a similar, but shorter effect (Fig. 1, lower panel). Levoprotiline was also effective in the cortex, where DOPA accumulation reflects NA rather than DA synthesis (not shown).

DISCUSSION

CGP 12104 and DMI, like levoprotiline, reduced 5-HT synthesis. The inhibitory effect of levoprotiline is not due to an interference with brain tryptophan levels nor to an impairment of the action of the decarboxylase inhibitor [6]. We have hypothesized that it could represent an indirect consequence of an interference with more fundamental process(es) of neuronal function, such as signal transduction, which might explain both reduction in 5-HT synthesis and increased functional responsiveness towards 5-HTP [2]. The fact that levoprotiline also reduced striatal DA and cortical NA synthesis strengthens the idea. Other antidepressants like DMI and the (+)-enantiomer of oxaprotiline seem to share the effect of levoprotiline which might suggest that it is rather nonspecific, perhaps the consequence of membrane effects caused by this type of chemical structure. However, the explanation is probably not so simple, since trimipramine, which does not differ markedly in this respect, had

Fig. 2 Effects of graded doses on cortical 5-HT synthesis: Groups of 6 rats (controls n = 12) were treated twice, at an interval of 16 h, with the compounds to be tested. Ninety min after the last treatment with levoprotiline, and 2 h after CGP12104 or DMI, 100 mg/kg NSD 1015 were injected i.p., and the rats were decapitated 30 min later. Accumulation of 5-HTP in cortex is given in percent of controls ± SEM.

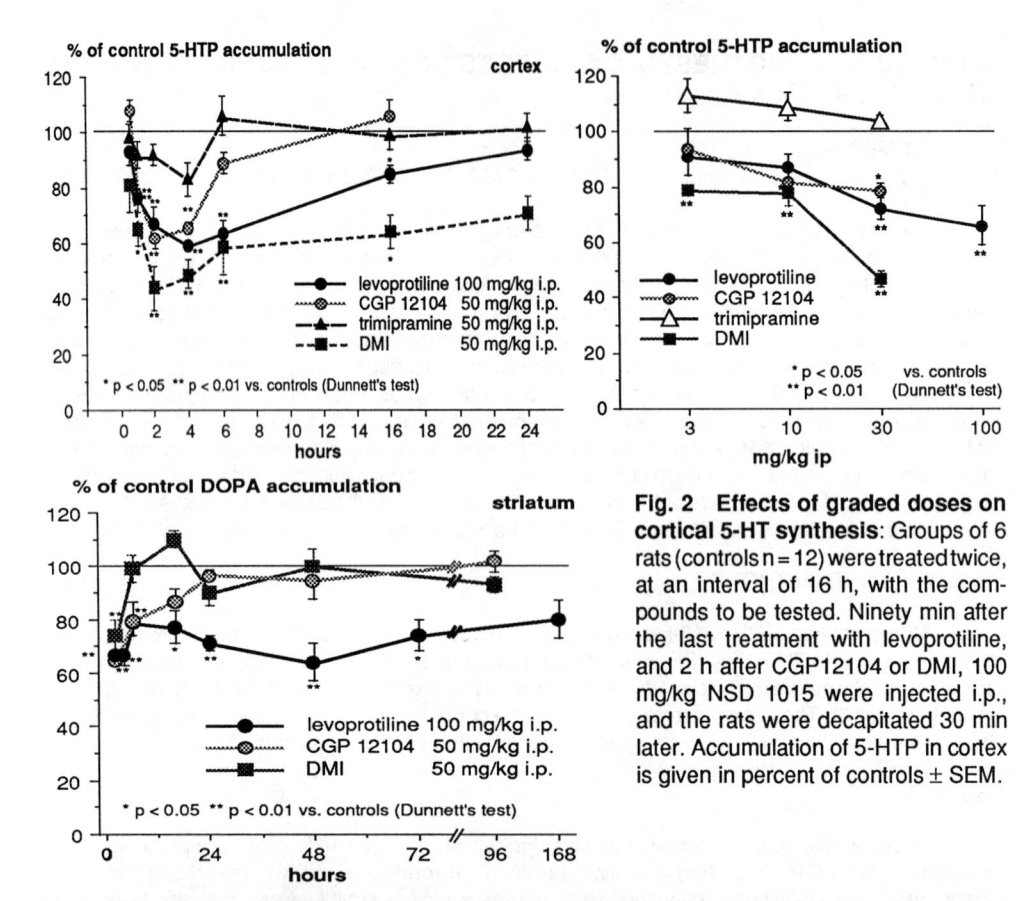

Fig. 1 Time course of effects on 5-HT and DA synthesis: Groups of 6 rats (controls n = 12) received the antidepressants at the intervals indicated before 100 mg/kg NSD 1015, and were decapitated 30 min later. Accumulation of 5-HTP in cortex (upper panel) or DOPA in striatum (lower panel) is given in percent of controls ± SEM.

no effect on 5-HT synthesis. This latter fact also suggests that we are not dealing with a property common to all antidepressants and essential for antidepressant activity. Instead, it may represent one of many mechanisms leading to therapeutic improvement. In any case, it may be premature to use the clinical efficacy of levoprotiline as an argument against the monoamine hypotheses of depression.

REFERENCES

1. Delini-Stula, A. and Mogilnicka, E. (1988): J. Neural Transm., 71: 91-98.
2. Delini-Stula, A. and Mogilnicka, E. (1989): J. Psychopharmacol., 3: 7-13.
3. Maj, J. and Wedzony, K. (1989): Eur. J. Pharmacol., 145: 97-103.
4. Waldmeier, P.C. (1987): Pharmacopsychiatry, 20: 37-47.
5. Waldmeier, P.C., et al. (1982): Biochem. Pharmacol., 31: 2169-2176.
6. Waldmeier, P.C. and Maitre, L. (1990). In: 5-Hydroxytryptamine and mental illness, A. Coppen, M. Sandler and S. Harnett, eds., pp. (in press). Oxford University Press, Oxford.
7. Waldmeier, P.C., et al. (1988): Naunyn-Schmiedeberg's Arch. Pharmacol., 337: 609-620.
8. Wolfersdorf, M., Wendt, G., Binz, U., et al (1988): Pharmacopsychiatry, 21: 203-207.

CORTICOTROPIN-RELEASING FACTOR (CRF) AND DEPRESSION: BEHAVIORAL, HORMONAL AND RECEPTOR CHANGES IN RATS FOLLOWING CHRONIC ADMINISTRATION OF CRF

M.E. ABREU, L.H. CONTI, D.G. COSTELLO AND S.J. ENNA
Nova Pharmaceutical Corporation, Baltimore, MD, U.S.A.

Corticotropin-releasing factor (CRF) has been implicated in the etiology of a number of stress-related diseases including anxiety and affective disorders (2,5,9). Major depression is associated with hypercortisolism, and clinical evidence indicates a dysfunction at or above the level of the hypothalamus with some patients displaying a blunted ACTH response to CRF or glucocorticoid administration (4,6). Additionally, depressed patients exhibit elevated levels of CRF in cerebrospinal fluid (1), and the number of CRF receptors is reduced in the frontal cortex of suicide victims (10). These data suggest a causal relationship between CRF release and depression.

Intracerebroventricular (icv) administration of CRF into animals elevates blood levels of ACTH and corticosterone and elicits a variety of behavioral and physiological responses similar to those induced by stress (3,8). Inasmuch as there appears to be a relationship among chronic stress, CRF release and some forms of depression, experiments were conducted to assess the effects of prolonged exposure to CRF on CRF receptor binding and function and on animal behavior.

METHODS

Male Sprague-Dawley rats were injected (icv) with CRF (1 ug) or vehicle (0.1 % bovine serum albumin in saline) once daily for 9 consecutive days. On the 10th day, half of the animals received an injection of CRF and half an injection of vehicle 30 min prior to monitoring grooming or footshock-induced (0.5 mA, 0.5 sec) immobility. Following these tests, the animals were sacrificed, plasma samples saved for measurment of ACTH and corticosterone, and cerebral cortex and pituitary removed for CRF binding experiments.

RESULTS

As reported previously (7), acute administration of CRF (icv) to naive animals nearly doubles the duration of footshock-induced immobility (Table 1). Animals receiving daily injections of CRF over 9 days also displayed an enhanced response to footshock 30 min after vehicle and up to 24 hrs after the last injection of peptide. No further increase in this response was seen in animals which had received an acute challenge with CRF following repeated administration of the peptide (Table 1.)

Administration of CRF 30 min before testing significantly increased the duration of grooming in animals which had been chronically treated with vehicle (Table 1). In contrast, the grooming response of animals treated chronically with CRF but challenged with vehicle was no different from that observed with control (vehicle/vehicle) subjects. Unlike chronic vehicle-treated animals, animals treated chronically with CRF did not display increased grooming 30 min after an acute challenge with the peptide.

Table 1. Behavioral and Hormonal Responses to CRF Administration.

Treatment Chronic/Acute	Footshock-Induced Immobility (min)	Grooming (min)	ACTH pg/ml	Corticosterone ng/ml
Vehicle/Vehicle	1.69 ± 0.51	0.16 ± 0.05	143 ± 25	117 ± 30
Vehicle/CRF	3.45 ± 0.56*	1.49 ± 0.30*	629 ± 111*	414 ± 30*
CRF/Vehicle	3.54 ± 0.65*	0.22 ± 0.07	261 ± 96	77 ± 18
CRF/CRF	3.58 ± 0.52*	0.42 ± 0.11	380 ± 77	407 ± 58*

* Significantly different from control (vehicle/vehicle) animals ($p \leq 0.05$). Values represent the mean ± SEM of 7-10 animals.

Rats treated chronically with CRF did not maintain elevated levels of either ACTH or corticosterone in plasma. Moreover, ACTH secretion in response to acute CRF injection was significantly attenuated in rats treated chronically with the peptide as compared to vehicle-injected animals (Table 1). In contrast, basal and stimulated corticosterone responses to CRF were essentially identical in both groups of rats (Table 1). Finally, CRF binding sites were decreased (15-25%) significantly in both pituitary and cerebral cortical tissue in animals treated chronically with the peptide.

DISCUSSION

The results of these experiments indicate that chronic administration of CRF leads to a reduction in CRF binding sites in brain and pituitary tissue and to functional alterations in this receptor system. Of particular interest was the finding that repeated treatment with CRF enhances a fear response (footshock-induced immobility), an action reminiscent of the behavioral sensitization produced by chronic exposure to stress. Thus it appears that chronic exposure to CRF mimics some of the clinical features of affective illness and therefore may provide a model for further investigating the neurochemical, pharmacological and behavioral characteristics of this disorder.

REFERENCES

1. Banki, C.M. et al., (1987): Am. J. Psychiatry, 144:873-877.
2. Bardelelben, U. Von and Holsboer, F. (1988): Prog. Neuro-Psychopharmacol. and Biol. Psychiat., 12:S165-187.
3. Fisher, L. (1988): Trends in Pharmacol. Sci., 10:189-193.
4. Gold, P.W. et al., (1986): New Engl. J. Med., 314:1329-1335.
5. Gold, P.W., Goodwin, F.K., and Chrousos, G.P. (1988): New Engl. J. Med., 319:413-420.
6. Holsboer, F. et al., (1984): Psychoneuroendocrinology, 9:147-160.
7. Kalin, N.H., Sherman, J.E. and Takahashi, L.K. (1988): Brain Res., 457:130-135.
8. Koob, G.F. and Bloom, F.E. (1985): Fed.Proc., 44:577-579.
9. Nemeroff, C.B. (1988): Pharmacopsychiat., 21:76-82.
10. Nemeroff, C.B. et al., (1988): Arch. Gen. Psychiatry, 45:577-579.

RODENT MODELS OF AGGRESSIVE BEHAVIOUR AND SEROTONERGIC DRUGS

B. OLIVIER and J. MOS
CNS-Pharmacology, Duphar b.v., P.O.B. 900, 1380 DA Weesp, Holland.

Rodent models of aggression have been frequently used to screen drugs on potential activity for psychiatric diseases, e.g., taming by benzodiazepines indicating anxiolysis or anti-muricidal effects for antidepressant potential. Although still in use for these applications, aggressive behaviour may offer far more to drug classification and may even lead to development of new drugs, specifically aimed at treatment of "aggressive" or "impulsive" disorders.

The study of aggressive behaviour has greatly benefited from the field of ethopharmacology, enabling the development of animal models to study offense, defense and flight. This distinction appeared important because in several models predominantly offense is generated and in others predominantly defense/flight. Effects of drugs have to be separated and measured in these different types of aggression models. Moreover, different neural substrates, each presumably with an own unique set of neurotransmitters, seem to underlie such different types of aggressive behaviours.

Several aggression models for offense are used to study drug effects, e.g., isolation-induced, social interaction, resident-intruder and maternal aggression in mice and rats. Adequate, but less often used models of offensive aggression are e.g., hypothalamically-induced aggression in rats or play-fighting in juvenile rats (4). Defensive models used are foot-shock induced biting, defensive behaviour of intruders when attacked or fear-induced flight (1).

We used both offensive and defensive animal models to study the anti-aggressive qualities of psychoactive drugs and focus here on the influence of the serotonergic (5-HT) systems in the CNS on aggressive behaviour. Although early work (2) suggested a simple inhibitory relationship between aggression and 5-HT, recent evidence on the distribution of 5-HT neurons in the CNS, the different types of 5-HT receptors (5-HT$_1$; 5-HT$_2$; 5-HT$_3$), their localization (pre-/postsynaptic, on cell body) and the coupling of the different receptor types to their respective second messenger-systems (e.g. c-AMP, phosphoinositol) makes it highly unlikely that such a simple hypothesis could hold.

The effects of drugs on aggression, exploration, social interest, avoidance and inactivity were measured. Several, if not all drugs decrease aggressive behaviour, but they do it in variable ways, including unwanted side-effects. By recording of all behaviour we were able to define a specific anti-aggressive profile of drugs: i.e. dose-dependent reduction of offensive behaviour, leaving social interactions and exploration intact. Moreover, no unwanted side-effects like sedation, muscle relaxation or psychostimulation should interfere with the proper performance of behaviour.

Extensive experimenting showed that it is feasible to develop and find such specific anti-aggressive drugs (3), which have been named "Serenics" (5). These drugs, represented by eltoprazine, appeared 5-HT$_1$ agonists with a high affinity for 5-HT$_{1B}$ and 5-HT$_{1A}$ receptor subtypes. Table 1 summarizes various serotonergic drugs in different offensive and defensive paradigms. 5-HT$_{1A}$-agonists either have no or nonspecific anti-aggressive effects. Due to the lack of specific drugs, no direct answers to the question of precise involvement of 5-HT receptor subtypes could be given. Indirect evidence strongly suggests that 5-HT$_2$ and 5-HT$_3$ receptors do not play a pivotal role in the modulation of offensive aggression (4).

Table 1: Effects of 5-HT drugs on 8 animal models for offensive and defensive aggression.

Drugs	IIA	SI	RI	EBS	MA	MK	DB	FS	Main serotonergic effect (affinities)
8-OH-DPAT	↓	↓	↓	o	↓	o	-	-	1A-agonist
Buspirone	↓	↓	↓	-	↓	↓	-	-	1A-agonist
Ipsapirone	↓	↓	↓	-	↓	o	-	-	1A-agonist
Flesinoxan	↓	↓	↓	-	↓	↓	-	-	1A-agonist
TFMPP	↓	ⓓ	ⓓ	ⓓ	ⓓ	ⓓ	o	o	1A,B,C-agonist
Eltoprazine	↓	ⓓ	ⓓ	ⓓ	ⓓ	ⓓ	o	o	1A,B,C ag.; 1C ant.
RU24969	↓	ⓓ	ⓓ	-	ⓓ	ⓓ	-	-	1A,B,C,D-agonist
5-MeODMT	o	o	(↓)	-	o	↓	-	-	1A,C; 2-agonist
DOI	o	-	(↓)	-	(↓)	o	-	-	1C,2-agonist
Ritanserine	o	o	o	-	o	o	-	-	2-agonist
MDL72222	o	o	-	-	o	o	-	-	3-antagonist
GR 38032F	o	o	-	-	o	o	-	-	3-antagonist
Mianserine	o	o	↓	↓	↓	↓	-	-	3-ant., 1C,2 ag.
Quipazine	↓	↓	↓	↓	↓	↓	-	-	3-ant., 1,2 ag.
Fenfluramine	↓	↓	↓	-	↓	↓	-	-	release
Fluvoxamine	↓	↓	↓	↓	↓	↓	o	o	reuptake block

- = not tested; ⓓ = specific antiaggressive effect; ↓ = nonspecific antiaggressive effect; o = no antiaggressive effect. ( ) = anti-aggressive, but interfering effects (serotonergic syndrome). IIA = isolation-induced aggression, SI = social interaction, RI = resident-intruder, EBS = hypothalamic aggression, MA = maternal aggression, MK = mouse killing, DB = defensive behaviour, FS = foot-shock defense.

The combination of ethopharmacological methods and testing of various 5-HT drugs leads to a picture of a heterogenous involvement of the serotonergic system in the CNS in aggressive behaviour. The available data suggest that in particular $5-HT_1$ receptors are involved in the modulation of offensive behaviour. Further work is needed to unravel the basic fundamentals of this neurobiological system. The use of ethopharmacology in aggression has led to a new class of serotonergic drugs, the serenics, which are now clinically tested in certain human psychiatric diseases.

REFERENCES
1. Blanchard, D.C. and Blanchard, R.J.: Ethoexperimental approaches to the biology of emotion. Ann. Rev. Psychol. 39: 43-68, 1988.
2. Miczek, K.A. and Donat, P.: Brain 5-HT system and inhibition of aggressive behaviour. In: Behavioural Pharmacology of 5-HT. Lawrence Erlbaum, New Jersey, 117-144, 1989.
3. Olivier, B. and Mos, J.: Serenics and aggression. Stress Medicine 2: 197-209, 1986.
4. Olivier, B. and Mos, J.: Serotonin, serenics and aggressive behaviour in animals. In: Depression, Anxiety and Aggression. Medidact, Houten, 133-165, 1988.
5. Olivier, B., Van Dalen, D. and Hartog J.: A new class of psychoactive drugs; Serenics. Drugs Future 11: 473-499, 1986.

SEROTONERGIC MECHANISMS AND IMPULSIVE AGGRESSION IN VERVET MONKEYS

MICHAEL J. RALEIGH and MICHAEL T. MCGUIRE

Dept. of Psychiatry, UCLA School of Medicine, Los Angeles, CA USA 90024

We have examined the contributions of serotonergic and other monoaminergic mechanisms to an animal model of both normative and impulsive aggression. These investigations have been conducted in vervet monkeys (<u>Cercopithecus</u> <u>aethiops</u> <u>sabaeus</u>). Phylogenetically, vervet monkeys are closely related to humans and they exhibit a rich repertoire of social and nonsocial behaviors that parallels many aspects of human nonverbal behavior. Thus, conclusions regarding the roles of monoaminergic mechanisms in promoting and constraining aggression are likely to generalize to humans.

We have used two approaches in our studies. One is correlational and examines the links between aggression and physiological functions. In these studies, we record the rate, intensity, antecedents, and consequences of aggression of subjects living in naturally constituted social groups. We have obtained repeated basal CSF 5-HIAA and HVA values from 62 adult males who were members of 17 social groups. CSF 5-HIAA and HVA are inversely related to spontaneous aggression ($r= -.84$, and $-.61$, respectively). CSF 5-HIAA is also inversely linked to more specific components of aggressive behavior including the likelihood of escalating fights ($r= -.73$); the probability of initiating unprovoked attacks ($r= -.84$); and the proportion of aggression directed toward inappropriate targets ($r= -.82$). When the association between 5-HIAA and HVA is partialled out, no significant correlations between HVA and these measures remain. These data support the view that diminished 5-HIAA is tied to heightened rates and maladaptive patterns of aggression, a finding compatible with studies of humans (2).

A second approach is experimental and involves pharmacologically manipulating serotonergic systems. We have employed compounds that diminish central serotonergic function including chronic PCPA, fenfluramine, ketanserin, and cyproheptadine. Each reduces serotonergic function but each also has a variety of other effects. However, the commonalities in the drugs behavioral effects are most parsimoniously attributed to their effects on serotonin.

parsimoniously attributed to their effects on serotonin. Treatments with these drugs produce dose-dependent increases in the rate and intensity of aggression, the probability of escalating aggressive encounters to the point where subjects are injured, and decrements in the likelihood of reconciliation occuring following a fight. We have also examined the effects of augmenting serotonergic function by chronic tryptophan, fluoxetine, or quipazine administration (1). These treatments alter maladaptive but not species typical appropriate aggression. Further, concurrent quipazine treatment eradicates heightened aggression produced by serotonergic antagonists. In addition, compounds whose effects are primarily on non-serotonergic systems may also increase aggressive behavior. These include phencyclidine (PCP) and amphetamine. Preliminary data suggest that the effects of these compounds on aggression can also be eradicated by concurrent administration of S_2 receptor agonists. These observations suggest that serotonergic systems diminish maladaptive aggression and that these effects may be largely mediated by actions at S_2 sites.

The robust relationship between diminished serotonergic function and heightened aggressivity is tempered by at least two social/environmental factors. One is social status. High ranking, or dominant individuals, are more sensitive to serotonergic agonists but less responsive to serotonergic antagonists than others. Thus, for example, a smaller dose of quipazine is required to ameliorate amphetamine-induced aggression in dominant than in subordinate males. The second factor is the stability of social relationships within a given group. In unstable social groups, both adult and adolescent males with low CSF 5-HIAA are particularly likely to engage in impulsive, unprovoked aggresssion that leads to severe injuries among group members.

Thus, in monkeys physiological and pharmacological data implicate serotonergic mechanisms in the expression of both normative and impulsive aggressive behavior. Many of the inhibitory effects of serotonergic mechanisms on aggression may be mediated largely through S_2 receptor sites. As in humans, social status and group stability can modify, but not eliminate, the links between serotonergic systems and aggression.

REFERENCES

1. Raleigh, M.J. et al., Dominant social status facilitates the behavioral effects of serotonergic agonists. Brain Res 348:274-282, 1985.

2. Virkkunen, M. et al., Psychobiological concomitants of history of suicide attempts among violent offenders and impulsive fire setters. Arch Gen Psychiatry 46:604-606, 1989.

PHARMACOLOGICAL MANIPULATION OF AGGRESSIVENESS AND IMPULSIVENESS IN HEALTHY VOLUNTEERS

A.J. BOND,
Department of Psychiatry, Institute of Psychiatry, University of London, U.K.

Clinically, many different psychotropic drugs have been used to treat aggressive and impulsive behaviour and many compounds have been claimed to be effective in its control, although none as yet has proved to be specifically anti-aggressive (3) and all have disadvantages. Although many compounds have been tested clinically (Table 1), there are few well-controlled, double-blind trials and the measurement of impulsive behaviour is fraught with difficulties. This is reflected in the paucity of studies in healthy volunteers.

Table 1: Psychotropic Drugs evaluated in Clinical Studies

Anti-Psychotics
Benzodiazepines
Lithium
B-blockers
Stimulants
Carbamazepine

In order to pharmacologically manipulate aggressiveness in healthy volunteers, it is necessary to develop techniques not just to measure but to elicit such behaviour without drugs. Although various rating-scales and verbal reports have been used, it is more valuable to have some behavioural measure (2). Various techniques have been developed and those which have been used alongside the psychotropic substances studied are listed in Table 2.

Table 2: Techniques used to elicit aggression in healthy volunteers and pharmacological manipulations tested.

Techniques	Psychotropic Substance
1. Group dynamics	Alcohol, Benzodiazepines
2. Teaching situation	Alcohol
3. Stooge intervention	Alcohol, B-blocker
4. Competition with provocation	Alcohol, Benzodiazepines Caffeine, Cannabis, Nicotine

From a swift perusal of tables 1 and 2, it can be seen that few of the drugs which are used clinically have been examined using specific techniques in volunteer subjects. The most widely tested substance has been alcohol because of its association with crime and violent behaviour. Alcohol has been shown to increase aggressive responding in the laboratory although its effects were moderated by certain methodological factors (1). Benzodiazepines have been tested using two of the techniques listed and have shown differing effects depending on the individual compound used: chlordiazepoxide, diazepam and lorazepam have all been shown to increase aggressive responding but oxazepam has not.

The other psychotropic compounds used: B-blockers, caffeine, cannabis and nicotine, have either not altered or decreased aggression in the situations in which they have been tested. Few drug combination have been examined but propranalol has been shown to attenuate and alprazolam to be additive with the effects of alcohol.

It seems now important to go on to try and link healthy volunteer studies with our knowledge of neurotransmitter involvement and clinical practice. The techniques exist and we know they can be manipulated pharmacologically. If central serotonin is lowered in patients with impulse control, then manipulating levels in volunteers and testing them with techniques designed to elicit aggression is one possible next step.

REFERENCES

1. Bushman, B.J. and Cooper, H.M. (1990): Effects of alcohol on human aggression: an integrative research review. Psychol. Bull. 107: 1-14.
2. Russell, G.W. (1981): A comparison of hostility measures. J. Soc. Psychol. 113: 45-55.
3. Sheard, M.H. (1988): Clinical pharmacology of aggressive behaviour. Clin. Neuropharm. 11:483-492.

SUICIDAL BEHAVIOR AND SEROTONIN

L. TRÄSKMAN-BENDZ[*], C. ALLING[**], G. REGNÉLL[*], P. SIMONS-SON[**], and R. ÖHMAN[*]
*Department of Psychiatry and **Department of Neurochemistry, University of Lund, Sweden.

By now, it is relatively well established that the serotonin (5HT)-system is important for suicidal behavior. Since the first findings of low CSF 5-HIAA (a 5HT-metabolite) in violent suicide-attempters and attempters later completing suicide (2), several studies have been performed, and with similar results. Apart from CSF-studies, 5HT-function could be estimated from platelet studies, whole blood-investigations, or challenge-tests.
Regardless of methodological approach, findings indicate an association between serotonin dysfunction and impulsivity and/or aggression directed outwardly or towards oneself (3).

The aim of our ongoing studies at the Lund Suicide Research Center are to get a detailed description of psychiatric patients at risk for repeated suicidal behavior, and to develop adequate treatment-strategies for suicide attempters.

PATIENTS AND METHODS

Suicide-attempters are recruited directly from the intensive care unit into our 13 bed research ward. They are offered an extensive multifactorial research program, which continues monthly or every three months 1-2 years after discharge.

Concerning 5HT, we study CSF 5-HIAA, platelet MAO-activity, platelet 5HT-2-receptor-function (hydrolysis of phosphatidyl-inositolphosphate), and whole blood serotonin. We compare clinical information acquired from ratings, inventories, and tests with various biochemical results.

RESULTS

Violent suicide-attempters tend to have lower CSF 5-HIAA than non-violent. Two patients have committed suicide within one year after discharge, and both had fairly low CSF 5-HIAA. In men, low CSF 5-HIAA is associated with various aspects of increased impulsivity.
In 14 suicide attempters, we found a significantly increased platelet 5HT-2 function in comparison with matched controls.

We have CSF follow-up data from 10 patients. Our preliminary findings show that low 5-HIAA suicide-attempters more often repeat their suicidal behavior than do high 5-HIAA suicide-attempters. Intra-individual follow-up CSF-data do not indicate seasonal variations of 5-HIAA.

DISCUSSION

Our CSF 5-HIAA-findings in drug-free suicide-attempters are congruent with other reports.

Our long-term studies confirm findings by Roy et al (4) of repeated suicidal behavior in low 5-HIAA depressed patients, and also observations by Virkkunen et al (6) of repeated violent behavior in former prisoners with low CSF 5-HIAA.

Other investigators have found increased binding to 5HT-2 receptors in frontal cortex of completed suicides (1, 5). Our platelet studies, which reflect dynamic 5 HT-2 receptor events, could also be interpreted as increased 5HT-2-receptor-sensitivity in suicidal people.

The implication of findings by us and others is that low CSF 5-HIAA is an important prognostic risk-factor for suicidal behavior. Possibly, future treatment strategies will include drugs specifically acting on the 5HT-2-receptor.

REFERENCES

1. Arora, R.C. and Meltzer, H.Y., (1989): Am. J. Psychiat., 146:730-736.
2. Åsberg, M., Träskman, L., and Thorén, P., (1976): Arch. Gen. Psychiat., 33:1193-1197.
3. Åsberg, et al.,(1987): In Psychopharmacology: The third generation of progress, Meltzer, H.Y. ed., pp. 655-668. Raven Press, New York.
4. Roy, A., de Jong, J. and Linnoila, M., (1989): Arch. Gen. Psychiat., 46:609-612.
5. Stanley, M., and Mann, J.J., (1983): Lancet, 1:214-216.
6. Virkkunen, et al., (1989): Arch. Gen. Psychiat., 46: 600-603.

VIOLENT BEHAVIOR, SEROTONIN AND GLUCOSE METABOLISM

M.Virkkunen*and M.Linnoila**
Psychiatric Clinic, Helsinki University Central Hospital*,
Laboratory of Clinical Studies,**DICBR, Bethesda, MD 20892,
U.S.A.

Until recently there have been very little evidence that man can predict violence; it means recidivist violent criminality. During the last years there have, however, been many findings to show that among the habitually violent and impulsive criminals who commit crimes under the influence of alcohol there are abnormal biochemical findings; especially low cerebrospinal fluid 5-hydroxy-indoleacetic acid level and the tendency to low blood glucose nadir in the glucose tolerance test (1,5). Glucose and brain serotonin metabolism are known to be connected with each other (3). This tendency to behave aggressively and impulsively under the influence of alcohol is usually connected with so called type 2 alcoholism of Cloninger et al. (2). Also peripheral indices of serotonin metabolism have been found to correlate with impulsive violence (1).

SUBJECTS AND METHOD

Recently we reported prospective follow-up studies of these habitually violent and impulsive offenders (4,6). Subjects included 58 men with a mean age of 30.2 ± 10.0 years. Of these 36 had either attempted or committed a manslaughter and 22 offenders were arsonists. The offense was categorized as impulsive if the victim was previously unknown to the offender and / or no or only minor provocation was evident and the attack did not represent an attempt to rob the victim. The nonimpulsive offenders knew the victim, and there was evidence of premeditation of the crime. All arsonists were selected to represent impulsive fire setters. The sample consisted of 46 impulsive and 12 nonimpulsive subjects. The impulsive violent offenders usually fulfilled the criteria of antisocial personality or intermittent explosive disorder and at the same time borderline personality disorder and alcohol abuse problems.

This report outcome data during a mean follow-up period of 35.6 ± 18.0 months after the release from prison. The criminal register was searched for repeated crimes at that time.

RESULTS

Thirteen of 58 offenders had committed new violent crimes under the influence of alcohol. Blood glucose nadir and low CSF 5-HIAA correctly classified the offenders as recidivists and nonrecidivists in 84.2 per cent of the cases. When the family histories of the violent offenders were studied, however, only the low CSF 5-HIAA was connected with alcoholism in the father.

DISCUSSION

Whether a low CSF 5-HIAA connection is characteristic of type 2 alcoholism with less-severe criminality than was typical for the present samples needs to be investigated further. The results suit to the idea that these impulsively violent persons may be treatable with serotoninergic drugs which could ameliorate the serotonergic deficit.

REFERENCES

1. Caccaro,E.F. (1989): Central serotonin and impulsive aggression. Br.J.Psychiat. Suppl.8:52-62.
2. Cloninger, et al.,(1981): Inheritance of alcohol abuse. Crossfostering analysis of alcoholic men. Arch. Gen. Psychiat. 38:861-868.
3. Fernström, J.D. and Wurtman, R.J. (1971): Brain serotonin content. Increase following ingestion of carbohydrate diet. Science 174:1023-1025.
4. Linnoila, et al. (1989): Family history of alcoholism in violent offenders and impulsive fire setters. Arch.Gen. Psychiat. 46:613-616.
5. Roy, et al., (1986): Indices of serotonin and glucose metabolism in violent offenders, arsonists, and alcoholics. In Psychobiology of Suicidal Behavior. J.J.Mann and M. Stanley, eds. Ann. NY Acad. Sci. 407:202-220.
6. Virkkunen, et al., (1989): Relationship of psychobiological variables to recidivism in violent offenders and impulsive fire setters. A follow-up study. Arch. Gen. Psychiat. 46:600-603.

DRUG TREATMENT OF SCHIZOPHRENIA: CURRENT CONCEPTS

D. NABER and H. HIPPIUS
Psychiatric Hospital, University of Munich, F.R.G.

It is widely accepted that typical neuroleptic drugs exhibit both their wanted antipsychotic action and their unwanted extrapyramidal effects via blockade of dopamine receptors within the CNS. Therefore, the relief of symptoms such as delusions and hallucinations seemed to be tightly coupled to unpleasant motor side-effects. Limitations of conventional neuroleptics are demonstrated by about 30% of schizophrenic patients, either therapy-resistant or too sensitive regarding side-effects, and by the only marginal improvement of negative symptoms.

However, there is evidence that the assumed close relationship between antipsychotic efficacy and extrapyramidal effects is not applicable for all neuroleptics and that pharmacotherapy of schizophrenia might change considerably. Clozapine with its antipsychotic action in the absence of marked motor side-effects and its efficacy in many patients resistant to classical neuroleptics was the first success in the search for more efficacious and better tolerated neuroleptics. Presently, promising approaches include sigma receptor blockade, 5-HT-2 or 5 HT-3 receptor blockade, selective D-1 or D-2 receptor blockade and partial agonism of D-2 receptor. These strategies have generated a number of compounds, but due to the scarcity of controlled studies, it is still too early to discuss their clinical usefulness.

Thus, clozapine is still the only atypical neuroleptic of clinical relevance. The growing interest in this drug prompted the present review, two naturalistic studies, to evaluate benefits and risks of clozapine treatment in a rather high number of in- and out-patients.

Medical charts of 503 in-patients (368 schizophrenics) were analyzed to document efficacy and side-effects of clozapine. Schizophrenic patients were previously treated for 3-7 weeks with 2-7 other neuroleptics and were either therapy-resistant (36%) or had too severe side-effects (64%). They were treated with clozapine for 47 ± 36 days; mean dosage was 208 ± 112 mg, maximal dosage 285 + 183 mg.

4% of patients showed worsening, 13% no change, 38% slight improvement, 42% marked improvement and 3% nearly total reduction of symptoms.

At least one major side-effect occured in 59% of patients. Most often were EEG-alterations (23%), sedation (17%), increase of liver enzymes (8%), hypotension (7%), hypersalivation (7%), fever (5%), ECG-alterations (4%), delirious states (4%), tachycardia (3%), gastro-intestinal symptoms (3%) and weight gain (3%). In none of these patients, irreversible complications occured. Only EEG-alterations were significantly related to clozapine dosage.

A gradual increase of dosage considerably reduced the incidence of sedation, hypotension and delirious states. There was no patient with leucopenia (WBC < 3.500 x 10 /ml) and no patient, whose neuroleptic treatment consisted of clozapine alone, showed major motor side-effects. A combination of psychotropic drugs such as typical neuroleptics, antidepressants or benzodiazepines with clozapine, administered in lower dosages than in monotherapy, did not result in increased side-effects.

At discharge, neuroleptic treatment consisted of clozapine alone in 60% of patients. In 19 %, clozapine was combined with conventional neuroleptics and only in 21%, clozapine treatment was discontinued. Reasons for discontinuation were insufficient efficacy (8%), severe side-effects (7%), non-compliance, mostly in hebephrenic patients because of the weekly hematological controls (5%) and refusal of private psychiatrists to prescribe clozapine (1%).

Effects of clozapine long-term therapy were, again retrospectively, evaluated in 78 schizophrenic out-patients, treated for 3 ± 4 years. Administered in monotherapy (67%), the daily dosage was 190 ± 105 mg; in combination with other neuroleptics (33%), it was 145 ± 110 mg. 36% of the patients improved slightly, 52% markedly and in 12% the symptoms nearly totally disappeared. Days of in-patient treatment as well as number of rehospitalization were significantly reduced under clozapine treatment.

Clinically relevant side effects occurred in 53% of patients. Sedation, EEG-alterations, hypotension, ECG alterations, increase of liver enzymes and weight gain were most often. Only 11% of patients were non-compliant, other reasons for discontinuation of clozapine treatment were insufficient efficacy (10%) and major side-effects (7%). One case of leucopenia with normalization of WBC after clozapine discontinuation, but no case of agranulocytosis occured.

These data indicate high compliance and a satisfactory benefit/risk ratio in most of the negatively selected patients. With regard to the low or non-existing risk of clozapine to induce tardive dyskinesia, further research should focus on criteria of indication. Is it justified to treat only those patients with clozapine where conventional neuroleptics have failed?

CLINICAL EFFICACY OF CLOZAPINE IN THE TREATMENT OF SCHIZOPHRENIA

H.Y. MELTZER*, L.D. ALPHS**, B. BASTANI*, L.F. RAMIREZ* and K. KWON**
Department of Psychiatry School of Medicine*, Case Western Reserve University, Cleveland, Ohio; Psychiatry Service, Veterans Administration Medical Center**, Brecksville, Ohio, U.S.A.

Clozapine is the first antipsychotic drug which has been shown to be significantly superior to typical neuroleptic drugs in the treatment of schizophrenic patients who do not respond satisfactorily to typical antipsychotic agents (3). Clozapine has also been shown to have much fewer extrapyramidal symptoms and not to produce a tardive dyskinesia.

As is well known, clozapine produces agranulocytosis in 1-2% of patients. For this reason, its use has been restricted to treatment-resistant patients and patients intolerant of typical neuroleptic drugs. Long-term effects must be considered in deciding upon a course of clozapine treatment.

There are a few retrospective long-term studies of clozapine treatment (2,4,5,6,8). In a preliminary report of a prospective study (7), clozapine was also found to produce significant improvement in positive and negative symptoms in subjects studied over a 6 week - 35 month period. This report will provide further data on that series of patients.

Eighty-five patients (60 M, 25 F) who met Research Diagnostic Criteria for schizophrenia or schizoaffective disorders and who began a trial of clozapine $\geq$ 12 months ago are reported herein. Their mean age was 34.6 ± 8.5 years.

Of the 85 patients, 57 remained on clozapine after 12 months. Twenty-eight patients dropped out for the following reasons: adverse reactions (N=8), non-compliance (N=9), inadequate response (N=8) and administrative reasons (N=3). Of the 57 patients still on clozapine, 46 had a decrease in BPRS score of $\geq$ 20% at various time points from 6 weeks to 12 months. Seventy of the patients had an admission Brief Psychiatric Rating Scale [BPRS (9)] score $\geq$ 36 (1-7 scale). Forty of these 70 patients had a decrease in BPRS of $\geq$ 20%, a total BPRS score $\leq$ 36 or a Clinical Global Impressions score of $\leq$ 3 over the course of the 12 months. Twelve of the 40 (30%) patients achieved this response by six weeks, the rest at later periods. The largest decrease in mean BPRS took place between baseline and six weeks. Significant improvement was noted in the BPRS and SADS-C Positive Symptom score as well as the SADS-C Negative Symptoms and Disorganization Subscales. The latter scale reflects hebephrenic-type symptoms. There was no difference in the response of paranoid, undifferentiated or disorganized schizophrenic patients. However, schizoaffective, mainly schizophrenic (N=14) and schizoaffective, mainly affective patients (N=5), tended to do less well or better than the schizophrenic patients, respectively.

Improvement in social function was demonstrated by significant changes in the Global Assessment Scale (GAS) and Quality of Life scale (1). Approximately half of the clozapine patients were able to hold volunteer jobs, work at paying jobs, or attend school.

Fifty-one of the 57 patients who remained on clozapine at 12 months had been hospitalized at least once in the 12 months before clozapine for a total of 77 hospitalizations. Only 8 patients were rehospitalized for psychiatric reasons a total of 8 times (an 89.6% decrease) in the 12 months after clozapine. Patients who were eventually rehospitalized did not differ from those who were not rehospitalized on sex, age, age of onset, number of previous hospitalizations, and baseline or discharge psychopathology.

Some of the patients remaining on clozapine showed dramatic improvement, moving into a clinical state close to residual schizophrenia. The majority of patients achieved a reduced level of psychopathology and improved social function. Because of low extrapyramidal symptoms, clozapine was well accepted.

In conclusion, the 12 month outcome of clozapine treatment indicates that it is a significant benefit in many but not all treatment resistant patients. Response may be delayed and is limited in most patients, but still clinically important. Together with psychosocial treatments, significant gains in social function can be achieved. A striking decrease in rehospitalization is possible.

REFERENCES:

1. Heinrichs, D.W., Hanlon, F.T., and Carpenter, W.T., Jr. (1984): Schiz. Bull. 10:388-396.
2. Juul-Povlsen, V.J., et al., (1985): Acta Psychiatr. Scand., 71:176-185.
3. Kane, J., et al., (1989): Psychopharmacology, 99:S60-S63.
4. Kuha, S., and Miettinen, E. (1986): Nord. Psychiatr. Tidskr., 40:225-230.
5. Leppig, M., et al., (1989): Psychopharmacology, 99:S77-S79.
6. Lindström, L.H. (1988): Acta Psychiatr. Scand., 77:524-529.
7. Meltzer et al., (1989): Psychopharmacology, 99:S68-S72.
8. Naber, D., et al., (1989): Psychopharmacology, 99:S73-S76.
9. Overall, J.E., and Gorham, D.R. (1962): Psychol. Rep., 10:799-812.

SIDE EFFECTS OF CLOZAPINE AND THEIR MANAGEMENT

L.D. Alphs, H.Y. Meltzer, B. Bastani and L.F. Ramirez
Department of Psychiatry, Case Western Reserve University, School of Medicine, Cleveland, Ohio and Cleveland VA Medical Center, Brecksville, Ohio 44141, USA

Clozapine has recently been demonstrated to offer considerable therapeutic promise for schizophrenic symptoms in patients who have heretofore been resistant to treatment (1). Despite its potential for improving therapy of schizophrenia, clozapine's use has been limited by a profile of side effects that is also atypical. Prominent among these are sedation, hypotension, tachycardia, sialorrhea, seizures, constipation, hyperthermia, weight gain and agranulocytosis. Understanding the management of these side effects is essential for the safe and skillful clinical use of this drug.

Sedation is the most common side effect. It occurred in 21% of the patients participating in the US multi-center study of treatment-resistant schizophrenics (1). Many patients tolerate to this effect, but, for those who do not, provision of the drug in divided doses with the larger dose given at bedtime, or reduction in dosage may be necessary.

Sialorrhea is reported to have an incidence of 5.7% worldwide (2), but, in our experience, it is considerably more common (about 20%). For many patients sialorrhea is benign and tolerable, but for others the constant excessive drooling is social embarrassing, and can result in complications from aspiration. Patients may tolerate to this side effect with prolonged treatment, but, for those who do not, lowering the dose of clozapine may be helpful. Some patients respond to treatment with anticholinergic medications.

Tachycardia is reported in over 5% of patients taking clozapine. It appears to be related to vagal inhibition secondary to clozapine-induced cholinergic blockade. If clinically significant, it is best managed by lowering the dose, adding adjunctive treatments (like propranolol), or, if necessary, stopping the drug.

Seizures have occurred among 4% of US-treated cases. This incidence is greater than that observed with typical neuroleptics and is considerably higher that observed worldwide (0.36%). This may be a consequence of the higher doses of clozapine used in the US. US experience suggests an incidence for seizures of 14% among patients taking more than 600 mg clozapine/day, and only 0.6% for patients taking less than 300 mg/day. Seizure management includes decreasing the dose of clozapine and using anticonvulsants as necessary.

Hypotension is commonly observed after initiating treatment with clozapine, but many patients develop tolerance to it. For this reason clozapine treatment is usually started at low doses tolerated by most patients (25 mg, once or twice daily). The dose is then elevated slowly until therapeutic response or side effects intervene.

Constipation is a common early side effect of clozapine treatment and can result in considerable discomfort if it is not promptly evaluated and treated. Most patients respond to treatment with a high fiber diet or bulk supplements. In our experience, patients usually tolerate to this side effect after a few weeks of therapy.

A mild hyperthermia frequently occurs in patients during the initial phases of treatment. Most often, it is not clinically significant, but because of the danger of agranulocytosis it can be disturbing and needs to be monitored. Severe hyperthermia and periodic cataplexy are much less common, but have been reported.

Weight gain is a common side effect that may necessitate termination of clozapine treatment. Dietary counseling and restriction are indicated, but are not always successful.

Agranulocytosis represents the most dangerous of the common side effects of clozapine. It occurs in 1-2% of patients with the risk being greatest during the second through fourth months of treatment. However, available data suggest that the risk is never reduced to zero. The limited data currently available fail to show a dose response relationship to this side effect. Patients who develop this side effect should be withdrawn from medication immediately. Their white blood cell (WBC) count should then be monitored daily until stable, while maintaining a careful watch for signs of infection. Such patients should not be re-challenged with clozapine after an initial occurrence of agranulocytosis as symptoms have been shown to recur when this is done. In the US, it is mandated that clozapine treatment be discontinued if the WBC count drops below 2000/mm^3 or 1000 granulocytes/mm^3.

REFERENCES

1. Kane, J. et al. Clozapine for the treatment-resistant schizophrenic. Arch Gen Psychiatry, 45:789-796, 1988.
2. Lieberman, J.A. et al. Clozapine: Guidelines for Clinical Management. J Clin Psychiatry, 50:329-338, 1989.

CURRENT VIEWS ON TARDIVE DYSKINESIA

J. Gerlach
Sanct Hans Hospital, Department P, Roskilde, Denmark.

Tardive dyskinesia (TD) is a syndrome of involuntary movements that develops in predisposed individuals during long-term neuroleptic treatment (2). In some patients the syndrome disappears within a few weeks or months after drug discontinuation, but in others it persists as irreversible TD. TD is therefore one of the most serious side effects of a traditional neuroleptic treatment.

CLINICAL ASPECTS

Different dyskinesia types. TD is a heterogeneous syndrome. The typical TD is mainly seen in elderly patients, most often as the bucco-linguo-masticatory (BLM) syndrome. Patients with this type of TD are not usually troubled by their syndrome, but is may embarrase the family. Usually it can be diminished by increased neuroleptic dosage and accentuated by reduced dosage or adjuvant anticholinergic medication.
About 10% of dyskinetic patients have a paradoxical TD syndrome, also called acute dyskinesia (2). These patients are often younger and clearly more disstressed than patients with the typical TD. Paradoxical TD is often accompanied by akathisia and/or dystonic features, and it is more wide spread in its localisation. Increased neuroleptic dosage aggravates,whereas dosage reduction improves the condition.
Finally, a few percent of the dyskinesia patients may suffer from a severe irreversible TD, which develops rapidly over a few months of treatment. This syndrome is also wide spread, involving ataxic and jerky movements of extremities and body. It is often
irreversible.

TD - parkinsonism. TD and parkinsonism has been shown to coexist i up to 70% of TD cases (3). This suggests that TD and parkinsonism are not reciprocal entities, but 2 aspects of the same "disease proces", i.e. the pharmacological blockade of D2 dopamine receptors.
Parkinsonism may be able to suppress TD more or less, just as sedation and improvement in the psychotic state may improve TD. However, TD is seldom completely suppressed, even with increasing dosages and induction of parkinsonism. In most cases neuroleptics cause a moderate suppression only, and in a few cases there is no change or even a TD aggravation (3). This is in accordance with the idea of a dual effect of neuroleptics: They induce not only parkinsonism (TD suppression), but also hyperkinetic movements (TD aggravation).

PATHOPHYSIOLOGICAL MECHANISMS

The pathophysiology of TD has only been partially elucidated. Available evidence suggests that the D2 dopamine receptor blockade and an individual vulnerability (old age and genetic constitution) represent the principal factors.

The traditional dopamine supersensitivity theory is no longer viable. Instead new hypotheses have been proposed: TD may be due to an increased ratio of D1/D2 receptor functions in the brain, or it may be related to a hypofunction in some GABA projections. Dopamine supersensitivity may precipitate or aggravate the syndrome by diminishing parkinsonism (2).

Recent studies have revealed that stimulation of D1 dopamine receptors causes tongue protrusions and chewing movements similar to TD. This has been shown in monkeys with D1 agonists such as SKF 81297, but also in rodents, especially when D2 receptor functions are inhibited.

With this background it is tempting to hypothezise that neuroleptics produce parkinsonism by blocking D2 dopamine receptors, but at the same time carry the potential to induce dyskinesia by dopamine stimulation of D1 receptors. The net result depends on the individual sensitivity and changes in the respective receptor groups.

PREVENTION OF TARDIVE DYSKINESIA

At present no causal treatment of TD is available. Traditional neuroleptics can only suppress the syndrome indirectly, via parkinsonism, sedation or mental improvement, but may aggravate the syndrome in th long run. Therefore, prevention becomes essential.

It follows from the pathophysiological mechanisms mentioned above that the only prophylactic measure is a limitation of the D2 blockade. This can be done by using the lowest possible dosages and the shortest possible treatment periods, but it can also be done by using antipsychotics with relatively low D2 receptor blocking capacity. At the moment clozapine is the only significant example, but by adding a benzodiazepine it might be possible to reduce the dose of a traditional neuroleptic.

Due to the weak dopamine receptor blocking capacity of clozapine (40-60% occupancy of D1 as well as D2 receptors) (1), this drug does not appear to induce TD. In cases where TD has already developed, clozapine may allow a spontaneous TD recovery, just as the D1 receptor blockade and the mental improvement/sedation produced by clozapine may contribute to a TD reduction.

REFERENCES

1. Farde, L. et al.: D1- and D2-dopamine receptor occupancy during treatment with conventionel and atypical neuroleptics. Psychopharmacology 99:S28-S31, 1989.
2. Gerlach, J. and Casey, D.C.: Tardive dyskinesia. Acta Psychiat, Scand. 77:369-378, 1988.
3. Gerlach, J. et al.: Effect of chlorprothixene,haloperidol, and perphenazine in tardive dyskinesia and parkinsonism. Psychopharmacology 90: 423-429, 1986.

MECHANISM OF ACTION OF ATYPICAL ANTIPSYCHOTICS

P.L. HERRLING, Sandoz Research Institute, CH-3001 Berne, Switzerland

INTRODUCTION

The following paper will give a definition of 'atypical antipsychotics' (AAPs) and discuss several hypotheses derived from preclinical findings thought to be relevant for the atypical nature of such compounds, taking clozapine, the prototypic AAP, as an example.

DEFINITIONS

For the purpose of this article those agents will be considered as **antipsychotics** (APs) that at least improve positive symptoms of schizophrenia. Agents improving only negative symptoms are considered complementary medication to existing classical APs. The terms 'positive' and 'negative' symptoms are used as described by Crow (1).

Atypical APs are agents i) improving the positive symptoms of schizophrenia; ii) causing only minimal acute and/or delayed extrapyramidal side-effects (EPS); iii) causing no elevation of serum prolactin levels following repeated administrations.

Further characteristics that might also contribute to an atypical profile could be a beneficial effect in a patient population resistant to treatment with classical APs as defined by Kane et al. (2) as well as an improvement of negative symptoms.

PRECLINICAL OBSERVATIONS WITH AN AAP (CLOZAPINE) POSSIBLY RELATED TO ITS ATYPICAL PROFILE IN MAN

1. Antipsychotic action (2): Similar to all clinically used APs and consistent with the dopamine (D) hypothesis of schizophrenia (3), clozapine has a D-2 antagonistic component (4). Although it is relatively weak, it can be assumed that this system is clearly inhibited at clinical doses (5).

2. Lack of acute EPS (2): This property might be due both to the relatively low affinity to D-2 receptors and to the relatively potent antimuscarinic component of this compound (6). Antimuscarinic agents are clinically used to overcome acute EPS caused by classical APs (7).

3. Lack of increase in serum prolactin levels (8): this might be due to an increase of dopamine release induced by clozapine in the tubero-infundibular system (9) and the relatively weak affinity for D-2 receptors.

4. Probable lack of tardive dyskinesia-inducing potential (10): this

aspect could be related to the observation that chronically administered clozapine does not induce depolarization inactivation of dopamine neurons of the substantia nigra as do classical APs (11,12). This may be due to clozapine's D-1 antagonistic properties: it is known that there are presynaptic D-1 receptors located on GABA-releasing striato-nigral terminals (13) and D-1 receptors have also been found in the substantia nigra pars compacta in man (14). Furthermore, chronic administration of a selective D-1 antagonist does not cause inactivation of substantia nigra dopamine neurons (15). GABA systems in the basal ganglia are thought to be involved in dyskinesias induced by chronic treatment with APs (16).

5. Beneficial effects on negative symptoms (2): this clinical observation could be resulting from clozapine's affinity to 5HT-2 receptors (17) because selective 5HT-2 antagonists tested in schizophrenic patients displayed the most pronounced effects on this type of symptoms (18).

REFERENCES

1. Crow, T.J. Schizophrenia Bull. 11:471-486, 1985
2. Kane, J. Arch.Gen.Psychiatr. 45:789-796, 1988
3. Meltzer, H.Y. ed. Psychopharmacology. The Third Generation of Progress. Raven Press, New York, 1987
4. Coward, D. et al. Psychopharmacology 99:S6-S12, 1989.
5. Farde, L. Psychopharmacology 99:S28-S31, 1989
6. Miller, R.J. and Hiley, C.R. Nature 248:596, 1974.
7. Rifkin, A. and Siris, S In:Psychopharmacology. The Third Generation of Progress. H.Y. Meltzer ed. pp. 1095-1102. Raven Press, New York, 1987.
8. Meltzer, H.Y. Am.J.Psychiatr. 136:1550 1555, 1979.
9. Gudelsky, G.A. et al. Psychopharmacol. Bull. 23:483-486, 1987.
10. Lieberman, J.A. et al. Psychopharmacol. Bull. 25:57-62, 1989.
11. Chiodo, L.A. and Bunney, B.S. J.Neurosc. 3:1607-1619, 1983.
12. Chiodo, L.A. and Bunney, B.S. J.Neurosc. 7:629-633, 1987.
13. Altar, C.A. and Marien, M.R. J.Neurosc. 7:213-222, 1987.
14. Cortes, R. et al. Neuroscience 28:263-273, 1989.
    Goldstein J.M. and Litwin L.C. Europ.J.Pharmacol. 155:175-180,1988.
16. Gunne, L.M. Nature 309:347-349, 1984.
17. Meltzer, H.Y. et al. J. Pharm.Exp.Ther. 251:238-246, 1989.
18. Gelders, Y.G. Brit.J.Psychiatry 155:33-36, 1989.

PHARMACOLOGICAL AND NON-PHARMACOLOGICAL MANIPULATION OF
CIRCADIAN RHYTHMS

F.W. TUREK, C. WICKLAND and O. VAN REETH*
Department of Neurobiology and Physiology, Northwestern University, Evanston, IL,
U.S.A. and Institute of Interdisciplinary Research*, Universite Libre de Bruxelles,
Brussels, Belgium.

Introduction
    A number of environmental and chemical stimuli that can induce phase shifts or changes in the period of the mammalian circadian clock have now been identified (4,6). Of particular interest is the observation that the phase response curves (PRC, i.e. the plot of the magnitude of the phase shift as a function of the circadian time of stimulus presentation) that have been generated to diverse stimuli fall into one of two general categories whereby the stimuli mimic either the effects of a short light pulse or a short dark pulse on the circadian clock. For the "light pulse type" PRC, exposure of free-running animals to the stimulus (e.g. 1 hr. pulse of light, electrical stimulation of the circadian clock in the hypothalamic suprachiasmatic nucleus, or treatment with a cholinergic agonist) in the early or late subjective night induces phase delays or phase advances, respectively, in circadian rhythms. In contrast, for the "dark pulse type" PRC, exposure of free-running animals to the stimulus (e.g. 3 hr. pulse of darkness on a background of constant light, exposure to a novel running wheel or injections of short-acting benzodiazepines or protein synthesis inhibitors) in the middle to late subjective day or late in the subjective night induces phase advances or phase delays, respectively, in circadian rhythms. These two classes of PRC's raise the possibility that diverse environmental and chemical stimuli may ultimately effect similar cellular or biochemical processes that are part of the circadian time-keeping mechanism.
    Recent studies indicate that the phase-shifting effects of many agents which induce a "dark pulse type" PRC may actually be due to changes in the activity-rest cycle of the animal. Evidence in support of the hypothesis that changes in the activity-rest cycle may have feedback effects on the the circadian clock regulating that cycle is briefly described below.

Feedback effects of activity-rest cycle on circadian clock
    A series of extensive studies in the golden hamster have demonstrated that treatment with short acting benzodiazepines, such as triazolam, can have pronounced phase shifting effects on the circadian clock regulating behavioral and endocrine rhythms in this species (8). Recent studies suggest that the effects of triazolam on the hamster circadian clock are due to an associated acute increase in locomotor activity when the hamsters are normally inactive since triazolam-induced phase shifts can be blocked if the acute increase in locomotor activity is prevented by confining the animal to a small chamber after treatment (9). Similarly, dark-pulse induced phase shifts are also blocked by preventing the associated hyperactivity (4, 5, 9). The effects of restraint on blocking phase shifts are specific to those stimuli that induce activity since restraint does not block phase shifts induced by light or the protein synthesis inhibitor,

cycloheximide, two agents that shift the clock without any associated acute increase in locomotor activity (unpublished results).

The hypothesis that an acute increase in locomotor activity during times of little or no activity can phase shift the circadian clock has been tested directly. Exposure of hamsters to a novel running wheel for a few hours during periods of low activity results in intense running behavior and an associated phase shift in the activity rhythm (4, 7). Similarly, preventing hamsters from being active during the time of intense activity also can induce phase shifts in the circadian clock (unpublished results). Taken together, these data indicate that feedback signals from the activity-rest cycle may influence the circadian clock controlling the timing of the cycle.

Clinical Significance

In animals, the light-dark cycle has been recognized as the primary environmental stimulus that synchronizes circadian rhythms, and until recently behavioral inputs to the circadian clock were thought to be of minimal importance. However, as noted above, changes in behavior can in fact have pronounced phase shifting effects on the circadian clock of animals. Interestingly, the evolution of our understanding of the regulation of human circadian rhythms has taken an opposite course. While for many years it was thought that social and behavioral stimuli were primarily responsible for the entrainment of human rhythms, more recent evidence indicates that the light-dark cycle can have pronounced phase-shifting and entraining effects in humans (1, 2, 3). Both animal and human studies have provided a number of approaches for inducing phase shifts in circadian rhythms, and it is anticipated that such approaches will be useful in the treatment of various mental and physical disorders that have been associated with either voluntary (e.g. shift-work, jet-lag) or involuntary (e.g. depression, aging) changes in biological time-keeping.

References

1. Czeisler, C.A. et al. Bright light induction of strong (Type O) resetting of the human circadian pacemaker. Science 244:1328-1333, 1989.
2. Eastman, C.I., Anagnopoulos, C.A. and Cartwright, R.D. Can bright light entrain a free-runner? Sleep Res. 17:372-377, 1988.
3. Hoban, T.M. et al. Entrainment of a free-running human with bright light? Chronobiol. International 6:347-353, 1989.
4. Mrosovsky, N. et al. Behavioural entrainment of circadian rhythms. Experientia 1C:000 70C, 1000.
5. Reebs, S.G., Lavery, R.J. and Mrosovsky, N. Running activity mediates the phase-advancing effects of dark pulses on hamster circadian rhythms. J. Comp. Physiol. A. 165:811-818, 1989.
6. Turek, F.W. Pharmacological probes of the mammalian circadian clock: use of the phase response curve approach. TIPS 8:212-217, 1987.
7. Turek, F.W. Effects of stimulated physical activity on the circadian pacemaker of vertebrates. J. Biol. Rhythms 4:135-147, 1989.
8. Turek, F.W. and Van Reeth, O. Altering the mammalian circadian clock with the short-acting benzodiazepine, triazolam. TINS 11:535-541, 1988.
9. Van Reeth, O. and Turek, F.W. Stimulated locomotor activity mediates phase shifts in the hamster circadian clock induced by dark pulses or benzodiazepines. Nature 339:49-51, 1989.

THE TWO-PROCESS MODEL OF SLEEP REGULATION: SIMULATING ULTRADIAN SLEEP DYNAMICS AND EFFECTS OF HYPNOTICS

A. A. BORBÉLY and P. ACHERMANN
Institute of Pharmacology, University of Zürich, CH-8006 Zürich, Switzerland

Sleep in humans exhibits global trends across the night as well as ultradian variations. One of the global trends is the progressive decline of EEG slow-wave activity (SWA; spectral power density in the 0.75-4.5 Hz band), an intensity parameter of nonREM sleep. In a recent model of sleep regulation, two processes (Process S and Process C) were postulated to account for the global changes of SWA as well as for the timing of sleep and waking (3, 5). The level of the sleep/wake-dependent, homeostatic Process S is assumed to rise during waking and to decline during sleep. Process C represents a sleep/wake-independent component of sleep regulation which is generated by a circadian pacemaker.

Whereas the two-process model is able to simulate the global trend of SWA, it does not account for the ultradian variations. Several mechanisms for the nonREM/REM sleep cycle have been proposed. McCarley and Hobson (6) advanced a model in which a Lotka-Volterra type of reciprocal interaction between two neuronal groups results in the ultradian oscillation underlying the nonREM/REM sleep cycle. More recently, McCarley and Massaquoi (7) proposed a limit cycle process to account for the sleep cycle. Whereas this model was able to explain changes of REM sleep latency and REM sleep episodes under various conditions, it did not take into consideration variations of nonREM sleep intensity. We therefore further elaborated the two-process model to incorporate these aspects.

ULTRADIAN DYNAMICS OF PHYSIOLOGICAL SLEEP

To simulate the ultradian dynamics we have analyzed the changes of SWA within nonREM sleep episodes (1). In each episode, SWA shows an initial buildup, then levels off, declines sharply several minutes before the onset of REM sleep, and remains at a low level during REM sleep. Mean SWA per nonREM/REM sleep episode exhibits typically a declining trend over the entire sleep period. For simulating these changes, the buildup of SWA is assumed to be determined by the combined action of an exponentially rising process and a saturation process. Initially, it is the former process that predominantly determines the buildup. As the level of SWA rises, the saturating process becomes increasingly influential. As a result, the rising part of the curve assumes a sigmoid shape. The activation of a REM sleep process by a REM trigger initiates an exponential process that predominantly determines the sharp decline of SWA at the end of a nonREM sleep episode. A noise variable is used to simulate the variability of the empirical SWA curves. The integrated value of SWA (Process S) represents the change in sleep need or "sleep pressure". The model has been applied for simulating the ultradian pattern of SWA in baseline nights as well as changes induced by a prolonged waking period, a day-time nap, a partial slow-wave sleep deprivation, or an antidepressant drug (2).

In a next step we incorporated a REM sleep generating process into the model. A Van der Pol oscillator was used to generate the REM trigger (REMT) signal. Whenever the oscillating variable is above a threshold the REMT signal is activated. REM sleep occurs whenever SWA falls below a second threshold.

The simulations can account for the typical lengthening of the REM sleep episodes and the stable cycle duration of a regular sleep period. Moreover, skipped first REM episodes and sleep onset REM episodes can be simulated.

EFFECTS OF HYPNOTICS

We have previously shown that various benzodiazepine (BDZ) hypnotics reduce SWA and enhance the activity in higher frequency bands (4). However, the drugs did neither abolish the typical declining trend of SWA nor disrupt the nonREM/REM sleep cycle. Abortive first REM sleep episodes characterized by a precipitous decline of SWA without rapid eye movements and/or muscle atonia, were more frequent in drug nights than in the pre- or post-drug nights. The results indicate that BDZ hypnotics depress SWA by affecting the EEG generating mechanisms, and that they inhibit a full manifestation of REM sleep by impeding EEG desynchronization. However, the basic homeostatic and ultradian sleep regulating processes are still operative. The typical BDZ-induced changes can be simulated by the extended version of the two-process model.

REFERENCES

1. Achermann,P. and Borbély,A.A.: Dynamics of EEG slow wave activity during physiological sleep and after administration of benzodiazepine hypnotics. Human Neurobiol. 6: 203-210, 1987.
2. Achermann,P. and Borbély,A.A.: Simulation of human sleep: ultradian dynamics of electroencephalographic slow-wave activity. J.Biol.Rhythms 5: in press, 1990.
3. Borbély,A.A.: A two process model of sleep regulation. Human Neurobiol. 1: 195-204, 1982.
4. Borbély,A.A., Mattmann,P., Loepfe,M., Strauch,I., Lehmann,D.: Effect of benzodiazepine hypnotics on all-night sleep EEG spectra. Human Neurobiol. 4: 189-194, 1985.
5. Daan,S., Beersma,D.G.M., Borbély,A.A.: Timing of human sleep: Recovery process gated by a circadian pacemaker. Am.J.Physiol. 246: R161-R178, 1984.
6. McCarley,R.W. and Hobson,J.A.: Neuronal excitability modulation over the sleep cycle: a structural and mathematical model. Science 189: 58-60, 1975.
7. McCarley,R.W. and Massaquoi,S.: A limit cycle mathematical model of the REM sleep oscillator system. Am.J.Physiol. 251: R1011-R1029, 1986.

DOSE-RELATED SUPPRESSION OF REM SLEEP
BY THE SEROTONIN-1 AGONIST ELTOPRAZINE

J. QUATTROCHI, D. BINDER, A. MAMELAK, J. WILLIAMS, and J.A. HOBSON
Laboratory of Neurophysiology, Department of Psychiatry, Harvard
Medical School, Boston, MA, U.S.A.

The role of serotonin in regulating sleep and waking remains controversial. Despite recent progress in delineating 5-HT receptor subtypes (1), there are surprisingly few reports in the literature of the effects of either centrally or peripherally administered serotonergic agonists on sleep. The reciprocal interaction model predicts that peripheral administration of a serotonergic agonist will suppress REM sleep via inhibition of REM-on cells in the distributed brainstem REM generator (2). We now report a dose-dependent relationship between parenteral administration of the $5-HT_1$ agonist eltoprazine and REM sleep suppression.

METHODS

We recorded continuously from 4 adult male cats prepared with EEG, EMG, EOG, and bilateral LGB electrodes. Seven eltoprazine doses were administered (0.0625 mg/kg, 0.125, 0.25, 0.5, 1.0, 2.0, and 4.0 mg/kg). The experimental protocol consisted of a control (2cc 0.9% saline i.p.) injection followed by eltoprazine administration (i.p.) on the next day, with a six-day washout period before the following control injection. Scoring of behavioral state and quantitative analysis of wave band activity was performed with a recently developed computer system (3). For each 24-hour recording period the following parameters were measured: percentage of time spent in REM (REM%), NREM (NREM%), waking (W%), latency to the first REM period (REM latency), and PGO wave activity (spikes/hr).

RESULTS

REM% decreased in a dose-dependent manner from a control mean of 14.4% to 0.4% at the 4.0 mg/kg dose ($F=19.11$, $df=3$, $p<.001$). Fig. 1 shows this dose-related decrease in REM%. Mean NREM% showed a dose-dependent increase from a control level of 45.7% to a 4.0 mg/kg mean of 58.7% ($F=15.20$, $df=3$, $p<.001$), while mean W% was unrelated to dose ($F=.08$, $df=3$, $p>.10$). REM latency increased in a dose-dependent fashion from a control value of 62.2 min to greater than 22 hr (>1320 min) at the 4.0 mg/kg dose ($F=311.17$, $df=3$, $p<.001$). PGO wave activity decreased in a dose-dependent manner from a control mean of 968 spikes/hr to a 4.0 mg/kg mean of 19 spikes/hr ($F=127.53$, $df=3$, $p<.001$).

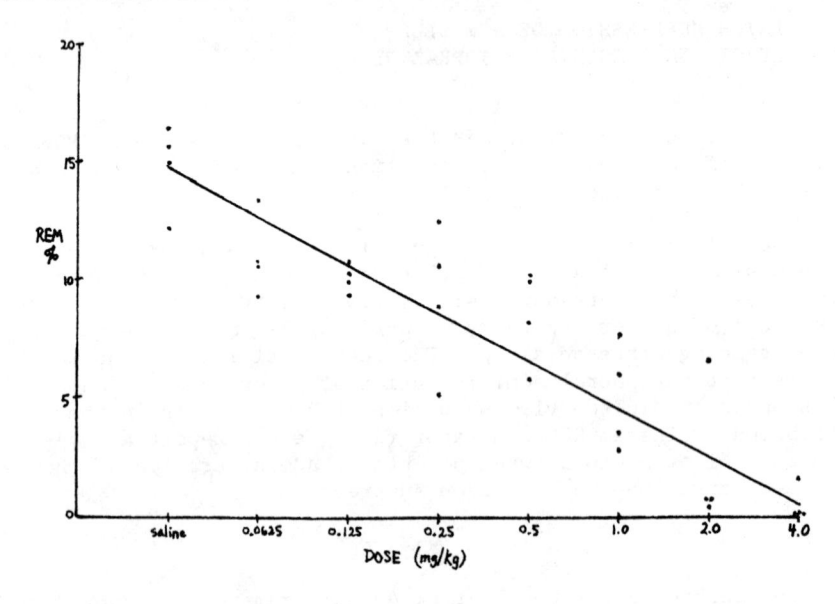

FIG. 1. DOSE-RELATED SUPPRESSION OF REM SLEEP BY ELTOPRAZINE

DISCUSSION

Our data demonstrate that peripheral administration of the 5-HT_1 agonist eltoprazine suppresses REM sleep in a dose-dependent manner, with almost total suppression (0.4% REM) at the highest dose. Concurrent with this dose-related suppression of REM is a dose-related increase in NREM and decrease in PGO activity, with no effect on W%. Our interpretation is based upon the assumption that parenterally administered eltoprazine stimulates 5-HT_1 receptors throughout the brain. It suppresses REM via the inhibition of the distributed brainstem generator. Complete suppression of PGO wave activity may be accomplished by inhibition of the PGO wave trigger zone in the dorsolateral pons. Increase in NREM could be due to direct serotonergic modulation of thalamocortical relay neurons. Because W% was unaffected, we postulate that 5-HT_1 receptors may be important in modulating the REM-NREM sleep cycle, but less important in modulating the sleep-wake cycle.

REFERENCES

1. Peroutka, S.J. 1988. *TINS* 11(1):496-500.
2. Hobson, J.A. et al. 1986. *Behav. Brain Sci.* 9:371-448.
3. Mamelak, A. et al. 1988. *Brain Res. Bull.* 21:843-849.

Supported by NIH grant MH 13,923 and Duphar, B.V.

SLEEP-EEG DATA AS IT RELATES TO THE CHOLINERGIC-AMINERGIC IMBALANCE THEORY OF AFFECTIVE DISORDERS

D. Riemann* and M. Berger**
* Central Institute of Mental Health, Mannheim and
** Psychiatric Clinic, University of Freiburg FRG

Desinhibition of REM sleep at the beginning of the night, i.e. shortening of REM latency, is the most robust and prominent biological marker of sleep in patients with a major depression. According to the reciprocal interaction model of NonREM-REM-regulation (1,2), REM sleep is triggered and maintained by cholinergic neurons mainly located in the pontine reticular formation, whereas aminergic neurons in the brain stem inhibit REM sleep. From that point of view REM sleep abnormalities in depression were interpreted as further evidence for the cholinergic-aminergic imbalance hypothesis of affective disorders (3), which postulates heightened central nervous cholinergic transmitter activity in relation to aminergic activity as causal for depressive disorders. We showed (4), that the cholinergic agonist RS 86 (which can be administered orally and has a half-life of 6 to 8 hours) provoked a highly significant induction of REM sleep in patients with major depression (MDD) compared to healthy controls (HC) and patients with other psychiatric disorders. Whereas 14 out of 16 depressed patients displayed SOREMPs (= sleep onset REM periods, REM latency $\leq$ 25 min.) after cholinergic stimulation, this happened only in 6 out of 36 healthy subjects. The present paper focusses on the question whether shortening of REM latency caused by administration of RS 86 is related to age in HC and patients with a MDD.

SAMPLES:
We investigated 36 healthy controls, (15 males; 21 females; 41.8 ± 15.6 years) and 38 patients with a primary major depressive disorder, (16 males; 22 females; 40.1 ± 12.0 years). For inclusion in the study, the 21 item Hamilton score had to be $\geq$ 18 pts. in the depressed patients. All subjects were administered 1.5 mg RS 86 and placebo prior to sleep in a randomized double blind order after one or two adaptation nights to the sleep laboratory. All subjects were free of psychoactive medication for at least 7 days prior to investigation.

RESULTS:
The results concerning mean REM latency are shown in fig. 1 when splitting both samples in three age groups.
As can been seen, RS 86 had a more pronounced effect on REM latency in patients with MDD compared to HC (p < 0.001). In HC, there was a slight age trend concerning the reagibility to the cholinergic stimulus. In contrast, in MDD REM latency values after cholinergic stimulation were similar in all three age groups. Concerning placebo values, REM latency did not discriminate between HC and MDD in the age range from 18 to 35 yrs. When considering single values after cholinergic stimulation in MDD, 12 out of 14 patients displayed SOREMPs in the young age group (18-35 yrs.), 12 out of 17 in the middle-age group (35-50 yrs.) and 5 out of 7 in the old age group (51-65 yrs.).

DISCUSSION:
In a recent evaluation of baseline sleep data comparing healthy controls and patients with MDD (5) we showed, that REM latency is not significantly shortened in depressives before the age of 35 yrs., whereas REM density was

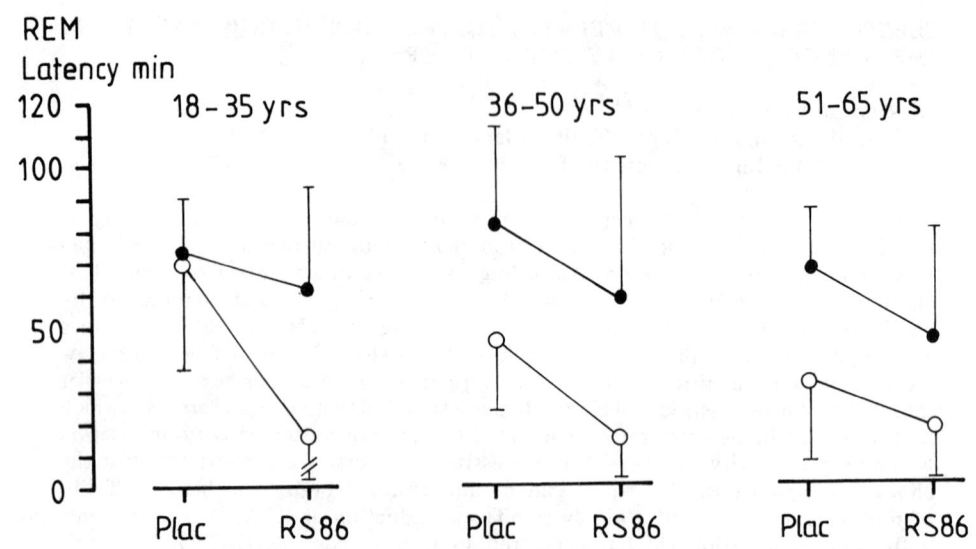

FIG.1: Influence of 1.5 mg RS 86 in comparison to placebo on mean REM latency (± SD). Black circles = HC; open circles = MDD. 18-35 yrs.: n= 13 HC; n= 14 MDD; 36-50 yrs.: n= 10 HC; n= 17 MDD; 51-65 yrs.: n = 13 C; n = 7 MDD.

heightened throughout the whole age range from 18 to 65 yrs. Furthermore we did not find shortened REM latency in nine remitted depressives (6). These results suggest, that shortened REM latency is not a trait-, but a state-marker of depression. Our data with the cholinergic REM induction test with RS 86 indicate, that additional cholinergic stimulation prior to sleep leads to a drastic reduction of REM latency at any age in MDD, thus demasking a cholinergic aminergic transmitter imbalance, which may be implied in the pathogenesis of the disorder.

Acknowledgement: Supported by a grant from the DFG (SFB 258, A 1)

REFERENCES:

1. Hobson, JA et al. Evolving concept of sleep cycle generation. Behav. Brain Sci. 9:371-448, 1986.
2. Mc Carley, RW. REM sleep and depression: Common neurobiological control mechanisms. Am. J. Psychiatry 139:565-570, 1982.
3. Janowsky, D. et al. A cholinergic-adrenergic hypothesis of mania and depression. Lancet 2:632-635, 1972.
4. Berger, M. et al. The cholinergic REM induction test with RS 86. Arch. Gen. Psychiat. 46:421-428, 1989.
5. Riemann, D., Lauer, Ch., Hohagen, F., Berger, M. Longterm evolution of sleep in depression. In: S. Smirne et al. (eds.) Sleep and aging. Masson (in press).
6. Riemann, D. and Berger, M. EEG sleep in depression and in remission and the REM sleep response to the cholingeric agonist RS 86. Neuropsychopharmacol. 2:145-152, 1989.

SLEEP-EEG AND NOCTURNAL HORMONAL SECRETION IN DEPRESSED PATIENTS AND UNDER PSYCHOACTIVE DRUGS

A. Steiger, U. von Bardeleben, C. Lauer, B. Rothe and F. Holsboer
Department of Psychiatry, University of Freiburg, D-7800 Freiburg, West Germany

In depressed patients changes of the sleep structure and of the hormonal secretion are robust findings (3,2). On the other hand it is known that most psychoactive drugs induce alterations of sleep-EEG pattern and of endocrine activity in patients and in controls. Sleep is a time of considerable activity in the endocrine system (6). Therefore it is an attractive approach to study simultaneously sleep-EEG and hormonal secretion simultaneously. We have performed a series of studies to investigate changes of sleep endocrine variables in depression and under various psychoactive drugs (antidepressants, neuropeptides and ligands of the GABA-benzodiazepine receptor complex).

SUBJECT AND METHODS

All studies were performed in male subjects in the sleep laboratory, where sleep-EEG and applying a "through-the-wall-technique" the secretion of cortisol and growth hormone (GH) and - partly - also of prolactin and testosterone were investigated as described in detail elsewhere (4), according to the following protocols:

1.) 12 patients with depression during a longitudinal study comparing acute illness before treatment and recovery after drug cessation,
2.) sleep-endocrine variables of 25 normal controls,
3.) normal controls during long-term-trials under consecutive administration of placebo (PL), various antidepressants (brofaromine, moclobemide, amitriptyline, clomipramine, trimipramine) and PL after withdrawal,
4.) effects of repetitive application of corticotropine releasing hormone (CRH) in 12 controls,
5.) sleep-endocrine changes under repetetive infusion of HOE-427, a ACTH (4-9) fragment analog in 10 controls and
6.) influences of ligands of the GABA-benzodiazipine-receptor-complex, the agonist midazolame (MID), the antagonist flumazenile (FLU), combined application of MID + FLU and PL in 10 controls.

RESULTS

In depressed patients sleep structure and GH secretion did not differ between the acute state and recovery, while cortisol concentration decreased and testosterone was enhanced in remission. No differences of prolactin concentration were evident between acute depression and recovery or between samples of depressed patients and controls. No systematic relationship was found between sleep structure and timing of the cortisol rise in patients and controls. The GH peak occurred before sleep onset in a subsample of 6 of 25 controls.

All investigated antidepressants, except of trimipramine, suppressed REM-sleep. Cortisol secretion was elevated under amitriptyline, clomipramine and moclobemide, while it was blunted under trimipramine in controls.

An elevated cortisol concentration, a blunted GH peak and a decrease of slow wave sleep (SWS) during the second half of the night were found under CRH.
Sleep period time decreased under HOE 427, sleep latency increased, wakefulness was enhanced, SWS diminished during the first third of the night, stage REM decreased during the second third, while endocrine variables remained unchanged.

Under MID sleep latency was shortened, while it was prolonged under FLU. Wakefulness was increased under FLU. The cortisol concentration was significantly diminished under FLU in comparison to MID. When sleep onset was elevated under FLU, the GH peak appeared delayed. However it was not advanced under MID.

DISCUSSION

Our data suggest that an enhanced cortisol secretion and a blunted release of testosterone are state markers of acute depression, while prolactin secretion is not affected by the disorder. The persistence of a disturbed sleep pattern and a blunted GH secretion after recovery may represent a "biological scar" due to metabolic aberrancies during acute illness.

The study results in controls suggest that relationships between sleep structure and hormonal secretion are less regular than previously suggested. Some of the sleep endocrine changes which are characteristical in acute depression can be induced by CRH acutely in controls. This finding gives further evidence that CRH mediates endocrine and behavioral phenomena in affective disorders (2).

The view that neuropeptides induce directly behavioral effects in the CNS is corroborated by the observation that the hormone peptide analog HOE 427 induces changes of the sleep structure, independently from challenges of peripheral hormonal secretion.

The results of long-term studies with antidepressants give no evidence for a systematic relationship between effects of drugs on the sleep structure and on endocrine activity. While most antidepressants may act by suppression of REM-sleep as hypothesized previously by Vogel et al. (5), we suggest, that suppression of cortisol release plays a role in the antidepressant action of trimipramine.

While MID has a sleep inducing effect, FLU delays sleep onset. The finding that - in comparison to MID - cortisol concentration is blunted under FLU, which enhances wakefulness, favours the view of Born et al. (1), that sleep stimulates cortisol secretion in contrary to wakefulness. It is also shown, that the timing of the GH surge can be delayed pharmacologically be deterioration of sleep under FLU.

REFERENCES

1.) Born, J. et al., (1988): Psychoneuroendocrinology, 13:233-243.
2.) Holsboer, F., (1989): Eur Arch Psychiatry Neurol Sci, 238:302-322.
3.) Reynolds, C.F. and Kupfer, D. J., (1987): Sleep, 10:199-215.
4.) Steiger, A. et al., (1987): Psychopharmacology, 92:110-114.
5.) Vogel, G.W. et al., (1975): Arch Gen Psychiatry, 32:765-777.
6.) Weitzman, E.D., (1976): Ann Rev Med, 27:255-243.

THE UNANSWERED QUESTIONS IN THE USE OF SELECTIVE SEROTONIN REUPTAKE INHIBITORS

F. S. ABUZZAHAB, Sr.
Departments of Psychiatry, Pharmacology, Family Practice & Community Health, University of Minnesota, Minneapolis, MN U.S.A.

The introduction of a new genre of antidepressant with selective serotonin reuptake inhibition properties has expanded psychopharmacological treatment into the obsessive compulsive disorders and depression non-responsive to the existing heterocyclic antidepressants or monoamino oxidase (MAO) inhibitors. In contrast to this therapeutic gain, the antidepressants have failed to produce higher therapeutic benefit than the existing antidepressants.

This short paper is concentrated on the unanswered questions raised by this new group of antidepressants. I shall restrict my comments to four drugs: zimeldine, indalpine, fluoxetine and sertraline.

Zimeldine, the forerunner of this new psychopharmacologic group, produced a Guillain-Barre like polyneuritis syndrome, and was taken off the market worldwide. So far, the existing selective serotonin reuptake inhibitors have not produced similar effects. This raises the question whether this rare neurologic complication of zimedline is due to the unique chemical structure of that compound, or to the general action of selective serotonin reuptake inhibition.

Indalpine has also been taken off the market worldwide due to agranulocytopenia. Since the existing selective serotonin reuptake inhibitors have not produced any significant amount of blood dyscrasias, most likely the agranulocytopenia is related to the unique chemical structure of indalpine rather than to the general process of selective serotonin reuptake inhibition.

Fluoxetine usage has raised issues mainly about dosage. In double blind investigations, antidepressant benefit was similar in patients who received 20 mg vs 60 mg. This raises the question whether doses below 20 mg should be tried. Tolerance to the therapeutic benefit of fluoxetine has been reported. The explanations offered include the possibility that fluoxetine induces its own metabolism. However, there is a need for well controlled studies which would include reliable blood levels to further clarify this question.

Several reports have appeared suggesting that fluoxetine, when given with other non-MAOI antidepressants impairs oxidative metabolism and results in higher therapeutic levels of the heterocyclic antidepressant. Such a combination has also produced therapeutic benefit leading to the possible explanation that fluoxetine produces a more rapid down regulation of postsynaptic beta adrenergic receptors, a putative mechanism of action of the heterocyclic antidepressants. These reports have included combinations of fluoxetine with amitriptyline, desipramine and trazodone.

The combination of fluoxetine with MAOI remains an extremely dangerous therapeutic excursion. The serotonergic syndrome from such a combination results in hyperthermia, hyperreflexia, coma, and death.

The combination of fluoxetine with benzodiazepines has also led to competitive liver enzyme inhibition since both fluoxetine and certain long-acting benzodiazepines, such as diazepam, undergo metabolism through demethylation. Due to the high therapeutic index of both the benzodiazepines and fluoxetine, no serious clinical consequences have emerged.

The combination of fluoxetine with other serotonin reuptake inhibiting antidepressants has not yet been fully explored. This is a fertile area for future clinical investigations. For example, combining fluoxetine with clomipramine might enhance the effectiveness of these compounds, especially in drug resistant disorders.

Fluoxetine might produce some benefit in negative symptoms of schizophrenia, however, this area has not been explored. The possibility of fluoxetine inhibiting the metabolism of neuroleptics has been reported, thus leading to the precipitation of parkinson side effects.

Finally, sertraline, a tricyclic, differs structurally from fluoxetine which is a bicyclic compound. However, all clinical studies reviewed indicate that sertraline has a similar psychopharmacologic profile to fluoxetine. Double blind studies of sertraline vs fluoxetine have not been done to elucidate the differences between these two compounds.

In conclusion, this new genre of selective serotonin reuptake inhibitors has raised issues regarding drug interaction with neuroleptics, heterocyclic antidepressants, benzodiazepines and the MAOI. Many questions regarding dosage, therapeutic effectiveness and long term tolerance await future clinical investigations.

1. Ciraulo, D and Shader, R.I. Fluoxetine drug-induced interactions: I. Antidepressants and antipsychotics. J.Clin.Psychopharmacol. 10(1): 48-50, 1990.

2. Doogan, D.P. and Caillard, V. Sertraline: a new antidepressant. J. Clin. Psychiat. 49 (Suppl) 46-51, 1988

3. Gastpar, M. and Wakelin, J.S. Selective 5-HT reuptake inhibitors: novel or commonplace agents? Advances in Biological Pyschiatry vol 17 Karger:Basel, 1988.

5HT$_2$ RECEPTOR SENSITIVITY AFTER CHRONIC ADMINISTRATION OF SERTRALINE AND OTHER SELECTIVE SEROTONIN UPTAKE INHIBITORS

Elaine Sanders-Bush
Department of Pharmacology, Vanderbilt University School of Medicine, Nashville, TN, USA

The regulatory influences of selective serotonin (5HT) uptake inhibitors on the density of brain 5HT$_2$ receptors have been studied by many laboratories; usually little or no change has been found. The present paper explores the hypothesis that selective 5HT uptake inhibitors regulate the 5HT$_2$ receptor by interacting at a site distal to the cell surface recognition site. This hypothesis was tested by examining the 5HT$_2$ receptor transmembrane signaling mechanism, phosphoinositide hydrolysis. Drugs were administered continuously to male rats for three weeks by subcutaneous implantation of Alzet minipumps. Forty-eight hours after pump removal, phosphoinositide hydrolysis was determined in slices of cerebral cortex, by measuring the formation of ^{3}H-inositol monophosphate (Berridge et al., 1982).

RESULTS AND DISCUSSION

The administration of large, daily doses of sertraline for four weeks caused a reduction in the 5HT$_2$ receptor-phosphoinositide hydrolysis signal with no detectable change in the density of 5HT$_2$ receptors (Sanders-Bush et al., 1989). Sertraline is a potent, highly selective 5HT uptake inhibitor; subsequent studies focused on the role of uptake inhibition in this postreceptor effect of sertraline. The onset of subsensitivity is delayed, requiring 2-3 weeks of treatment. Thus, the change does not reflect the initial acute effects on 5HT uptake, but may be secondary to uptake inhibition. In order to investigate this possibility, fluoxetine, another selective 5HT uptake inhibitor, was investigated. Ten mg/kg was administered daily for four weeks. This treatment regimen did not alter 5HT-mediated phosphoinositide hydrolysis in cerebral cortex slices. It was assumed that this dose of fluoxetine would maintain a blockade for the entire 24 hours between doses. If so, the response to chronic administration of sertraline must not reflect an adaptive response to chronic inhibition of 5HT uptake. To investigate this further, a continuous release paradigm was used so that a given drug level could be maintained throughout the course of treatment.

Sertraline elicited a decrease in 5HT$_2$ receptor-mediated phosphoinositide hydrolysis when administered continuously for three weeks (Fig. 1). This subsensitivity was not detected 7 days after the initiation of treatment (Sanders-Bush et al., 1989). The continuous release of fluoxetine caused a comparable

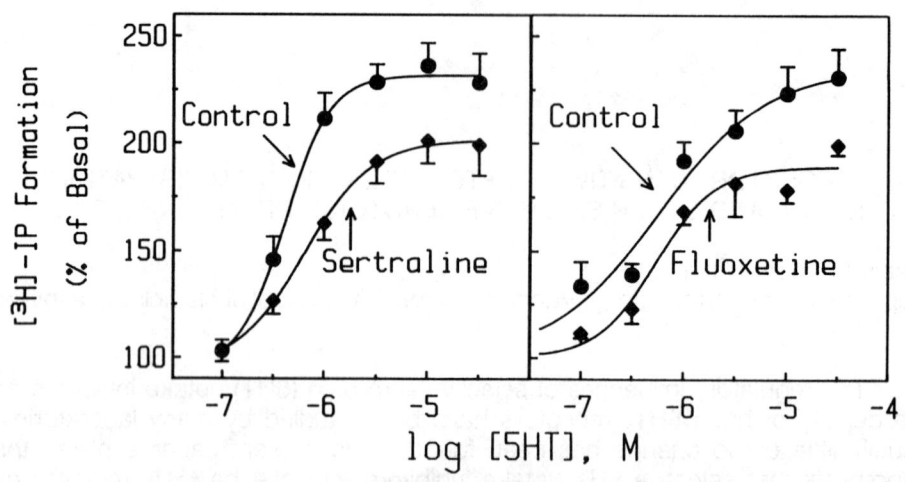

FIG. 1. Effects of chronic administration of selective 5HT uptake inhibitors on $5HT_2$ receptor sensitivity. Sertraline (1 mg/kg/day) or fluoxetine (5 mg/kg/day) was administered continuously for three weeks. Serotonin (5HT)-elicited [^{3}H]-inositol monophosphate (IP) in cerebral cortex slices was used as an index of $5HT_2$-receptor mediated phosphoinositide hydrolysis. The values plotted are the mean of 4-5 animals $\pm$ standard error of mean. The curves were generated using the equation for a sigmoid curve. The data for sertraline are a modification of Figure 2 of Sanders-Bush et al. (1989).

decrease (Fig. 1). The change in the phosphoinositide hydrolysis response elicited by both drugs was manifested as a decrease in the maximum response, with no change in the EC50 of 5HT. In order to determine if these treatments were in fact inhibiting 5HT uptake, prevention of p-chloroamphetamine-induced depletion of brain 5HT was examined. Six days after pump implantation, p-chloroamphetamine was administered and the brain level of 5HT determined. Both sertraline and fluoxetine completely prevented the depletion of 5HT, suggesting that 5HT uptake was profoundly inhibited during the course of these treatments.

In conclusion, two drugs that are selective 5HT uptake inhibitors elicit an adaptive decrease in the sensitivity of $5HT_2$ receptors in cerebral cortex. This effect is important in light of the evidence that other antidepressant drugs (tricyclic antidepressants, monoamine oxidase inhibitors and atypical antidepressants) decrease $5HT_2$ receptor density. Thus, $5HT_2$ receptor signaling is uniformly reduced by drugs used in the treatment of depression, albeit by interaction at different sites along the signal cascade.

REFERENCES
1. Berridge, M.J., Downes, P. C. and Hanley, M.R. (1982): Biochem. J. 206: 578-595.
2. Sanders-Bush, E., Breeding, M., Knoth, K. and Tsutsumi, M. (1989): Psychopharmacology, 99: 64-69.

THE NEURONAL TRANSPORT OF SEROTONIN AS A TARGET OF ACTION OF ANTI-DEPRESSANT DRUGS

S.Z. LANGER, H. ESNAUD AND D. GRAHAM
Department of Biology, Synthélabo Recherche (L.E.R.S.), 58, rue de la Glacière, 75013 Paris, France

A number of studies have suggested that changes in serotonergic neurotransmission are associated with the pathophysiology of depression (1, 2). Moreover, it is well established that the tricyclic and non-tricyclic serotonin uptake inhibitors whose primary target site is the plasmolemmal sodium-dependent serotonin transporter are effective antidepressant drugs. Given the important role that active transport systems for serotonin play in the homeostasis of this biogenic amine, it is, therefore, interesting to note that modifications at the level of the sodium-dependent serotonin transporter have been reported to coincide with, and possibly act as a state-dependent marker of, depressive states (3). As such, characterization of this serotonin transporter at the molecular level could help to advance our understanding of the mechanisms involved in serotonin uptake inhibitor antidepressant action. In this context, we report recent work directed towards purification of the serotonin transporter protein.

METHODS

Crude membranes from rat cerebral cortex were solubilized with the detergent, digitonin, as described previously (4). The detergent extracts were passed over an agarose support to which a citalopram derivative had been covalently coupled. This affinity-chromatographic support was extensively washed and then the serotonin transporter eluted in the presence of the selective serotonin uptake inhibitor, SL 81.0385. The eluted fractions were subjected to gel-exclusion chromatography and assayed for [^{3}H]paroxetine binding activity.

RESULTS

Solubilized sodium-dependent serotonin transporter preparations were chromatographed on a column containing a citalopram based agarose support. Under the conditions chosen, the bulk of the protein applied was unretarded by the support, whereas 60-80% of the [^{3}H]paroxetine binding activity was retained. After extensive washing of the support, elution with the selective serotonin uptake inhibitor, SL 81.0385, led to a > 3,000 fold enrichment of [^{3}H]paroxetine binding activity. The K_d value for [^{3}H]paroxetine binding to this affinity-purified preparation was 0.15 nM with a B_{MAX} value of greater than 1,962 pmol/mg of protein. In addition, citalopram, SL 81.0385 and imipramine inhibited [^{3}H]paroxetine binding with K_i values in the low nanomolar range (Table 1).

Table 1 : PHARMACOLOGICAL PROFILE OF [^{3}H]PAROXETINE BINDING TO SODIUM-DEPENDENT SEROTONIN TRANSPORTER PREPARATIONS

AGENTS	K_d/K_i (nM) OF TRANSPORTER PREPARATION	
	AFFINITY-PURIFIED	MEMBRANE-BOUND
[^{3}H]PAROXETINE	0.15	0.15
CITALOPRAM	7	1.00
SL 81.0385	8	3
IMIPRAMINE	64	41
5-HT	2500	700

DISCUSSION

Radiolabelled forms of selective 5-HT uptake inhibitors, such as [^{3}H]paroxetine, have been used as highly specific markers of the sodium-dependent serotonin transporter in both membrane and detergent-solubilized preparations (4,5). In the present study, an affinity-chromatographic protocol was used to provide an extensive purification of this transporter, as judged by retention of the pharmacological profile of [^{3}H]paroxetine binding to the purified preparation (Table 1). This purification of the serotonin transporter now opens up the possibility to analyse further the biochemical properties of this protein and to apply molecular biological techniques to elucidate its primary structure.

REFERENCES

1. Shopsin, B. et al. Parachlorophenylalanine reversal of tranylcypramine effects in depressed patients. Arch. Gen. Psychiat. 33:811-819, 1976.
2. Price, L.H. et al. Effects of desipramine and fluvoxamine treatment on the prolactin response to tryptophan. Arch. Gen. Psychiat. 46:625-631, 1989.
3. Langer, S.Z. et al. Association of [^{3}H]-imipramine and [^{3}H]-paroxetine binding with the 5HT transporter in brain and platelets : relevance to studies in depression. J. Rec. Res. 7:499-521, 1987.
4. Habert, E. et al. Solubilization and characterisation of the 5-hydroxytryptamine transporter complex from rat cerebral cortical membranes. Eur. J. Pharmacol. 122:197-204, 1986.
5. Habert, E. et al. Characterization of [^{3}H]paroxetine binding to rat cortical membranes. Eur. J. Pharmacol. 118:107-114, 1985.

THE CLINICAL PHARMACOLOGY AND PHARMACOKINETIC ASPECTS OF SELECTIVE SEROTONIN UPTAKE INHIBITORS

Louis Lemberger, Ph.D.,M.D.
Lilly Laboratory for Clinical Research, Lilly Research Laboratories, Eli Lilly and Company, Indianapolis, IN 46285.

The ability of antidepressant drugs to affect the uptake of serotonin has been known for several years. The tricyclic antidepressant drugs imipramine and chlormipramine can affect serotonin reuptake and neurotransmission; however, they also have a marked effect on the uptake of the catecholamine norepinephrine. In the early 1970s with the discovery of fluoxetine and zimelidine, it became clear that it was possible to inhibit the uptake of serotonin without affecting the uptake of norepinephrine. Thus, these agents, which were structurally unrelated to the tricyclic antidepressants, became the prototype drugs of this class. These agents and a variety of newer drugs, including citalopram, fluvoxamine, paroxetine, indolapine, femoxetine and sertraline, have been shown to share this property. Several of these drugs have been shown to be clinically effective in the treatment of major depressive illness as well as a variety of other disorders thought to be related to a deficiency of serotonin.

The clinical pharmacologic studies conducted with this class of drugs have basically been a confirmation of those effects seen in animals. Thus using fluoxetine as a prototype was shown to be an inhibitor of the uptake of tritiated serotonin in platelets harvested for normal volunteers who received the drug (3). Moreover, fluoxetine did not affect the expected blood pressure elevations produced by infusions of norepinephrine or bolus injections of tyramine, indicating its selectivity for serotonin reuptake. Similarly, fluoxetine did not produce anticholinergic effects in this population. Zimelidine (4) and fluvoxamine (5) shared a similar pharmacological profile in humans, i.e., they were selective reuptake inhibitors of serotonin without affecting norepinephrine uptake and they did not produce significant anticholinergic effects in man.

The pharmacokinetics of these agents are drug specific and are in part responsible for the clinical doses necessary for treating the various diseases. Thus, the clinical dose of fluvoxamine can be 300 mg b.i.d. or t.i.d.; that for zimelidine has ranged from 150 to 300 mg daily in divided doses, usually b.i.d.; and the dose of fluoxetine administered is 20 mg daily in a single daily dose, although doses up to 60 mg have been used in certain clinical conditions.

After the oral administration of fluvoxamine to normal, healthy volunteers, the plasma pharmacokinetics were characterized by a plasma half life of about 15 hours and a peak plasma concentration (tmax) occurring at 1 1/2 to 8 hours. The drug was excreted in urine with about 95 percent of the dose being recovered in about 48 hours. Fluvoxamine is extensively metabolized and its major metabolites are inactive with respect to inhibiting the uptake of serotonin and norepinephrine (5).

Zimelidine pharmacokinetics have been studied after oral and intravenous administration (1). After oral administration, the peak plasma concentration of the drug occurs at 3 hours and its bioavailability is about 28 percent. This probably simply represents the first-pass conversion to norzimelidine, its pharmacologically active metabolite. After intravenous administration, the elimination half life of zimelidine is approximately 5 hours, whereas that for norzimelidine is about 15 hours (1).

Fluoxetine's pharmacokinetics can explain its ability to be dosed once daily after oral administration. Fluoxetine peak plasma concentration occurs at 6 to 7 hours. The plasma eliminations of fluoxetine and one of its metabolites norfluoxetine (also an active compound) are approximately 2 days and 7 days, respectively. Fluoxetine is excreted primarily via the renal system following its degradation to more polar metabolites in the liver (2). Metabolism by the liver is an important aspect of its elimination since in patients with cirrhosis, the half life of fluoxetine is prolonged.

All of the selective serotonin reuptake inhibitors have been demonstrated to be efficacious. The acceptability of these drugs will depend upon their individual side effect profile.

REFERENCES

1. Brown D, Scott DHT, Meyer M, Westerlund D, and Lundstrom J: Eur. J. Clin. Pharmacol. 17:111-116,1980.
2. Lemberger L, Bergstrom RF, Wolen RL, Farid NA, Enas GG, and Aronoff GR: J. Clin. Psychiatry, 46:14-19, 1985.
3. Lemberger L, Rowe H, Carmichael R, Horng J, Bymaster F, and Wong D.: Science 199:436-437, 1978.
4. Ogren SO, Ross SB, Hall H, Holm AC, Renyi AL: Acta Psychiatr. Scand. 290:127-151, 1981.
5. Wakelin JS. In: Frontiers in Neuropsychiatric Research, ed: E Usdin, M Goldstein, A J Friedhoff and A Georgotas, Macmillan Press (London) 1983, pp. 159-173.

CLINICAL EFFICACY OF 5-HT UPTAKE INHIBITORS

STUART A. MONTGOMERY
Dept. Psychiatry, St Mary's Hospital, London W2, UK

The requirements for establishing the efficacy of potential new antidepressants have become more demanding in recent years than was formerly the case. The Committee on Proprietary Medicinal Products (CPMP) guidelines on the investigation of antidepressant drugs in the EEC require that efficacy is demonstrated in comparison with placebo in syndromally defined depression using recognised diagnostic and assessment scales. The studies of many of the new 5HT uptake inhibitors have largely been carried out to standards equivalent to those in these newer guidelines so that it is possible to be more confident of efficacy of these drugs than of some older antidepressants which have not yet been adequately tested.

The 5-HT uptake inhibitors as a class have a stronger claim to be regarded as effective antidepressants than any other class of antidepressants. The efficacy studies of newer antidepressants such as fluvoxamine, fluoxetine, paroxetine, sertraline and, to a lesser extent, citalopram, have been conducted at the new more rigorous standard required by recent guidelines. There can be little doubt that 5-HT uptake inhibitors are effective compared with placebo but that they also appear to have similar levels of efficacy to reference antidepressants such as imipramine.

A characteristic side effect of 5HT uptake inhibitors is an increase in nervousness or anxiety which is sometimes quite marked early in treatment. There was some concern that this increase in anxiety might prejudice an antidepressant effect, particularly in depressed patients with agitation. It has also been a commonly held, though inadequately tested, belief that the sedative effect of older TCAs such as amitriptyline was required in treating agitated patients. The 5HT uptake inhibitors differ in this respect from the earlier TCAs as they are not sedative drugs. In some studies the 5HT uptake inhibitors produced a better improvement in the anxiety symptoms of depression than the reference TCAs and they may even be the preferred treatment for depressed patients where the anxiety component is marked. A specific analysis of subgroups of depressed patients with agitated depression showed that these patients responded better to the 5HT uptake inhibitor fluoxetine than to the reference tricyclics (Montgomery 1989) (3). A similar metanalysis found fluvoxamine to be superior to imipramine in the treatment of anxiety symptoms within depression (Wakelin 1988) (4). In this context it is interesting to note the successful use of drugs affecting serotonin in patients with various anxiety disorders. There are positive reports of treatment of phobic and panic patients with zimelidine and in panic patients with fluvoxamine (den Boer et al 1987) (1) which showed a selective advantage compared with the noradrenaline uptake inhibitor maprotiline.

Theoretically drugs affecting serotonin might be expected to improve aggression and suicidal behaviour. Sporadic reports have shown 5-HT uptake inhibitors to have an advantage in reducing suicidal thoughts and a metanalysis (Wakelin 1988) (4) has shown fluvoxamine to have a clinical advantage compared with both imipramine and placebo.

The more exacting standards now required in demonstrating the efficacy of a new antidepressant include the need to establish long term efficacy. As a result the 5HT uptake inhibitors have been subjected to properly conducted studies in long term and in prophylactic treatment which is not the case for many of the older antidepressants. The prophylactic efficacy of zimelidine was shown in 1981; since then the efficacy of fluoxetine in reducing the risk of new episodes in recurrent depression has been demonstrated in a large placebo controlled study (Montgomery et al 1988) (3) and also that of sertraline in a study of maintenance treatment.

REFERENCES

1. den Boer J.A. Serotonergic mechanisms in anxiety disorders. (1987) CIP-Gegevens Koninklijke Bibliotheek, den Haag
2. Montgomery S.A., Dufour H., et al. The prophylactic efficacy of fluoxetine in unipolar depression. B.J. Psychiat. 153 (1988) Suppl. 3, 69-76
3. Montgomery S.A. The efficacy of fluoxetine as an antidepressant in the short and the long term. Int. Clin. Psychophar. 4 (1989) Supp. 1 113-119
4. Wakelin J. S. The role of serotonin in depression and suicide: do serotonin reuptake inhibitors provide a key? Advances in Biological Psychiatry 17 (1988) 70-83

THE EFFECT OF SEROTONIN REUPTAKE INHIBITORS ON SOME PERIPHERAL MARKERS OF THE SEROTONERGIC SYSTEM IN DEPRESSED PATIENTS

B.E. LEONARD
Department of Pharmacology, University College, Galway, Ireland.

The platelet has a number of anatomical and biochemical features in common with the nerve terminal. Such features include an active transport system for serotonin, the presence of alpha 2 adrenoceptors and 5HT2 receptors that are functionally involved in aggregation and specific storage sites for serotonin. Serotonin re-uptake inhibitors reduce the transport of 3H-5HT into platelets from control subjects, and have a quantitatively and qualitatively similar effect on the uptake of this amine into synaptosomes isolated from the rat brain (1, 2). To what extent can the effects of serotonin reuptake inhibitors on isolated platelets from control subject be extrapolated to their effect on platelet serotonin transport in patients with major depression. The purpose of this presentation is to consider the differences between platelet serotonin transport in depressed patients compared to their age and sex matched controls.

PLATELET 3H-5HT UPTAKE IN DEPRESSED PATIENTS.

Over the period 1976-1990, some 16 adequately controlled studies have shown that the V max of serotonin reuptake is significantly decreased in untreated patients diagnosed with major depressive disorder (see 3 for details); this change is not present in patients with minor depressive disorder nor in those with delusions asociated with major depression. Only 2 studies have reported no change in 3H-5HT uptake in major depression. Apart from panic attack (4), no reduction in serotonin uptake has been reported in schizophrenia or mania. It would therefore appear that a reduction in 3H-5HT uptake is a marker of major depressive disorder and would not appear to be attributable to a reduction in the platelet serotonin content (5) or to the presence of antidepressants that could impede the serotonin transport. Thus the reported changes in the V max probably reflect a change in the number of transport proteins in the platelet membrane.

EFFECT OF CHRONIC ANTIDEPRESSANT TREATMENT ON 3H-5HT UPTAKE INTO PLATELETS OF DEPRESSED PATIENTS

Some 11 controlled studies have reported that effective antidepressant treatment is associated with a normalisation of the 3H-5HT utpake in patients with major depression (see 3). In 5 of these studies, selective serotonin reuptake inhibitors (e.g. dothiepin, sertraline, fluvoxamine and trazodone) were used to treat the patients. Thus it would appear that antidepressants that selectively inhibit the re-uptake of 3H-5HT into platelets from control subjects actually facilitate serotonin uptake in those depressed patients that show a beneficial response to treatment; patients failing to respond do not show a normalisation of serotonin uptake despite the presence of an adequate plasma concentration of the drug.

ENDOGENOUS FACTORS WHICH MAY AFFECT THE TRANSPORT OF SEROTONIN INTO PLATELETS OF DEPRESSED PATIENTS

Despite the initial evidence that the 3H-imipramine binding site on the platelet serotonin transporter is reduced in depressed patients, recent evidence suggest that the evidence implicating such an abnormality is equivocal (see 3) and may reflect the hypercortisolaemia which characterizes depressed patients. There is no evidence that raised cortisol levels decreased 3H-5HT transport. One possible explanation is that the lowered 3H-5HT uptake in depression reflects a disturbed circadian rhythm and that the function of all effective antidepressant treatments, including ECT, is to normalize the disturbed circadian rhythm (6).

CONCLUSION

Studies in depressed patients have implicated a lesion in the transport of 3H-5HT into the platelets which is corrected by effective antidepressant treatment irrespective of the nature of the drugs used to treat the patient. Whether a similar change occurs in the serotonergic nerve terminals in the brain of the depressed patient is presently uncertain. There is experimental evidence from an animal model of depression that the synaptosomal serotonin transport is also abnormal but is corrected by chronic antidepressant treatment (7). Thus a defective platelet serotonin tranport would appear to be a state marker of depression; selective serotonin re-uptake inhibitors would appear to facilitate and not inhibit serotonin re-uptake in depressed patients!

Acknowledgement
Partly supported by funding from the Health Research Board of Ireland Unit for Affective Disorders.

REFERENCES
1. Lemberger, L. et al. Use of specific serotonin uptake inhibitors as antidepressants. Clin. Neuropharmacol. 8 (4): 299-317, 1985.
2. Manies, D. and Taylor, D.A. Inhibition of in vitro amine uptake into rat brain synaptosomes after an in vivo administration of antidepressants. Eur. J. Pharmac., 95: 305,-309, 1983.
3. Healy, D. and Leonard, B.E. Monoamine transport in depression : Kinetics and dynamics. J. Affect. Dis., 12: 91-103, 1987.
4. Butler, J. et al. (1988). Functional changes in the adrenergic and serotonergic systems in patients with panic disorder. Prog. Catecholamines Res. Part C. Belmaker et al. ed., pp. 399-407, Alan Liss, Inc., New York.
5. Stahl, S.M. et al. (1983). Platelet serotonin in schizophrenia and depression. In Serotonin in Biological Psychiatry, T. Ho, ed., pp. 183-198, Raven Press. New York. 1983.
6. Healy, D. et al. Variations in platelet 5-HT uptake in control and depressed populations. J. Psychiat. Res., 20: 345-354, 1986.

DOSAGE SCHEDULES IN THE TREATMENT OF MOOD DISORDERS WITH LITHIUM

P. Plenge*, E.T. Mellerup*, H.V. Jensen**, K. Olafsson**, A. Bille** and J. Andersen**.
Psychochemistry Institute, Rigshospitalet, Blegdamsvej 9, Copenhagen, DK-2100*. Department B, Vordingborg Psychiatric Hospital, Vordingborg, DK-4760**. Denmark

"All good drugs have side effects", a quotation which also covers treatment with lithium in the prophylaxis of manic-depressive mood-swings. As lithium treatment due to the lifelong course of the illness is often given to a patient throughout most of his life, the question of side effect reduction is more pertinent in lithium treatment than in most other pharmacological treatments.

Side effects in prophylactic lithium treatment primarily depend on the daily amount of lithium consumed. Two alternative strategies have been investigated in attempts to reduce side effects. One method is to reduce the two daily lithium doses, and thus also the serum lithium concentration, to the lowest possible level where prophylaxis is preserved (5). The other method has focused on prolonging the interval between intakes of lithium by reducing the number of daily doses from two (or three) to one, larger dose, given in the evening (4). Following this second idea of prolonging the interval between intake of lithium, we have been investigating the prophylactic efficacy and side effects of lithium treatment in manic-depressive patients when lithium was given every second day, in the evening (2).

Subject and Method:

The patient population consisted of 13 manic depressive patients (3 men and 10 women) in neutral phase and in continuous lithium treatment. The study was scheduled to last 2 years for each patient. After about 2 month in the study, then blind to both the patient and the psychiatrist, the lithium intake (Lithiumcarbonate, Priadel[R]) was changed from lithium every day to lithium-every-second-day. To change only one parameter, i.e. the interval between lithium intakes we wanted to keep the 12 hour serum lithium concentration unchanged. This meant a 40-50% increase in the lithium dose every second day as the half-life period of lithium in man is about 24 hours (3). The patients met a psychiatrist every second month to receive prepackage medicine, to have the serum lithium concentration checked and to answer different questionnaires regarding side effects as well as the prophylactic effect of the lithium treatment.

RESULTS

The median 12 hour serum lithium concentrations in the patients were the same at the entry and the end of the study, namely 0.7 mM (range 0.5 - 1.0 mM). This corresponded to median doses of lithiumcarbonate of 900 mg/day and 1200 mg/second day. The median duration of treatment with lithium every second day was 20 month, and in this period no relapses occurred. Two patients left the study for personal reasons after about one year. One have continued with lithium every second day by her self, and have stayed well, the other stopped medication and went into mania within three month. Regarding side effects no general side effects were observed during the treatment period. However several lithium related side effects were much reduced or disappeared, when lithium was given every second day. In one patient edema disappeared, in an other weight gain decreased. Two patients, artists, who had stopped painting and writing respectively during conventional lithium therapy, again took up their creative work. Two patients reported less frequent nocturnal diuresis, and in one patient tremor disappeared. The complain of "lack of emotional color" which is common among lithium treated patients in conventional treatment, disappeared in the period with lithium every second day. No lithium induced side effects worsened during the lithium-every-second-day regiment.

DISCUSSION

The study was an open study comprising relatively few patients. With such reservations the treatment period with lithium-every-second-day could be considered long enough to verify the prophylactic effect of lithium in this new treatment schedule, as relapses probably would have occurred during the two years if its prophylactic efficacyhad disappeared (1). The reduction in side effects were very convincing, and often reported spontaneously by the patients themselves. There may however be other advantages than the reduction in side effects in "normal lithium responders" when considering a lithium-every-second-day regime: 1: The risk of lithium intoxication is considerably reduced because most of the previous dose of lithium is excreted when the next dose is given. This may make it possible to spread the cheap and efficient lithium prophylaxis to areas in the world where laboratory facilities are scarce and serum lithium control therefore is difficult, and 2: Treatment of "lithium non-responders" who may belong to a subgroup of patients needing particularly high lithium concentrations. If such high lithium concentrations were reached every day side effects would be intolerable, but giving lithium every second day may overcome this problem.

These questions together with an extended investigation of both prophylaxis and reduction in side effects may be answered in the just started WHO multicenter study where 12 centers each with 10 patients have joined a protocol where the prophylactic effect of lithium given every second day will be investigated for 2 years.

REFERENCES

1. Gelenberg, A.J., Kane, J.M., Keller, M.B. et al.: Comparison of standard and low serum lithium for maintenance treatment of bipolar disorder. N. Engl. J. Med. 321:1490-1493, 1989.
2. Jensen, H.V., Olafsson, K., Bille, A., Andersen, J., Mellerup, E. and Plenge, P.: Lithium every second day. A new treatment regiment? Lithium In press.
3. Plenge, P. and Rafaelsen, O.J.: Lithium effects on calcium, magnesium and phosphate in man: Effects on balance, bone mineral content, faecal and urinary excretion. Acta Psychiatr. Scand. 66:361-373, 1982.
4. Plenge, P. and Mellerup E.T.: Lithium and the kidney: Is one daily dose better than two? Compr. Psychiatry 27:336-342, 1986.
5. Vestergaard and Schou, M.: Prospective studies on a lithium cohort. Acta Psychiatr. Scand. 78:421-426, 1988.

THE RELATION BETWEEN ANTIMANIC AND PROPHYLACTIC ACTION OF LITHIUM

A. KOUKOPOULOS M.D., D. REGINALDI M.D., A. TUNDO M.D., L. TONDO M.D.
Centro "Lucio Bini" - 4, Via Crescenzio 00193 Roma, Italy

While the antimanic action of lithium is proven by many trials and everyday clinical experience, the antidepressant effect of lithium remains controversial and for many Clinicians very doubtful.
Yet lithium exerts its prophylactic effect both against manic and depressive episodes.
The following clinical observations and studies suggest that lithium prevents the depressive episodes by suppressing the manic episodes or the excitatory phenomena that are present in mixed states or in the temperament of affective patients.

1- In cases with a regular course, it can be observed that a depressive episode is usually prevented or attenuated by lithium if the preceding manic or hypomanic episode has been prevented or attenuated by the treatment (3). When lithium is started during the manic episode, and after some time the mania abates, the depression will still take place even if lithium is continued.

2- It is well known and accepted that response to lithium of rapid cyclers greately improves when antidepressants are suspended. This could be seen as a failure of lithium to suppress manic processes that are activated by antidepressant drugs.

3- In a study published in 1980 (4) the response to prophylactic lithium was investigated according to the sequence of the polarity of the episodes of the manic-depressive cycle. The patients with MDI course i.e. starting with a mania which is followed by a depression and then a free interval were much better responders (60% good responders, 19% partial responders, 21% poor responders) than the patients with the DMI course i.e. starting with a depression which is followed by a hypomania or a mania and then a free interval. They had a good response in 33% of the cases, 40% had a partial response and 27% had a poor response.
This finding was replicated by H. Haag et al. in 1986 (2), E. Grof et al. in 1987 (1) and M. Maj et al. in 1989 (5).
This finding may be interpreted in many ways. Our explanation is that lithium acts more effectively upon a gradually rising mania of the MDI patients than upon the rapidly onsetting mania which follows a depression in the DMI patients. The antidepressants given during the depression probably make the mania or hypomania more resistant to lithium. Indeed if antidepressants are not used in the depression, the response to lithium greatly improves.

4- Many affective patients have temperaments of the hyperthymic, irritable, or cyclothymic type. During lithium treatment they become calmer more even tempered, and some complain of having become more passive, less sensitive, less creative and less able to enjoy aesthetic pleasures. Mogens Schou (6) reported that "responsiveness to environmental stimuli was diminished, the subjective experience was primarily one of indifference".

It is probably not too speculative to assume that the tempering of the hyperthymic temperament of many unipolars (the so called BP III) and of the cyclothymic or hyperthymic temperament of the BP II is responsible for the stabilizing prophylactic effect of lithium in these patients. The main objection to the assumption that lithium achieves prophylaxis through a direct antimanic action is its prophylactic efficacy in unipolar depressive patients. But bipolarity is a more complex phenomenon than the occurrence of clear episodes of opposite polarity. Mild hypomanias and mild mixed states that may pass unnoticed, periods of particular tension and irritability, rapid mood changes, are probably bipolar manifestations. Furthermore, the basic temperament of many patients is of a type that could be considered the opposite polarity of their morbid affective episodes as in BP II, BP III and in many BP I who have a dysthymic temperament.

REFERENCES

1. Grof E. et al. (1987): Lithium response and the sequence of episode polarities: preliminary report on a Hamilton sample. Prog. Neuro - Psychopharmacol. and Biol. Psychiat. 11: 199–203.
2. Haag H. et al. (1986): Response to stabilizing lithium therapy and sequence of affective polarity. Pharmacopsychiatry 19: 278–279.
3. Kukopulos A. and Reginaldi D. (1973): Does lithium prevent depressions by suppressing manias? Int. Pharmacopsychiat. 8: 152–158.
4. Kukopulos A. and Reginaldi D. (1980): Recurrences of manic-depressive episodes during lithium treatment. In: Handbook of Lithium Therapy. F.N. Johnson ed., pp 109–117. MTP Press, Lancaster.
5. Maj M., Pirozzi R. and Starace F. (1989): Previous pattern of course of the illness as a predictor of response to lithium prophylaxis in bipolar patients. Journal of Affective Disorders 17: 237–241.
6. Schou M. (1968): Lithium in psychiatric therapy and prophylaxis. J. Psychiat. Res. 6: 67–69.

THE TREATMENT OF AFFECTIVE DISORDERS WITH CARBAMAZEPINE

A. KISHIMOTO.
Department of Neuropsychiatry, Tottori University School of Medicine, Yonago 683 Japan

Considering the recurrent nature of course in bipolar affective disorders, the impotance of prophylactic treatment with drugs can not be minimized. In this point of view, recently, it seems that the clinical position of carbamazepine (CBZ) is being recognized to be more important. One of the merits of CBZ in the episode prophylaxis is due to the safety in long-term use [1]. In this paper, the prophylactic effects of CBZ in long-term clinical practice was compared with those of lithium (Li).

SUBJECTS AND METHODS

Patients satisfying the following criteria were included as subjects: 1) the duration of regular medication exceeded 24 months, 2) the period of CBZ and Li use was long enough in comparison with the mean duration of lucid intervals and 3) in the Li group the blood level was meaintained above 0.3mEq/L. The mean duration of therapy was 64.5 months in the CBZ therapy(n=41), and 58.8 months in the Li therapy (n=42). Prophylactic effects were determined by comparing the affective episodes before therapy with episodes during therapy. To evaluate the effectiveness of therapies, the frequency and duration of hospitalization and additional use of psychotropic drugs were considered. All manic and depressive episodes that occurred more than two weeks after the start of therapy, as well as the episodes lasting for more than one week were investigated.

RESULTS AND DISCUSSION

Incidence of episode

Fig. Comparison of two therapies for episode incidence (mean number of episodes for two yrs.). Vertical bars indicate standard error of means. ** $p < 0.01$, *** $p < 0.001$, during treatment as compared with pretreatment incidence.

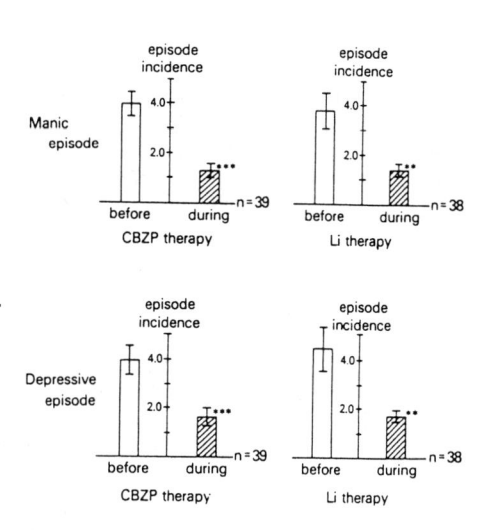

Table Changes in episode incidence
and symptom severity during CBZP therapy and Li therapy

Incidence of episodes	Decreased*	Unchanged	Unchanged	Increased**
Symptom severity or episode duration	Decreased†	Decreased†	Unchanged	Unchanged
Manic episode				
CBZP group (n = 41)	29	1	9	2
Li group (n = 41)	21	5	9	6
Depressive episode				
CBZP group (n = 36)	23	2	9	2
Li group (n = 37)	16	7	8	6

* "Decreased" means episode incidence was reduced to less than 50% that of pretherapeutic incidence.

** "Increased" means episode incidence increased by more than 50% that of pretherapeutic indicence.

† "Decreased" means a decrease in symptom severity or episode duration was confirmed for most morbid episodes during therapy.

As results, the frequencies of episode recurrence for two years before and during the period of prophylatic therapy were compared in both groups. These two therapies equally siginificantly (P<0.01-0.001) reduced both manic and depressive episode recurrences (Fig.). No significant difference in episode incidence was found between the two therapies.

Severity of symptoms

When a comparison was made of the changes in symptom severity between the two therapies (Table), there was a parallel reduction in symptom severity and episode incidence in the majority of cases in both theapies. In the Li group, however, five to seven cases showed a decrease in manic or depressive symptom severity without a decrease of incidence of manic or depressive episode. Moreover, in Li therapy, six cases showed an increase of manic or depressive episode incidence by more than 1.5 times that of the pretherapeutic episode incidence. This phenomenon was observed in only two cases in the CBZ therapy.

In this study, comparison of prophylactic effects of CBZ and those of Li was based on an observation extending over a mean period of five years (minimum two years). The prophylactic efficacy obtained by CBZ therapy in this study is almost comparable to Li therapy and parallel to some results [2,3,4] reported recently in which the episode prophylaxis by CBZ was compared with that by Li. These results susggest the usefulness of CBZ for long-term episode prophylaxis of bipolar disorders.

REFERENCES

1)Kishimoto,A., etal.,(1983):Br.J.Psychiatry,143:327-331.
2)Watkins,S.E.,et al.,(1987):Br.J.Psychiatry,150:180-182.
3)Placidi,G.G., et al.,(1986):J.Clin.Psychiatry,47:490-494.
4)Lusztnut,R.M., et al.,(1988):Br.J.Psychiatry,153:198-204.

PHARMACOKINETICS OF CARBAMAZEPINE IN THE TREATMENT OF MOOD DISORDERS

MARTIN J. BRODIE

Epilepsy Research Unit, University Department of Medicine and Therapeutics, Western Infirmary, Glasgow, Scotland.

INTRODUCTION

Carbamazepine (CBZ) is a first-line anticonvulsant for the prophylaxis of generalised tonic-clonic and partial seizures and the drug of choice for trigeminal neuralgia (2). Over the past decade its psychotropic properties have come to be recognised, particularly as a treatment for acute mania and in the prophylaxis of bipolar affective disorder (3).

PHARMACOKINETICS

The pharmacokinetics of carbamazepine are of substantial relevance to its optimal clinical use. Oral absorption is slow and bioavailability has been estimated at 80-90%. Peak levels occur around 4 hours after dosing. The drug is eliminated by hepatic metabolic processes down a number of pathways, the most important being epoxidation to the active metabolite CBZ 10,11 epoxide.

CBZ is a powerful enzyme inducer which accelerates its own metabolism as well as that of endogenous hormones and other lipid soluble drugs. The elimination half-life, initially 24-48 hours, is reduced to as little as 12 hours on chronic dosing. Towards the end of the first month of treatment, apparent steady-state levels can fall by as much as 30%. The extent of auto-induction contributes to a three-fold variation in trough and peak concentrations in patients taking the same CBZ dose.

CONCENTRATION-EFFECT-TOXICITY RELATIONSHIPS

The relationship between serum CBZ concentrations and clinical response is complicated by varying degrees of conversion to its active metabolite, as well as individual pharmacodynamic variability. In epilepsy, maximum therapeutic therapeutic benefit is generally obtained with CBZ levels above 6mg/L (25 umol/L), although some patients require concentrations of 12mg/L (51 umol/L) or more. This concentration-effect relationship need not be applicable to its use in psychiatric disorders. Circulating CBZ levels around 8mg/L (34 umol), especially in the naive patient, can lead to mild neurotoxic symptoms including nausea, headache, drowsiness, diplopia and ataxia which can be overcome in some patients by dividing the daily dose into 3 or 4 increments. These intermittent side-effects, however, reflect the large diurnal variation in CBZ concentrations and provide the rationale for the introduction of a controlled-release formulation.

CONTROLLED-RELEASE CARBAMAZEPINE

A controlled-release formulation of CBZ in a crystalline matrix has been marketed recently in Europe (CBZ-CR, Tegretol Retard, Ciba-Geigy). This provides substantial reduction in intra-dose fluctuation of CBZ concentrations which has been quantified at 50% in a double-blind comparison with conventional CBZ (4). Its improved pharmacokinetic profile makes CBZ-CR less likely to impair psychomotor function (1).

In a recently completed double-blind, double-dummy random order comparison of conventional CBZ versus CBZ-CR in 21 epileptic patients, fluctuation around the mean concentration over 12 hours was significantly less with the new formulation (CBZ 41 ± 3%; CBZ-CR 29 ± 2%; $p<0.01$). Indeed, lower fluctation was found with CBZ-CR given twice daily than during a dosage interval in patients taking conventional CBZ 3 or 4 times daily. Peak concentrations were lower and times to peak longer with CBZ-CR. The new preparation also resulted in slightly lower mean levels when given in the same total daily dose as conventional CBZ - a probable consequence of reduced bioavailability. Monitoring circulating concentrations, therefore, is advised when changing a patient from one form of CBZ to another.

The new controlled-release formulation is a pharmacokinetically attractive way of providing CBZ. Twice daily dosing is suitable for all patients and once daily administration may be possible for some. CBZ-CR allows "gentler" introduction of the drug and is associated with fewer neurotoxic side-effects in patients established on chronic treatment. Theoretically, this preparation may also permit higher CBZ doses to be tolerated.

CONCLUSION

CBZ is an important pharmacological agent with a widening range of neurological and psychiatric indications. It has a narrow therapeutic index and its pharmacokinetics are complex. The new controlled-release formulation holds out the possibility of fewer side-effects and increased therapeutic potential and is clearly the one to use.

REFERENCES

1. Aldenkamp, A.P. et al. Controlled release carbamazepine: cognitive side effects in patients with epilepsy. Epilepsia 20:507-514, 1987
2. Editorial. Carbamazepine update. Lancet ii:595-597, 1989
3. Elphick, M. Clinical issues in the use of carbamazepine in psychiatry: a review. Psychol. Med. 19:591-604, 1989
4. Larkin, J.G. et al. A double-blind comparison of conventional and controlled-release carbamazepine in healthy subjects. Br. J. Clin. Pharmacol 27:313-322, 1989

VALPROATE - TREATMENT OF PSYCHOTIC DISORDERS IN COMPARISON WITH CARBAMAZEPINE - THERAPY

H.M. Emrich* and M. Dose**
*Max Planck Institute for Psychiatry, Munich, FRG, and **District Hospital, Ansbach, FRG

Our interest in the therapeutic effects of the GABAergic anticonvulsant valproate was raised from pharmacopsychiatric investigations pointing to the view that mania results from a dysfunction of inhibitory neurotransmitters in the CNS. Using a double-blind, placebo-controlled trial, it has been demonstrated that valproate exerts a rather specific antimanic action, a finding which has been replicated in the meantime by several groups. Also long-term prophylactic medication using valproate was efficacious in 12 lithium nonresponders, in 11 cases in combination with low doses of lithium. It could be demonstrated that the character of the phase-chart is greatly improved during the valproate-prophylaxis: the average relapse-free time increased from 10.0 ± 4.3 months up to 41.2 ± 18.5 months during valproate treatment (cf. 3, 4), which is highly significant ($p < .005$).

Regarding the anticonvulsants carbamazepine and oxcarbazepine, an acute double-blind, placebo-controlled ABA design demonstrated an acute antimanic effect of oxcarbazepine (5). In the meantime a larger number of studies have been performed regarding the acute antimanic effect of oxcarbazepine (Trileptal) (for a review cf. 1) and an antimanic action, similar to that of carbamazepine, has been demonstrated. In carbamazepine-prophylaxis of affective and schizoaffective psychoses, another sample of 12 patients, poorly responding to lithium prophylaxis, were treated with carbamazepine. In a similar fashion as with valproate, carbamazepine long-term treatment resulted in an about 4-fold increase of the relapse-free time during treatment (2). Interestingly, a comparison regarding the psychopharmacological profile of action of carbamazepine in comparison to valproate showed a more pronounced prophylactic therapeutic effect of carbamazepine in schizoaffective psychoses, whereas valproate appears to be more effective in the pure mood disorders without schizophrenic symptomatology.

This finding is plausible, bearing in mind the study by Dose et al. (7) which showed that carbamazepine is an effective adjuvant to neuroleptic therapy of schizophrenic psychoses. Recently, it could be demonstrated (8) that in acute schizophrenic psychoses, under double-blind conditions, carbamazepine revealed a more pronounced adjuvant effect in comparison to the adjuvant treatment with valproate. On the other hand, chronic-defectuous schizophrenic psychoses, which represent especially difficult problems in pharmacopsychiatry of schizophrenia and in which monotherapy with neuroleptics often induces a deterioration of defectuous symptoms, showed, in a pilot investigation, some improvement as the result of valproate medication: in these open trials, 8 severely ill patients with chronic-defectuous psychoses were treated with valproate as an adjuvant. In 2 cases a very pronounced therapeutic effect was observed, and in 4 cases a slight improvement occurred (6). As a consequence of this, double-blind studies as to the possible beneficial effects of valproate in chronic defectuous psychoses should be performed.

REFERENCES

1. Emrich, H.M. (1990a): Studies with oxcarbazepine (Trileptal^R) in acute mania. *Intern. Clin. Psychopharm.* 5(suppl.1):83-88

2. Emrich, H.M. (1990b): Alternatives to lithium prophylaxis for affective and schizoaffective disorders. In: *Affective and Schizoaffective Disorders*, A. Marneros and M.T. Tsuang, eds. Springer-Verlag, Berlin (in press)

3. Emrich, H.M. and Wolf, R. (1989): Valproate and mania. In: *Fourth International Symposium on Sodium Valproate and Epilepsy*, D. Chadwick, ed, pp. 217-224. Royal Society of Medicine Services Ltd., London-New York

4. Emrich, H.M., von Zerssen, D., Kissling W., et al. (1980): Effect of sodium valproate on mania - The GABA hypothesis of affective disorders. *Arch. Psychiatr. Nervenkr.* 229:1-16

5. Emrich, H.M., Altmann, H., Dose, M., et al. (1983): Therapeutic effects of GABA-ergic drugs in affective disorders. A preliminary report. *Pharmacol. Biochem. & Behav.* 19:369-372

6. Emrich, H.M., Weber, M.M., Garcia-Borreguero, D. (1990): Neuere systemtheoretische Konzepte zur Therapie chronisch defektuöser Psychosen. In: *Proceedings of the 1st Bonner Kraepelin-Symposium*, H.-J. Möller and E. Pelzer, eds. Springer-Verlag, Berlin (in press)

7. Dose, M., Apelt, S., Emrich, H.M. (1987): Carbamazepine as adjunct of antipsychotic therapy. *Psychiatry Res.* 22:303-310

8. Dose, M., Hellweg, R., Loycke A., et al. (1990): Combined treatment of schizophrenic psychoses with haloperidol and anticonvulsants. *Biol. Psychiatry* (submitted)

ANTIMANIC EFFECT OF ZOTEPINE, A NEW THIEPIN DERIVATIVE - ACUTE AND LONG-TERM TREATMENT

T. HARADA
Department of Neuropsychiatry, Okayama University Medical School, Okayama 700, Japan

We investigated the antimanic effect of zotepine(ZTP), a new antipsychotic belonging to the thiepin group. The antimanic effect was observed both in the acute treatment for acute manic onset or recurrence and in the long-term treatment for the prophylaxis of recurrence of mania.

THE ACUTE TREATMENT

In the acute treatment, ZTP markedly improved manic symptoms in 12 patients(75%) of all the 16 manic patients within a week, and afforded at least slight improvement in all patients. In most of patients, ZTP was used concomitantly with Lithium(Li), but two patients started taking Li midway into the treatment period. The two patients slightly improved when they received ZTP alone, but markedly improved by combined use with ZTP and Li. As shown on Table 1, when the two patients were added to the Li group and Li-free group respectively, the rating of markedly improved tended to be higher in the Li group than in the Li-free group. Concerning the adverse effects of ZTP, ZTP caused the change from mania to depression in 50%. The other frequent adverse effects were dysarthria(50%), parkinsonism(33%), dry mouth(28%) and sleepiness (28%). The noteworthy adverse effects were EEG abnormalities (paroxysmal changes)(22%). There were great differences in the maximum dosage (50-600 mg/day) among individual patients.

THE LONG-TERM TREATMENT

In the long-term treatment, 12 patients of all were able to be followed up over one year. Figure 1 shows the clinical courses of the patients. ZTP tended to be used whenever recurrence of mania and not to be used continuously. In only 3 patients(case 2,3,4), ZTP was used continuously over one year and ZTP prevented the recurrence of mania (Case 2,3) or reduced the severity of recurring

TABLE 1. IMPROVEMENT RATING OF MANIC SYMPTOMS(GLOBAL IMPROVEMENT)

GROUP	MARKEDLY IMPROVED	MODERATELY IMPROVED	SLIGHTLY IMPROVED	TOTAL
LI GROUP	10(77)	2(15)	1(8)	13
LI-FREE GROUP	2(40)	1(20)	2(40)	5
TOTAL	12(67)	3(17)	3(17)	18

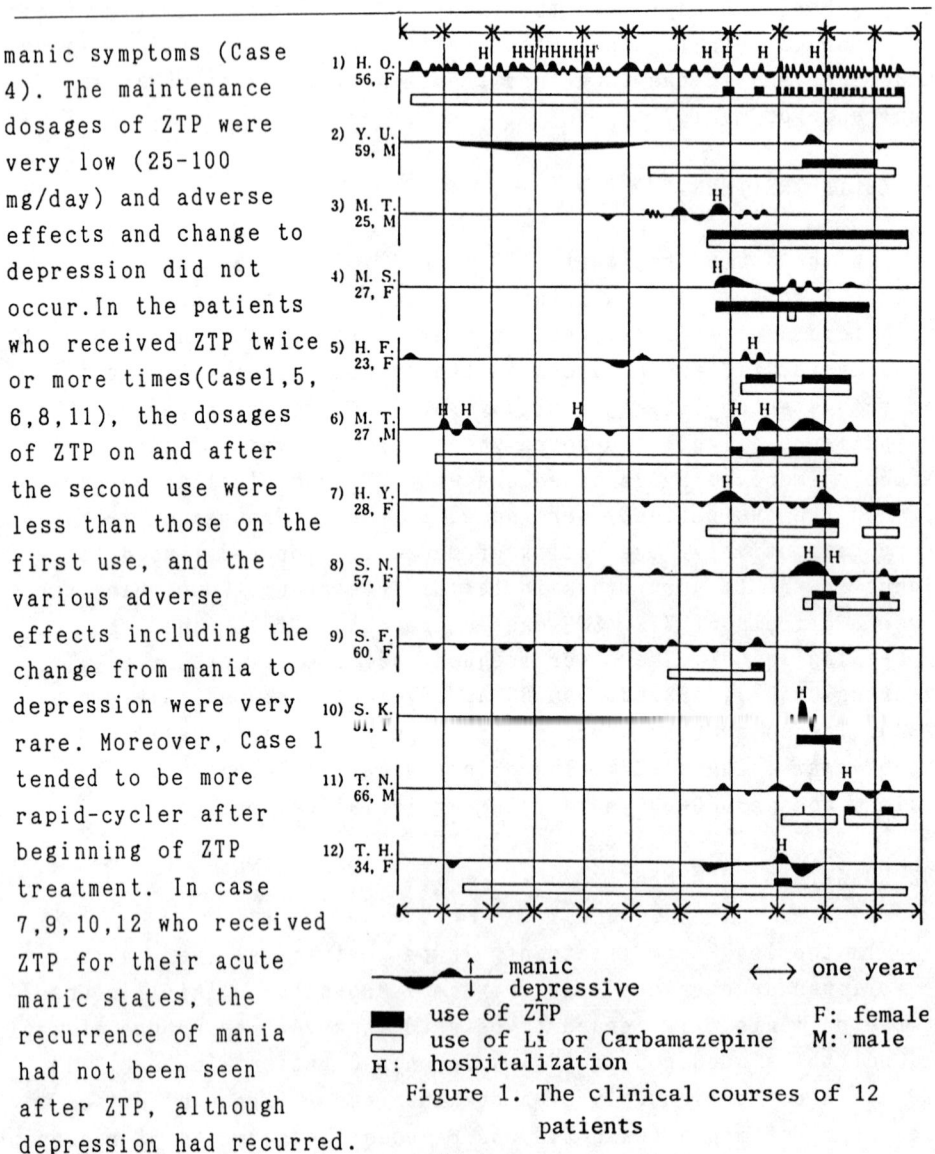

manic symptoms (Case 4). The maintenance dosages of ZTP were very low (25-100 mg/day) and adverse effects and change to depression did not occur. In the patients who received ZTP twice or more times(Case1,5,6,8,11), the dosages of ZTP on and after the second use were less than those on the first use, and the various adverse effects including the change from mania to depression were very rare. Moreover, Case 1 tended to be more rapid-cycler after beginning of ZTP treatment. In case 7,9,10,12 who received ZTP for their acute manic states, the recurrence of mania had not been seen after ZTP, although depression had recurred.

Figure 1. The clinical courses of 12 patients

ENDOGENOUS EXCITOTOXINS AND NEUROPSYCHIATRIC DISORDERS

JOHN W. OLNEY
Department of Psychiatry, Washington University, St. Louis, MO. USA

Significant progress has been made recently in understanding the neurotoxic (excitotoxic) properties of glutamate (Glu) and related excitatory amino acids (EAA). Three EAA receptor subtypes [N-methyl-D-aspartate (NMDA), kainic acid(KA), quisqualic acid (Quis)] have been identified, drugs with anti-excitotoxic actions have been discovered and evidence for the potential complicity of both exogenous and endogenous excitotoxins in neurodegenerative disorders has begun to unfold. There now is substantial evidence for the involvement of each EAA receptor subtype in at least one human neurodegenerative syndrome, and recent findings suggest that EAA receptors are sensitive mediators of excitotoxicity at both ends of the age spectrum.

NMDA RECEPTOR-MEDIATED SYNDROMES

Excessive activation of NMDA receptors may play a critical role in acute neuronal degeneration associated with hypoxia-ischemia, hypoglycemia and epilepsy (5). These conditions cause excessive release of endogenous excitotoxins (Glu and aspartate) from the intra to extracellular compartment of brain which brings these excitotoxins in direct contact with EAA receptors through which they can induce excitotoxic neuronal death. It has been shown in animal studies that NMDA receptor antagonists can mitigate brain damage associated with each of these three conditons. However, as discussed below, NMDA antagonists may prove more effective in preventing hypoxic/ischemic brain damage in the immature than mature CNS, the postulated reason being that hypoxic/ischemic damage may be mediated almost exclusively by NMDA receptors in the immature CNS but by all three EAA receptor types in the adult CNS (2-4).

NON NMDA RECEPTOR-MEDIATED SYNDROMES

In addition to the possible involvement of both KA and Quis receptors in hypoxic/ischemic brain damage in adulthood, there is evidence for selective involvement of each of these non NMDA receptor subtypes in at least one other adult human neurodegenerative syndrome. BOAA (B-N-oxalylamino-L-alanine), an environmental excitotoxin implicated in neurolathyrism, exerts excitotoxic activity exclusively through Quis receptors (7). Domoic acid, an environmental excitotoxin implicated in a recent food poisoning incident that killed some individuals and left others demented, exerts its excitotoxic activity exclusively at KA receptors (8). It is noteworthy, however, that domoic acid, like KA, is a powerful convulsant that induces brain damage primarily by a seizure mechanism, and that seizure-mediated brain damage of the type induced by KA can be largely prevented by blockade of NMDA receptors (1). The postulated basis for this is that, although KA receptor activation is the mechanism by which domoic acid induces persistent seizure activity, much of the ensuing brain damage stems from seizure-mediated release of endogenous Glu at NMDA receptors. While BOAA and domoic acid are exogenous rather than endogenous excitotoxins, research focusing on the neurotoxic syndromes induced by specific interaction of these agents with Quis and KA receptors respectively, provides examples of the types of neurodegenerative syndromes that might occur if endogenous excitotoxins became aberrantly active at these receptors. For example, since neurolathyrism is a disease specifically affecting motor neurons, evidence that this motor neuron disease may be caused by BOAA, a Quis receptor agonist, suggests the possibility that other motor neuron diseases, such as amyotrophic lateral sclerosis, might be explained in terms of an endogenous excitotoxin acting at Quis receptors.

Speculation that endogenous excitotoxins might play a role in Parkinson's and Huntington's diseases was recently strengthened by the finding (6) that L-DOPA and its ortho-hydroxylated derivative 6-OH-DOPA have excitotoxic activity. This activity is mediated specifically at non NMDA receptors. Thus, it is reasonable to propose that L-DOPA, or one of its derivatives, acting as endogenous excitotoxins at non NMDA receptors, may be responsible for neuronal degeneration in either Huntington's or Parkinson's disease.

EXCITOTOXIC MECHANISMS OPERATIVE IN YOUTH AND OLD AGE

Recent evidence (2,3) suggests that the developing CNS is much more sensitive than the adult CNS to the neurotoxic effects of NMDA and that the converse is true for KA or Quis neurotoxicity. If NMDA receptors are relatively hypersensitive, and non NMDA receptors relatively hyposensitive, to excitotoxic stimulation during development, it follows that NMDA receptors may be the exclusive mediators of excitotoxic neuronal degeneration in the immature CNS, and that NMDA antagonists may be particularly effective in preventing such degeneration. This may have practical significance in relation to the hypothesis that several CNS disorders, including cerebral palsy and schizophrenia, might be causally linked to subtle brain damage occuring in utero due to an excitotoxic mechanism. The basis for postulating a link between developmental excitotoxic cytopathology and schizophrenia will be discussed at the meeting.

Involvement of EAA receptor systems in neuropsychiatric disorders of old age may be postulated based on evidence pertaining to domoic acid poisoning. Although individuals poisoned by domoic acid ranged in age from 20 to 89, severe neuropsychological impairment (profound anterograde amnesia) occurred only in those over 60 years of age. This suggests that KA receptors, and probably also NMDA receptors, are sensitive mediators of excitotoxic neuropathology in the aging human brain, and presumably either receptor system would be sensitive to pathological stimulation by endogenous as well as exogenous excitotoxic agents.

REFERENCES

1. Clifford DB, Olney JW, Benz AM et al. Ketamine, phencyclidine and MK-801 protect against kainic acid induced seizure related brain damage. Epilepsia (in press).
2. Ikonomidou C et al. Sensitivity of the developing rat brain to hypobaric/ischemic damage parallels sensitivity to NMDA neurotoxicity. J Neurosci 9, 2809-2818, 1989.
3. McDonald, J. W., Silverstein, F. S. and Johnston, M. V. Neurotoxicity of NMDA is markedly enhanced in developing rat CNS. Brain Res. 459:200-03, 1988.
4. Mosinger JL and Olney JW. Combined treatment with MK-801 and CNQX prevents ischemic neuronal degeneration in the in vivo rat retina. Soc. Neurosci Abst 15, 45, 1989.
5. Olney JW. Excitatory amino acids and neuropsychiatric disorders. Biol Psychiatry 26, 505-525, 1989.
6. Olney, JW, Zorumski CF, Stewart GR et al. Excitotoxicity of L-DOPA and 6-OH-DOPA: Implications for Parkinson's and Huntington's Diseases. Exp Neurol, (in press).
7. Ross SM, Allen C and Spencer PS. Biochemical and electrophysical studies on the Neurotoxic Action of β-N-oxalylamino-L-alanine, In: Neurotoxicology and Epidemiology of ALS, F. Norris, Editor, (in press)
8. Stewart GR, Zorumski CF, Price MT and Olney JW. Domoic acid: A dementing excitotoxic food poison with kainic acid receptor specificity. Exp Neurol. (in press).

MECHANISMS OF PHENCYCLIDINE (PCP) - N-METHYL-D-ASPARTATE (NMDA) RECEPTOR INTERACTION: IMPLICATIONS FOR PSYCHIATRIC DISORDERS

STEPHEN R. ZUKIN and DANIEL C. JAVITT
Departments of Psychiatry and Neuroscience, Albert Einstein College of Medicine/Montefiore Medical Center and Bronx Psychiatric Center, Bronx, NY, U.S.A.

Phencyclidine (1,1-phenylcyclohexylpiperidine; PCP; "angel dust") was originally developed as a general anesthetic in the late 1950's. Subanesthetic doses (0.1 mg/kg i.v.) doses were subsequently found to induce psychotic episodes in normal volunteers and to rekindle presenting symptomatology in recompensated schizophrenic subjects (Rosenbaum et al., 1959). In addition, subanesthetic doses of PCP, but not LSD, amobarbital or amphetamine, could induce abnormalities in tests of abstract reasoning, cognitive processing, attention, motor function and proprioception in normal volunteers which closely resembled those seen in patients with chronic schizophrenia. These findings led to the proposal that the mechanisms of action of PCP may be relevant to the pathogenesis of schizophrenia. PCP binds with high affinity to a specific brain PCP receptor which is a site within the ion channel gated by the NMDA-type excitatory amino acid receptor. Thus, NMDA and PCP receptors represent distinct sites associated with a supramolecular NMDA receptor complex. The identification of noncompetitive inhibition of NMDA receptor function as the mechanism underlying the psychotomimetic effects of PCP suggests that elucidation of the functioning of the NMDA receptor complex may reveal mechanisms relevant to the pathogenesis and treatment of schizophrenia.

METHODS

In order to elucidate mechanisms underlying NMDA receptor activation, binding of the selective PCP receptor ligand [^{3}H]MK-801 was determined in the presence and absence of L-glutamate and glycine, agents which stimulate ligand binding to PCP receptors. L-glutamate has been shown to mediate its actions as an agonist at the NMDA recognition site while glycine mediates its actions at a non-strychnine sensitive glycine recognition site associated with the NMDA receptor complex. Specific binding of [^{3}H]MK-801 to extensively washed, frozen-thawed rat forebrain homogenate was determined at 12 - 16 time points between 5 min and 24 hr using a filtration radioreceptor assay in the presence of a 5 mM Tris buffer system adjusted to pH 7.4 and a low (30 μM) concentration of Mg^{2+} (Javitt and Zukin 1989, Javitt et al., 1990).

RESULTS

These studies resulted in three novel findings. First, analysis of association curves using a computer-assisted, non-linear curve fitting technique revealed the presence of two distinct components of [^{3}H]MK-801 binding: a fast component with a $t_{1/2}$ of approximately 5 min and a slow component with a $t_{1/2}$ of approximately 3 hrs. This suggests that PCP-like agents do not gain access to their receptor only via open channels, since channel-blocking drugs which interact exclusively with open channels should manifest single exponential association and dissociation. A model of PCP-NMDA receptor interaction consistent with bi-exponential association of [^{3}H]MK-801 would be one in which PCP-like agents can gain access to their recognition site via two distinct paths, each corresponding to one of the observed kinetic components of binding. When channels were maximally activated in the presence of combined L-glutamate and glycine, we found that >90% of [^{3}H]MK-801 binding displayed fast kinetics of association (Javitt and Zukin, 1989), suggesting that the fast path represents binding of [^{3}H]MK-801 to its receptor following diffusion to the binding site via a path corresponding to the open NMDA receptor channel. In the absence of added L-glutamate or in the presence of D(-)AP5, >99% of [^{3}H]MK-801 binding displayed slow kinetics of association, suggesting that the slow path represents binding of [^{3}H]MK-801 following diffusion to the binding site via a path associated with closed NMDA receptor channels. Bi-exponential kinetics of association of [^{3}H]MK-801 in the presence of L-glutamate alone indicate that association via fast and slow paths can occur simultaneously, indicating that different underlying processes are involved. The ability of PCP-like agents to reach their binding site within closed NMDA channels over the course of hours may be relevant to course of PCP intoxication since it suggests that PCP can reach its site of action even in the absence of NMDA receptor activation.

A second finding of these studies (Javitt and Zukin, 1989) was that L-glutamate significantly increased total steady-state [^{3}H]MK-801 binding while D(-)AP5 significantly decreased total steady-state [^{3}H]MK-801 binding, presumably by displacing endogenous agonists from the NMDA receptor. A third finding of our studies (Javitt et al., 1990) was that the Hill coefficient for stimulation of [^{3}H]MK-801 binding by L-glutamate was 2.06 ± 0.08, significantly greater than unity, suggesting that more than one molecule of agonist is required to induce NMDA channel activation.

DISCUSSION

A model of NMDA receptor functioning which can account for these findings postulates the existence of two independent sets of agonist recognition sites within each functional NMDA receptor complex. Occupation of both sets by agonist would be required for channel activation and fast [^{3}H]MK-801 binding. Partial activation would not permit channel opening but would permit slow diffusion of [^{3}H]MK-801 to its binding site via a hydrophobic path. In the total absence of agonist, however, the channel would remain closed and in a conformation to which PCP receptor ligands could not bind. This model is similar to models which have been proposed to account for the functioning of nicotinic acetylcholine receptors (Hess et al., 1983). NMDA receptors thus may be structurally homologous to receptors of the Class I superfamily of ligand-gated channels, which includes nicotinic, GABA$_A$, and strychnine-sensitive glycine receptors as well (Barnard et al., 1987).

The ability of PCP-like agents to bind with high potency to a site within the NMDA channel suggests that PCP-induced NMDA channel blockade may be relevant to the clinical effects of PCP. The abilities of PCP receptor ligands to evoke PCP-like behavioral effects correlate with their affinities for the PCP receptor, but not with their affinities for other sites such as the σ receptor or the DA reuptake carrier. Furthermore, PCP-induced psychosis has been found to be associated with serum concentrations of PCP as low as 20 nM, at which only PCP receptors would be significantly occupied by drug. In summary, PCP induces psychotomimetic effects that closely resemble those of schizophrenia. Our experimental data from experiments measuring the effects of NMDA receptor activation on binding of [^{3}H]MK-801 to PCP receptors support a model of NMDA receptor functioning in which two molecules of agonist are required for NMDA receptor activation. This model is similar to models which have been proposed for the nicotinic acetylcholine receptor, suggesting the possibility of functional and structural homology between NMDA receptors and members of the Class I superfamily of ligand-gated channels. The psychotomimetic effects of PCP are observed at serum concentrations similar to the concentration at which PCP binds to the NMDA-associated PCP receptor. These findings suggest that endogenous dysfunction or dysregulation of NMDA receptor-mediated neurotransmission may contribute to the pathogenesis of schizophrenia, and that novel agents influencing NMDA receptor functioning could prove of interest as potential treatments for schizophrenia.

Acknowledgements - This work was supported in part by USPHS grants DA-03383 to SRZ and MH-00631 to DCJ, grants from the Ritter Foundation and the David Berg Family Fund for Research in Manic Depressive Illness to SRZ, and by the generous support of the Department of Psychiatry of the Albert Einstein College of Medicine, Herman M. van Praag, M.D., Ph.D., Chairman.

REFERENCES

1. Barnard EA, Darlison MG and Seeburg P: Molecular biology of the GABA$_A$ receptor: the receptor/channel superfamily. Trends Neurosci 10:502-509, 1987.
2. Hess GP, Cash DJ and Aoshima H: Acetylcholine receptor-controlled ion translocation: chemical kinetic investigations of the mechanism. Ann Rev Biophys Bioeng 12:443-473, 1983.
3. Javitt DC, Frusciante MJ and Zukin SR: Rat brain N-methyl-D-aspartate (NMDA) receptors require multiple molecules of agonist for activation. Mol Pharmacol in press.
4. Javitt DC, Zukin SR. Bi-exponential kinetics of [^{3}H]MK-801 binding: evidence for access to closed and open N-methyl-D-aspartate receptor channels. Mol Pharmacol 35:387-393, 1989.
5. Rosenbaum G, Cohen BD, Luby ED, et al.: Comparison of sernyl with other drugs. AMA Arch Gen Psychiatry 1:651-656, 1959.

MODULATION OF NMDA RECEPTORS BY ACh IN THE CENTRAL NERVOUS SYSTEM

N. AKAIKE and N. TATEISHI
Department of Neurophysiology, Tohoku University School of Medicine, Sendai 980, Japan

The nucleus basalis of Meynert (NbM) provides the major souce of cholinergic input to the cerebral cortex in mammals (1). In the cholinergic complex of rat basal forebrain, the extensive lesions of the neocortex by cortical injection of excitatory amino acids such as kainate and N-methyl-D-aspartate (NMDA) induced retrogradely the cell shrinkage (2). While the glutaminergic system could participate in the plasticity of synapse and play an important role on the learning and memory (3). In the present study, therefore, the pharmacologic properties of the acetylcholine (ACh)- and NMDA-induced currents and the modulatory action of ACh on the NMDA response were investigated in the NbM neurons freshly isolated from the young and adult rats by the use of conventional patch-clamp technique.

METHODS

Isolated NbM neurons were prepared from young (1-2 week-old) or adult (8-10 week-old) Wistar rats by enzymatically and mechanically dissociation. Electrical measurements were performed with the conventional patch-clamp technique in whole-cell or outside-out mode. External solution was changed by 'Y-tube' method allowing for exchange of the external solution surrounding the entire cell including the processes within 10-20 msec.

RESULTS

At a holding potential (V_H) of -50 mV, ACh (10^{-4}M) evoked a transient inward current (I_{nACh}), mimicked by nicotine, followed by a sustained outward current (I_{mACh}), mimicked by carbamylcholine (CCh). The K_D and Hill coefficient were 10^{-5}M and 1.3 for I_{nACh} and 8.3×10^{-7}M and 1.0 for I_{mACh}. The reversal potentials of I_{mACh} and I_{nACh} were close to the E_K and 0 mV respectively, suggesting that I_{mACh} is passing through K$^+$ channels and I_{nACh} is carried through large cation channels. The I_{mACh} was inhibited cholinergic antagonists in the order of atropine > AF-DX-116 > pirenzepine in a concentration-dependent manner, indicating that I_{mACh} is mediated by ACh receptors of muscarinic M$_2$ type.
The NMDA-induced current (I_{NMDA}) was suppressed by the low concentrations of ACh (10^{-15} to 10^{-5}M) and facilitated by the high concentrations of ACh over 10^{-4}M only in the NbM neurons isolated from the adult rats. ACh had no effect on the NMDA response in the NbM neurons of young rats. The low concentrations of CCh and nicotine also could suppress the I_{NMDA}.

Fig.1: Modulation of I_{NMDA} by ACh. All points are normalized to 10^{-4}M NMDA-induced peak response. Inset: effects of ACh on I_{NMDA} in the NbM neurons isolated from young (a) and adult (b) rats.

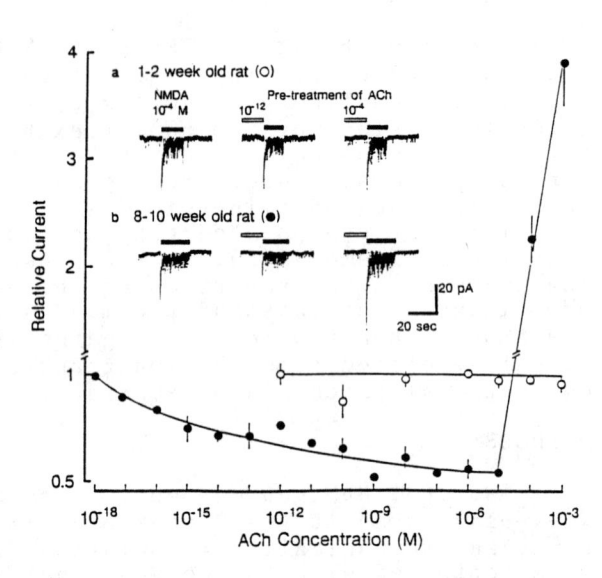

DISCUSSION

The inhibitory effect of ACh on NMDA response was maintained for a few minutes even after washing out ACh from bathing medium. Moreover, this suppression was also observated in outside-out excised membrane. Thereby, the results suggest a possibility that the inhibitory effects of cholinergic agonists on I_{NMDA} seem to be mediated by G-protein associated with the ACh receptor.

ACh suppressed the NMDA response at 10^{-15} to 10^{-5}M, but facilitated it at the high concentrations over 10^{-4}M. This phenomenon was observed only neurons isolated from adult rats, indicating developmental change in an interaction between ACh and NMDA receptors. It might be reflexed to the functional change in learning and memory with aging.

REFERENCES

1. Johnston, M.V. et al. Evidence for a cholinergic projection to neocortex from neurons in basal forebrain. Proc. Natl. Acad. Sci. USA. 76:5392-5396, 1979.
2. Sofroniew, M.V. and Pearson, C.A. Degeneration of cholinergic neurons in the basal nucleus following kainic or N-methyl-D-aspartic acid application to the cerebral cortex in the rat. Brain Res. 339:186-190, 1985.
3. Mattson, M.P. Neurotransmitters in the regulation of neuronal cytoarchitecture. Brain Res. Rev. 13:179-212, 1988.

RELATION BETWEEN AN EXCITATORY AMINO ACID, ACETYLCHOLINE AND CA CHANNEL IN THE CEREBELLAR GRANULE CELL

Y. Wanatabe and T. Shibuya. Dept. of Pharmacol., Tokyo Med. Col., Tokyo 160 Japan

It is well-documented that the cerebellar granule cells are regulated mainly by excitatory neurons, of which glutamic acid (Glu) is the major neurotransmitter. For instance, exposure of primary cultured cerebellar granule cells to increased extracellular K^+ or veratridine results in a dose-dependent increase in glutamate release. These results were obtained using either the radiolabelled glutamine or an HPLC method. In general, however, excessive accumulation of Glu in extracellular spaces damages neurons, and this toxicity of Glu may be mediated by the NMDA receptors (1). In this study we examined the inhibitory effects of Ca channel- and ACh antagonists on Glu- induced accumulation of intracellular Ca^{++} ($[Ca^{++}]_i$) levels in cultured granule cells.

MATERIALS AND METHODS

Cerebellar granule cells were obtained from 8 day old rats using the tissue culture method of Gallo et al(2). These cells (2.5×10^6 cells/35mm dish) were resuspended and incubated in Basal Modified Eagle's Medium(25 mM KCl and 2 mM glutamine) for 10 days in vitro. In order to differentiate between neurons and glia cells, 10 μM of cytosine arabino furanoside (Ara-C) was not added to some of dishes within 16 hr after resuspension. For measurement of $[Ca^{++}]_i$ levels, we incubated the cultured granule cells with 5 μM fura-2 for 30 min at 37°C. Fluorescence of the fura-2 was then measured by a computer-controlled dual-wavelength microfluorimeter using the modified method of Becker and Fay (3) (Fig-1). Each drug and the 2 mM Glu were applied to the cells through a Y-shaped tube, as shown in Fig-1.

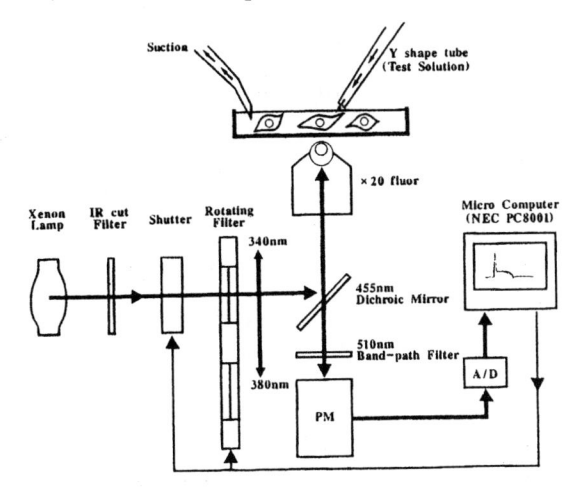

Fig-1 : Schematic diagram of computer-controlled dual-wavelength microfluorimeter for measurement of intracellular Ca^{++} levels

Table-1 : Inhibitory effects of Ca antagonists and a cholinergic antagonist on glutamate accumulated intracellular Ca^{++} levels

Drugs	IC_{50} values (micromole ; mean±S.E.)
flunarizine	2.63 ± 0.12
nicardipine	8.41 ± 0.11
nifedipine	12.42 ± 0.32
verapamil	28.62 ± 0.28
diltiazem	54.14 ± 0.48
scopolamine	51.92 ± 0.39

Table-2 : Comparative effects of Ca antagonists on Ca^{++} movement in the the cerebellar granule cells with or without Ara C treatment

high K +flu (1 μM)	+Ara C $\geq$ -Ara C
glutamic acid +flu (1 μM)	+Ara C $<$ -Ara C
high K +nic (2 μM)	+Ara C $\geq$ -Ara C
glutamic acid +nic (2 μM)	+Ara C $\leq$ -Ara C
high K +dil(30 μM)	+Ara C $\geq$ -Ara C
glutamic acid +dil(30 μM)	+Ara C $=$ -Ara C

RESULTS AND DISCUSSION

In the microspectrofluorimetric studies fluorescence of fura-2 was recorded only from neurons, but not from glia cells. The IC_{50} values of flunarizine(flu) and nicardipine(nic) for inhibiting glutamate-induced Ca^{++} accumulation were about 20 and 6 times less than that of diltiazem, respectively. Micromolar concentrations of scopolamine also blocked Glu-enhanced $[Ca^{++}]_i$ accumulation (Table-1). In addition, this Glu effect and its inhibition by Ca antagonists were influenced by the population of glia cells present (Table-2). Thus, the flu and nic sensitive channels appear to be associated with a NMDA-linked channel and the ACh receptors. Moreover, these associations were modified by the presence of glia cells. In future studies, we plan to measure concentrations of Ach in cultured granule cells using a new improved pyrolysis gas chromatography/mass spectrometry system.

REFERENCES

1. Michaels, R.L. and Rothman, S.M. Glutamate neurotoxicity in vitro :Antagonist pharmacology and intracellular calcium concentration. J.Neurosci. 10(1) : 283~292, 1990.
2. Gallo, V.M. et al. Selective release of glutamate from cerebellar granule cells differentiating in culture. Proc. Natl. Acad. Sci. U.S.A. 79 : 7919~7923, 1982.
3. Becker, P.L. and Fay, F.S. Photobleaching of fura-2 and its effect on determination of calcium concentrations. Am. J. Physiol. 253 (Cell Phsiol. 22) : C613~C618, 1987.

EXOGENOUS EXCITATORY AMINO ACIDS (EAAs) IN NEURODEGENERATIVE DISORDERS

P.S. SPENCER, C. ALLEN, R. ALLEN, G. KISBY, A.C. LUDOLPH, S.M. ROSS AND D.N. ROY
Center for Research on Occupational and Environmental Toxicology, Oregon Health Sciences University, Portland, OR, U.S.A.

There is interest in the possibility that elevated levels of *endogenous* excitatory amino acids (behaving as excitotoxins) are involved in the etiopathogenesis of certain neurodegenerative disorders, such as amyotrophic lateral sclerosis (ALS) and Alzheimer's disease. This paper summarizes evidence linking three other diseases with neuronal degeneration to *exogenous* EAA excitotoxins of plant or animal origin.

LATHYRISM AND BETA-N-OXALYLAMINO-L-ALANINE (BOAA)

BOAA is a stereospecific EAA and excitotoxin present in low (1-2%) concentrations as a non-protein amino acid in the seed of <u>Lathyrus sativus</u> (grass or chickling pea). In humans and animals, prolonged heavy consumption of this legume causes dysfunction and degeneration of the central motor pathway culminating in permanent spastic paraparesis (lathyrism). Recognized since antiquity and still prevalent in Bangladesh, China, Ethiopia and India, lathyrism is the best studied human excitotoxic disorder. In heavily poisoned subjects, the early reversible symptoms of global muscle cramping, urgency and frequency of micturition, nocturnal erection and ejaculation, suggest diffuse and transitory CNS excitation of somatic motor and autonomic function likely associated with the pharmacological actions of BOAA. Myoclonic-like movements are rarely reported and seizures are not described, probably because L-BOAA crosses the blood-brain barrier with difficulty and, consequently, CNS extracellular concentrations of the EAA remain sub-convulsive. Continued intake of <u>L. sativus</u> leads to loss of cortical motoneurons and degeneration of pyramidal pathways, with associated weakness and increased muscle tone of the legs. Pyramidal signs in the upper extremities are found in only the most severely affected subjects. While some degree of increased clinical deficit may appear years or decades after cessation of intoxication, lathyrism (unlike ALS) is a largely self-limiting disease and therefore does not follow an aggressive downhill course.

Several lines of evidence suggest that BOAA has a high affinity for the quisqualate receptor which mediates both its excitatory and excitotoxic actions. BOAA-activated ion currents in isolated hippocampal neurons show a concentration-dependent desensitization which is consistent with activation of an ion channel by quisqualate. Additionally, the rank order of BOAA potency in displacing specific radioligand binding in mouse synaptic membranes is quisqualate ($[^3H]$AMPA: IC_{50} 0.94 µM) > kainate (40 µM) > N-methyl-D-aspartate (NMDA). The IC_{50} value is lower for cortex (0.79 µM) than for hippocampus (3.82 µM) or cerebellum (5.9 µM), and there is sparse AMPA binding to spinal cord. If, like the mouse, cortical quisqualate receptors of other species possess the highest affinity for BOAA, this may explain the preferential involvement of cortical (motor) neurons in lathyrism. Intracerebroventricular (i.c.v.) administration of BOAA in mice elicits seizures that are temporally attenuated by prior administration of cis-2,3-piperidine dicarboxylic acid (PDA), a non-specific quisqualate and kainate antagonist. Similarly, pretreatment with PDA (but not the NMDA antagonist AP7) largely blocks induction of post-synaptic vacuolation (superficial layers) and neuronal degeneration (deep layers) in mouse cortical explants treated with BOAA. Taken together with the clinical picture of lathyrism, these data raise the possibility that quisqualate receptors on the dendritic arborization of human cortical motoneurons represent the principal target of BOAA. The earlier and greater clinical involvement of the lower relative to the upper extremities might reflect a differential organization of quisqualate receptors on upper motoneurons supplying the legs versus the arms, a larger reserve of neurons regulating the function of the latter, or a more expansive dendritic arborization (i.e. a greater neuronal surface membrane target for BOAA) of motoneurons projecting to the lumbosacral cord relative to those with axons terminating in the cervical region.

AMNESTIC SHELLFISH POISONING AND DOMOIC ACID

The potent kainate agonist domoic acid (DOA) is held responsible for a 1987 outbreak of 140 cases of neurological disease among Canadian consumers of DOA-contaminated mussels. Detailed information on the human neurotoxic action of DOA is currently awaiting publication (Cashman, N., personal communication to A.C.L.). Acute signs of neuroexcitation included seizures, myoclonic-like movements of the face and autonomic hyperactivity. Organic pyschosyndrome, fever, nausea, vomiting, headache and ophthalmolplegia were also seen. Weakness was common, and hyperreflexia (positive Babinski sign), hemiparesis, diploplia and fasciculations were noted in a few subjects. Residual signs six months after intoxication included varying degrees of memory deficit (impaired or delayed recall), mild weakness and distal muscle atrophy, cramping and fasciculation. Electrophysiological studies revealed widespread denervation and nerve conduction deficits with reduced amplitudes, and examination by positron emission tomography showed hypometabolism of the amygdala and hippocampus. Damage to hippocampus, amygdala, thalamus (medial dorsal nucleus), insula, claustrum and nucleus accumbens was noted in autopsy studies of subjects who died from mussel poisoning. DOA induces scratching motions, convulsions and death in mice, and its neurotoxic effects in hippocampus and spinal cord are likely mediated by kainate receptor activation. Thus, while DOA and BOAA both elicit acute neuroexcitatory phenomena at disease onset, the pattern of acute dysfunction and permanent deficits are markedly different. This disparity presumably reflects the differential distribution of kainate and quisqualate receptors in the human brain.

ALS/PARKINSONISM-DEMENTIA (P-D) AND BETA-N-METHYLAMINO-L-ALANINE (BMAA)

BMAA is a low-potency, stereospecific EAA and excitotoxin found in low concentrations (~0.02%) in cycads, a family of ancient neurotoxic plants (gymnosperms) whose members have been used for food and medicine in various cultures, including the Chamorros of Guam, the Japanese of the Kii Peninsula, and the Auyu and Jaqai linguistic groups of west New Guinea. In these areas, heavy use of Cycas spp. for food or medicine (or both) in the first part of life has been proposed as the cause of a long-latency, progressive neurodegenerative disorder with the clinical features of ALS, often combined with parkinsonism and dementia. Pathological studies of middle-aged subjects reveal widespread neurofibrillary tangles of the Alzheimer type, as well as multinucleated and displaced Purkinje cells and other neurons that are suggestive of a developmental perturbation. Although prolonged treatment of primates (but not rodents) with huge oral doses of BMAA elicits a disease with pyramidal, extrapyramidal and behavioral features, there are many additional chemical components of cycad seed, including cycasin (2%), the glycone of methylazoxymethanol (MAM). Cycad seed and cycasin both induce neuromuscular disease in grazing animals; MAM reacts with physiological amino acids to generate additional excitotoxins and also arrests neuronal mitosis and migration during development. Cycasin, MAM, and BMAA are under study to determine whether they initiate a pathological process that culminates in progressive neuronal degeneration unlike that associated with BOAA or DOA. A "slow toxin" of this type is needed to explain the latent period of years or decades that intervenes between cycad exposure and the clinical expression of ALS/P-D. While such an agent potentially could employ a cell surface receptor to gain access to neurons, its toxic activity is more likely to be expressed intracellularly, perhaps by altering genomic expression or some other critical function.

BMAA lacks the dicarboxylic acid structure of most EAA excitotoxins but nevertheless activates ion currents in isolated hippocampal neurons (both in the presence and absence of bicarbonate). While specific NMDA antagonists (APV and ketamine) block currents generated by either NMDA (500 µM) or BMAA (500 µM) in this system, the channel activated by BMAA (unlike that by NMDA) is neither blocked by Mg^{2+} nor modulated by glycine. Low concentrations of BMAA also fail to displace ligands for NMDA and non-NMDA receptors. BMAA elicits an AP7-sensitive hyperexcitable state in i.c.v-treated mice, and the selective NMDA antagonists AP-7 and MK-801 also block BMAA-induced post-synaptic vacuolation and neuronal degeneration in murine cortical explants. Thus, at certain concentrations, BMAA's excitotoxic activity is somehow linked to the NMDA receptor complex. While the EAA action(s) of BMAA explain its seizuregenic effects in rodents, the mechanism underlying its chronic effects in macaques is unknown.

NEUROPSYCHOLOGICAL INDICATORS OF THE VULNERABILITY TO SCHIZOPHRENIA

W. MAIER *, CH. HAIN *, F. RIST **
* Department of Psychiatry, University of Mainz, Untere Zahlbacher Str. 8, D-6500 Mainz, West-Germany
** Department of Psychology, University of Konstanz, D-7750 Konstanz, West-Germany

INTRODUCTION

The majority of family and twin studies in schizophrenia is in agreement with a transmission due to major gene(s) (with polygenetic background) in families. However, the penetrance of the major gene(s) must be assumed to be rather low. Under this hypothesis a substantial proportion of first degree relatives of schizophrenic probands carrying the major gene(s) but without psychopathological signs is to be expected. This consequence is provoking studies in healthy first degree relatives of schizophrenics trying to identify healthy carriers of the major gene(s) by non-psychophathological means. Especially neuropsychological methods are promising in this respect. Reaction time trials with either varying the intrastimulus intervals or varying stimulus modality were able to provide two major paradigms contrasting schizophrenic patients from healthy controls: the cross-over effect and the modality shift effect. The hypothesis will be tested, that healthy first degree relatives of schizophrenic patients are located between patients and healthy controls with respect to both effects.

PROCEDERE AND SAMPLE

Cross-over paradigm: Six blocks à 25 were presented; a trial is consisting of a stimulus (i.e. a bright square presented on a monitor); the intrastimulus intervals (ISI) are varying in a systematic manner: in the first three blocks the ISI are fixed (one block for 1,5 sec, one for 3,5 and one for 5,5 sec); in the subsequent three blocks the ISI are varying randomly with the mean ISI identical to block 1 to 3. Cross-modality-paradigm: Six blocks à 55 trials were presented; the trials of the first four blocks are simple reaction tasks the proband is asked to respond with a button press as soon as the auditory or the visual stimulus appears; followed by two blocks with choice reaction tasks.

Patients, Siblings and Controls: 18 inpatients (mean age 25 years) with schizophrenia (RDC) 1 to 6 days after admission; the patients were free of any drugs for at least two weeks. 20 siblings to the patient group (mean age 28 years) without any psychiatric disorder by RDC or DSM-III (axis I or axis II). 20 healthy controls recruited in the general population without any RDC- or DSM-III diagnosis (axis I or axis II) matched to the siblings of the patients by age (± 2 years), sex and education status. All diagnoses mentioned were evidenced by a SADS-LA interview.

RESULTS

1. Cross-over: A cross-over effect (i.e. reaction times for irregular presentation of stimuli) are longer for shorter ISI and smaller for longer ISI compared to the regular presentation of stimuli) was found in the majority of schizophrenic patients and only in a minority of healthy controls; the healthy siblings are in between:
  schizophrenic patients 60 %   healthy siblings 48 %
        healthy controls 38 %

2. Modality shift: The reaction times to tone (T) were proposed in the previous literature to measure the modality shift effect by "reaction time under cross-modal condition "LT" minus reaction time under ipsimodal condition "TT"". Using a simple reaction time setting a trend to a significant difference (p ≤ .10) was observed for the variable "LT-TT" between the schizophrenic patients and the healthy controls; the healthy siblings were located in between (table 1). In a choice reaction time setting a significant difference (F-tests for matched pairs p = .05) was observed.

CONCLUSION

The cross-over effect as well as the modality shift effect was apparent in drug-free schizophrenic patients compared to healthy controls. The most significant finding discriminating healthy siblings of patients and healthy controls became apparent by comparing the modality shift effect with choice reaction. The reaction times received by variation of the intrerstimulus interval (cross-over effect) was not able to discriminate healthy siblings of schizophrenic probands and healthy controls significantly, although there was a clear trend in the hypothesized direction.

TABLE 1: MODALITY SHIFT EFFECT

	patients (drug free)	healthy siblings	healthy controls
SIMPLE r.t.(msec)			
LT (crossmodal)	418,2	338,2	334,7
TT (ipsimodal)	358,0	270,7	294,0
LT - TT	60,2	67,5	40,7
CHOICE r.t. (msec)			
LT (crossmodal)	516,3	438,3	414,4
TT (ipsimodal)	455,5	389,3	409,1
LT - TT	60,8	49,0	5,3

VARIABLE EXPRESSIVITY OF THE PHENOTYPE IN THE
RELATIVES OF SCHIZOPHRENIC PATIENTS

PHILIP S. HOLZMAN
Department of Psychology and Department of Psychiatry,
Harvard University, Cambridge, MA, U.S.A.

Family, twin, and adoption studies have produced strong evidence that genes play a major role in schizophrenic conditions. These conventional approaches, however, are not able to reveal anything about the way in which genes influence that disease except that the family prevalence of schizophrenia is too low to fit a classical Mendelian transmission mode. New molecular biological techniques (including restriction fragment length polymorphisms) offer bright possibilities for identifying the chromosomal loci of genetic diseases, but these techniques rely for their effectiveness on a Mendelian distribution of the trait under investigation. Psychological methods can play a decisive role in making these new biological techniques available for the study of schizophrenia by expanding the phenotype (schizophrenia) to include associated behaviors that fit a model of transmission by major loci.

In following such a program of experimentation, one behavior we have investigated is a disorder of smooth pursuit eye movements, which occurs in about two-thirds of schizophrenic patients and about half of their first-degree relatives. Recent studies strongly suggest that these eye movement abnormalities can illuminate the biology and particularly the genetics of schizophrenia.

A second behavior is the existence of mild but significant thought disorder in the first-degree family members of schizophrenic patients. The quality of thought disorder seems to "run true" in families.

We have formulated a model to account for these and other characteristics of the distribution of these traits within families. We postulate that there is a latent trait which is not directly observable, but which can cause either schizophrenia, eye movement dysfunctions, thought disorder, or all three. Indeed, there may be other traits that are caused by the latent trait. But it is the latent trait that is to be regarded as transmitted genetically, rather than the manifest traits of schizophrenia, bad eye tracking, or thought disorder, and the transmission pattern of the latent trait may be closer to that of a Mendelian gene with high penetrance than any of the manifest traits alone.

This model highlights the potential value for studying the mildly-affected and clinically asymptomatic members of the families of schizophrenic probands. These family members have been a neglected resource for psychobiological investigation. Thus, we show the value of studying each of the relatives of a family in which there is schizophrenia, including those who seem well.

^{3}H-SPIPERONE BINDING CAPACITY IN LYMPHOCYTES: A FAMILY STUDY

B. BONDY*, M. ACKENHEIL*, R.R. ENGEL*, M. ERTL, G. MINELLI*, C. MUNDT**, G. SCHLEUNING**
* Psychiatric Hospital, University of Munich, Nussbaumstraβe 7, D-8000 Munich 2, FRG; ** Psychiatric District Hospital, D-8013 Haar, FRG

An increased morbidity risk for psychiatric disorders in relatives of schizophrenic probands is well established (4). However, so far it is not possible to identify individuals being at risk for developing psychiatric disturbances. Investigations of biological markers on a phenotypic level could be very fruitful in two aspects. First, vulnerable persons might be identified on a status even without clinical symptoms, and secondly, these parameters could also discriminate phenocopies, thus being able to address the problem of heterogeneity of psychiatric disorders.
Increased binding capacity of the dopamine antagonist 3H-spiperone to lymphocytes could be one of the parameters worth being investigated. Recently we and others reported studies that the ^{3}H-spiperone binding capacity in lymphocytes is fulfilling the criteria for vulnerability markers (1,2,5,6). Increased binding capacity was found to be associated with schizophrenia with high sensitivity and specifity and was furthermore not influenced by treatment or the actual state of the disease.

SUBJECTS AND METHOD

Our family study comprises 220 relatives of 17 indexprobands with either schizophrenia (n=12) or schizoaffective disorder (n=5). The clinical investigations and were carried out using the SADS-LA semistructured interview, including the schizophrenia part of the CIDI and the personality part of the SCID. Blood samples (50 ml) were taken from all probands on the day of the interview to evaluate the 3H-spiperone binding capacity in lymphocytes with a radioreceptor method (3). The laboratory personel was blind against clinical diagnosis. According to our earlier results with spiperone binding capacity in lymphocytes we obtained a clear distinction between patients and controls, with a cut off point at 3,7 fmol/10^6 cells. The B_{max} values for schizophrenics was in the range from 4 to 30 fmol/10^6 cells.

RESULTS

Concerning clinical results we could establish psychiatric disorders in 53 of the 220 relatives: schizophrenia was diagnosed in 10, schizoaffective disorder in 8, bipolar I disorder in 9, unipolar affective disorder in 23 and borderline personality disorder in 3 of the probands.
The results with spiperone binding assay in lymphocytes have shown that in 14 of the 17 families an increased lymphocyte spiperone binding capacity was obtained in the index probands and in all

relatives with psychiatric disturbances. Interestingly binding was elevated not only in schizophrenics but also in probands with other psychiatric diagnoses. In these families increased binding was also found in several healthy probands. In contrast to that spiperone binding was within normal ranges in 3 nuclear families where none of the probands, neither the indexproband nor any of the relatives had incresed binding.

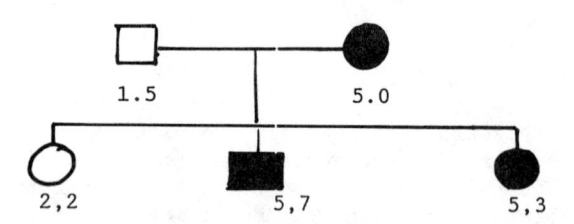

Fig. 1: Maximal binding capacity of ^{3}H-spiperone to lymphocytes (in fmol/10^6 cells) in a family. Values above 4 are "pathological". o female, ◻ male, not affected; ● female, ■ male, affected

DISCUSSION

These findings stronly suggest that elevated lymphocyte spiperone binding is valuable as vulnerability marker in schizophrenia. One can assume, that at least within some families this assay could indicate persons being vulnerable to develop psychiatric disturbances. Secondly, our results further indicate, that it might be possible to distinguish biologically homogenous groups amongst the schizophrenics on basis of an biological investigation. This would be of further extreme importance in genetic studys on a DNA basis.

REFERENCES

1.   Bondy, B. et al. Catecholamines and their receptors in blood: evidence for alterations in schizophrenia. Biol. Psychiat. 19(10):1377-1390, 1984
2.   Bondy, B. and Ackenheil, M: 3H-spiperone binding in lymphocytes as possible vulnerability marker in schizophrenia. J. psychiat. Res. 21(4):521-529, 1987
3.   Bondy, B. et al. Methodology of ^{3}H-spiperone binding to lymphocytes. J. psychiatr. res., in press, 1990
4.   Crow, T.J. The continuum of psychosis and its implication for the structure of the gene. Brit. J. Psychiat., 149:419-429, 1986
5.   LeFur, G. et al. 3H-spiroperidol binding in lymohocytes:changes in two different groups of schizophrenic patients and effect of neuroleptic treatment. Life Sci. 32:249-255, 1983
6.   Rotstein, E. et al. Lymphocyte 3H-spiroperidol binding in schizophrenia: preliminary findings. Progr. Neuro. Psychopharmacol. & Biol. Psychiat. 7:729-732, 1983

PSYCHOMETRIC, POLYSOMNOGRAPHIC, AND NEUROENDOCRINE FINDINGS IN SUBJECTS AT HIGH RISK FOR PSYCHIATRIC DISORDERS

J.-C. KRIEG, C.J. LAUER and F. HOLSBOER
Department of Psychiatry, University of Freiburg, Freiburg, F.R.G.
now at: Max-Planck-Institute for Psychiatry, Munich, F.R.G.

Several neuroendocrine and polysomnographic abnormalities are alleged to be neurobiological markers for depression, especially a hyperactivity of the limbic-hypothalamic-pituitary-adrenocortical (LHPA)-axis (1) and alterations of REM sleep parameters (2). In the remitted state the secretion pattern of the LHPA axis usually normalizes, whereas the persistence of an altered function seems to signalize the reoccurrence of a depressive episode (1). Polysomnographic studies performed on patients remitted from a depressive episode yielded conflicting results: thus, a normalization as well as a persistence of the EEG sleep stigmata of depression have been reported. In a recent study, however, a high risk for relapse was found in those patients displaying a short REM latency during depression as well as in the remitted state (3).
In order to determine biological markers indicating vulnerabilty for affective illness or - more general - for psychiatric disorders, investigations have to be extended to healthy subjects with a risk of developing a psychiatric illness. The described ongoing study presents psychometric, polysomnographic, and neuroendocrine data of healthy subjects with a hereditary disposition for a psychiatric disorder.

SUBJECTS AND METHODS

Twelve 1st degree relatives (HRP; 5 female, 7 male; mean age 29 ± 9 (SD) yrs) of 12 patients with an affective disorder, who had at least one further 1st degree relative with either an affective or schizophrenic disorder, took part in the study. Ten healthy subjects served as a control group (CP; 4 female, 6 male; age: 26 ± 5 yrs). All study participants were interviewed by means of the Structured Clinical Interview according to DSM-III-R (SCID) in order to verify the absence of a current and lifetime psychiatric disorder. The psychometric assessments included personality traits (MP-T), vegetative lability (BL), and stress coping behavior (SCOPE). The EEG sleep was registered and visually scored according to standard criteria. For assessing LHPA-axis function, a combined dexamethasone-corticotropin releasing hormone (DEX/CRH)-test was performed (4).

RESULTS

Age and gender distribution of the HRP and the CP were similar. In the HRP psychometric measurements revealed an elevated score on the neuroticism scale (MP-T: 10 ± 5 vs 6 ± 2 pts., $p<0.05$) and an increased vegetative lability (BL: 13 ± 7 vs 6 ± 6 pts., $p<0.05$). Regarding stress coping behavior (SCOPE), the HRP displayed increased values on the scales 'stress reaction' (2.4 ± 0.5 vs 1.9 ± 0.5 pts., $p<0.08$), 'negative life experience' (2.1 ± 0.6 vs 1.7 ± 0.7 pts., $p<0.05$), 'emotional restraint' (3.2 ± 1.2 vs 2.3 ± 0.8 pts., $p<0.08$), and on the second-order factor 'stress' (2.3 ± 0.4 vs 1.8 ± 0.5 pts, $p<0.05$). No group differences were found regarding the measurements assessing extraversion, frustration tolerance, rigidity (all MP-T), pursuit of success and restraint (all SCOPE). The polysomnographic measurements assessed in the HRP and the CP showed no significant group differences in the parameters describing either total sleep or single sleep cycles. However, clear trends ($p \leq 0.15$) became obvious: as compared with the CP, the HRP more frequently displayed nocturnal awakenings (9 ± 8 vs 4 ± 3), their sleep efficiency index was lowered (87 ± 9 vs $94 \pm 3\%$), and they spent less time in slow wave sleep during the 2nd sleep cycle (20 ± 13 vs $35 \pm 16\%$). The REM latency was, on average, slightly prolonged in the HRP (110 ± 62 vs 85 ± 46 min). However, in the HRP, this parameter was characterized by an extremely high variablity (range: 39-262 min). The

REM density measurements also did not differ between groups.
In the DEX/CRH-test neither significant nor tendentious group differences were observed regarding basal plasma cortisol levels after DEX adminstration (7.6 ± 6.2 vs 7.9 ± 5.1 ng/ml), CRH-stimulated cortisol release (net area: 4.2 ± 5.3 vs 2.8 ± 1.4 ng x min x 10^3/ml), and the delta values of the CRH induced plasma cortisol rise (31.8 ± 44.8 vs 19.1 ± 12.0 ng/ml).
To characterize each HRP on an individual level, several scores alleged to mirror conspicuousness were computed by taking pattern from the distribution of the respective measurements assessed in the CP. Regarding psychometrics, 5 HRP were rated to be conspicuous, 4 HRP showed signs of EEG sleep stigmata of depression (but only one had a REM latency < 60 min), and the DEX/CRH-test was classified to be conspicuous in 4 HRP (in one HRP the test result was abnormal). 2 HRP reached scores mirroring conspicuousness in at least 2 of these areas.

DISCUSSION

The advantage of the conservative recruiting procedure applied in the present study (only subjects with at least 2 psychiatrically ill family members entered the study protocol) is an increased likelihood of gaining a true high risk study sample.
On the psychometric level, the subjects at high risk displayed elevated scores on the neuroticism scale, an increased vegetative lability, and - when condensing the measurements of the SCOPE - an accentuated 'stress-personality' pattern. These observations are in agreement with other reports (5). The polysomnographic part of the study yielded some obvious trends pointing towards a more shallow and fragmented sleep in the high risk probands. Furthermore, 4 of these subjects displayed features of EEG sleep stigmata of depression. The assumed link between a shortened REM latency and high risk (3), however, is yet not supported by our observations. In the combined DEX/CRH-test, one high risk proband displayed an abnormal result and 3 further subjects were rated to be conspicuous. These observations, however, did not result in significant group differences.
Regarding the dissimilar patterns of conspicuousness observed on the individual level, it may be speculated that vulnerability for psychiatric disorders expresses itself differently in different individuals. Although in the present study conservative inclusion criteria were applied, one has to keep in mind that the observations reported are drawn from a sample in which high risk probands who will develop a psychiatric disorder were pooled with those who will remain healthy. Thus, at this point of the study, a clear statement about a true marker for vulnerability is rendered more difficult.

REFERENCES

1. Holsboer, F Implications of altered limbic-hypothalamic-pituitary- adrenocortical activity. Eur. Arch. Psychiatr. Neurol. Sci. 238:302-322, 1989.
2. Reynolds, C.F., Kupfer, D.J. Sleep research in affective illness: state of the art circa 1987. Sleep 10:199-215, 1987.
3. Giles, D.E. et al. Reduced rapid eye movement latency: a predictor of recurrence in depression. Neuropsychopharmacol. 1:33-39, 1987.
4. von Bardeleben, U., Holsboer, F. Cortisol response to a combined dexamethasone-human corticotropin-releasing hormone challenge in patients with depression. J. Neuroendocrinol. 1:485-488, 1989.
5. Angst, J., Clayton, P. Premorbid personality of depressive, bipolar, and schizophrenic patients with special reference to suicidal issues. Compr. Psychiatry 27:511-532, 1986.

AGING EFFECT ON RESPONSE TO NORTRIPTYLINE IN DEPRESSED PATIENTS

S. KANBA*, K. MATSUMOTO**, G. YAGI*.
Department of Neuro-psychiatry, Keio University School of Medicine, 35 Shinanomachi, Shinjuku-ku, Tokyo 160*.
Department of Clinical Chemistry, Toho University School of Pharmacy, 2-2-1 Miyama, Funabashi, Chiba**.

It is well known that depressed geriatric patients are more susceptible to side effects. They are sometimes difficult to treat with antidepressants. However, it is not clear if this is due to the side effects or poor responsivity to antidepressants. Little is known about pharmacokinetics and pharmacodynamics of antidepressants in this population. We examined effects of aging on bioavailability and hydroxylation of nortriptyline, and on clinical response as well as propensity for side effect. We also describe an automated column-switching HPLC, a simple, rapid and cost-effective method, to determine antidepressants, which we have established.

SUBJECTS AND METHODS

We examined serum level of nortriptyline (NT) and 10-OH-NT, an active metabolite, in 30 depressed out patients (53 +/- 15, 23-79 years old) who met the diagnosis of major depression by DSM-III-R and all patients were treated with nortriptyline, p. o. with a flexible dosing method. For the last two weeks, NT dose was fixed to obtain steady state level. The severity of depression was rated with Hamilton Depression Scale on the first day and the day of week 6. A rater was blind to the treatments. At 10 am on the day of week 6, blood samples were obtained and serum level of NT and 10-OH-NT was measured by a column switching HPLC (1).

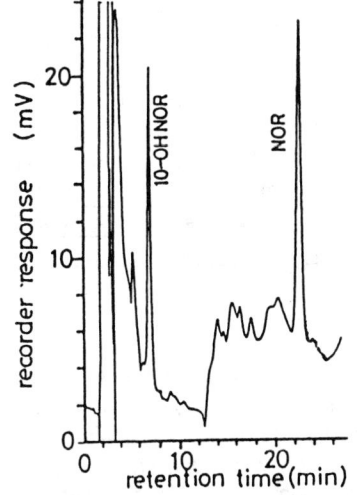

Fig. 1 Typical chromatogram for NT and 10-OH-NT in serum.
Recovery and reproducibility of NT were 99.7-100.6 % and 1.21-1.49 % (within-run CV) and 0.91-3.51 % (day to day CV).

RESULTS

The automated column-switching method could determine nine antidepressants and their metabolites within 30 min with the analytical recoveries of 95-100%, reproducibilities (within-run CV < 3 %), and detection limits (10 µg/ml).

Briefly described, a 200 µL serum is directly injected onto the precolumn (Fig. 1).

After washing the serum proteins with potassium buffer, the precolumn connection is switched to introduce the retained substances onto analytical column. The compounds are then eluted with an acetonitrile/potassium phosphate buffer mixture containing sodium 1-heptanesulfonate.

There was no significant relationship between age and bioavailability of NT (NT level/NT dose/kg), age and apparent rate of hydroxylation of NT (10-OH-NT level/NT level), or age and clinical response (% improvement of Hamilton Scores).

When divided the group into two groups, a younger group (39 +/- 8 years old) and an elderly group (64 +/- 8 years old) with a cut off age of 50, each group comprised almost equal number of patients (Table 1). We compared several variables between the two groups. NT dose and NT capacity (NT dose/kg) were significantly lower in the elderly group, and the elderly group had tendency to have lower serum level of NT as well as 10-OH-NT.

However, bioavailability or apparent rate of hydroxylation of NT was not significantly different between the two groups. No significant difference was found in improvement scores, % improvement of depression, but the elderly patients had tendency to have higher propensity for side effects(χ^2, p<o.1) than the younger patients.

TABLE 1: PHARMACOKINETIC FACTORS AND CLINICAL RESPONSE

	Elderly (16)	Younger (14)	T value	Prob.
Age	64.4 +/- 8	39.1 +/- 8	8.45	0.0001
NT Dose, mg/day	58.8 +/- 32.2	96.4 +/- 25.7	3.51	0.0016
NT Capacity	1.15 +/- 0.65	1.74 +/- 0.65	2.47	0.019
NT Level	90.9 +/- 71.2	140.2 +/- 70.9	1.89	0.068
10-OH-NT Level	75 +/- 49.8	103.9 +/- 45.7	1.64	0.111
NT Level / Capacity	82.6 +/- 52.2	81.6 +/- 33.8	0.06	0.95
10-OH-NT / NT	0.93 +/- 0.41	0.88 +/- 0.48	0.32	0.75
Improvement Score	15 +/- 8.6	16 +/- 5	0.33	0.75
% Improvement	58.4 +/- 31.8	66 +/- 16.6	0.8	0.43
Side Effect Rate(%)	43.8	14.3	3.09*	0.08

* χ^2

DISCUSSION

Our results suggest that depressed geriatric patients may well respond to nortriptyline (NT) at lower serum level than the younger patients, although they have higher propensity to develop side effects. Since there was no significant age-related change in bioavailability or apparent rate of hydroxylation of NT, the increased sensitivity of the geriatric patients to NT may not be explained by alternation in pharmacokinetics, but by pharmacodynamic factors. It is known that sensitivity of benzodiazepine receptors is increased in elderly people. Similarly, sensitivity of central receptors involved in pharmacodynamic actions of antidepressants such as β-, α-adrenergic or 5-HT receptors might be increased in the geriatric patients. Basic research on this possiblity may be of great interest and value for clinicians in the treatment of geriatric depressed patients.

REFERENCE

1. Matsumoto, K. et al. Automated determination of drugs in serum by column-switching high-performance liquid chromatography. Clinical Chemistry, 35, 453-456, 1989.

CENTRAL NORADRENERGIC FUNCTION IN DEPRESSION AND
ANTIDEPRESSANTS

O. TAJIMA and K. KAMIJIMA
Department of Neuropsychiatry, School of Medicine
Kyorin University, Tokyo Japan

Since the original"cathecholamine hypothesis" of
depression has been proposed about 20 years ago, a large
number of sturdies have been done to elucidate the possible
involvement of central noradrenergic and/or serotonergic
dysfunction in affective disorder. Clinically, the levels of
monoamine metabolites in body fluid such as urine, CSF,
plasma in patients with affective disorders were studied.
Collaborative studies of CSF monoamine metabolites which
have been done in USA and Europe suggest that CSF levels
of MHPG and 5-HIAA were not decreased in most depressive
patients. These findings are not consistent with the
monoamine deficiency hypohtesis.

Along with rapid progress of neurochemistry and the
developement of new generation antidepressants which have
different phamacologic and chemical profiles from tricyclic, many
researchers have tried to find the final common pathway of
action of antidepressants including ECT. These studies
suggest that the down-regulation or desensitization of
B-adrenergic receptor may be the final common pathway of
effective antidepressant treatments. Normal or high levels
of CSF monoamine metabolites in depressive patients and
B-receptor down-regulation following chronic antidepressant
treatment have led to the reformulation of monoamine
hypothesis. Several lines of second generation
cathecholamine hypothesis were proposed ;"noradrenergic
dysregulation hypothesis", reverse cathecholamine hypothesis
which postulates the noradrenergic hyperactivity in
depression ;" 1-adrenoreceptor theory", revision of the
noradrenaline deficiency hypothesis.

It is not clear whether B-receptor down-regulation
following chronic antidepressant treatment means a net
decrease of noradrenergic neurotransmission or only adaptive
changes associated with a net increase of synaptic
noradrenaline. Recent explosive progess in research of
intracellular signal transduction systems are expected to
clarify these questions on mode of action of
antidepressants. Neverthless, there are many theoretical
deficiency in biological hypothesis of affective disorders,
mainly based on pharmacologic action of antidepressants and
"reserpine model". Affective disorders are considered to be
a heterogeneous group of disorders which have different

genetic predisposition, longitudinal course and treatment response. The etiological model of affective disorders are needed to explain these questions. "Kindling model" of affective disorders which is based on the effectiveness of anticonvulsants as mood stabilizer could explain the spontaneous reccurence or rapid cycling following stress-induced onset of depression and the response to various treatment modalities.

We have been studied the central noradrenergic function in affective disorders and the mode of action of antidepressants. We have reported that plasma levels of MHPG in pretreatment depressive patients were not significantly different from controls, but the changes in MHPG during antidepressants treatment were dependent on their pharmacologic profiles. From these results, we have postulated a net decrease of noradrenergic neurotransmissions in depression. In order to elucidate our hypothesis, the effects of acute and chronic antidepressants on the locus coeruleus-hippocampal noradrenergic activity were studies by single-unit electrophysiologic recordings and in vivo brain microdialysis methods.

Recently several researchers suggest that the action of different neurotransmitters may converge to common postsynaptic ion channels. We have interested in the effects of antidepresants on Ca^{2+}-activated K^+ channels which regulate the spike frequency adaptation. We have reported the inhibition of slow afterhyperpolarization and spike frequency accommodation in hippocampal pyramidal cells following acute and chronic antidepressant treatments. Antidepressants enhance the signal/noise ratio of hippocampal neurons to exitatory neurotransmitters systems such as glutamate. These results suggest that S/N ratio of cortical neurons may be decreased in some of depression, probably due to the net decrease of noradrenergic neurotransmission, and chronic antidepressant treatments may improve the S/N ratio of postsynaptic neurons via inhibition of Ca^{2+}-activated K^+ channels.

CLINICAL SIGNIFICANCE OF RECEPTOR EFFECTS OF ANTIDEPRESSANTS

E. RICHELSON
Departments of Psychiatry and Pharmacology, Mayo Clinic Jacksonville, Jacksonville, FL, U.S.A.

The degree to which various antidepressant drugs antagonize neurotransmitter receptors reflects their relative abilities to produce certain adverse effects. Such antagonism may be a useful predictor of side effects for newly introduced agents and guide the clinician in choosing suitable drugs that may improve patient compliance. Certain antidepressants are more potent *in vitro* than others in blocking these receptors (1,2). Some of these data are presented in Table 1.

In general, the most potent interaction of antidepressants is at the histamine H_1 receptor (Table 1). Their next most potent effect is at the muscarinic receptor. Monoamine oxidase inhibitors have very weak effects on these two receptors and are practically devoid of clinically significant pharmacologic activity on them.

Some antidepressants are exceedingly potent histamine H_1 antagonists (Table 1). As a result clinicians are using them to treat allergic and dermatological problems. However, this effect likely causes sedation and drowsiness, among other adverse effects.

Muscarinic acetylcholine receptors are the predominant type of cholinergic receptors in brain. In that organ they may be involved with memory and learning. Antidepressants have a broad range of affinities for human brain muscarinic receptors (Table 1). This blockade likely causes blurred vision, dry mouth, urinary retention, and memory dysfunction in patients.

Antidepressants are also weak competitive antagonists of dopamine (D_2) receptors (Table 1). The most potent compound, amoxapine, is a demethylated derivative of the neuroleptic, loxapine. It is very likely that this in vitro activity of amoxapine explains its extrapyramidal side effects and its ability to elevate prolactin levels in patients. Because of this dopamine receptor blocking property of amoxapine, some clinicians are using it in psychotic depressions.

Some antidepressants are quite potent at blocking $5-HT_2$ receptors relative to methysergide, a drug sometimes used to treat migraine headaches prophylactically (Table 1). Most are weak at blocking other subclasses of the serotonin receptors.

In general, newer generation antidepressants (for example, bupropion and fluoxetine) have lower potencies at blocking all these receptors relative to the older drugs (for example, amitriptyline and imipramine). This information predicts that newer antidepressants have side effect profiles that are different from the first generation compounds.

TABLE 1: POTENCIES* OF ANTIDEPRESSANTS AT BLOCKADE OF SOME NEUROTRANSMITTER RECEPTORS

DRUG	NEUROTRANSMITTER RECEPTOR BLOCKADE**			
	H_1	Muscarinic	$5\text{-}HT_2$	D_2
Antidepressants				
amitriptyline	91	*5.5*	3.4	0.10
amoxapine	4.0	0.1	*170*	*0.62*
bupropion	*0.015*	0.0021	*0.0011*	*0.00048*
desipramine	0.91	0.50	0.36	0.030
doxepin	*420*	1.2	4.0	0.042
fluoxetine	0.016	0.050	0.48	0.015
imipramine	9.1	1.1	1.2	0.050
maprotiline	50	0.18	0.83	0.28
nortriptyline	10	0.67	2.3	0.083
protriptyline	4.0	4.0	1.5	0.043
trazodone	0.28	*0.00031*	13	0.026
trimipramine	370	1.7	3.1	0.56
Reference Compounds				
diphenhydramine	7.1			
atropine		42		
methysergide			15	
haloperidol				26

*Data can be compared both vertically and horizontally to find the most potent drug for a specific property and to find the most potent property of a specific drug. **$10^{-7} \times 1/K_D$, where K_D = equilibrium dissociation in molarity. Data from references (1) and (2). In each column, the highest and lowest numbers are emphasized for the antidepressants.

REFERENCES

1. Richelson, E. and Nelson, A. (1984): J. Pharmacol. Exp. Ther., 230:94-102.
2. Wander, et al: Eur. J. Pharmacol. 132:115-121, 1986.

FROM RAT 5-HT NEURONS TO THE STRATEGY OF LITHIUM AUGMENTATION IN REFRACTORY DEPRESSION

C. de MONTIGNY
Neurobiological Psychiatry Unit, Department of Psychiatry, McGill University, Montréal, Québec, CANADA H3A 1A1

It is generally estimated that approximately a third of patients suffering from a major depression do not respond satisfactorily to tricyclic antidepressant (TCA) drugs, as well as to newer antidepressant drugs (8).

As we had observed that long-term administration to TCA drugs induced a sensitization of postsynaptic neurons to serotonin (5-HT) in the rat forebrain (2), we proposed that this property of TCA drugs could be related to their antidepressant activity. This was based on the pharmacological specificity of this effect, on the congruence of its time course with that of the therapeutic activity of these drugs, as well as on the previously reported reversal of the therapeutic effect of TCA drugs by the 5-HT synthesis inhibitor para-chlorophenylalanine (10).

Our first lithium augmentation trial in TCA refractory depression was devised to put to the test the hypotheses: 1) that a similar sensitization to 5-HT was also induced in man by TCA drugs; and 2) that it was related to their therapeutic effect. The rationale for choosing lithium as an adjunct to the TCA drug was the available evidence that lithium, at low plasma levels, could rapidly increase the efficacy of 5-HT neurons themselves (6). Hence, our reasoning was that lithium addition, by augmenting the function of 5-HT neurons, should unveil the sensitization of postsynaptic neurons to 5-HT and, if our hypothesis was corrected, alleviate depression.

Since our initial report of the efficacy of this strategy (3), numerous reports have confirmed its efficacy not only in depression resistant to a TCA drug, but also to an amazingly wide variety of antidepressant treatments such as MAOI's, 5-HT reuptake blockers, trazodone, mianserine, maprotiline and carbamazepine (see ref. 6 for a recent review). Lithium has even been shown to potentiate sleep deprivation (1). The lithium augmentation strategy has been shown to be as efficacious in adolescents (9) and in the elderly (5) than in adults. A recent prospective controlled study has shown lithium addition to be as efficacious, and even more rapidly acting, than ECT in TCA-refractory depression (4).

Hence, this exemplifies quite dramatically how much fundamental research in animals can contribute directly to the advancement of therapeutics in Psychiatry.

REFERENCES

1. Baxter, J.R. et al.: Prolongation of the antidepressant response to partial sleep deprivation by lithium. Psychiat. Res. 19:17-23, 1986.

2. de Montigny, C. and Aghajanian, G.K.: Tricyclic antidepressants: long-term treatment increases responsivity of rat forebrain neurons to serotonin. Science 202:1303-1306, 1978.
3. de Montigny, C. et al.: Lithium induces rapid relief of depression in tricyclic antidepressant drug non-responders. Br. J. Psychiatry 138:252-256, 1981.
4. Dinan, T.G. and Barry, S.: A comparison of electroconvulsive therapy with a combined lithium and tricyclic combination among depressed tricyclic nonresponders. Acta Psychiat. Scand. 8:97-100, 1989.
5. Finch, E.J.L. and Katina, C.L.E.: Lithium augmentation in the treatment of refractory depression in old age. Int. J. Ger. Psychiatry 4:41-46, 1989.
6. Grahame-Smith, D.G. and Green, A.R.: The role of brain 5-hydroxytryptamine in the hyperactivity produced in rats by lithium and monoamine oxidase inhibition. Br. J. Pharmacol. 52:19-26, 1974.
7. Kramlinger, K.G. and Post, R.M.: The addition of lithium to carbamazepine. Antidepressant efficacy in treatment-resistant depression. Arch. Gen. Psychiat. 46:794-800, 1989.
8. Thase, M.E. and Kupfer, D.J.: Characteristics of treatment-resistant depression. In: Treating Resistant Depression. J. Zohar and R.H. Belmaker, eds., pp.23-45. PMA, New York, 1987.
9. Ryan, N.D. et al.: Lithium antidepressant augmentation in TCA-refractory depression in adolescents. J. Am. Acad. Child Adolesc. Psychiatry 27:371-376, 1988.
10. Shopsin, B. et al.: Use of synthesis inhibitors in defining a role for biogenic amines during imipramine treatment in depressed patients. Psychopharmacol. Commun. 1:239-249, 1975.

THE SELECTIVE SEROTONIN REUPTAKE INHIBITORS

J.P. FEIGHNER and W.F. BOYER
Feighner Research Institute, La Mesa, CA, USA

In this paper we will very briefly summarize the current state of five of the most important selective serotonin reuptake inhibitors (SSRIs), fluoxetine, sertraline, citalopram, fluvoxamine and paroxetine.

Most authorities agree that the SSRIs are at least as effective as earlier antidepressants in alleviating depression. They are often useful in patients with severe, long-lasting or treatment-refractory depressions. They are ideal for maintenance because they remain effective and are generally well tolerated.

The SSRIs offer no advantage in latency to onset. Although some studies showed significant differences from placebo as early as one or two weeks in others the SSRI was not superior to placebo or equivalent to the TCA until six weeks or more.

The SSRIs have been used in a number of studies of elderly patients. The results have been positive, both in terms of antidepressant effect and patient acceptance. Fluoxetine is also being prescribed for some younger patients with clinical depression or obsessive-compulsive disorder (OCD), although there is much less data available about its use in this age group.

Early clinical studies of fluoxetine used doses of 60 to 80 mg per day. More recent studies indicate that 20 mg a day is usually effective and causes fewer side effects. Increasing the dose above 20 mg a day is rarely helpful. Similarly, paroxetine doses above 40 mg a day or more than 50 mg a day of sertraline are not associated with significantly superior results. Use of higher doses may still have value with some patients.

Unfortunately plasma levels can not serve as a guide to proper dosing. There is also no relationship between inhibition of platelet serotonin uptake and response, although the number of studies in this area is smaller.

Biological measures, including the DST and CSF monoamine metabolites have generally been unsuccessful in predicting differential response to the SSRIs. However two recent studies have shown that blunted prolactin or melatonin response to fenfluramine may predict good response to fluvoxamine.

Some data suggests that the SSRIs may have special value in the treatment of depression with anxiety or atypical features. Montgomery recently presented a meta-analysis of several fluoxetine studies which suggests that this SSRI is significantly superior to TCAs in patients with anxiety and psychomotor agitation. Reimherr found that patients with atypical features may be especially responsive to fluoxetine. The concept of atypical depression may be central, since it is linked with anxiety and other psychiatric disorders which improve with SSRIs.

Panic disorder is one such illness. Several open and double-blind studies show it is responsive to SSRI treatment, although there may be an initial period of increased anxiety. There are also reports of the SSRIs efficacy in OCD. Research suggests that the SSRIs may be more effective than noradrenergic compounds in panic and OCD.

A large amount of data indicates that suicidal ideation and attempts are linked to serotonin dysfunction. Several studies have found that fluoxetine, fluvoxamine, and citalopram are more effective than a comparison TCA in reducing suicidal ideation. This is especially important because the SSRIs are generally much safer than TCAs in overdose.

The SSRIs may also be helpful in addictive behaviors. Several studies have shown the SSRIs reduce alcohol consumption in animals and man. Because the SSRIs generally do not potentiate the effects of alcohol they may be indicated in depressed patients with alcohol abuse. Animal data suggests that fluoxetine may also be helpful in the treatment of stimulant abuse. Research is also being conducted into the efficacy of the SSRIs in smoking cessation.

The SSRIs are often associated with loss of appetite or anorexia in proprotion to their potency in blocking serotonin reuptake. Several of the SSRIs have been studied for weight reduction in depressed and nondepressed obese subjects. They were found superior to placebo and were generally well tolerated. Weight loss does not depend on nausea, one of the more common side effects. Instead it appears related to whether the patient has carbohydrate craving, which itself may be a sign of serotonergic dysfunction.

Other areas in which the SSRIs may prove useful include bulimia, chronic pain, cataplexy, dementia, impulsivity, aggressiveness, and some personality disorders.

As the SSRIs come into wider use it is likely that some side effects may become important issues. Fluoxetine has been reported to produce or aggravate extrapyramidal reactions in a few individuals. A few patients experienced marked increase in suicidal ideation. Adverse effects on sexual function are being reported as well.

More data is emerging about the use of SSRIs in combination with other medications. Coadministration with warfarin may increase bleeding tendency. Cimetidine may impair first-pass metabolism, leading to build-up of higher SSRI plasma levels.

It is not uncommon in our practice to combine fluoxetine with TCAs. There may be a theoretical basis for this combination since animal studies indicate that coadministration of desipramine and fluoxetine results in more rapid down-regulation of beta-adrenergic receptors than either drug alone.

Several reports have appeared of increased tricyclic plasma levels when a TCA is given with fluoxetine. In some cases this has lead to increased tricyclic side effects and worsening of depression. There have also been reports of significant negative interactions between fluoxetine and lithium. However lithium augmentation has helped some patients who did not respond to fluoxetine or fluvoxamine alone. Other succesful combinations have been reported with clomipramine, trazodone, neuroleptics, buspirone, and amphetamine.

A potentially serious interaction occurs with monoamine oxidase inhibitors. We have seen a number of patients develop a "serotonergic syndrome" with this combination. This is characterized by myoclonus, diarrhea, tremor, and mental status changes which include hypomania, racing thoughts and confusion. Death has occured with combination of fluoxetine and tranylcypromine. Although the only human data so far involves fluoxetine, a similar syndrome has been reported in rats treated with paroxetine plus phenelzine or nialimide.

There are likely to be significant clinical differences between the SSRIs. One should remember that the chemical structure of the TCAs differ very little from each other, yet there are significant clinical differences. The chemical structures of the SSRIs are very different, which suggests even greater clinical differences. Experience with these compounds already points to some meaningful distinctions. The very long half-lives of fluoxetine and norfluoxetine make it possible to treat patients every few days. However side effects may be more prolonged. Somnolence may be more common with fluvoxamine and paroxetine. We have also observed more nausea with fluvoxamine and a lower incidence of weight loss with paroxetine.

REFERENCE

Feighner, J.P. and Boyer, W.F. (1990): Clinical use of the selective serotonin reuptake inhibitors. (in press).

PSYCHOENDOCRINOLOGY AND PHARMACOTHERAPY OF PTSD

E.L., GILLER, JR. * R.T. KOSTEN **, R.YEHUDA *, B.D. PERRY ***,
S. SOUTHWICK **, J.W. MASON **

* University of Connecticut Health Center, Farmington, CT; ** Yale West Haven VAMC, West Haven, CT; *** Harris Center, University of Chicago, Chicago, IL, USA

Posttraumatic stress disorder (PTSD) has been a known syndrome, characterized by fairly specific cognitive, anxiety and autonomic nervous system (ANS) symptoms for many years (1). Consequently, alterations in catecholamine metabolism would be expected, reflecting a state of increased arousal and sympathetic nervous system functioning, and changes in cortisol metabolism are often found in acute and chronic stress responses. Previous psychoendocrine research has suggested that twenty-four hour urine excretions of catecholamines and cortisol are a more stable, integrated measurement of metabolism than plasma samples, which can vary markedly from moment to moment. In addition, the efficacy of medications capable of modulating anxiety and ANS symptoms were studied.

Inpatients with PTSD showed higher twenty-four hour urinary excretion of norepinephrine (76.0 $\pm$ 10.4 ug/day, mean $\pm$ SE) and epinephrine (22 $\pm$ 2.3 ug/day) than comparison groups of other psychiatric patients (2). Further support for a hyperadrenergic state in PTSD is that subjects with PTSD showed a significant reduction in total platelet alpha$_2$ receptor binding sites, and an increase in the ratio of low affinity to high affinity sites, compared to controls (2). This findings that the platelet alpha$_2$ receptor sites show both downregulation (decreased Bmax) and desensitization (increased ratio of low affinity to high affinity sites). Also, alpha$_2$ receptor sites on platelets from PTSD subjects, when incubated with epinephrine in the test tube, showed a significantly more rapid and more extensive downregulation than sites on platelets from controls (2).

Cortisol output can be increased during acute stress, but chronic stress may be associated with low, rather than high, cortisol levels (2), though acute superimposed stress can increase cortisol levels. In two studies PTSD subjects showed relatively low twenty-four hour urinary excretion of free cortisol compared to other patient groups and controls (2).

Antidepressants and benzodiazepines have shown efficacy in in the treatment of PTSD. In a randomized clinical trial sixty outpatient male combat veterans with chronic PTSD participated in an eight week comparison of phenelzine (n=19), imipramine (n=23), and placebo (n=18). The three treatment groups were similar in sociodemographic variables, rates of comorbidity, comorbid psychopathology and baseline symptoms. No subject met criteria for major depressive disorder although twenty-eight (47%) had RDC minor depression. Mean (± SD) dose of imipramine was 225 ± 55 mg with a mean blood level of imipramine plus desipramine of 184 ± 80 nanograms/ml., mean dose of phenelzine 68 ± 20 mg with mean platelet MAO activity inhibition 94% ± 7%. IES scores dropped 45% from baseline in the phenelzine group compared to 25% in the imipramine and 5% in the placebo group. This was primarily in intrusive symptoms, though avoidant symptoms also showed improvement. While anxiety and depression ratings did not show a statistically significant decrease, the reduction in symptoms was greater in the groups receiving medication that placebo.

Clinical experience in a medication clinic (N=29) supports the efficacy of antidepressants. In addition, 52% of patients benefited from a benzodiazepine (primarily alprazolam), either alone or with an antidepressant. In a pilot inpatient study, alprazolam appeared to reduce PTSD symptoms more quickly and to a greater extent than other medications during the initial stages of hospitalization.

The brain noradrenegrgic system (NS) is a major component of the fight or flight alarm reaction. If similar long-term receptor changes also occur in the NS, it may render this system more sensitive to and less able to damp excitatory and possibly inhibitory inputs. Specifically, if $alpha_2$ receptors on the NS are significantly downregulated, firing of these cells would be disinhibited. Since both antidepressants and benzodiazepines inhibit NS firing, the efficacy of these compounds in PTSD is consistent with the hypothesis that dysregulation of the NS contributes to the pathophysiology of PTSD.

1. Da Costa, J.M. (1871): Am. J. Medical Sci. 71, 17-52.
2. Giller, E. (1990): Biological Assessment and Treatment of PTSD, APA Press, Washington, DC

RESPONSE TO TRICYCLIC THERAPY IN PTSD

J. Davidson [1], H. Kudler [1,2], R. Stein [1,2], L. Ericksen [2], R. Smith [1], Department of Psychiatry, Duke University and Durham VA Medical Center, Durham, NC, USA.

Over sixty veterans of combat, carrying a diagnosis of chronic PTSD, were enrolled in a treatment protocol which compared amitriptyline and placebo in double blind fashion. These individuals were veterans of World War II, Korea and Vietnam. Inpatients and outpatients were included in the sample, most of whom exhibited other psychiatric comorbidity.

Assignment to treatment was randomized, taking into account military conflict, inpatient/outpatient status and presence or absence of comorbidity.

Duration of treatment ranged up to 12 weeks, with eight weeks constituting the endpoint in this set of analyses.

Assessments included the SADS-LA, a structured interview for PTSD (SI-PTSD), the Hamilton scales, measures of personality, global severity and improvement scales, and PTSD self-ratings. Measures of combat experience (i.e. trauma "dose") were also obtained.

Out of the above variables, we will be conducting multivariate analyses to examine possible predictors of outcome, including those which are specific predictors of drug effect.

REFERENCES

1. Davidson JRT, Kudler HS, Smith RD, et al. Treatment of post-traumatic stress disorder with amitriptyline and placebo. Arch Gen Psychiatry. 47: 259-266, 1990.
2. Davidson JRT, Smith RD, Kudler HS. Validity and reliability of the DSM-III criteria for posttraumatic stress disorder: experience with a structured interview. J. Nerv. Ment. Dis. 177: 336-341, 1989.

POSTRAUMATIC STRESS DISORDER AND MAJOR DEPRESSION: AN INTEGRATED PERSPECTIVE

B. LERER*, A.DOLEV**, A.BLEICH**, R.P.EBSTEIN*
*Yaacov Herzog Research Center and Dept. Psychiatry, Hebrew University, Jerusalem **Dept. of Mental Health, IDF Medical Corps Israel

The long-term psychological sequellae of traumatic stress are classified under the DSM III-R category of chronic Posttraumatic Stress Disorder (PTSD). Items contributing to this diagnosis overlap substantially with those of other entities in the anxiety disorder and depression categories. In the U.S.A particularly, alcoholism and substance abuse are frequently observed concommitants of the syndrome.

We have obtained evidence that in Israeli combat veterans with long-standing, chronic PTSD, clinical, biochemical and psychopharmacological overlap with major depression is so substantial as to raise the possibility that these two entities may be closely interlinked from the standpoint of pathophysiology and even predisposition.

(1) Structured clinical interviews (SADS-L) with a series of 50 sequential referrals fulfilling DSM III-R criteria for chronic PTSD, revealed a concomitant RDC diagnosis of Major Depressive Disorder (MDD) in 46 cases. In 50% of interviewees, Panic Disorder or Obsessive Compulsive Disorder were additional co-diagnoses. In all cases the PTSD diagnosis preceded the appearance of MDD. However, in 50% of subjects MDD criteria were fulfilled while significant PTSD symptomatology was no longer present.

(2) In two separate medication-free samples with chronic PTSD, drawn from the same population, we have observed abnormally low cyclic AMP signal transduction in lymphocytes and platelets (3,4). Similar findings have been obtained in patients with major depressive disorder (3) and alcoholism. Detailed studies in the PTSD subjects suggest that a defect at the level of the catalytic subunit or G-protein-catalytic subunit coupling may underly this abnormal responsiveness (4).

(3) Treatment with antidepressant medication (particularly tricyclic antidepressants) frequently yields a positive response of depressive symptomatology

while symptoms specific to PTSD are variably altered if at all. Similarly, a focussed effect on anxiety symptoms was observed in a double blind comparison between alprazolam and placebo while core PTSD symptoms were unaffected (1)

It should be stressed that these findings relate to subjects with long-standing symptomatology (5-8 years since the traumatic exposure) and may not be referable to patients with acute or subacute PTSD. They suggest that the chronic form of this syndrome may be closely linked to major depression beyond the level of a simple overlap in terms of items contributing to the diagnosis. They warrant consideration of the possibility that predisposition to the development of chronic posttraumatic morbidity may be linked to a predisposition to major depression, the traumatic event serving as a psychological trigger. However, the presence of core PTSD symptoms specific to the syndrome and not observed in non-traumatic major depression requires separate explanation. The differential incidence of alcoholism and substance abuse in Israeli and U.S. populations with PTSD should also be addressed. That clinical major depression and the biochemical correlates observed may be a secondary consequence of chronic PTSD and not the product of a shared predisposition, must be considered as an alternative hypothesis. In either case, the striking degree of comorbidity demands appropriate consideration in the planning of therapeutic intervention with a specific focus on antidepressant medication.

REFERENCES

(1) Braun, P., Greenberg, D., Dasberg, H. and Lerer, B.: Core PTSD symptoms unimproved by alprazolam treatment. J Clin Psychiatry (In Press).
(2) Ebstein, R.P., Lerer, B., Shapira, B., Kindler, S. and Shemesh, Z.: Cyclic AMP second messenger signal amplification in depression. Br J Psychiatry 152:665-669,1988.
(3) Lerer, B., Ebstein, R.P., Shestatzky, M., Shemesh, Z. and Greenberg, D.: Cyclic AMP signal transduction in posttraumatic stress disorder. Am J Psychiatry 144:1324-27, 1987.
(4) Lerer, B., Bleich, A., Bennett, E.R., Ebstein, R.P.: Platelet adenylate cyclase and phospholipase C activity in posttraumatic stress disorder. Biol Psychiatry (In Press)

PSYCHO-NEURO-PHYSIOLOGIC CHARACTERISTICS OF COMBAT VETERANS WITH POSTTRAUMATIC STRESS DISORDER

A. BLEICH[*], Y. ATTIAS[**], Y. DAGAN[***], P. LAVIE[***], A. SHALEV[*], B. LERER[*]
Department of Mental Health[*] and Institute for the Research of Noise Hazards and Brain Potentials[**], IDF Medical Corps, Sleep Laboratory, Hatechnion - Medical School[***], Haifa, Israel.

The demonstration of psychoneurophysiologic findings which accompany a mental disorder, complements assesment of the psychological and behavioral aspects, provides data that may be more objective and accurate than self-reported complaints, and contributes to understanding the underlying pathophysiology of the disorder.

The few studies of this type which have been done in relation to Posttraumatic Stress Disorder (PTSD) have shown that combat veterans with PTSD are characterized by physiologic hyperreactivity (expressed by **peripheral** measurements such as tachycardia, increased blood pressure, increased muscle tension and decreased skin conductance) to combat related stimuli. The stimuli used were noises or sights of combat, and in one case a taped script of a traumatic combat experience (1).

CEREBRAL MEASUREMENTS

We report here on **cerebral** measurements in the psychoneurophysiologic assesment of nonalcoholic, medication-free combat veterans with PTSD as opposed to matched normal control:
I) In the evoked potentials laboratory we found physiologic hyperreactivity to pictures of combat, as expressed by recording P-300 potentials. This was absent in the controls, while response to neutral, targeted visual stimuli was equivalent in the two groups.
II) Audiological evaluation, using neutral stimuli, did not reveal a decreased audiological threshold, as tolerance of intense auditory stimuli by patients was similar to that of controls. Significant differences in central audiological functions were found between PTSD and controls and, within a subgroup of PTSD subjects, between the right ear and the left ear. These differences suggest a cerebral asymetry, favoring the dominant hemisphere, in processing verbal stimuli (2).
III) In the sleep laboratory: a) an increased intensity of neutral audiological stimuli (and an increased reaction time) were needed in order to awake combat veterans with PTSD as compared to normal controls. Thus audiological

threshold which was not found to be decreased during wakefulness - in these subjects, was shown to be increased during sleep. b) No correlation has been found between the subjects' report of nightmares and their REM elicited dream recall. Combat veterans with PTSD, while complaining of frequent nightmares, had great difficulties in recalling dreams (including nightmares) even when they were awakened during REM sleep, compared to normal controls.

COMMENT

Based on the aforementioned findings the following assumptions may be considered:
I) PTSD can be characterized by specific psychoneurophysiologic findings.
II) The physiologic hyperreactivity to various stimuli, found in PTSD combat veterans, is probably related to the meaning of the stimuli and not to their physical components.
III) As an adaptive response to the continuous sensation of threat, originating from internal and external stimuli as well, PTSD patients use suppressing mechanisms, which may cause impaired perceptual discrimination. This may explain frequently reported subjective complaints, e.g. hypersensitivity to noises, difficulties in sleep, frequent nightmares, and various somatic complaints (3), which can not be supported by direct "objective" findings.

REFERENCES

1. Pitman, R.K., Orr, S.P., Forgue, D.F., et al.: Psychophysiological assesment of posttraumatic stress disorder imagery in Vietnam combat veterans. Arch. Gen. Psychiatry. 44:970-975, 1987.
2. Shalev, A., Attias, Y., Bleich, A., et al.: Audiological evaluation of nonalcoholic, drug-free posttraumatic stress disorder patients. Biol. Psychiatry. 24:522-530, 1988.
3. Shalev, A., Bleich, A., and Ursano, R. Posttraumatic stress disorder: Somatic comorbidity and effort tolerance. Psychosomatics. In press.

BEHAVIOR THERAPY AND PSYCHOPHYSIOLOGICAL ASSESSMENT OF PTSD: CONTROLLED TRIALS

TERENCE M. KEANE, PH.D.*
*National Center for PTSD - Boston
Boston VA Medical Center and Tufts University School of Medicine

Recent epidemiological work has indicated that 15% of all Americans who served in Vietnam have sufficient symptoms today to warrant the diagnosis of PTSD (1). Given that nearly 3.2 million American men and women fought in that war, the problems of Vietnam veterans represent a major challenge to public health in the United States. The problem is further magnified if one considers that nearly twice as many veterans have met diagnostic criteria at one time since their return from Vietnam and that twice the number of current cases of PTSD have symptoms of anxiety and depression that constitute the label "partial PTSD" (1). Large numbers of veterans are today seeking psychological assistance from the many programs developed by the U.S. Department of Veterans Affairs to help these veterans readjust to nonmilitary life. Unfortunately, there are few empirical data available to guide clinicians in the assessment and treatment of PTSD. The purpose of the present paper is to describe a program of research directed at understanding and treating the problems of veterans with PTSD.

PSYCHOPHYSIOLOGICAL ASSESSMENT

Perhaps most noticeable among the many symptoms of PTSD in combat veterans is a persistent level of autonomic arousal that is manifested in behavioral, psychological, and psychophysiological measurement channels. Several research laboratories have begun to quantify this autonomic arousal and have reached the following conclusions (2,3,4).

1. This psychophysiological arousal is apparent across measurement systems including heat rate, skin conductance, blood pressure, and Frontalis EMG.

2. This psychophysiological arousal is most evident when cues associated with the original traumatic conditioning experience are presented to the patients.

3. Cue presentation can be either audiovisual, auditory alone, or in imagery. Each evokes significant psychophysiological reactivity.

4. Recent research indicates that veterans without PTSD cannot fake the physiological arousal even when instructed to do so.

5. In addition to consistent physiological reactivity to trauma cues, there may also be baseline differences in arousal among PTSD patients. Several studies addressing this topic will be reviewed.

6. Psychophysiological reactivity has been able to correctly classify seventy percent of subjects in some studies to nearly ninety percent in others.

CONCLUSIONS

Clearly the study of the psychophysiology of PTSD has raised many questions for researchers and clinicians alike. Research now underway (5) in a VA Cooperative Study at fifteen sites across the USA will determine the extent to which this psychophysiological arousal is a marker for the disorder. Moreover, studies in different laboratories are investigating the basic mechanisms underlying this psychophysiological arousal and reactivity from both a pathophysiological standpoint and a psychological standpoint. In addition, treatment strategies, both behavioral and psychopharmacological, are directly addressing the issue of psychophysiological arousal and reactivity. Future research directions will be presented.

REFERENCES

1. Blanchard, E.B. et al. (1982): Psychiat. Quart. 54:220-229.
2. Kulka, R.A. et al. (1988): National Vietnam Veterans Readjustment Study, Research Triangle Institute, Research Triangle Park, North Carolina.
3. Keane, T.M., Malloy, P.F. and Fairbank, J.A. (1984): JCCP, 52:888-891.
4. Pitman, R.K et al. (1987): Arch Gen Psychiat. 44:970-975.

DREAMS' REPRESSION IN ADJUSTED HOLOCAUST SURVIVORS.

Peretz Lavie and Hanna Kaminer
Sleep Laboratory, Faculty of Medicine
Technion - Israel Institute of Technology, Haifa, Israel.

The long-term effects of massive traumatic events can affect survivors for the rest of their lives. Some survivors present a clinical picture consistent with post-traumatic stress disorder (PTSD) many years after the trauma. Much effort has been invested in trying to understand what differentiates survivors who have succeeded in freeing themselves from the terrors of the past, from those who have never been able to do so. Since sleep disturbances and disturbed dreaming are among the hallmarks of the long-term effects of traumatic events, we compared sleep structure and dreaming in holocaust survivors as a function of the success by which they had readjusted to post-war life.

Method and design

Thirty-three subjects (23 holocaust survivors plus 10 controls) participated in the study. Eleven were survivors of Nazi concentration camps, while 12 had spent most of the time in hideouts, or constantly on the move. All survivors were free from major physical or mental illnesses, and were able to abstain from taking drugs. Division of survivors into those who have successfully adjusted to post-war life, and those who were less successfully adjusted, was based on clinical interviews regarding the following 6 areas of life: Problems at work, marital and familial problems, social relations, somatic complaints, mental problems, and general satisfaction in life. Those complaining of at least 3 of the 6 above were included in the less-adjusted group. This group included 11 survivors (5 male, 6 female) with a mean age of 57.5 ± 5.7 yrs. They had a mean number of 3.8 ± 0.98 complaints. The well-adjusted group included 12 survivors (5m and 7f) with a mean age of 62.7 ± 4.4. They had a mean of 0.9 ± 1 complaints. This division based on the clinical interview was further validated with the 'Structured and Scaled Interview to Assess Maladjustment' - SSIAM by Gurland, which revealed a highly significant difference between the groups. The control group included 10 (5m and 5f) Israeli-born age matched normals (mean age 61.1 ± 5.4 yrs). The sleep study included 4 whole-night conventional sleep recordings. Two nights were scheduled consecutively, and two separately. During the first, third and fourth nights, subjects were awakened from all REM periods, starting from the second REM period for dream recall.

Awakenings were done approximately 15-20 min after the beginning of each of the REM periods. After each awakening subjects were asked to report everything that went on in their mind just before the awakening. Reports were taped, and later typed and coded for content analysis. During the second night, there were no awakenings.

Results

Sleep data showed significant differences between groups in the direction of more disturbed sleep in the less-adjusted group vs. the controls and well-adjusted group. Less-adjusted had less sleep time ($p < .001$), had longer sleep latency ($p < .0001$), and had more stage wake during sleep ($p < .001$). Consequently, they had lower sleep efficiency index ($p < .01$). There were no significant differences between the groups with respect to REM percent, REM latency, and percentages of sleep stages 3/4 and 2.

Dream Recall, calculated as the percent of positive dream recalls per total number of REM awakenings for each subject, was significantly different among the three groups. The well-adjusted had the lowest rate of dream recall - 34%; the less-adjusted and controls had 51% and 78%, respectively. (chi squar = 38.1, df = 2; $p < .00001$). Upon awakening most of the well-adjusted survivors often not only did not recall any dream content; they did not recall having dreamed at all. Furthermore, even the few dreams recalled by the well-adjusted survivors were qualitatively different from those of the other two groups. They were characterized by being shorter, devoid of emotional content and dealing with trivial everyday matters. There were no between-group differences in the physiologic characteristics of the REM periods.

Discussion

The present results reveal a dramatic lack of dream recall in a group of survivors who showed outstanding adjustment to post-War life. A survey of literature showed no comparable findings of such low REM-elicited dream recall in a group otherwise having normal sleep parameters. Based on the complete clinical evaluation, we suggest that the lack of dreaming in the well-adjusted group complemented their waking coping style. To avoid the risk of intrusion of distressing memories and thoughts on past events, the well-adjusted survivors had developed massive dream suppression which led to almost complete amnesia regarding dreaming in general.

ETIOLOGY, DIAGNOSIS, AND COURSE OF PANIC DISORDER

R.M.A. Hirschfeld
Mood, Anxiety, and Personality Disorders Research Branch
National Institute of Mental Health, Rockville, MD, U.S.A.

Although there were lucid descriptions of the syndrome of panic disorder dating back to the Nineteenth Century, panic disorder as a distinct clinical syndrome has not been included in the official nomenclatures until very recently. Panic disorder first appeared in the Diagnostic and Statistical Manual of the American Psychiatric Association in its third revision published in 1980 (1). It has never been included in the International Classification of Diseases (10), but is proposed for inclusion in the tenth revision.

Panic disorder frequently presents with a dramatic episode involving sudden, intense, unprovoked attacks of anxiety, shortness of breath, palpitations, trembling, sweating, chest pain, and often fear of dying. A continuation of the syndrome can lead to profound influences on the quality of life, limiting such normal activities as driving, shopping, going to restaurants, or using elevators.

Panic disorder is a frequent psychiatric illness, the one-month prevalence being approximately 1 in 200 and lifetime prevalence being slightly less than 2 percent. It occurs twice as frequently in women as in men. Its onset is usually in adolescence and early adulthood, and occurs throughout adulthood, although it is most common between ages 25 and 44. Its frequency decreases substantially following age 65.

The consequences of this disorder are pervasive and far-reaching. In a community based study conducted by Markowitz et al. (5), consequences included subjective feelings of poor physical and emotional health, alcohol and other drug abuse, financial dependency, and marked impairments in interpersonal functioning. Furthermore, subjects showed increased use of psychoactive medications, and increased use of general medical, psychiatric, and emergency room services.

The relationship between panic disorder and depression has been increasingly documented in the recent literature (3,4,6,7), with the comorbidity indicating a greater risk for increased severity and diminished response to treatment. Data indicate that the association between panic disorder and depression is even greater than the association between other forms of anxiety disorder and depression (2,8). Panic disorder is often associated with mitral valve prolapse, and because many medical conditions, such as myocardial infarction, pheochromocytoma, and drug reactions can cause a similar syndrome, a comprehensive medical examination is essential.

In contrast to depressive disorders, relatively little research has been done on the long-term course of panic disorder. Weissman et al. (9), however, in a random sample of adults from the N.I.M.H. Epidemiologic Catchment Area study, found that 20 percent of the subjects with panic disorder had made suicide attempts. Subjects with panic disorder had more suicide attempts and more suicidal ideation than those with other psychiatric disorders, including major depression.

REFERENCES

1. American Psychiatric Association (1980): <u>Diagnostic and Statistical Manual of Mental Disorders, 3rd Revision</u>. American Psychiatric Association, Washington, D.C.
2. Boyd, J.H., Burke, J.D. Jr., Gruenberg, E. et al., (1984): Exclusion criteria of DSM-III. A study of co-occurrence of hierarchy-free syndromes. <u>Arch. Gen. Psychiatry</u>, 41: 983-989.
3. Coryell, W., Endicott, J., Andreasen, N.C. et al., (1988): Depression and panic attacks: the significance of overlap as reflected in follow-up and family study data. <u>Am. J. Psychiatry</u>, 145: 293-300.
4. Grunhaus, L., Harel, Y., Krugler, T. et al., (1988): Major depressive disorder and panic disorder. Effects of comorbidity on treatment outcome with antidepressant medications. <u>Clin. Neuropharmacol.</u>, 11: 454-461.
5. Markowitz, J.S., Weissman, M.M., Ouellette, R., et al., (1989): Quality of life in panic disorder. <u>Arch. Gen. Psychiatry</u>, 46: 984-992.
6. Maser, J.D., and Cloninger, C.R. (1990): <u>Comorbidity of Mood and Anxiety Disorders</u>, American Psychiatric Press, Inc., Washington, D.C.
7. Thompson, A.H., Bland, R.C., Orn, H.T., et al., (1989) Relationship and chronology of depression, agoraphobia, and panic disorder in the general population. <u>J. Nerv. Ment. Dis.</u>, 177: 456-463.
8. Vollrath, M., Koch, R., Angst, J. (1990): The Zurich Study. IX. Panic disorder and sporadic panic: symptoms, diagnosis, prevalence, and overlap with depression. <u>Eur. Arch. Psychiat. Neurol. Sci.</u>, 239: 221-230.
9. Weissman, M.M., Klerman, G.L., Markowitz, J.S. et al. (1989): Suicidal ideation and suicide attempts in panic disorder and attacks. <u>N. Eng. J. Med.</u>, 321: 1209-1214.
10. World Health Organization (1977): <u>International Classification of Diseases, 9th Revision</u>. World Health Organization, Geneva.

FAMILY GENETIC STUDIES IN PANIC DISORDER

Myrna M. Weissman, Ph.D.
Columbia University Department of Psychiatry, Division of Clinical-Genetic Epidemiology; New York State Psychiatric Institute, 722 West 168 Street, Box 14, NY, NY 10032, USA

While there is good evidence that panic disorder is a familial disease, data on the extent to which the transmission among family members is genetic has not been resolved. There are at least 4 types of evidence that genes contribute to a disorder of unknown etiology: 1) increased rate of the disorder among biological relatives (Family Studies); 2) a higher concordance among monozygotic (MZ) than among dizygotic (DZ) twins (Twin Studies); 3) a higher rate of the disorder among biological as compared to adoptive relatives of an ill person (Adoptive Studies); 4) genetic linkage of the disorder with an allele at a marker locus on a chromosome (Linkage Studies). Limited data for panic disorder is emerging from all but the Adoptive Studies.

FAMILY STUDIES: While there are a number of family studies of anxiety disorders, most have not separated out panic from other anxiety disorders, and some use family history, not direct interview methods (7,8). There have been 3 family studies that include probands with panic disorder, and use direct interviews and specified diagnostic criteria (2,3,6). These studies confirm the highly familial nature of panic disorder. The rates of illness obtained were higher than those reported in the earlier family history studies (1,9), but the patterns were similar. The relatives of probands with panic disorder have markedly elevated rates of panic disorder in their first-degree relatives. There have been attempts to explain the familial patterns of panic disorder using genetic models. However, no specific patterns of genetic transmission have been conclusively or consistently established (10).

TWIN STUDIES: There has been only one twin study of anxiety disorders using DSM-III criteria (11). In a study of 29 adult twins of the same sex, monozygotic twins had a significantly higher rate of panic disorder or agoraphobia with panic attacks than did dizygotic twins. The monozygotic concordance rate was 31%, compared to no concordance in dizygotic twins.

LINKAGE STUDIES: Recent advances in molecular genetics

have led to a growing number of genetic markers which can be used to examine linkage of a disorder to a marker on a chromosome. The ultimate goal is the eventual identification and study of the gene itself. In November 1897, Crowe and the Iowa groups reported preliminary findings from a linkage study of panic disorders using red cell antigens and protein polymorphisms as genetic markers (4,5). Twenty-nine markers in 26 families with panic disorder provided suggestive linkage at one locus mapped to chromosome 16 or 22. The maximum lod score for haptoglobin was 2.27 at a recombinant fraction of 0.0. Linkage was excluded at 18 loci. Currently, at least three groups -- Crowe, Fryer, Weissman -- have ongoing linkage studies in panic disorder using modern DNA techniques.

In addition to reviewing available family and twin studies, this paper will present preliminary findings from a large ongoing family study of panic disorder.

REFERENCES

1. Carey, G. and Gottesman, I.I. (1981). Twin and family studies of anxiety, panic and obsessive disorders: In Anxiety: New Research and Changing Concepts, D.F. Klein and J.G. Rabkin, eds. Raven Press, New York.
2. Cloninger, C.R. et al., (1981). A blind follow-up and family study of anxiety neurosis: Preliminary analysis of the St. Louis 500: In Anxiety: New Research and Changing Concepts, D.F. Klein and J.G. Rabkin, eds., pp. 137-154. Raven Press, New York,.
3. Crowe, R.R., et al., (1984): Arch Gen Psychiatry, 41(9):919.
4. Crowe, R.R., et al., (1987): J Affective Disord, 12:23-87.
5. Crowe, R.R., et al., (1987): Arch Gen Psychiatry, 44:933-937.
6. Harris, E.L., et al., (1983): Arch Gen Psychiatry, 40:1061-1064.
7. Hopper, J.L., et al., (1987: Genet Epidemiol, 4:33-41.
8. Moran, C. and Andrews, G. (1985): Br J Psychiatry, 146:262-267.
9. Pauls, D.L., Noyes, R. Jr., and Crowe, R.R., (1979): J Affective Disord, 1:279-285.
10. Pauls, D.L., et al., (1980): J Hum Genet, 32:639-644.
11. Torgersen, S. (1983): Arch Gen Psychiatry, 40:1085-1089.

PSYCHOLOGICAL TREATMENTS OF PANIC DISORDER

DAVID M CLARK and MICHAEL GELDER
Department of Psychiatry, University of Oxford, Warneford Hospital, Oxford, England

WHY PSYCHOLOGICAL TREATMENT?

Several medications have significant anti-panic effects. However, not all patients are willing to take, or respond to, medication and there are grave doubts about the long-term efficacy of pharmacological interventions (5, 7). It may be that psychological treatments, which aim to teach patients coping strategies, may be more effective in producing the sustained change which appears to elude drug treatment.

THE COGNITIVE THEORY AND THE TREATMENT OF PANIC

Recently considerable progress has been made in developing effective psychological treatments for panic. Most of these treatments are based on the cognitive theory of panic (2). This theory proposes that individuals who experience panic attacks do so because they have a relatively enduring tendency to interpret a wide range of bodily sensations as indicative of an immediately impending physical and mental catastrophe (e.g. interpreting palpitations as evidence of an impending heart attack). If this theory is correct, it should be possible to treat panic attacks in two ways. First, patients could be taught an effective relaxation technique which would directly modify the bodily sensations experienced in an attack and indirectly counteract patients catastrophic interpretations by showing that the attacks are controllable. Second, therapy could aim to directly modify a patient's interpretations and in this way prevent attacks.

REVIEW OF OUTCOME STUDIES

The first approach, of attempting to control the problematic bodily sensations, has been adopted by Ost who has developed a special form of relaxation called applied relaxation. In a recent controlled trial (6) applied relaxation was compared with traditional relaxation training and found to be significantly more effective at reducing panic frequency, with most patients becoming panic free.

Cognitive therapy adopts the second approach, that of teaching patients to identify and challenge their misinterpretations of bodily sensations. In the first evaluation of cognitive therapy (3) a consecutive series of patients was treated. All the panic disorder patients became panic-free and gains were maintained at two year follow-up. In a subsequent controlled trial, Beck and colleagues (6) found cognitive therapy was significantly more effective than supportive psychotherapy. Most recently, Clark, Salkovskis, Gelder et al (4) compared cognitive therapy with applied relaxation and with imipramine. Preliminary results indicated that all three treatments were effective in the short-term. There were no significant differences between applied relaxation and imipramine. However, on several measures cognitive therapy was more effective than either alternative treatment.

CONCLUSION

Recent research has led to the development of two distinct psychological treatments for panic, applied relaxation and cognitive therapy. Both of these treatments have been shown to be significantly more effective than a no treatment control or an alternative, plausible, psychological treatment and both are associated with extremely high response rates with between 80-100% of patients becoming panic free at the end of treatment. In the case of cognitive therapy, one study (3) has reported a long-term follow-up, and it would appear that the gains obtained in treatment are maintained for at least two years. Further research needs to directly compare the long-term efficacy of pharmacological and psychological treatments and to investigate the advantages and disadvantages of combined treatment.

REFERENCES

1. Beck, A.T. (1988): In Panic: Psychological Perspectives, S. Rachman and J.D. Maser eds., p.p. 91-110. Erlbaum, New Jersey
2. Clark, D.M. (1986): Behav. Res. Ther., 24, 461-470
3. Clark, D.M., Salkovskis, P.M. and Chalkley, J. (1985): J. Behav. Ther. Expt. Psychiat., 16, 23-30
4. Clark, D.M., Salkovskis, P.M. and Gelder, M.G. (1989): Presented at World Congress of Cognitive Therapy, Oxford, England. 28 June - 2 July
5. Fyer, A.J. (1988): In Panic and Phobias II, I. Hand and H. Wittchen eds., pp 47-53. Springer-Verlag, Heidelberg.
6. Ost, L.G., (1988): Behav. Res. Ther., 26, 13-22
7. Sheehan, D.V. (1986): Psychosom., 27, 10-16.

EMERGING CONSENSUS FOR TREATMENT OF PANIC DISORDER

L.L. JUDD and A.H. ROSENFELD
National Institute of Mental Health
Rockville, MD, U.S.A.

Growing scientific evidence indicates that panic disorder responds well to specific pharmacological and psychotherapeutic approaches. Medications successfully used include imipramine (IMI) and other tricyclic antidepressants; phenelzine and other MAOIs; and alprazolam and other high-potency benzodiazepines. Effective psychotherapies include in vivo and imaginal exposure, relaxation training, and cognitive therapy. Controversy continues, however, concerning the most appropriate treatment. No treatment, used alone, is ideal in addressing all the symptom clusters of panic disorder (4), and none is free of potentially adverse effects.

For many patients, a combination of somatic and nonsomatic treatments may prove to be synergistic. This brief overview, drawn largely from reviews by Telch (4) and Barlow (1), will focus on relatively recent studies combining and contrasting IMI and behavioral exposure. In the early 1980s, Zitrin et al. (5) found that the combined treatment (particularly in vivo exposure plus IMI) showed a strong advantage over medication or exposure alone. Marks et al. (2) used a 2x2 design of IMI plus therapy or assisted exposure, singly and in combination, for agoraphobia. Panic attacks responded equally well to all treatments; IMI conferred no added advantage to the effects of exposure alone (possibly because of low drug dosage). Mavissakalian and Michaelson (3), using a similar design, found an IMI-plus-exposure effect, but it ended 1 month posttreatment.

Telch et al. (4) randomly assigned 37 severe agoraphobics with panic attacks to IMI alone (with no-practice instructions), IMI plus intensive in vivo exposure, or placebo plus intensive in vivo exposure. At 8-week assessment, the IMI group had improved little on phobic anxiety and avoidance, heart rate, or panic, but depressed mood was significantly improved. Patients in the two exposure conditions (but especially IMI plus exposure) improved markedly on measures of phobic anxiety and avoidance, self-efficacy, and depression. At 26 weeks, only the combined-treatment group showed antipanic effects. Phobia measures in the IMI group improved significantly between weeks 9 and 26 once the no-practice instructions were removed, apparently in response to self-directed exposure practice. Although depressed mood improved in all groups at 8 weeks, by week 26 only the combined-treatment group showed further mood improvement.

Much larger carefully designed prospective studies on combined vs. single treatments for panic disorder are needed to clarify short-term treatment efficacy and long-term outcome, to identify specific patient groups most responsive to specific treatment types, and to tease apart the components of panic disorder itself and its treatments. Exploring the many somatic and nonsomatic treatments to be combined and compared, their most effective sequencing and duration, and the role of patient and site variables represents a substantial research agenda for the field that promises many benefits for panic disorder patients.

A number of new activities by the National Institute of Mental Health (NIMH) should help to clarify the treatment of panic disorder and encourage greater consensus among researchers and practitioners. These initiatives include the first study designed to assess the relative efficacy of a pharmacologic treatment, a cognitive/behavioral panic control treatment (PCT), and their combination for panic disorder patients. In this four-site collaborative study, a 12-week acute treatment trial will be followed by 6 months of maintenance treatment and 6 months of follow-up. A total of 600 patients, enrolled over 4 years, will be randomly assigned to one of five treatment cells: IMI with medical management, pill placebo with medical management, PCT alone, PCT with IMI, or PCT with placebo. The IMI and placebo treatment conditions will use a double-blind, fixed flexible dose design. In 1991, NIMH will cosponsor with the National Institutes of Health (NIH) the Consensus Development Conference on the Treatment of Panic Disorder. NIMH has also initiated a national public/professional education program to improve recognition and treatment of panic disorder.

In summary, steady and appreciable gains are being made in identifying and refining effective somatic and nonsomatic treatments for panic disorder, both singly and in combination. At the same time, many controversies remain concerning the relative merits of various treatment approaches that can only be resolved through further treatment research. In fact, the most important emerging consensus to date may well be the recognition that such research is essential.

REFERENCES

1 Barlow, D. (1988): Anxiety and its Disorders: The Nature and Treatment of Anxiety and Panic. The Guilford Press, New York.

2. Marks, I., et al. (1983): Imipramine and brief therapist-aided exposure in agoraphobics having self exposure homework: a controlled trial. Arch. Gen.Psychiat. 40: 153-162.

3. Mavissakalian, M., and Michelson, L. (1986): Two-year follow-up of exposure and imipramine treatment of agoraphobia. Am. J.Psychiat. 143: 1106-1112.

4. Telch, M. (1988): Combined pharmacological and psychological treatments for panic sufferers. In Panic: Psychological Perspectives, S. Rachman and J. Maser, eds., Erlbaum, Hillsdale, New Jersey.

5. Zitrin, C., Klein, D., and Woerner, M. (1980): Treatment of agoraphobia with group exposure in vivo and imipramine. Archives of General Psychiatry 37: 63-72.

PSYCHOSIS AND THE GENETICS OF BRAIN ASYMMETRY

T. J. CROW
Division of Psychiatry, Clinical Research Centre, Northwick Park Hospital, Harrow, HA1 3UJ, U.K.

Three findings suggest that the genetic contribution to the aetiology of schizophrenia is greater than is often thought - (i) in pairs of siblings illness occurs at the same age and not at the same time[10]. (ii) adoption away from a family with the disease does not reduce risk[12]. (iii) incidence is approximately constant across populations with widely differing social, geographical and industial environments[15].

CLUES TO THE NATURE OF THE PSYCHOSIS GENE

The finding of a degree of enlargement of the lateral ventricle in schizophrenia[11] is now generally accepted. The nature and location of the brain changes are elucidated by two recent post-mortem studies. In the first[1] brains of patients with schizophrenia and affective disorder were assessed on a photograph of a coronal brain section at the level of the interventricular foramina. The main findings were that (i) brain weight was reduced (by 5 to 6%) in the patients with schizophrenia, (ii) lateral ventricular area was modestly (by 15%) but not significantly increased, (iii) temporal horn area was significantly ($p<0.01$) increased, the relative increase being over 80%, and (iv) the width of the parahippocampal gyrus was reduced ($p<0.01$). Of particular interest[1] was a diagnosis by side interaction, the differences between the groups being significantly ($p<0.02$) greater on the left side.

In the second post-mortem study[7] of brains of patients with schizophrenia and age-matched controls the components of the lateral ventricle were assessed on X-ray images after formalin fixation. The posterior and particularly the temporal horn of the lateral ventricle was increased in patients with schizophrenia, in the latter case by a factor of 80% relative to the control group. Of particular interest was the finding that the change in schizophrenia was selective to the left side of the brain (ANOVA $p<0.001$), while in the Alzheimer cases there was no such lateralisation. The findings support the view[4] that the disease process in schizophrenia is associated with the mechanisms that determine the asymmetries in the human brain.

LOCATION OF THE CEREBRAL DOMINANCE GENE

A clue to the location of the cerebral dominance gene[6] comes from studies of the neuropsychology of Turner's and Klinefelter's syndromes. On IQ tests they have reciprocal deficits - in Turner's there is a performance deficit[13] and in Klinefelter's a verbal deficit[14]. A possible explanation is that the cerebral dominance gene is located in the pseudo-autosomal region, that region of the short arms of the X and Y chromosomes within which recombination occurs in male meiosis[2]. A pseudoautosomal locus for psychosis has been tested by examining whether concordance by sex is associated with paternal transmission In a series of 120 pairs of siblings with schizophrenia[8,9] and in a molecular study with a telomeric probe[3]. Siblings with schizophrenia or schizoaffective illness were found to share alleles at the DXYS14 locus above chance expectation, a finding that suggests linkage between psychosis and this locus.

CONCLUSIONS

Structural brain changes in schizophrenia are greater on the left, consistent with the view that schizophrenia is an anomaly of development of cerebral asymmetry. Evidence from sex chromosome aneuploidies suggests that the cerebral dominance gene is located in the pseudoautosomal region of the X and Y chromosomes. That the psychosis locus is also here is supported observations that in sibling pairs with schizophrenia i) concordance by sex is associated with paternal transmission, and ii) alleles at a telomeric locus are shared above chance expectation.

REFERENCES

1. Brown R, et al (1986) Arch. Gen. Psychiatry, 43: 36-42.
2. Burgoyne PS (1986) Nature, 319: 258-259.
3. Collinge J, et al., (1989) Cytogenet. Cell Genet., 51: 978.
4. Crow TJ (1984) Brit. J. Psychiatry, 145: 243-253.
5. Crow TJ (1988) Brit. J. Psychiatry, 153: 675-683.
6. Crow TJ (1989) Lancet, 2: 339-340.
7. Crow TJ, et al., (1989a) Arch. Gen. Psychiatry, 46: 1145-1150.
8. Crow TJ, DeLisi LE, Johnstone EC (1989b) Brit. J. Psychiatry, 154: 92-97.
9. Crow TJ, DeLisi LE, Johnstone EC (1990) Brit. J. Psychiatry, 156: 416-420.
10. Crow TJ, Done DJ (1986) Psychiatry Res., 18: 107-117.
11. Johnstone EC, et al., (1976) Lancet, 2: 924-926.
12. Karlsson J. (1970) Biol. Psychiatry, 2: 1013-1020.
13. Netley CT, Rovet J (1987) Brain & Cognition, 6: 153-160.
14. Netley CT, Rovet J (1982) Cortex, 18: 377-384.
15. Sartorius N, et al., (1986) Psychol. Med., 16: 909-928.

POSSIBLE NEUROTRANSMITTER IMBALANCES IN SCHIZOPHRENIA

A. CARLSSON AND M. CARLSSON
Department of Pharmacology, University of Gothenburg, Gothenburg, Sweden

Recent animal experiments have disclosed that dopamine plays a less decisive role than formerly supposed, in the regulation of psychomotor activity. Thus, even in the virtually complete absence of dopamine in the brain, resulting in an almost complete immobility of experimental animals, motility can be induced by manipulating non-dopaminergic mechanisms. Drugs acting as antagonists on NMDA receptors (one of the major subtypes of glutamatergic/aspartergic receptors; NMDA = N-methyl-D-aspartic acid), such as MK-801 or AP-5, are capable of inducing motility under such conditions (2, 5). These observations indicate that a glutamatergic/aspartergic mechanism exerts a powerful inhibitory influence. A reasonable candidate for such activity is the corticostriatal pathway (1). The striatal complexes appear to serve a powerful inhibitory function on their major targets, that is the thalamus and the mesencephalic reticular formation, and this inhibition is reinforced by the corticostriatal pathway. According to our hypothesis this inhibition will serve to restrict the sensory information relayed from the thalamus to the cortex. Likewise, the arousal induced by stimuli from the outer world and from the various parts of the body is dampened, partly by an action on the mesencephalic reticular formation. The mesostriatal dopamine pathways exert an inhibitory influence on the striatum and thus allow for more information to reach the cortex and to induce arousal. If the flow of information reaching the cerebral cortex is allowed to become excessive, the integrative capacity of the cortex breaks down, and psychosis or delirium may arise.

Phencyclidine (PCP, angel dust) is an NMDA-receptor antagonist acting on the same site as MK-801. PCP has been found to be capable of inducing disease states mimicking schizophrenia perhaps even more faithfully than amphetamine. Also MK-801 appears to be psychotogenic. PCP also has affinity for so-called sigma sites, but this appears to be less important for its pharmacological profile.

From these observations and interpretations it is inferred that the glutamatergic/aspartergic corticostriatal pathway could be involved in the pathogenesis of schizophrenia and other psychotic conditions, as well as in mania and various confusional states. The development of an NMDA-receptor agonist with satisfactory selectivity for the functions being discussed here might turn out to have considerable clinical utility. Antagonists, on the other hand, might find use in Parkinson's disease, provided that psychotogenic activity can be avoided.

A dramatic potentiation of the motility-inducing action of MK-801 by the alpha-2-receptor agonist clonidine has been discovered. This effect was found to be resistent against classical neuroleptics, but could be blocked by the "atypical" neuroleptic agent clozapine (3). The remarkable efficacy and profile of clozapine, with but few extrapyramidal side effects, may thus in part be explained by its well-established anti-adrenergic action, which may be assumed to potentiate its dopamine-receptor blocking action.

Another remarkable recent observation is the ability of clonidine in combination with atropine to induce motility in dopamine-depleted mice. The motility thus induced differs from that evoked by MK-801 (4). Whereas the latter motility is clearly abnormal, allowing almost exclusively for forward locomotion in the mouse, the latter looks like normal exploratory activity. These observations suggest that the glutamatergic/aspartergic system serves to select behavioral programs, adequate for the actual situation, by releasing its tonic inhibitory influence on these particular programs.

Moreover, these observations draw attention to both adrenergic and cholinergic mechanisms. Maybe the potential of manipulating these mechanisms in the treatment of psychiatric disorders, including schizophrenia, should be revisited in light of recent evidence.

REFERENCES

1. Carlsson, A.: The current status of the dopamine hypothesis of schizophrenia. Neuropsychopharmacology 1:179-186, 1988.
2. Carlsson, M. and Carlsson, A.: The NMDA antagonist MK-801 causes marked locomotor stimulation in monoamine-depleted mice. J. Neural Transm. 75:221-226, 1989.
3. Carlsson, M. and Carlsson, A.: Dramatic synergism between MK-801 and clonidine with respect to locomotor stimulatory effect in monoamine-depleted mice. J. Neural Transm. 77:65-71, 1989.
4. Carlsson, M. and Carlsson, A.: Marked locomotor stimulation in monoamine-depleted mice following treatment with atropine in combination with clonidine. J. Neural Transm. (P-D Section) 1:317-322, 1989.
5. Carlsson, M. and Svensson, A.: Interfering with glutamatergic neurotransmission by means of MK-801 administration discloses the locomotor stimulatory potential of other transmitter systems in rats and mice. Pharmacol. Biochem. Behavior 36, 1990 (in press).

POSSIBLE INVOLVEMENT OF NEUROPEPTIDES IN CHRONIC SCHIZOPHRENIA

H. SHIBUYA
Department of Neuropsychiatry, Tokyo Medical and Dental University, Tokyo, Japan

Schizophrenic symptoms such as hallucinations, delusions, thought disorder and psychomotor excitation which appear during the acute state of this disease are potentially responded to neuroleptics and may be related to dopaminergic hypertransmission in the brain. The symptoms such as flattening of affect, poverty of speech and aspontaneity typically seen in the chronic state of the disease, however, show generally poor response to anti-psychotics. It is now known that neuropeptides play important roles as neurotransmitters or neuromodulators in the brain and many kinds of neuropeptide change their concentration in the brain and the body fluid at the psychotic state or by the administration of antipsychotic drugs. Biochemical approaches to the chronic schizophrenia from various points of view would contribute to develop new therapeutic agents for such chronic defective state.

In this study, we measured neuropeptides and their receptors in the postmortem brain areas of chronic schizophrenic patients.

MATERIALS AND METHODS

The postmortem brain samples were obtained from 14 schizophrenics (9 males and 5 females, mean age 57.9+3.5) and 10 controls (7 males and 3 females, mean age 66.7+2.7). The age did not statistically differ between schizophrenics and controls. The diagnosis of schizophrenia was categorized according to DSM-III. "Off-drug" cases were arbitrarily defined as those who had not received antipsychotics more than 40 days before death.

Frontal cortex, temporal cortex, parietal cortex, basal ganglia, limbic brain area, thalamus and brain stem were dissected. These brain tissues were divided into small areas based on the difference of the architecture of neurons.

Methionine-enkephalin like immunoreactivity and opioid receptor binding such as mu-opioid receptor and delta opioid receptor were measured with RIA and RRA respectively. Besides, cholecystokinin like immunoreactivity in water extract and that in acid extract and cholecystokinin receptor binding were assayed.

RESULTS

Significantly high values of methionine-enkephalin like

immunoreactivity were found in the medial frontal cortex, eye-movement area and orbital cortex of schizophrenics. At the same time, mu-opioid receptor binding with 3H-DAGO was significantly increased in the medial frontal cortex and the eye-movement area, delta-opioid receptor binding with 3H-DADLE was increased in the medial frontal cortex and the orbitofrontal cortex compared to those of control.

With respect to cholecystokinin, abnormal findings were mainly found in the limbic brain area and the temporal cortex. Cholecystokinin like immunoreactivity in water extract was mainly composed of cholecystokinin-8 and that in acid extract was mainly cholecystokinin-33. Cholecystokinin like immunoreactivity in water extract from schizophrenic brains showed the tendency to be high in general. On the other hand, cholecystokinin like immunoreactivity in acid extract was significantly low in the subiculum of the hippocampus, the corticomedial nuclei of amygdala, the posterior portion of the pyriform cortex and the lateral occipitotemporal cortex of schizophrenia. Particularly in the subiculum and the posterior portion of the pyriform cortex, there was a significant decrease even in the "off-drug" schizophrenic group. Significantly low cholecystokinin like immunoreactivity in acid extract was noticed in the lateral occipitotemporal cortex of the "off-drug" and "on-drug" schizophrenics. Cholecystokinin receptor binding with 3H-cholecystokinin-8 showed no difference in the lateral occipitotemporal cortex, the medial and inferior temporal cortex, the superior temporal cortex and the posterior portion of the temporal cortex between schizophrenia and cotrol.

DISCISSION

These findings in peptide immunoreactivities and their receptors may suggest that the etiology of schizophrenia could not be caused by a single substance in the small brain area. Opioid dysfunction in the prefrontal cortex and the abnormal cholecystokinin metabolism in the limbic brain area and the temporal cortex might be involved in schizophrenic pathology. The relationship between these peptide changes and alterations of classical neurotransmitters or excitatory amino acids and clinical features of schizophrenia are remained to be dissolved.

REFERENCE

Toru, M. et al., (1988):Neurotransmitters, receptors and neuropeptides in post-mortem brains of chronic schizophrenic patients. Acta Psychiatr Scand. 78:121-137.

FUNCTIONAL SUBTYPING OF SCHIZOPHRENIC PATIENTS

E. R. JOHN, L. PRICHEP, J. VOLAVKA, J. BRODIE, K. ALPER, R. CANCRO.
NYU Medical Center, N.Y., N.Y. 10016 and Nathan S. Kline Institute
for Psychiatric Research, Orangeburg, N.Y. 10962

Since Eugen Bleuler, various observations have forced the students of the schizophrenic disorders to the conclusion that they are heterogenous as to etiology, pathogenesis, and clinical manifestations. While this statement has been repeated for over eighty years, efforts to reduce the heterogeneity have been largely ineffective. There is an obvious need to create a typology that is useful for enhanced clinical care or for better understanding of etiopathogenesis or, ideally, for both.

An effort is underway to approach the problem of typology from the vantage of functional imaging of the brain. Initial data have been obtained on grouping chronic schizophrenics utilizing quantitative electrophysiologic assessments of spontaneous brain electrical activity (neurometrics). Initial data have also been obtained on subtyping schizophrenic subjects utilizing measures of deoxyglucose metabolism by positron emission tomography (PET). Finally, data are being collected on schizophrenic subjects who will be classified through the combined use of neurometrics and PET.

Subjects and Method

A cohort of forty nonmedicated schizophrenics was classified using neurometrics, into five groups. These groups are electrophysiologically quite different from each other, although they have enough commonalities to be easily separable from normals and dementias. The addition of evoked electrical brain activity measures to the spontaneous activity measures further improved the separation of schizophrenics from normal and demented subjects.

A major problem in interpreting PET data has been the failure to normalize metabolic rates in healthy subjects. This deficiency has led to group comparisons made between various study populations and small individual normal control groups. Much information is lost because of this methodologic failure. Twenty-five normal subjects were studied with deoxyglucose, utilizing absolute metabolic activity, on a PET-VI machine. Fourteen slices were made with ten-thousand pixels per slice, for a total of 140,000 pixels per head. The mean and standard deviation for each group pixel was calculated, allowing thereby a Z-transformation of the individual pixel against the group data. This method allows the comparison of the activity of any individual pixel against the norms to be expressed in color-coded standard deviation units above and below the normal subject mean for that pixel. Ten normal subjects who were not used to construct the norms were tested and they showed no deviation from expected levels of metabolic activity.

FUNCTIONAL SUBTYPING

Results

The BPRS had been administered to the schizopherenic subjects at baseline and four BPRS factors derived. These were active behavioral symptoms (ABS), mood related symptoms (MRS), passive behavioral symptoms (PBS), and evidence of reality distortion (ERD). All patients were medicated with haloperidol, and the BPRS was readministered. The ERD factor improved in four out of the five neurometric groups, but significant improvement in ABS occured only in group two, while significant improvement in PBS occured only in group one. In other words, only two groups showed more than a general antipsychotic effect of the haloperidol. It was of particular interest that the group one subjects showed improvement in emotional withdrawal, blunt affect, and posturing. Of further interest was the finding that haloperidol administration worsened six out of a possible sixteen BPRS factor scores in four groups of patients. The hints of a more rational and selective basis for neuroleptic administration begin to emerge from this effort at subtyping.

Thirty-five schizophrenic subjects were studied by the PET method described earlier. Their absolute metabolic activity for seven levels was transformed against the norms, and color maps of deoxyglucose activity were produced. Three judges independently visually inspected the thirty-five maps and classified them into five groups of patterns with excellent interrater agreement. What is clear from these five different groups of Z-transformed maps is the metabolic variability of the picture, again suggesting several different diseases or else a variably placed "lesion" in the brain stem and/or midbrain that expresses itself differently as a function of the exact location and extent of that "lesion."

Discussion

The need to merge these functional imaging approaches, i.e., neurometrics and PET, on the same set of schizophrenic subjects is apparent and presently underway. The resulting unified functional subtypes will then have to be evaluated to assess their clinical correlates and clinical utility.

The assumption underlying this line of investigation is that the schizophrenic disorders share certain core, genetically-controlled, biochemical abnormalities in common which are located in deep brain structures. This commonality permits the separation of these disorders by functional imaging from other psychiatric disorders. Furthermore, differences in the localization and extensiveness of the biochemical abnormalities and differences in brain compensatory mechanisms result in different functional and clinical patterns. The identification of these patterns should contribute not only to enhanced care, but to a better appreciation of etiopathogenic factors.

TESTING NEURAL MODELS OF SCHIZOPHRENIA WITH POSITRON EMISSION TOMOGRAPHY

M.S. BUCHSBAUM, R. HAIER, M. KATZ, R. TAFALLA, S. LOTTENBERG
S. POTKIN AND W.E. BUNNEY, Jr.
Department of Psychiatry, University of California, Irvine, California, USA.

Three brain areas are the current scientific targets in schizophrenia research: the frontal lobes, the basal ganglia and the temporal lobe, especially the hippocampus. Reduced frontal lobe function, supported by blood flow, PET and EEG studies, is consistent with behavioral deficits in executive functions in schizophrenia, but less directly compatible with information about the distribution of dopamine receptors and medication effects. Basal ganglia dysfunction is consistent with the dopamine hypothesis, some autopsy and PET studies of receptor density, and with neuroleptic response, but less easily related to the symptoms of thought disorder, hallucinations, and social withdrawal. Temporal lobe dysfunction is supported by MRI imaging studies, some CT studies, and EEG studies, and is consistent with sensory and verbal symptoms but less closely linked to dopamine receptor change.

Are there three distinct types of schizophrenia, frontal, basal ganglia and temporal lobe illness, with possibly differing etiology, course and treatments? Or are there varying degrees of a deficit in a single frontal-striatal or even fronto-striatal-temporal neural system? Positron emission tomography with fluorodeoxyglucose (FDG) as a tracer of metabolic rate provides a method to evaluate the activity of all three areas simultaneously, in life, in the behaving patient.

SUBJECT AND METHODS

Eighteen male patients (mean age 29.6, SD=7.2) recruited from referral through the clinical aqnd research programs of the University of California at UC Irvine, UCLA and UCSD served as subjects. No patient had a history of having received neuroleptic medication before scanning. The average age of onset was 24.9, SD=7.0, range 13-40. The average duration of illness was 4.6 years, sd=5.9. Nine patients had been ill one year or less. Three patients had never been hospitalized, and 12 were currently hospitalized. All patients were in good health based on medical history, physical examination and laboratory measures.

Patients were diagnosed using DSM-III criteria by interviewers entirely independent of brain imaging data. The control subjects (20 men, mean age 27.1, sd=6.4) were screened with the same physical and laboratory examination as the patients. None had a history of psychiatric illness in themselves or in first-degree relatives and none were taking psychoactive medications by history or urine screen.

RESULTS

Frontal lobe. The frontal/occipital ratio for the right inferior frontal gyrus was significantly lower in never-medicated schizophrenics (mean 1.01, sd=.07) than in normal controls (1.07, sd=.10, t=1.91, p=0.027, 1-tailed in replication of our earlier study (Buchsbaum et al., 1990) on unmedicated patients). Areas of the medial frontal cortex, frontal white matter were also reduced in patients with schizophrenia. Other medial areas including the precuneus, posterior corpus callosum, and the upper frontal lobe were not significantly different.

Basal ganglia. Patients were 5.4 micromoles lower than normals in the right caudate. Using the right caudate (34%slice) cutoff of 23.6 identified 14 of 18 schizophrenics and 11 of 20 patients; in this distribution there are five schizophrenics lower than any normal and eight normals higher than any schizophrenic.

Temporal lobe. Patients had higher left than right metabolic rates in the temporal lobe; normals had higher right than left metabolic rates in all gyri. Averaging across the frontal and temporal lobe, normals had 23.7 on the left and 24.7 on the right; schizophrenics had 21.6 on the left and 21.9 on the right (group by hemisphere interaction, F=8.77, df=1,36, p=0.005).

DISCUSSION

Low metabolic rates were seen in frontal, striatal, and left temporal areas of the brain in schizophrenics. Both the significant correlation coeficients between the three areas and the results of cluster analysis are more consistent with a model of combined fronto-striatal or fronto-striatal-temporal pattern of dysfunction than the model of three separate subtypes.

REFERENCES

1. Buchsbaum, M.S., DeLisi, L.E., Holcomb, H.H., Cappelletti, J., King, A.C., Johnson, J., Hazlett, E., Dowling-Zimmerman, S., Post, R.M., Morihisa, J., Carpenter, W., Cohen, R., Pickar, D., Weinberger, D.R., Margolin, R., & Kessler, R.M. (1984) Anteroposterior gradients in cerebral glucose use in schizophrenia and affective disorders. Arch. Gen. Psychiat. 41, 1159-1166.

2. Buchsbaum, M.S., Nuechterlein, K.H., Haier, R.J., Wu, J., Sicotte, N., Hazlett, E., Asarnow, R., Potkin, S. & Guich, S. Glucose metabolic rate in normals and schizophrenics during the continuous performance test assessed by positron emission tomography. Brit. Jour. Psychiat. 156, 216-227, 1990.

BASIC MECHANISMS OF REFRACTORY EPILEPSIES

B.S. MELDRUM
Department of Neurology, Institute of Psychiatry,
London SE5 8AF, U.K.

Over the last decade hypotheses concerning the pathogenesis of refractory epilepsy have emphasised loss of inhibitory function, but definitive data are lacking. Recently evidence has been produced showing that there are abnormalities in excitatory neurotransmission that could account for some of the features of refractory epilepsy. These abnormalities have been described in an experimental model of chronic epilepsy (kindled seizures in the rat) and in refractory complex partial seizures (in specimens removed by anterior temporal lobectomy). Two types of change have been described, one is in the number or sensitivity of post-synaptic excitatory receptors, particularly those of the NMDA preferring subtype. The other is the abnormal growth of terminals ("sprouting") providing an excitatory feedback within the hippocampus.

ENHANCED NMDA RECEPTOR SENSITIVITY

In vitro electrophysiological studies comparing responses in hippocampal slices from kindled and non-kindled rats provide clear evidence for enhanced post-synaptic responses to NMDA. Thus in the kindled rat the decrease in extracellular [Ca++] induced by the iontophoretic application of NMDA is enhanced in stratum oriens and radiata (7). In the dentate gyrus NMDA receptors contribute to post-synaptic potentials after kindling but not before (3). These functional changes could explain the induction of sustained burst discharges by initially subthreshold stimuli.

Similar data have been obtained in _in vitro_ studies using slices from focal epileptic cortex obtained during cortical resection for refractory focal seizures (2). Measurements of decreases in extracellular [Ca++] induced by iontophoretic application of NMDA show the largest responses in superficial laminae in control cortex, but markedly enhanced responses in the deeper laminae in epileptic cortex.

SPROUTING OF THE HIPPOCAMPAL MOSSY FIBRE SYSTEM

Lesions producing partial deafferentation of the hippocampus are followed by growth of nerve terminals to occupy vacated areas. Sprouting of the mossy fibre system in the hippocampus can be studied by Timm's staining, by kainate receptor autoradiography or by dynorphin immunoreactivity (1,4,6). Such studies in the rat show that kindling is associated with an abnormal dense mossy fibre input to the inner molecular layer (5). It is not yet clear whether this is a consequence of hilar cell loss or of abnormal electrical activity. Nevertheless it appears to provide a recurrent excitatory input to the granule cells. Studies in temporal lobectomy specimens and in post mortem material from various childhood epilepsies indicate that there is a similar process occurring in human epilepsy. Here also the relationship to prior cell loss or abnormal electrical activity is not clear, but the abnormal synapses may contribute importantly to refractoriness of seizures.

REFERENCES

1. Houser, C.R. et al. Altered patterns of dynorphin immunoreactivity suggest mossy fiber reorganization in human hippocampal epilepsy. J. Neurosci. 10(1):267-282, 1990.

2. Mody, I., Stanton, P.K. and Heinemann, U. Activation of N-methyl-D-aspartate receptors parallels changes in cellular and synaptic properties of dentate granule cells after kindling. J. Neurophysiol. 591:1033-1053, 1988.

3. Louvel, J. and Pumain, R. N-methyl-D-aspartate-mediated responses in epileptic cortex in man : an in vitro study. In Neurotransmitters, Seizures and Epilepsy IV, edit. Engel J. et al. Raven Press, 1990.

4. Represa, A. et al. Hippocampal plasticity in childhood epilepsy. Neurosci. Lett. 99:351-355, 1989.

5. Sutula, T. et al. Synaptic reorganization in the hippocampus induced by abnormal functional activity. Science 239:1147-1150: 1988.

6. Sutula, T. et al. Mossy fiber synaptic reorgazation in the epileptic human temporal lobe. Ann. Neurol. 26(3):321-330, 1989.

7. Wadman, W.J. and Heinemann U. Laminar profiles of [K+]o in region CA1 of the hippocampus of kindled rats. In: Kessler M et al (eds) Physiology and Medicine. Berlin : Springer-Verlag, 1985:221-228.

Diagnostic Evaluation of Uncontrolled Epilepsy

William H. Theodore M.D.
Clinical Epilepsy Section, National Institutes of Health
Bethesda Maryland, USA

The diagnosis of uncontrolled epilepsy must take into account not only seizure frequency but severity of the episodes, possibility of injury, effect on employment, education, and social status, and the reaction of friends and family members. Persistent seizures are associated with serious adverse consequences. The standardized mortality ratio is increased for all patients with epilepsy (2.3:1), especially in the first ten years after diagnosis (3).

Patients who will not respond to conventional antiepileptic drug therapy can usually be chosen within two years of seizure onset. High pretreatment seizure frequency, abnormal neurologic examination, structural lesions (excluding the regions of focal gliosis now identified by increased signal intensity on MRI), a history of repeated or complicated febrile seizures, frequent generalized tonic clonic seizures, generalized EEG abnormalities, family history of epilepsy, and psychiatric, or social problems predict a poor response to AED therapy (1, 4). Drug toxicity, early onset and frequent seizures predict IQ decline (1).

The first step in identifying patients for experimental drug trial or surgery is to confirm the diagnosis of epilepsy and establish that the seizures cannot be controlled by medication. Prolonged video-EEG monitoring, combined with frequent measurement of AED blood levels is essential. Non-epileptic attacks are diagnosed in as many as 22 % of patients admitted to monitoring units for uncontrolled epilepsy. Psychiatric episodes are most common, but cardiovascular and sleep disorders may be misdiagnosed as epilepsy as well (6). A minority of patients may have both pseudoseizures and real epilepsy (8). In these cases it is essential to try to determine the frequency of each type of episode and their relation to the patient's overall function.

Although no single criterion unequivocally differentiates pseudoseizures from epilepsy, pseudoseizures do not conform to the clinical patterns of recognized seizure types. True seizures impair normal neurologic function, especially acts involving high degrees of coordination. Suspicious events include elaborate behavioral patterns which could not be performed without normal control over motor function. EEG recordings should show neither epileptiform discharges during, nor slow activity after, pseudoseizures.

Unfortunately, there are no physical or historical findings which exclude cardiogenic syncope, and seizures themselves may evoke arrythmias capable of producing loss of consiousness (2). In order to be implicated as the cause of a neurological event, the arrythmia must be shown reliably to precede clinical and electrographic signs of 'seizure onset.' History and physical examination, as well as routine EEG, may suggest the diagnosis in about 50% of patients with cardiogenic syncope. If a cardiac etiology is suspected when these tests are negative, 24-72 hours of ambulatory EEG monitoring should be enough to detect an arrythmia (2). ECG and video-EEG recording can easily be combined in an epilepsy monitoring unit.

Once the diagnosis of epilepsy is established, it is important to review the patient's clinical seizure classification. CPS are often confused with absence or Petit Mal seizures. In addition to EEG patterns, they may be distingushed by clinical characteristics, including longer duration, presence of an aura, and postictal confusion (6). Other seizure types which have a good prognosis, such benign rolandic epilepsy, which may be confused with partial seizures of temporal origin, need to be identified.

In addition to video-EEG monitoring, neuroimaging tests are part of the evaluation of uncontrolled seizures. MRI is more valuable than CT (7) in detecting focal lesions, especially in patients with CPS. SPECT and PET can show functional abnormalities when structural studies are normal, helping either to identify surgical foci or exclude patients who have widespread pathology. PET in particular can be used for quantitative studies to evaluate the effect of antiepileptic drugs, neuropsychological function, and neurotransmitter receptor binding (7). At present, these are research procedures, and not of proven clinical value. The presence of an MRI lesion or PET hypometabolism is not an indication of intractable epilepsy, since both may occur in patients with well-controlled, and be absent in patients with frequent, seizures (7).

It is important to make sure patients have had an adequate AED trial. Patients with uncontrolled epilepsy should have blood levels maintained at the upper end of the therapeutic range or beyond. Patients with uncontrolled partial seizures should receive at least two drugs, preferably CBZ and PHT, in combination, before considering experimental drugs or surgery. Phenobarbital and primidone, only marginally less effective, but associated with greater neuropsychological toxicity, are useful alternatives. The role of VPA in the treatment of CPS is uncertain. The management of patients, often children, with atonic and myoclonic seizures may be more difficult. VPA appears to be the most effective drug, although only 20% of patients are well-controlled. Benzodiazepines have limited usefulness due to sedation, intellectual impairment, and tolerance (9).

Uncontrolled epilepsy is a severe medical and social problem. If progressive deterioration of quality of life is to be avoided, patients should not be followed in the hopes that seizures will resolve spontaneously. Instead, a vigorous attempt should be made in each case to find a new therapeutic approach.

References

1. Brorson LO and Wranne L (1987): Epilepsia 28: 424-430
2. Dohrmann ML, Cheitlan MD (1986): in Epilepsy Porter RJ, Theodore WH eds pp 531-48. WB Saunders Philadelphia
3. Hauser WA, Annegers JF, Elveback LR (1980): Epilepsia 21: 399-412
4. Schmidt D (1984): J Neurol Neurosurg Psychiatr 47: 1274-1278
5. Theodore WH, Porter RJ, Penry JK (1983): Neurology 33: 1115-1121
6. Theodore WH, Schulman EA, Porter RJ (1983): Epilepsia 24:336-343
7 Theodore WH (1988): in Clinical Neuroimaging Theodore WH ed pp 183-210. Alan R. Liss NY
8. Trimble MR (1986): in Epilepsy Porter RJ, Theodore WH eds pp 531-548. WB Saunders Philadelphia
9. Vining EPG (1986): in Epilepsy. Porter RJ, Theodore WH (eds). pp 617-632. W.B. Saunders, Philadelphia

Single or Polytherapy for Refractory Epilepsy

A. Sengoku
Kansai Regional Epilepsy Center, Utano National Hospital, Kyoto, Japan

The superiority of single-drug therapy (monotherapy) to multiple-drug therapy (polytherapy) has been suggested since the monitoring of plasma concentration was used for the treatment of epilepsy.
Schmidt(3)(4) also supported the advantage of monotherapy through a series of prospective clinical studies. His method of monotherapy is to increase the dose until the seizure is controlled or toxic manifestations occurred. This method is excellent to evaluate the efficacy of the anticonvulsant drug for intractable epilepsy. Of those who could not be controlled with the maximal dosage of a single drug, only a few patients respond to the add-on therapy of the second drug. Lesser(1) also supported the high-dose monotherapy in treatment of intractable epilepsy.
We (2)(5) have been studying the efficacy of monotherapy for refractory epilepsies with the same method as Schmidt, and through the studies, various problems about monotherapy arose. They are: 1) can the maximal dose without toxicity be easily determined, 2) is the impairment of smooth-pursuit eye movement helpful for the earlier detection of toxicity, 3) do chronic adverse effects, such as psychoses, occur during maintenance of high-dose monotherapy, and 4) whether the monotherapy is possible for patients with more than two types of seizures or not.
In the following, these four problems are discussed.
1. Monotherapy for intractable temporal lobe epilepsy
Thirty four patients with intractable temporal lobe epilepsy who had complex partial seizures (CPS) more than once a month were subjected to treatment with monotherapy of phenytoin(PHT) or carbamazepine (CBZ). The method of dosage is principally the increase in dose until CPS is controlled for longer than one month or toxic manifestations occurred. Treatment was effective in 13 patients with a mean plasma concentration of $26.9 \mu g/ml$, and ineffective in 15 patients with a mean plasma concentration of $35.9 \mu g/ml$. CBZ monotherapy was effective in 3 patients with a mean plasma concentration of $9.6 \mu g/ml$, and ineffective in 15 patients with a mean plasma concentration of $12.3 \mu g/ml$. The mean effective plasma concentration of both antiepileptics was lower than the ineffective concentration. There were a few patients who showed no acute toxic manifestations despite extremely high plasma concentration. Because there is a risk of sudden and unexpected occurrence of toxicity, and we abandoned to obey the principle of increasing the dose until occurrence of toxic manifestations.
2. The smooth-pursuit eye movement (SPEM) with monotherapy and combination therapy of PHT and CBZ
Adverse effect of PHT and CBZ, alone and in combination, to the patients with temporal lobe epilepsy, was studied. Impairment of SPEM was used as an indicator for the adverse effect of the antiepileptic drug. SPEM was examined simultaneously with measurement of serum concentration of PHT or CBZ at more than three different time points in each patient. The mean correlation rate between serum level and

threshold of SPEM was -0.94 in 6 cases with PHT, and -0.55 in 4 cases with CBZ monotherapy. Despite inter-individual variation, there was a positive inverse-correlation between SPEM threshold and serum level of the antiepileptic drug in each individual. The degree of impairment of SPEM was nearly parallel with increase of serum level, and it was impossible to determine the maximal dose of monotherapy in each patient from the evaluation of impairment of SPEM. In combination therapy with PHT and CBZ, impairment of SPEM occurred additively.

3. Episodic psychotic state by PHT monotherapy

Among 1207 patients older than 15 years of age at the first examination at our clinic, 26 patients(2.2%) had acute psychotic episodes during follow-up. Of them, 4 cases were treated by PHT monotherapy. Three cases had a plasma level over $20\mu g/ml$ for longer than one month until occurrence of psychoses, and during this period the seizures were suppressed. Thus, the maintenance of a high level of PHT monotherapy appeared to cause psychoses, although seizures are controlled. High dose monotherpy of PHT is advantageous for the control of seizures, but it is accompanied by the risk of the occurrence of psychoses.

4. One drug for one seizure type

We have cases with temporal lobe epilepsy whose CPSs were controlled with PHT monotherapy, but secondarily generalized tonic-clonic seizures (grand mal) were not controlled. By addition of phenobarbital, both seizures were controlled. Thus, some patients with temporal lobe epilepsy who had both CPS and grand mal are better treated by combination therapy. The patients with Lennox-Gastaut syndrome also had various seizure types and as the antiepileptic drugs, for example, the absence seizures are indicated for valproic acids or ethosuximide, on the other hand the tonic seizures are indicated for phenobarbital or phenytoin. From this point, polytherapy appeared to be advantageous in patients with more than one seizure types, and we will propose here " one drug for one seizure type".

Monotherapy is known to be advantageous for treatment of epilepsy. High-dose of monotherapy for refractory epielpsies is often effective, but it is difficult to maintain the dose, because the maximal dose is difficult to determine, and chronic adverse effects, such as psychoses, occur. We propose not to adhere to monotherapy for refractory epilepsies, especially for the patients with various seizure types.

REFERENCES
1. Lesser RP, Pippenger CE, Lueders H, Dinner DS. High-dose monotherapy in treatment of intractable seizures. Neurology 34:707-711,1984.
2. Naruto T, Sengoku A, Kawai I. Monotherpay and combination therapy with phenytoin and carbamazepine -- smooth-pursuit eye movement and serum level of antiepileptics. J.Jpn.Epil.Soc. 7:132-138,1989.
3. Schmidt D. Reduction of two-drug therapy in intractable epilepsy. Epilepsia 24:368-376,1983.
4. Schmidt D. Single drug therapy for intactable epilepsy. J.Neurol.229:221-223,1983.
5. Sengoku A, Kanazawa O, Kawai I. Monotherapy for intractable temporal lobe epilepsy. J.Jpn.Epil.Soc.5:19-23,1987.

METHODOLOGICAL REQUIREMENTS FOR CLINICAL TRIALS IN REFRACTORY EPILEPSIES
- OUR EXPERIENCE IN ZONISAMIDE -

K. YAGI and M. SEINO
National Epilepsy Center, Shizuoka Higashi Hospital, Urushiyama 886,
Shizuoka 420, Japan

The authors investigated significant factors in clinical evaluation of a new antiepileptic drug, Zonisamide (ZNS), originally developed in Japan and released in 1989. ZNS was administered to a total of 1008 patients with various epilepsies during a 7-year trials from phase 1 to phase 3, in that ZNS was evaluated as effective if the baseline seizure frequency was reduced by over 50%.

I. Number of concomitantly used antiepileptic drugs (AED) and efficacy of ZNS

There were 55 cases where no concomitant AEDs were administered (ZNS monotherapy, or ZNS-0); 121 cases using one AED (ZNS-1); 256 cases using two AEDs (ZNS-2); and 576 cases using three or more AEDs (ZNS-3). Their respective efficacies were found to be 72%, 52%, 48% and 43%. In other words, the fewer the number of concomitant AEDs, the higher the rate of efficacy.

II. Seizure frequency and efficacy

When the seizure frequency was rated as more than once a day, more than once a week, more than once a month and more than once a year, ZNS efficacy was 42% in 362 cases with daily seizures; 48% in 386 cases with weekly seizures; 59% in 165 cases with monthly seizures; and 93% of 90 cases with yearly seizures. It was clearly shown that the higher the frequency of seizures, the lower the efficacy.

III. Seizure types and efficacy

Efficacies in terms of seizure types, as classified by the International Classification of Epileptic Seizure (1981), were: efficacy was 57% in 63 cases with simple partial seizures, 50% in 82 with simple partial onset followed by impairment of consciousness, 50% in 362 with complex partial seizures, 60% in 168 with partial seizures evolving to secondarily generalized seizures, 59% in 46 with generalized tonic-clonic seizure, 26% in 74 with generalized tonic seizures, 67% in 9 with atypical absences, 50% in 10 with atonic seizures, 43% in 7 with myoclonic seizures, and 41% in 129 with mixed seizures.

IV. Epilepsy types and efficacy

ZNS was effective in 54% of 428 cases with temporal lobe epilesy (TLE); in 51% of 224 cases with partial epilepsy other than TLE (NTLE); in 57% of 21 cases with partial epilepsy of either TLE or NTLE; in 66% of 411 cases with primary generalized epilepsy; in 22% of 9 cases with West syndrome; in 32% of 132 cases with Lennox-Gastaut syndrome; in 47% of

Table 1: Types of Epilepsies and Number of Concomitantly used Antiepileptic Drugs

	ZNS-0	ZNS-1	ZNS-2	ZNS-3
TLE	29(53)	60(50)	123(48)	236(40)
NTLE	11(20)	36(30)	78(30)	111(20)
PE	1	3(2)	7(3)	11(2)
PGE	8(16)	8(7)	4(2)	25(4)
West	0	4(3)	3(1)	2
L-G	1(2)	6(5)	17(7)	110(19)
SGE	5(9)	3(2)	22(9)	79(14)
Other	0	1	2	2
Total	55(100%)	121(100%)	256(100%)	576(100%)

TLE: temporal lobe epilepsy, NTLE: partial epilepsies other than TLE
PE: localization undetermined partial epilepsy, West: West syndrome
L-G: Lennox Gastaut syndrome, SGE: other secondary generalized epilepsies

100 cases with other symptomatic generalized epilepsies; and in 25% of 4 cases with other unclassifiable epilepsies. Thus, ZNS seems to exert effectiveness to a certain extent on symptomatic generalized epilepsies including West and Lennox-Gastaut syndromes.

V. Epilepsy types and numbers of concomitant AEDs

It was clearly shown that the higher the frequency of seizures, the lower the efficacy. Also, ZNS efficacy varied according to individual seizure types as well as epilepsy classification. The efficacy of ZNS was unequivocally higher in cases using fewer concomitant drugs and highest in ZNS monotherapy cases. The epilepsy types in relation to the number of concomitant AEDs are shown in Table 1. Partial epilepsies, i.e. TLE, NTLE and PE occupied about 80% of the 3 groups except for ZNS-3. In ZNS-3 group the ratios of partial epilepsies to generalized epilepsies were about 60% and 40%, respectively. The patient population was markedly inclined to cases with partial epilepsies, in spite of the fact that those placed on one or two concomitant AEDs were selected prior to administration of ZNS.

Summarizing, the guidelines for AED evaluation proposed by ILAE (1989) were scrutinized through our experiences in clinical trials for ZNS. Seizure type, seizure frequency, number of concomitant AEDs, and type of epilepsy were found crucial factors to determine the rate of efficacy of the new drug. If we select the patients conforming to the guidelines, they should be those with active seizures in spite of taking one or two conventional AEDs, and with one or two seizure types. Our results indicate that the majority of such patients thus selected are inevitably occupied by those with partial seizures with or without secondary generalization. In order to avoid such predilection, we should arrange to include those with generalized epilepsies at least 30 to 40% in the whole population.

NEW DRUGS FOR REFRACTORY EPILEPSIES

D. SCHMIDT and S. RIED
Department of Neurology, Klinikum Rudolf Virchow, Free University of Berlin,
Berlin, West-Germany

Patients with symptomatic generalized epilepsies and patients with complex partial seizures form the majority of patients with refractory epilepsies. A quantitative score to is useful to determine the response to previous drug therapy (Table 1)

Table 1: Drug Treatment of Refractory Epilepsy: A quantitative score for the assessment of treatment failures

Index of intractability	Seizures persist despite treatment with
0	Other than primary drug regardless of its daily dose
1	Primary drug below the recommended daily dose
2	Primary drug within the recommended daily dose
3	Primary drug with plasma concentrations within the recommended "therapeutic range"
4	Primary drug with maximum clinically tolerable daily dose
5	More than one primary drug with maximum clinically tolerable daily dose in subsequent single-drug therapy

In about twenty percent of all patients with chronic epilepsy seizures are not controlled by current antiepileptic drugs (Schmidt, 1986), approximately further twenty percent suffer from moderate to severe side effects during chronic antiepileptic drug therapy (Schmidt, 1986). Fortunately, life-treatening side effects such as hypersensitivity reactions, hepatic coma or aplastic anemia are extremely rare. In summary, approximately forty percent of all treated patients could potentially benefit from new antiepileptic drugs.

The new antiepileptic drugs are usually tested in double-blind placebo-controlled add-on designs in non-responders to standard antiepileptic drugs. In this classic design addition of a standard antiepileptic drug can be expected to achieve a reduction in the number of seizures of more than 50 percent in approximately 30 percent of cases including a reduction of 75 percent or more in 15 percent. New agents should be compared to results achieved by standard drugs. The new antiepileptic drugs can be classified in GABA-ergic agents e.g. the GABA-transaminase inhibitor vigabatrin and the 1.5-benzodiazepine clobazam and those with various other putative mechanisms of action e.g. lamotrigine, gabapentin, topiramate, felbamate and zonisamide. For this brief survey vigabatrin and clobazam have been selected because we recently performed clinical trials with these GABA-ergic agents.

Vigabatrin

GABA-transmission plays a critical role in controlling seizures. The precise nature of its antiepileptic effect depends on the particular location in the brain and the pathway involved. Animal studies have suggested specific brain regions such as the substantia nigra and area tempestas. Vigabatrin, a drug rationally developed to treat resistant epilepsy can enhance GABA transmission in these regions and may therefore afford seizure protection (Gale, 1989). In fact, in four large trials half of the patients in each trial had a more than 50 percent reduction in seizure frequency when vigabatrin was added (Treiman, 1989). In our single-blind add-on trial a reduction of that seizure frequency of thirty percent was observed when vigabatrin was added to 18 patients with drug refractory partial seizures (Fig. 1).

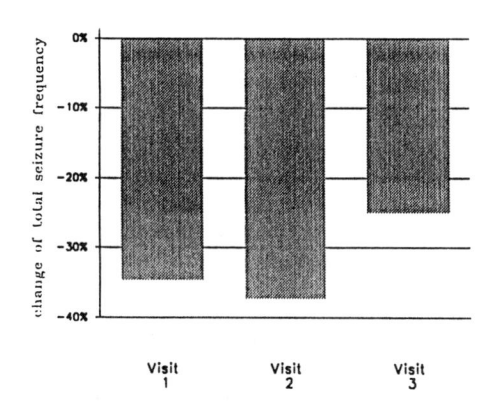

Figure 1
Relative change of total seizure frequency (mean) under vigabatrin compared to baseline after 1 month treatment (visit 1, 18 patients 2 g/day), after 2 months (visit 2 15 patients, 2,6 g/day) and after 3 months (visit 3, 10 patients, 2,9 g/day). A clear decrease of seizure frequency around 30 percent could be observed.

Because of the potential efficacy of vigabatrin in controlling previously refractory epilepsy and of the absence of evidence of significant toxicity in humans, the addition of vigabatrin is very useful in patients with drug-refractory partial epilepsy

Clobazam

We assessed the 1,5-benzodiazepine clobazam in a double-blind add-on trial in 20 patients with chronic complex partial seizures uncontrolled by maximally tolerable daily dosages of primary antiepileptic drugs. The number of seizures was lowered compared to placebo ($p < 0.01$). At the end of the 3 months 20 percent of the patients had a seizure reduction of more than 75 percent, and 20 percent were completely controlled. Unfortunately, tolerance to the antiepileptic effect of clobazam was noted in 56 percent. Mild sedation occurred in 40 percent. Despite these drawbacks, clobazam is an effective add-on drug for some patients with refractory focal epilepsy (Schmidt, et al, 1986)

Conclusions and summary

Vigabatrin and clonazepam effectively reduce the number of seizures in patients with refractory partial epilepsy. Each agent can be recommended for add-on treatment when standard drugs have failed. Previously intractable cases have become tractable when these drugs were added. Further progress can be expected with the introduction of available experimental models for intractable partial epilepsy in the evaluation of new compounds (Löscher and Schmidt, 1988).

1) Gale,K.: GABA in epilepsy: The pharmacologic basis. Epilepsia 30 Suppl.: 1-11,1989.
2) Löscher,W., Schmidt,D.: Which animal models should be used in the search for new antiepileptic drugs? A proposal based on experimental and clinical considerations. Epilepsy Research 2 :145-181,1988.
3) Schmidt,D.: Diagnostic and therapeutic management of intractable epilepsy :237-258,1986. in: Schmidt,D., Morselli, P.L.: Intractable Epilepsy: Experimental and Clinical Aspects, Raven Press, New York
4) Schmidt,D., Rhohde,M.,Wolf,P. et al.:Clobazam for refractory focal epilepsy. A controlled trial. Arch.Neurol.,43:824-826,1986.
5) Treiman,D.M.: Gamma vinyl GABA: Current role in the management of drug resistant epilepsy. Epilepsia 30 Suppl.:31-35,1989.

THE NATURE OF ADDICTION, WITH SPECIAL REFERENCE TO ALCOHOL

H. KALANT
Department of Pharmacology, University of Toronto, and Addiction Research Foundation of Ontario, Toronto, ON, Canada

Addiction has recently been defined as "a strongly established pattern of behaviour characterized by (i) the repeated self-administration of a drug in amounts which reliably produce reinforcing psychoactive effects, and (ii)great difficulty in achieving long-term voluntary cessation of such use, even when the user is strongly motivated to stop" (8). In this view, the essence of addiction lies in the pattern of drug use and the motivation for it; physical dependence, and harm to the user and to society, are seen as *consequences* of addiction, rather than as essential and defining features of it. Recent research has therefore focused on the mechanisms responsible for the reinforcing effects of such drugs.

Reinforcement or "reward" by drugs is thought to depend upon the same neuronal circuits that give rise to reinforcement by food, water, sex, and other factors essential for survival of the individual and the species (10). The same circuits are involved in the phenomenon of intracranial self-stimulation (ICSS) via implanted electrodes, and various addictive drugs have been found to lower the threshold current required to elicit ICSS. More commonly, however, reinforcement is studied in models involving either intravenous or intracerebral self-administration of drugs, or conditioned preferences for novel tastes or places that have been paired with the drug (4).

A large body of evidence supports the hypothesis that dopaminergic (DA) neurons with cell bodies in the ventral tegmental area A10, and axons projecting to the N. accumbens(NAcc), form a central link in the reinforcement circuit (11). However, there is also much evidence that there may be more than one circuit, mediating the reinforcing effects of different drugs (4). In addition, the activity of the DA neurons is either modulated by, or summated with, that of neurons releasing other transmitters, including norepinephrine (7), serotonin (1), endogenous opioids, angiotensin (3) and prostaglandins (2). The fact that cocaine and amphetamines are the most strongly reinforcing drugs, in animal models, is attributed to their ability to enhance DA release directly at the receptor sites in the NAcc. However, the very strong reinforcing action of heroin and morphine suggests that opioid receptors directly affect DA release, or interact strongly with DA receptors.

Unfortunately these concepts, developed largely on the basis of work with opiates and cocaine, do not apply nearly as well to alcohol. Ethanol is one of the most widely used psychoactive substances, and alcoholics outnumber opiate and cocaine addicts in North America by at least 10:1 (6). Yet animal studies have consistently shown that it is a weak reinforcer. It is extremely difficult to induce a rat to self-administer ethanol intravenously, in contrast to the ease with which cocaine or heroin self-injection is acquired. Most strains of rat will work (e.g., bar-pressing) to obtain ethanol by mouth (4), but place-conditioning studies show that the rat develops an aversion to the environment in which it voluntarily consumes the alcohol (9). Therefore the development of alcohol addiction must require the operation of other factors in addition to this weak pharmacological reinforcing action.

One factor is probably the development of greater tolerance to the aversive than to the reinforcing effects of the drug, so that even a weak reinforcing effect can become predominant (4). This is reflected by the gradual increase in alcohol preference, even in strains that originally reject alcohol, when they are exposed to it over prolonged periods. Another factor is a genetic predisposition (5) that may consist of relative resistance to the aversive effects of alcohol, or of relatively stronger reinforcing action than in most individuals. In addition, very important influences are exerted by social factors. For example, social approval for using alcohol may provide the main initial reinforcement until such time as tolerance permits the pharmacological mechanism to predominate. Relative price, ease of availability, and other environmental influences also contribute importantly to the probability of initiating or continuing the use of alcohol, as of any other drug, and they affect alcoholics as well as social drinkers (4).

Moreover, reinforcement operates in the social drinker as well as in the addict, yet the former is able to abstain voluntarily. Some additional factor must account for the transformation of reinforced behavior into addiction. Neither genetic nor social factors have so far explained the difference. Whether Pavlovian or operant conditioning principles can do so remains to be demonstrated.

REFERENCES

1. Carboni, E. et al. (1989): Psychopharmacology 97:175-178.
2. George, F.R. (1989): Ann. NY Acad. Sci. 559:382-391.
3. Grupp, L.A. (1988): Med. Hypoth. 24:11-19.
4. Kalant, H. (1989): In Molecular and Cellular Aspects of the Drug Addictions, A. Goldstein, ed., pp. 1-28. Springer-Verlag, New York.
5. Kiianmaa, K., Tabakoff, B. and Saito, T., eds. (1989): Genetic Aspects of Alcoholism, Finnish Foundation for Alcohol Studies, Helsinki.
6. NIDA Household Survey on Drug Abuse, Population Estimates (1988).
7. Opitz, K. (1990): Drug Alcohol Depend. 25:43-48.
8. Royal Society of Canada (1989): Tobacco, Nicotine, and Addiction. Royal Society, Ottawa.
9. Stewart, R.B., and Grupp, L.A. (1986): Pharmacol. Biochem. Behav. 24:1369-1375.
10. White, N.M., and Franklin, K.B.J., eds. (1989): The Neural Basis of Reward and Reinforcement (Special Issue), Neurosci. Biobehav. Rev. 13:59-186.
11. Wise, R.A. (1987): Pharmacol. Ther. 35:227-263.

NEUROCHEMISTRY OF OPIOID ADDICTION

A. HERZ, R. BALS-KUBIK, R. SPANAGEL and T.S. SHIPPENBERG
Department of Neuropharmacology, Max-Planck-Institute for
Psychiatry, Am Klopferspitz 18a, D-8033 Planegg, FRG.

The abuse liability of morphine and heroin, prototypic
μ-opioid receptor agonists, is well documented. These
agents produce euphoria in humans and function as positive
reinforcers in varies species. In contrast, κ-receptor
agonists and opioid antagonists such as naloxone lack such
effects and induce aversive states. Although both motivational effects of opioids appear to be centrally mediated,
the substrates mediating such actions are unclear.

This paper will review recent behavioral and biochemical
studies which have sought to identify the sites of action
and neurochemical substrates underlying the motivational
effects of opioids. Studies employing the conditioned place
preference paradigm, an animal model which permits the
detection of drug-induced motivational states, have shown
that selective μ- (DAMGO, morphine) or δ- (DPDPE) agonists
function as positive reinforcers, producing preferences for
an environment previously paired with their administration.
In contrast κ-agonists (U-50,488H, U-69593) and the dynorphin analog E 2078 produce place aversions. Aversive
effects are also observed in response to naloxone or the
selective μ-antagonist CTOP, whereas the blockade of δ- or
κ-receptors is without effect. The doses producing such
motivational effects are significantly lower following
intracerebroventricular as compared to systemic injection,
indicating a cerebral site of action.

Mapping studies in which opioids were microinjected into
discrete brain areas suggest an involvement of the mesolimbic dopamine (DA) system in both opioid-induced reward and
aversion. Injection of DAMGO into the ventral tegmental
area (VTA), the site of origin of the A10 DAergic system,
produces place preferences, whereas injection of κ-agonists
into the VTA or the n. accumbens (NAC) and the medial prefrontal cortex, major projection areas of the A10 neurons,
produces aversive effects. Injections of opioids into other
areas (striatum, substantia nigra) were without effect.
Further evidence for a role of this DA system in the motivational effects of opioids is suggested by studies using
6-OHDA and selective DA-receptor antagonists. Thus, 6-OHDA
lesions of NAC or the blockade of NAC D-1 by SCH-23390 but
not D-2 DA receptors abolish both the reinforcing and aversive effects of opioids.

Biochemical data also suggest a critical role of the
mesolimbic DA system in the motivational effects of opioids. In vivo microdialysis studies have shown that μ- and
δ-agonists increase the release of DA and its metabolites
from the NAC. The effective doses are those which produce

reinforcement in the place conditioning paradigm. In contrast, κ-agonists as well as E-2078, which induce aversive effects, markedly decrease the release of DA and its metabolites.

Taken together such data suggest that the mesolimbic DA system and, in particular the D-1 receptor, are critical for the expression of both opioid reward and aversion. In view of the opposing effects of opioids on DA-release it is suggested that an increase in DA release and a subsequent increase in D-1 DA receptor activity underlies the reinforcing and addictive properties of opioids. In contrast, a decrease in release, and a resulting decrease in D-1 DA receptor activity leads to aversive states.

TABLE 1   DOPAMINERGIC TRANSMISSION-RELATIONSHIP

Motivation

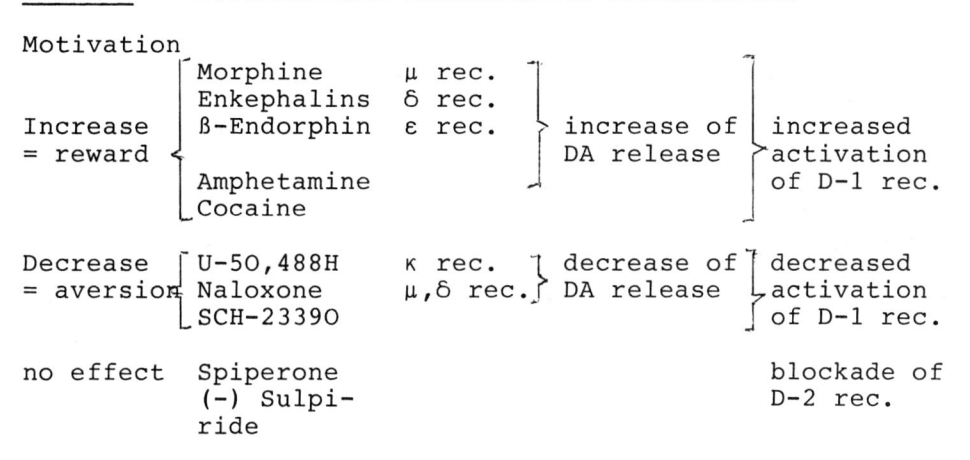

Increase = reward	Morphine Enkephalins ß-Endorphin Amphetamine Cocaine	μ rec. δ rec. ε rec.	increase of DA release	increased activation of D-1 rec.
Decrease = aversion	U-50,488H Naloxone SCH-23390	κ rec. μ,δ rec.	decrease of DA release	decreased activation of D-1 rec.
no effect	Spiperone (-) Sulpiride			blockade of D-2 rec.

Table 1 summarises these results. It includes also the psychostimulants D-amphetamine and cocaine. Amphetamine also increases DA release, whereas cocaine increases dopaminergic transmission by other mechanisms. The final result is an activation of D-1 DA receptors, giving rise for a general theory on the common mechanisms of action of addictive drugs (Wise and Bozarth, 1987).

READING LIST
1. Herz, A. and T.S. Shippenberg: Neurochemical aspects of addiction: opioids and other drugs of abuse. In: Molecular and Cellular Aspects of the Drug Addictions, Ed. A. Goldstein, Springer-Verlag New York 1989, 111-141.
2. Herz, A.: Bidirectional effects of opioids in motivational processes and the involvement of D-1 dopamine receptors. In: Problems of Drug Dependence, 1988. Ed. L.S. Harris, NIDA Research Monograph 90:17-26, 1989.
3. Wise, R.A. and Bozarth, M.A.: Psychomotor stimulant theory of addiction. Psychol. Rev. 94:469-492, 1987.

THE INVOLVEMENT OF ENDORPHINS IN DRUG SELFADMINISTRATION

J.M. VAN REE, M. KORNET and N. RAMSEY
Department of Pharmacology, Rudolf Magnus Institute, Medical Faculty, University of Utrecht, Vondellaan 6, 3521 GD Utrecht, The Netherlands

Endorphins (endogenous morphine-like substances) mimic opiates in inducing a variety of effects ranging from antinociception to behavioral activation. The presence of these peptides in pituitary and brain has raised the question whether these entities are involved in dependence on opiates and other addictive drugs. The dependence creating properties of drugs can reliably be determined by the procedure of drug selfadministration in experimental animals, establishing the reinforcing efficacy of drugs. It was found that β-endorphin is selfadministered in opiate-naive animals when administered intracerebroventricularly (4). This and other studies indicate that endorphins and especially β-endorphin have intrinsic rewarding properties. The involvement of endorphins in reward is supported by the attenuating influence of opiate antagonists on intracranial electrical selfstimulation, a procedure used to explore brain reward mechanisms. The inherent rewarding properties of endorphins and their modulatory role in brain reward have led to the idea that these peptides may be critical endogenous factors in addictive behavior in general. To gather information on this subject we have performed some studies in monkeys drinking alcohol and in rats selfadministering cocaine. We selected these drugs because they share with opiates the high abuse potential, but they are otherwise lacking the typical opiate-like effects.

ALCOHOL DRINKING IN MONKEYS

Male adult rhesus monkeys were given continuous access to three drinking bottles, two containing water/ethanol solutions with different concentrations and one always contained drinking water (2). The subjects started with drinking from the alcoholic beverages within 3 days and maintained alcohol drinking throughout the whole experimental period. After one year of uninterrupted drinking, the involvement of opioids in their drinking habit was assessed, by investigating the effect of naltrexone treatment under two experimental conditions. The two conditions were unrestricted access to the water/ethanol solutions and imposing a 2 days period of interruption in the supply of alcohol. Such a deprivation period led to an increase in ethanol consumption shortly after renewal of the alcohol supply ('catch-up drinking'). Graded doses of naltrexone, ranging from 0.02 to 1.5 mg.kg^{-1}, were tested under both conditions. In the unrestricted alcohol access condition naltrexone reduced ethanol intake during the first 2 hours after injection as well as during the next period of 17 hours. After interruption of alcohol supply, naltrexone reduced the observed increase in ethanol intake during the first hours after the renewed alcohol supply. Under this last condition the subjects were somewhat more sensitive to naltrexone. Clear differences were present between the effects of naltrexone on water drinking and ethanol intake.

COCAINE SELFADMINISTRATION IN RATS

Male Wistar rats equipped with a jugular cannula and partially food deprived, were tested for intravenous cocaine selfadministration. The animals could inject themselves by pressing a lever in an operant chamber during 6 hours per day for 5 consecutive days. Cocaine selfadministration was reliably acquired under the present conditions. Daily pretreatment with naltrexone decreased acquisition of cocaine selfadministration, when the rats had access to an intermediate unit dose of cocaine (1). The effect of naltrexone was not present in case of a high unit dose of cocaine. When rats were pretreated with naltrexone for 2 weeks before the start of the experimental sessions, the acquisition of cocaine selfadministration was enhanced. To further explore the significance of endorphins for drug dependence, the levels of β-endorphin immunoreactivity (βE-IR) were measured in plasma and parts of pituitary and brain of rats selfadministering cocaine or heroin as compared to animals offered saline (3). When rats were sacrificed immediately after the 5th experimental session, no marked and consistent changes in βE-IR were observed. But rats that were decapitated 18 h after this session, showed an increased concentration of βE-IR in plasma and decreased concentrations in the anterior lobe of the pituitary and in specific areas of the anterior limbic system of the brain. No differences were found between rats selfadministering cocaine or heroine.

CONCLUDING REMARKS

The present studies provide evidence that endorphins are involved in alcohol drinking in monkeys and in cocaine and heroin intravenous self-administration in rats. The data suggest that the endorphins play a modulatory role in the rewarding effects of addictive drugs. This may be expressed particularly under conditions of acquisition of drug dependence. The biochemical findings reveal that β-endorphin and related peptides in limbic brain regions may represent a neurochemical correlate for psychic dependence, a common feature of dependence on different addictive drugs and habits.

REFERENCES

1. De Vry, J., Donselaar, I. and Van Ree, J.M. (1989): Food deprivation and acquisition of intravenous cocaine self-administration in rats: Effect of naltrexone and haloperidol. J. Pharmacol. Exp. Ther., 251(2): 735-740.
2. Kornet, M., Goosen, C., Ribbens, L. and Van Ree, J.M. (1987): In New Perspectives in Pharmacological Sciences, F. Drago and J.M. Van Ree, eds., pp. 98-100, Italian Pharmacological Society.
3. Sweep, C.G.J., Wiegant, V.M., De Vry, J. and Van Ree, J.M. (1989): β-Endorphin in brain limbic structures as neurochemical correlate of psychic dependence on drugs. Life Sci., 44: 1133-1140.
4. Van Ree, J.M., Smyth, D.G. and Colpaert, F.C. (1979): Dependence creating properties of lipotropin C-fragment (β-endorphin): evidence for its internal control of behavior. Life Sci., 24: 495-502.

COCAINE ABUSE AND DEPENDENCE: PHARMACOLOGICAL EXPLORATIONS AND INTERVENTIONS

JEROME H. JAFFE, M.D.
National Institute on Drug Abuse, Rockville, Maryland, U.S.A.

In the United States, the cocaine epidemic of the past decade and the possibility of a new epidemic of amphetamine use has led to a significant increase in research funding aimed at advancing knowledge about the mechanisms by which these two classes of drugs produce their reinforcing and toxic effects, and developing pharmacological agents that might be useful in treating or preventing problems caused by their use. Research groups at the NIDA Addiction Research Center in Baltimore have employed a variety of methods to further these objectives, including studying the effects in rats and monkeys of pretreatment with potential therapeutic agents on patterns of self-administration of cocaine, cocaine congeners, and amphetamine-like drugs; receptor-binding assays; and combinations of these approaches. Clinical research included studies of the effects of cocaine on brain glucose metabolism as measured by positron emission tomography, observations of mood and endocrine effects during withdrawal, blind and double-blind clinical trials of amantadine, desipramine, and fluoxetine on cocaine users seeking treatment in an outpatient setting, and studies involving administration of cocaine to cocaine abusers. Only the latter will be summarized in this abstract.

In a series of studies with cocaine abusers who volunteered to be hospitalized on a research ward, Kumor and coworkers (1) found that the response to intravenous cocaine consists of two overlapping but separable subjective experiences - the "rush", a relatively intense but brief experience which decays within minutes even if plasma levels are maintained, and a longer lasting "high" (consisting of feelings of well being, a sense of increased power and sexuality) which generally persists if plasma levels are maintained, although it may be associated with increasing levels of anxiety and dysphoria. In double-blind studies we found that pretreatment with oral bromocriptine even at relatively high doses (5 mg) had very little effect on either the intensity of "rush" or the more persistent positive feelings of euphoria. However, we observed that although the subjects had relatively little "craving" for cocaine prior to the experimental session, the administration of cocaine (40 mg) resulted in increased craving for cocaine that seemed to peak at about 15 minutes after the cocaine, an effect not seen following the administration of saline. Cocaine-induced craving returned to baseline levels over the next 1 1/2 to 2 hours. Pretreatment with 2.5 mg of bromocriptine appeared to attenuate this cocaine-induced craving (2).

In another series of experiments, intramuscular haloperidol (8 mg 20 min prior to intravenous cocaine) produced only a modest attenuation of the "high" (feeling good, powerful, etc.) and had virtually no effect on "rush", although it did attenuate some of the cardiovascular actions of cocaine (3). This lack of effect may be related to too short an interval between pretreatment and cocaine challenge.

In a third series of studies, pretreatment with 10 mg of the calcium channel blocker nefedipine produced statistically significant reduction in the intensity of the "rush" but less marked reduction in the longer lasting euphoric effects. More interestingly, this dose of nefedipine appeared to attenuate the cocaine-induced craving.

In addition to its capacity to induce a pleasurable "rush", feelings of euphoria, and increased sense of power and sexuality, cocaine stimulates the urge to immediately repeat its use. This appears to be in contrast to drugs such as the opioids which at least for a brief period after use appear to induce satiation. After repeated use, some users develop still another motive for continued use - the avoidance of the fatigue, dysphoria, and depression associated with cessation ("crashing"). Thus more than one action of cocaine may be causally linked to its repetitive, compulsive use.

The findings in this short series of studies in which different drugs altered the effects of cocaine in distinct ways argue for examining a diverse range of agents for potential utility as therapeutic agents. Some of these may alter aspects of the acute reinforcing effects; others may affect the acute sense of craving; still others may attenuate the withdrawal syndrome; and still others may alter its toxicity without significantly affecting its reinforcing properties.

A summary of the potential therapeutic agents now under investigation by NIDA supported researchers will be presented.

REFERENCES:

1. Kumor, et al. Lack of cardiovascular tolerance during intravenous infusions of cocaine in man. Life Sciences 42:2063-2071, 1988.
2. Sherer, M.A. et al. Effects of intravenous cocaine are partially attenuated by haloperidol. Psychiat. Res. 27:117-125, 1989.
3. Jaffe, J.H. et al. Cocaine-induced cocaine craving. Psychopharmacology 97:59-64, 1989.

IS IT POSSIBLE TO DISSOCIATE MORPHINE ANALGESIA, TOLERANCE AND DEPENDENCE?

H. KANETO
Department of Pharmacology, Faculty of Pharmaceutical Sciences, Nagasaki University, Nagasaki 852, Japan.

Because of the tolerance/dependence liability, use of the drugs of clinical importance, such as morphine, barbiturates, ethanol, benzodiazepines, are strictly restricted. The aim of the present study is to search for the possibility to dissociate the analgesic action of morphine from its side effects, tolerance/dependence liability, and to extend the possibility to all the dependence liable drugs.

We have reported that daily concomitant treatment with morphine and a small dose of reserpine or adrenergic blockers, which neither affect the analgesic effect of morphine nor modify the brain level of catecholamines, completely suppressed the development of analgesic tolerance as long as the combined treatment was continued (4,5).

MATERIALS AND METHODS

Male mice of ddY strain weighing 23 -25 g were used. The analgesic effect was assessed by the tail pinch method, and the degree of tolerance was evaluated by comparing the daily changes in the analgesic effect of the test dose of morphine with that on the initial day. The degree of dependence was estimated by measuring the intensity of naloxone precipitated withdrawal signs according to the method of Kaneto et al. (2).

RESULTS

1. Dissociation of tolerance from physical dependence:
    In the animals treated daily with 10 mg/kg of morphine plus 10 mg/kg of phentolamine or propranolol for 5 days, in which the development of tolerance was completely suppressed, the withdrawal signs were precipitated as in the animals treated with morphine alone.

2. Dissociation of dependence from analgesic effect:
    To mask the analgesic effect of morphine, 1 mg/kg of naloxone was daily given 5 min prior to the injection of 10 mg/kg of morphine for 5 days. On the 6th day, 1 hr after the final dose of 10 mg/kg of morphine, animals were challenged with 1 mg/kg of naloxone. No significant difference in the intensity of the withdrawal signs was found between

the groups which were treated with morphine alone and morphine plus naloxone.

3. Dissociation of analgesic effect from tolerance:

Besides adrenergic blockers, the suppressive effect of cycloheximide on the development of tolerance has been reported by Cox et al. (1), and we also reconfirmed the effect (3). Recently, we are trying another approach to the phenomenon.

a) Stress exposure

In the animals daily exposed to electric foot shock stress (0.2 mA, 1 sec duration, 0.2 Hz for 15 min) 5 min after injection of morphine, the development of tolerance was suppressed without influencing the analgesic effect.

b) Anti-arginine vasopressin (AVP) antiserum

Intracerebroventricular injection of anti-AVP antiserum (100 fold diluted serum, 0.1 ul/mouse) 30 min prior to morphine injection did not affect the analgesic effect but completely suppressed the development of tolerance.

CONCLUSION

In addition to the previous finding that the analgesic effect of morphine is separable from tolerance liability, by reserpine, adrenergic blockers, cycloheximide etc, in the present experiments, the dissociation was demonstrated by stress exposure and by the i.c.v. injection of anti-AVP antiserum. Similarly, the dissociation of analgesic action from dependence, and also tolerance from physical dependence have been suggested.

Thus, the possibility to dissociate the principal action of morphine from its side effects, tolerance/dependence liability, and the similarity and discrepancy of the underlying mechanisms of the effects, and also the extension of the possibility to other dependence liable drugs will be discussed.

REFERENCES

1. Cox, B. M. et al. (1968): Br. J. Pharmac. Chemother., 33: 245-258.
2. Kaneto, H. et al. (1973): Japan. J. Pharmacol., 23: 701-707.
3. Kaneto, H. et al. (1982): Life Sci., 31: 2351-2354.
4. Kaneto, H. and Kihara, T. (1986): Japan. J. Pharmacol., 42: 169-173.
5. Kihara, T. and Kaneto, H. (1986): Japan. J. Pharmacol., 42: 419-423.

STRESS-INDUCED CHANGES IN BRAIN NORADRENERGIC SYSTEM AND EMOTIONS: NEUROCHEMICAL MECHANISM OF ANXIOLYTIC DRUGS

M. TANAKA, Y. YOSHIDA, H. YOKOO, T. TANAKA and A. TSUDA
Department of Pharmacology, Kurume University School of Medicine, Kurume 830, Japan.

A variety of stressful stimuli have been well known to cause increases in noradrenaline (NA) release in the brain regions of the rodents (1, 5). A hypothesis has been proposed that neuronal activation of the brain NA system, in particular, the locus coeruleus (LC), has an important role for provocation of anxiety and/or fear (4, 5). This report focuses on characterizations of increases in NA release in the rat brain regions caused by several different stresses and their pharmacological modifications by anxiolytics.

SUBJECT AND METHOD

Male Wistar rats were subjected to the study excluding the two behavioral studies, where male PVG/c hooded rats or Sprague-Dawley (SD) rats were used. In the neurochemical studies, levels of NA and its major metabolite, 3-methoxy-4-hydroxyphenylethyleneglycol sulfate (MHPG-SO4) in the brain regions of the rats exposed to various stresses and treated with the drugs related to anxiety, were measured by the fluorometric method developed by us (2). In the intracranial microdialysis study, the probe, the tip of which consisted of a U-shaped dialysis membrane was implanted into the anterior hypothalamus under pentobarbital anesthesia and the microdialysis was performed 24 hrs after operation. NA levels in the dialysates collected for every 20 min were determined by the HPLC-ECD system (8).

RESULTS AND DISCUSSION

Immobilization stress for 1 hr caused significant increases in MHPG-SO4 levels in the extended brain regions including the hypothalamus, amygdala and LC region, which accompanied the reductions of NA levels in most regions. The result suggests that increases in NA release occur in these regions by the stress. This was confirmed by the fact that NA contents in the dialysates were significantly elevated by the same stress. Diazepam at 2.0 or 5.0 mg/kg, an anxiolytic of benzodiazepines, injected i.p. before stress exposure, significantly attenuated not only increases in the metabolite levels in the hypothalamus, amygdala, hippocampus, cerebral cortex and LC region but also emotional responses of stressed rats such as vocalization and defecation. These attnuating effects were antagonized by Ro 15-1788 at 10 mg/kg, an antagonist of benzodiazepines. The intracranial microdialysis study also exhibited that increases in NA contents in the dialysates caused by stress were significantly attenuated by pretreatment with diazepam at 5.0 mg/kg, which did not affect the basal NA levels in the dialysates by itself.

Although pretreatment with naloxone at 5.0 mg/kg injected s.c., an antagonist of opioids, resulted in enhancement of both increases in NA release in the hypothalamus, amygdala and thalamus and emotional responses such as defecation and struggling, morphine at 6.0 mg/kg injected s.c. and β-endorphin at 10 μg and Met-enkephalin at 100-200 μg injected i.c.v. significantly attenuated both neurochemical and behavioral changes caused by stress. Furthermore, by the two emotional stresses, where emotional factors rather than physical ones were more predominantly involved, i.e., psychological stress where the rats were exposed to emotional responses shown by other electrically-shocked rats and the conditioned fear where the rats were replaced in the box where they had received electric shock 24 hr before, increases in NA release occurred preferentially in the hypothalamus, amygdala and LC region. An α2-antagonist, yohimbine at 0.5-2.0 mg/kg, which caused increases in NA release in the extended brain regions, and ethyl-β-carboline-3-carboxylate (β-CCE), which possess anxiogenic actions, increase the conditioned defensive burying of PVG/c hooded rats and the straw-climbing behavior of SD rats in Porsolt's forced swimming test modified by us (3). These two behavioral parameters are cosidered to be closely related to anxiety of the animals (3, 7). Furthermore, β-CCE at 10 mg/kg injected twice i.p., significantly increased NA release in the brain regions such as the hypothalamus, amygdala and LC region. Furthermore, our recent study indicates that there exists a critical period of the drug administration for appearance of attenuating effects of Met-enkephalin; the peptide injected, only immediately before but not 10 min after stress exposure, could attenuate stress-induced increases in NA release and emotional responses (6).

Together with these findings, the marked increases in NA release in such brain regions as the hypothalamus, amygdala and LC region, lead to, in part, provocation of hyperemotional responses of the animals such as anxiety and/or fear. Anxiogenic drugs such as β-carbolines and yohimbine also increase NA release in these regions via benzodiazepine receptors and α2-adrenoceptors, respectively, which results in induction of anxiety and/or fear. In contrast, anxiolytic drugs of benzodiazepines, morphine, and some of opioid peptides such as β-endorphin and Met-enkephalin, attenuate increases in NA release in these regions caused by stress or anxiogenic drugs via bezodiazepine receptors and opioid receptors, respectively, which results in the relief of anxiety and/or fear in the animals exposed to stress or treated with anxiogenic drugs.

REFERENCES

1. Glavin, G.B., (1985): Behav. Neurosci. Rev., 9: 233-243.
2. Kohno, Y., et al., (1979): Anal. Biochem., 97: 352-358.
3. Nishimura, H., et al., (1988): Physiol. Behav., 43: 665-668.
4. Redmond, D.E.Jr. (1987): Psychopharmacology: The Third Generation of Progress; H.Y. Meltzer, ed., pp. 967-975, Raven Press, New York.
5. Tanaka, M., et al., (1983): Brain Res., 275: 105-115.
6. Tanaka, M., et al., (1989): Pharmacol. Biochem Behav., 32: 791-795.
7. Tsuda, A., et al., (1988): Psychobiology, 16: 213-217.
8. Yokoo, H., et al., (1990): Experientia, 46: 290-292.

CENTRAL DOPAMINE INVOLVEMENT IN STRESS-INDUCED GASTRIC PATHOLOGY

G.B. Glavin*
Department of Pharmacology and Therapeutics and Department of Surgery
University of Manitoba, Winnipeg, Manitoba, CANADA, R3E 0W3

We report herein new evidence that dopamine (DA) exerts gastroprotection specifically through peripheral DA1 and central D1 receptor subtypes. A role for DA in the pathogenesis of ulcer disease was suggested by others (1,2,3). DA and its agonists protect the gut while DA antagonists exacerbate gastric ulcers and acid secretion. Further evidence suggests that DA1 receptors are involved in these effects, since Sandrock (4) showed DA receptors in rat gut but no [3H]haloperidol (DA2) binding. Hernandez et al. (3) showed DA receptors in human stomach and, using competition binding studies found a higher affinity for SKF38393 (DA1) than for DA2 ligands. Our work with selective DA agonists and antagonists in vivo further supports DA1 receptor mediation of these effects and are shown in Table 1. That DA2 receptors are minimally involved in the gastrointestinal effects of DA is suggested by comparing relative potencies:

Agonists: SKF38393 >>> DA >N0437 > N0434 > Quinpirole
Antagonists: SCH23390 >> Domperidone >>> Eticlopride = YM09151-2 = sulpiride

We conclude that compounds active at the DA1 subtype are more effective at reducing (agonists) or exacerbating (antagonists) gastric ulcers than are compounds selective for the DA2 subtype. Evidence also exists for central DA receptor involvement in mediating peripheral gastroprotection and suggests D1 receptor mediation. DA compounds were given icv and Table 2 shows larger effects when the compounds were given icv than peripherally, with the exception of l-dopa. SKF38393 (D1 agonist) and SCH23390 (D1 antagonist) were more potent at reducing and worsening, respectively, ulcers that were D2 compounds. We suggest that D1/DA1 receptors are the functionally important species mediating gastroprotection.   *SUPPORTED BY THE MRC.

REFERENCES

1. Glavin, G. Activity of selective dopamine DA1 and DA2 agonists and antagonists on experimental gastric lesions and gastric acid secretion. J. Pharmacol. Exp. Ther. 251(2): 726-730, 1989.
2. Glavin, G. et al. Effects of dopamine agonists and antagonists on gastric acid secretion and stress responses in rats. Life Sci. 41: 1397-1408, 1987.
3. Hernandez, D. et al. Increased dopamine receptor binding in duodenal mucosa of duodenal ulcer patients Dig. Dis. Sci. 34: 543-547, 1989.
4. Sandrock, A. Identification and binding properties of dopamine receptors in the rat gut: Possible role in experimental duodenal ulcerogenesis. Gastroenterol. 80: 1362, 1981.

TABLE 1: Dopaminergic Compounds Tested for Activity in the Gut

COMPOUND	ROUTE OF ADMINISTRATION	EFFECT ON STRESS ULCERS	EFFECT ON ETHANOL ULCERS	EFFECT ON GASTRIC ACID SECRETION
dopamine	ip	↓	↓	↓
domperidone	icv,ip	↑	0	↑
SKF 38393	icv,ip,intra-nigral intra-mesocortical	↓	↓	↓
SCH 23390	icv,ip,intra-nigral intra-mesocortical	—	↑	↑
N 0434	ip	↓	↓	↓
N 0437	ip	↓	↑↓	↓
YM 09151-2	ip	-	-	-
eticlopride	ip	-	-	-
quinpirole (LY17155)	ip	-	-	-
SKF 83566	ip	↑	↑	↑
sulpiride	ip	↑	-	-
haloperidol	ip	↑	↑	↑
pimozide	ip	↑	↑	↑
l-deprenyl	icv,ip	↓	↓	↓
l-dopa	icv,ip	↓	↓	↓
bromocriptine	ip	↓	↓	↓
bupropion	ip	↓	↓	↓
metoclopramide	ip	-	0	↑
methylphenidate	ip	↓	↓	↓
p-hydroxymethylphenidate	icv,ip	↓	↓	↓

ip = intraperitoneal; icv = intracerebroventricular; ↑ = increased;
↓ = decreased; - = no effect; 0 = not studied; ↑↓ = biphasic effect

TABLE 2: Central Versus Peripheral Effects of Dopaminergic Compounds on Gastric Ulcerogenesis

Compound	Site of Action	Percent Change in Ulcer Length-icv	Percent Change in Ulcer Length-ip
l-deprenyl	MAO$_B$ inhibitor	94.3% ↓	81.4% ↓
l-dopa	precursor	74.4% ↓	73.1% ↓
SKF38393	D$_1$/DA$_1$ agonist	94.6% ↓	69.9% ↓
SCH23390	D$_1$/DA$_1$ antagonist	165.8% ↑	133.5% ↑
N-0437	D$_2$/DA$_2$ agonist	7.1% ↓	18.2% ↓
Eticlopride	D$_2$/DA$_2$ antagonist	11.3% ↓	21.1% ↓
p-hydroxymethyl-phenidate	release enhancer	68.9% ↓	57.6% ↓

THE IMPACT OF STRESS AND INJURY ON CENTRAL DOPAMINERGIC ACTIVITY

MICHAEL J. ZIGMOND, KRISTEN A. KEEFE, GRETCHEN L. SNYDER, EDWARD M. STRICKER and ELIZABETH D. ABERCROMBIE

Department of Behavioral Neuroscience and Center for Neuroscience, University of Pittsburgh, Pittsburgh, PA 15260, U.S.A.

It generally is assumed that catecholamines play an important role in the physiological and behavioral responses to stress. This relation is best documented for the peripheral nervous system. However, supporting evidence exists for the CNS, as well. For example, the noradrenergic neurons that project to forebrain appear to respond to stressful stimuli with an increase in firing rate and norepinephrine turnover (1,5,9). In addition, stress-induced changes occur within the dopamine (DA)-containing neurons of the mesocortical and mesolimbic projections. In contrast, both electrophysiological and biochemical data suggest that stress does not affect DA neurons within the nigrostriatal bundle (13,15).

Partial injury to catecholaminergic neural systems also affects activity in residual neurons. Thus, lesions of both peripheral and central catecholaminergic systems result in an apparent increase in catecholamine turnover within those neurons that remain (2,6,7,12). Since the capacity of neurons to increase their release of transmitter may be limited, animals whose release of catecholamine is elevated in response to injury may be unable to respond normally to a physiological or behavioral challenge. This may explain the familiar observation that animals that have sustained lesions of the sympathoadrenal system are vulnerable to stress (7).

Like sympathectomized animals, rats with lesions of the nigrostriatal bundle are impaired in their response to stressors (10,14). This finding raises the possibility that nigrostriatal DA neurons indeed are affected by stress, despite previous findings to the contrary. In this report we summarize our recent observations (8, 11) concerning the interaction between stress and injury on dopaminergic activity in the striatum.

METHODS

<u>Animals</u>: Adult male Sprague-Dawley rats were used throughout this series of experiments. They were housed one per cage and provided with food and water ad libitum. Lesions were produced using 6-hydroxydopamine (6-HDA) placed along the medial forebrain bundle or into the lateral ventricles at least 1 mo prior to biochemical measurements.

<u>In vivo dialysis</u>: Dialysis probes were constructed and implanted unilaterally into the medial portion of the rostral striatum (1). CSF was perfused through the probes (1.5 ul/min) and samples were analyzed for DA by HPLC with electrochemical detection.

<u>In vitro efflux</u>: Coronal slices (350 um) of striatum were superfused (100 ul/min) with a modified Krebs bicarbonate buffer and effluent was analyzed for DA (12). After a baseline was established, slices were exposed to electrical field stimulation at 2-12 Hz using a constant current, bipolar pulse.

RESULTS

<u>In vivo studies</u>: The DA content of extracellular fluid under basal conditions was 38 $\pm$ 4.3 pg per 20 ul fraction as determined by microdialysis. Intermittent tail shock (1 mA) delivered for 30 min increased DA overflow in striatum by 25% (to 47.5 pg/20 ul). Animals with 6-HDA-induced brain lesions had tissue DA levels that were only 12% of control; however, extracellular DA values were 26% of control (10 pg/20 ul). This

resulted in a 2-fold increase in the ratio of extracellular DA to tissue DA. Since tissue DA content appears to reflect the number of DA terminals present, these results suggest an increase in the net contribution of transmitter to extracellular fluid by each remaining DA terminal. As in the case of intact animals, tail shock increased extracellular DA in the striatum of lesioned animals. The increase was significantly larger than observed in intact animals when it was expressed as a percent of pre-stress baseline (67% increase; from 10 to 17 pg/20 ul). However, the increase failed to raise extracellular DA levels to the range seen in control animals subjected to the same stressor.

In vitro studies: DA was released spontaneously from superfused striatal slices at a rate of $0.8 \pm .1$ ng/mg protein per 15 min. Fifteen min of field stimulation at 2 Hz increased DA efflux 4-fold resulting in a total DA overflow above baseline of $2.3 \pm .3$ ng/mg protein. Increasing stimulation frequency up to 12 Hz caused a linear increase in the rate of DA efflux. 6-HDA treatment reduced striatal DA content to 15% of control but reduced stimulation-evoked overflow of striatal DA to 58% of control, resulting in a 4-fold increase in fractional DA overflow. The relative increase in fractional DA overflow remained constant up to 8 Hz; however, at 12 Hz stimulation the higher rate of DA overflow could no longer be sustained.

DISCUSSION

These results suggest that the net amount of DA released in striatum can be increased in vivo by exposing animals to an environmental stressor. The failure of previous investigations to reveal this phenomenon may reflect the increased sensitivity obtained by measuring changes in extracellular DA concentration rather than by utilizing conventional post-mortem indices of DA turnover.

Efflux per terminal also appears to increase after partial damage to these neurons as well as by environmental stimulation. However, the capacity of individual terminals to respond to an environmental stimulus as measured by microdialysis did not appear to be compromised by lesioning. In fact, the stress-induced change in extracellular DA was increased in lesioned animals. On the other hand, high affinity reuptake of DA, which is a major determinant of in vivo extracellular DA concentration, is greatly reduced by 6-HDA (4,12). Thus, after 6-HDA-induced lesions, the fraction of the DA released in vivo that is collected via the microdialysis probe is greatly increased (4), and this may account for the apparent increase in the responsiveness to stress. It remains possible, therefore, that stress-induced impairments in behavioral function may reflect a failure of residual DA neurons to increase their release of transmitter by an amount comparable to that observed in control animals.

REFERENCES

1. Abercrombie E.D., Keller, R.W., & Zigmond, M.J. (1988): Neurosci., 27: 897-904.
2. Abercrombie, E.D. et al. (1989): J. Neurochem., 52: 1655-1658.
3. Abercrombie, E.D. & Zigmond, M.J. (1989): J. Neurosci., 9: 4062-4067.
4. Abercrombie, E.D. Bonatz, A.E., & Zigmond, M.J. (1990): Brain Res., in press.
5. Abercrombie, E.D. & Jacobs, B.L. (1987): J. Neurosci., 7: 2837-2843.
6. Acheson, A.L. & Zigmond, M.J. (1981): J. Neurosci. 1: 493-504.
7. Fluharty, S.J. et al. (1985): J. Pharmacol. Exp. Ther., 235: 354-360.
8. Keefe, K.A. et al. (1989): Soc. Neurosci. Abstract. 15: 558.
9. Korf, J. Aghajanian, G.K., & Roth, R.H. (1973): Neuropharmacol., 12: 933-938.
10. Snyder, A.M., Stricker, E.M. & Zigmond, M.J. (1985): Ann. Neurol. 18: 544-551.
11. Snyder, G.L., Keller, R.W., & Zigmond, M.J. (1990): J. Pharm. Exp. Ther., in press.
12. Stachowiak, M.K. et al. (1987): J. Neurosci. 7: 1648-1654.
13. Strecker, R.E. & Jacobs, B.L. (1985): Brain Res., 361: 339-359.
14. Stricker, E.M. & Zigmond, M.J. (1974): J. Comp. Physiol. Psychol. 86: 973-994.
15. Thierry, A.M. Tassin, J.P., Blanc, G., and Glowinski, J. (1976): Nature, 263: 242-244.

THE ACTION OF STRESS ON GABAERGIC TRANSMISSION

A. CONCAS, M. SERRA, E. SANNA and G. BIGGIO
Department of Experimental Biology, Chair of Pharmacology,

University of Cagliari, Italy

The discovery that anxiolytic and anxiogenic drugs such as benzodiazepines and ß-carbolines have specific recognition sites at the level of the $GABA_A$ receptor complex has allowed to suggest that GABAergic synapses play a major role in the physiopathology of stress and anxiety (1). Accordingly, a stressful condition decreases the density of low affinity $GABA_A$ receptors (2) and alters the function of the GABA dependent chloride channel (3,4,5). In particular, we found that the binding of t-butylbicyclophosphorothionate (^{35}S-TBPS) to the GABA-dependent chloride channel is increased in the cerebral cortex of rats exposed to foot-shock stress. This effect is mimicked by the "in vitro" addition to cortical membrane preparations of anxiogenic ß-carbolines and GABA antagonists and reversed by anxiolytic benzodiazepines and GABA mimetics. These findings suggest that the stress-induced increase of ^{35}S-TBPS binding in the rat cerebral cortex may reflect a decrease in the function of the GABA-dependent chloride channel. To further verify this conclusion we studied the effect of foot-shock stress on ^{35}S-TBPS binding in the brain of rats previously treated with isoniazid or with the ß-carboline derivative FG 7142, two inibitors of the GABAergic transmission known to decrease the availability or the interaction of GABA at the receptor site, respectively.

METHODS

Male Sprague Dawley rats weighing 180-200 g were used. Isoniazid, FG 7142, alprazolam and ethanol were given 60, 15, 30 and 40 min before sacrifice, respectively. Foot-shock (0.2 mA every 500 ms with 500 ms duration) was delivered continuously for 5 min before sacrifice. ^{35}S-TBPS binding was performed in unwashed cortical membrane preparation as previously described (3).

RESULTS

Foot-shock stress like the "in vivo" administration of isoniazid and FG 7142 increased ^{35}S-TBPS binding in the rat cerebral cortex. When foot-shock was delivered to rats previously injected with isoniazid or FG 7142 ^{35}S-TBPS bin-

TABLE 1: ACTION OF GABAERGIC DRUGS ON STRESS-INDUCED INCREASE OF ^{35}S-TBPS BINDING IN THE RAT CEREBRAL CORTEX

TREATMENT	^{35}S-TBPS BINDING (% OF CONTROL)	
	Control	Foot-shock
Solvent	100 ± 4	130 ± 7*
Isoniazid (300 mg/kg s.c.)	136 ± 8*	173 ± 5**
FG 7142 (12.5 mg/kg i.p.)	128 ± 6*	168 ± 8**
Alprazolam (0.5 mg/kg i.p.)	78 ± 5*	105 ± 6**
Ethanol (1 g/kg p. os)	71 ± 5*	106 ± 7**

*$p < 0.05$ vs control.
**$p < 0.05$ vs foot-shock.

ding was increased by 73 and 68% above the control value, respectively. On the other hand, the effect of foot-shock was completely abolished by pretreatment of rats with alprazolam or ethanol which per se enhanced ^{35}S-TBPS binding.

DISCUSSION

The present study provides additional insights into the molecular events involved in the action of stress on the function of the GABA$_A$ receptor complex. The results showing that the increase of ^{35}S-TBPS binding elicited by both isoniazid and FG 7142, is enhanced and not reduced by foot-shock stress indicate that this treatment has an inhibitory influence on the function of GABAergic synapses. This conclusion is supported by the finding that the effect of stress is completely antagonized by the previous administration to rats of alprazolam and ethanol. Our data demonstrate that the increase of ^{35}S-TBPS binding in the rat brain is a sensitive biochemical marker of a functional inhibition of the GABAergic synapses.

REFERENCES

1. Biggio, G. and Costa, E. (1983) Benzodiazepine Recognition Site Ligands: Biochemistry and Pharmacology. Raven Press, New York.
2. Biggio, G. et al., (1981) Brain Res. 229: 363-369.
3. Concas, A. et al. (1988) J. Neurochem. 51: 1868-1876.
4. Serra, M. et al. (1989) Neurosci. Res. Comm. 4: 41-50.
5. Drugan, R.C. et al. (1989) Brain Res. 487: 45-51.

DOPAMINE AND NEUROPEPTIDES INTERACTIONS IN SLEEP DEPRIVATION

W.FRATTA, P.FADDA, M.C.MARTELLOTTA AND G.L.GESSA
"B.B.Brodie" Department of Neuroscience, University of Cagliari, Italy.

Several evidence indicate that sleep deprivation causes behavioral changes in animals and humans. The platform technique, which consists of keeping the animals on a small platform (7 cm diameter) surrounded by water for 72h is the most widely used sleep deprivation method in the rat. Besides its specific action on sleep, this method involves several factors such as isolation, immobilization, falling into the water, soaking and others which produce a heavy stress in the animals. This experimental model must therefore be considered mainly as a stress model of which sleep deprivation is one factor. A peculiar feature of this model in that, following the period of sleep deprivation, the rat does not fall asleep once returned to its home cage as could be expected but shows a constant period of wakefulness. This period which lasts 30-35 min. under our experimental conditions is characterized by a high degree of motor activity and exploratory behavior, increased alertness and reativity toward enviromental stimuli. For all the above reasons we have regarded this particular feature as a model of stress-induced insomnia (1). In order to understand the possible biochemical mechanisms involved in this phenomenon, we have investigated whether different treatments known to affect opiatergic, dopaminergic neurotrasmission could specifically interfere with this behavior.

RESULTS

As shown in table 1, the administration of Naloxone to rats at the end of 72 h. of sleep deprivation significantly reduced the sleep latency. On the contrary, the administration of morphine, ß-Endorphine and DADLE markedly increased the sleep latency. L-Sulpiride did not produce any significant effect, while SCH 23390 induced a great reduction in the sleep latency. On the contrary the administration of SKF 38393 markedly prolonged sleep latency.

DISCUSSION

The present resuls indicate that excitement and insomnia wihich immediately follow sleep deprivation in rats are related to hyperactivity of opiatergic and dopaminergic

TABLE 1: EFFECT OF DIFFERENT TREATMENTS ON SLEEP LATENCY IN SLEEP DEPRIVED RATS

Treatment	Dose (mg/Kg)	Sleep latency (min.)
Saline	--	32.4 ± 0.9
Naloxone	1	22.0 ± 3.5*
Naloxone	10	14.7 ± 3.1*
Morphine	1	71.2 ± 4.3*
Morphine	5	112.3 ± 5.0*
β-Endorphin	0.002 ~	83.7 ± 5.3*
DADLE	0.001 ~	51.8 ± 5.2*
CRF	0.001 ~	60.1 ± 1.9*
L-Sulpiride	25	29.0 ± 1.8
SCH 23390	0.003	21.0 ± 0.6*
SCH 23390	0.010	16.0 ± 1.0*
SCH 23390	0.030	13.0 ± 0.7*
SKF 38393	10	109.0 ± 4.1*

Sleep latency: time from the end of sleep deprivation period to the first episode of sleep.* $P < 0.01$ in respect to saline values (student's "t" test) ~ mg/rat i.c.v.

systems. Dopaminergic control, specifically mediated through D_1 type receptors, was evident. In fact, L-Sulpiride, a selective receptor blocker, was ineffective up to 25 mg/Kg while the D_1 selective antagonist SCH 23390 seemed to be the most potent among the drugs tested since as little as 3 µg/Kg was significantly active. Further evidence for a specific role of the D_1 receptor is given by the results obtained with the selective D_1 agonist SKF 38393 which markedly prolonged the sleep latency in sleep deprived rats showing that the opposite effect induced by SCH 23390 could be obstained by stimulation of the D_1 receptors. Furthermore we found (2) that an increased number of D_1 receptors associated with an increased Dopamine-stimulated adenylate cyclase activity was present in the limbic system of rats immediatly after the sleep deprivation period. These data suggest an active role of opioids and limbic D_1 receptors in the generation of arousal and behavioral changes related to sleep deprivation induced stress.

REFERENCES

1. Fratta W., Collu M., Martellotta M.C., Pichiri M., Muntoni F. and Gessa G.L.; Stress-induced insomnia: opioid-dopamine interactions. Eur. J. Pharmacol. 142,437-440; 1987

2. Demontis M.G.,Fadda P.,Devoto P.,Martellotta M.C.,and Fratta W., Sleep deprivation increases ³[H] SCH 23390 binding and DA-stimulated adenylate cyclase in the rat limbic system. Neurosc. Lett. 1990 (Submitted)

CNS TARGETS FOR ACTH: THEIR POTENTIAL ROLE IN STRESS RESPONSES

J.A.D.M. TONNAER, W.J. FLORIJN*, T. DE BOER and D.H.G. VERSTEEG*
Scientific Development Group, Organon International B.V., Oss;
*Rudolf Magnus Institute, State University, Utrecht, The Netherlands

Activation of the hypothalamic-pituitary-adrenocortical (HPA) system is considered a major component of the stress response as classically defined by Selye. Noxious sensory stimuli are conveyed to the paraventricular nucleus of the hypothalamus via spinal and cranial fibers, whereas emotional stimuli reach the hypothalamus through limbic forebrain projections (6). Catecholaminergic mechanisms in the paraventricular nucleus mediate the release of CRF into the portal vessels of the median eminence which, in turn, facilitates the release of the POMC-derived peptide ACTH from the pituitary. ACTH's endocrine function involves the release of glucocorticoids from the adrenal cortex. The corticoids shut off the HPA activation via feedback mechanisms at the level of the pituitary, hypothalamus and higher CNS circuitries.

Widespread POMC- and ACTH-containing projections in the CNS are found in and outside the hypothalamus. The cerebral ACTH levels appear to be regulated independently of the HPA-axis as they are unaltered following hypophysectomy or adrenalectomy. Moreover, chronic treatments with corticosterone or dexamethasone do not affect ACTH concentrations in the CNS (see 1). Reports on the effects of stress on brain ACTH are scarce and inconsistent. Acute stress depletes ACTH levels in the origin of the major CNS projections, i.e. the arcuate nucleus of the hypothalamus. This has been interpreted to reflect extensive ACTH release (5). The suggestion of stress-induced release of brain ACTH is supported by behavioural syndromes such as the grooming response. Grooming, stretching and yawning constitute a behavioural repertoire which is markedly elicited by ICV injections of ACTH (see 1). The short latency to the induction of grooming following local application in the brain, the lack of grooming after systemic administration, and the grooming-inducing potential of ACTH fragments which have lost steroidogenic properties suggest that a brain-specific mechanism mediates this behaviour. The striking similarity between the ACTH-evoked syndrome and novelty-induced grooming points to a role of endogenous brain ACTH in the latter stress-related behaviour. This is further strengthened by the observation that novelty-induced grooming is inhibited by ICV injections of antiserum against ACTH (1).
Brain ACTH-peptides may also influence the regulation of the HPA axis at the level of the hippocampus. Thus, chronic treatment of aged rats with a non-steroidogenic ACTH analogue influences the balance of hippocampal gluco- and mineralocorticoid receptors, which is thought to be involved in the disturbed HPA activity of these animals (7).

The molecular mechanisms by which ACTH might affect brain processes are far from understood but various possibilities have been proposed. Early work has pointed to influences on RNA synthesis. However, these studies are inconclusive as they did not differentiate between nuclear, ribosomal or messenger RNA. Structure-activity relationship studies and behavioural observations suggest effects on protein synthesis as a common link in ACTH- and stress-induced grooming. In vitro studies indicate that ACTH-derived peptides exhibit potential to modulate the phosphorylation of the phosphoprotein B50, probably via a direct inhibition of protein kinase C. The structure-activity relationship closely resembles that of the ACTH-related grooming response. Similar structure-activity relationships and pharmacological evidence point to the involvement of opiate, cholinergic and dopaminergic mechanisms in ACTH-induced grooming and yawning (see 1,8).

Various reports suggest that dopaminergic mechanisms are activated under acute stress conditions (2,4). Thus, both ACTH- and stress-induced grooming are inhibited by DA antagonists (see 1). A potentially direct influence on DA systems by ACTH is evidenced by our work showing that ACTH-derived peptides interfere with the in vitro binding of DA ligands to D2 receptors. These effects are found in various brain regions which contain D2 sites, and are independent of variables such as membrane lipid fluidity and the coupling state of the receptor. The structure-activity relationship resembles that seen in ACTH-induced grooming, but is clearly distinct from the structure-activity relationship as found for binding to recently discovered brain binding sites for radiolabelled ACTH (3). The interaction of ACTH with D2 binding sites is of higher potency than that with D1, 5-HT, muscarinic or histaminergic binding sites. We conclude from these studies that direct interference with dopaminergic binding sites may mediate the central actions of ACTH in acute stress responses.

REFERENCES

1. Dunn, A.J. (1984): In Peptides, Hormones and Behavior, C.B. Nemeroff and A.J. Dunn, eds., pp. 273-348. Spectrum Publications, Inc, New York.
2. Dunn, A.J. (1989): In Stress: Neurochemical and Humoral Mechanisms, G.R. Van Loon et al., eds., pp. 79-97. Gordon and Breach Science Publishers, New York.
3. Hnatowich, M.R. et al. (1989): Can. J. Physiol. Pharmacol. 67: 568-576.
4. Nagatsu, T. et al. (1989): In Stress: Neurochemical and Humoral Mechanisms, G.R. Van Loon et al., eds., pp. 43-51. Gordon and Breach Science Publishers, New York.
5. Palkovits, M. (1984): In Stress: The Role of Catecholamines and Other Neurotransmitters, E. Usdin, R. Kvetnansky and J. Axelrod, eds., pp.75-80. Gordon and Breach Science Publishers, New York.
6. Palkovits, M. (1989): In Stress: Neurochemical and Humoral Mechanisms, G.R. Van Loon et al., eds., pp.31-42. Gordon and Breach Science Publishers, New York.
7. Reul, J.M.H.M., Tonnaer, J.A.D.M. and De Kloet, E.R. (1988): Neurobiol. Aging. 9: 253-260.
8. Tonnaer, J.A.D.M., Van Vugt, M. and De Graaf, J.S. (1986): Peptides 7: 425-429.

GABA$_B$ RECEPTORS IN BRAIN FUNCTION

N.G. Bowery, Department of Pharmacology, The School of Pharmacy, University of London, 29/39 Brunswick Square, WC1N 1AX, U.K.

It is now ten years since GABA$_B$ receptors were originally detected in the mammalian brain [4;11]. Since then much progress has been made. They have been assigned a physiological role [7] and present data indicate that the receptors may even be heterogeneous [2;8;10;18].

Receptor distribution and channel coupling. GABA$_B$ sites were initially demonstrated on peripheral autonomic nerve terminals and central aminergic processes [3;4]. On activation by GABA or the selective ligand (-)baclofen, a reduction in neurotransmitter release occurred. Subsequent studies have revealed that GABA$_B$ sites function as autoreceptors [15;20] and are also present on post-synaptic membranes within the brain [see 8]. Unlike GABA$_A$ receptors, which gate Cl$^-$ channels, GABA$_B$ receptors are coupled to either K$^+$ or Ca^{++} channels, depending on the tissue, via G-proteins [1;6;9].

The overall distribution of GABA$_B$ sites differs from that of GABA$_A$ sites in the brain. In many regions both receptor types are present but in certain areas such as the inter-peduncular nucleus, GABA$_B$ sites predominate [5]. Within the spinal cord a very high density is present in laminae II & III and at least 50% of the sites appear to be present on afferent terminals [16]. Their activation in the cord may modulate the release of primary afferent transmitters such as substance P [17] and this may explain, in part, the analgesic action of baclofen.

Biochemical Events. Opposing biochemical effects have been attributed to GABA$_B$ receptor activation in neuronal tissue, namely - inhibition of adenylyl cyclase and potentiation of cAMP generation by e.g. β-adrenoceptor agonists, and inhibition of stimulated phosphoinositide (PI) turnover as well as a small direct stimulation of PI turnover [see 2]. The relevance of any of these to the functional role of GABA$_B$ sites is not clear, however an increase in the potentiation of cAMP generation in frontal cortex has been reported following chronic antidepressant administration and this appears to be allied to an increase in GABA$_B$ receptor binding in this same region [14;19]. These different biochemical phenomena associated with GABA$_B$ site activation may provide the basis for heterogeneity of GABA$_B$ sites. Pre- and post-synaptic electrophysiological events have already been considered to reflect separate receptor mechanisms [8;10].

Pharmacological Aspects. Pharmacological characterisation of $GABA_B$ sites has recently benefited from the advent of selective antagonists as well as agonists. Phaclofen and 2-hydroxy saclofen are selective antagonists [12;13] but neither readily crosses the blood brain barrier. By contrast CGP 35348 appears to be active after parenteral administration (Bittiger and Olpe, this symposium).

Numerous pharmacological effects are produced by $GABA_B$ receptor agonists [see 2] and some of these must surely be of physiological importance particularly in diseased states. $GABA_B$ antagonists may then have a significant role in therapeutics. At present we can only make informed guesses but it is possible that such antagonists may be effective in cognitive disorders, depression and even anxiety.

References

1. Andrade R. et al. (1986) Science 234, 1261-1265.
2. Bowery N.G. (1989) Trends Pharmacol.Science 10, 401-407.
3. Bowery N.G. et al. (1981) Eur.J. Pharmacol. 71, 53-70.
4. Bowery N.G. et al. (1980) Nature 283, 92-94.
5. Bowery N.G. et al. (1987) Neuroscience 20, 365-383.
6. Dolphin A.C. & Scott R.H. (1987) J.Physiol.(Lond.) 386, 1-17.
7. Dutar P. & Nicoll R.A. (1988) Nature 332, 156-158.
8. Dutar P. & Nicoll R.A. (1988) Neuron 1, 585-598.
9. Feltz A. et al. (1987) Biochemie 69, 395-406.
10. Harrison N.L. (1990) J.Physiol.(Lond.) 422, 433-446.
11. Hill D.R. & Bowery N.G. (1981) Nature 290, 149-152.
12. Kerr D.I.B. et al. (1987) Brain Res. 405, 150-154.
13. Kerr D.I.B. et al. (1988) Neurosci.Lett. 92, 92-96.
14. Lloyd K.G. et al. (1985) J.Pharmacol.Exp. Ther. 235, 191-199.
15. Pittaluga A. et al. (1987) Eur.J.Pharmacol. 144, 45-52.
16. Price G.W. et al. (1987) Synapse 1, 530-538.
17. Ray N.J. et al. (1989) Br.J.Pharmacol. 97, 562P.
18. Scherer R.W. et al. (1988) Brain Res. Bull. 21, 439-443.
19. Suzdak P.D. & Gianutsos G. (1986) Eur.J.Pharmacol. 131, 129-133.
20. Waldmeier P.C. et al. (1988) Naunyn-Schmiedeberg's Arch.Pharmacol. 337, 289-295.

PARTIAL PURIFICATION OF γ-AMINOBUTYRIC ACID $_B$ RECEPTOR FROM BOVINE BRAIN

Y.OHMORI and K.KURIYAMA
Department of Pharmacology, Kyoto Prefectural University of Medicine, Kyoto, JAPAN.

γ-Aminobutyric acid (GABA)$_B$ receptor in the brain has been found to be coupled with adenylate cyclase (4), phosphatidylinositol turnover (3) and calcium ion channel. It is not yet clear, however, whether these reactions occur sequentially or independently and which component is directly coupled with GABA$_B$ receptor. In order to clarify these unknown characteristics of cerebral GABA$_B$ receptor, the purification of GABA$_B$ receptor must be important. Recently affinity chromatography has proven to be a successful technique for the purification of membrane-bound neurotransmitter receptors such as muscarinic cholinergic (1) and α-adrenergic receptors (2). In this study, we have, therefore, attempted to develop an affinity gel useful for the purification of GABA$_B$ receptor and to examine pharmacological properties of GABA$_B$ receptor using these purified fractions.

METHOD

Affinity gels were obtained by the coupling of various compounds having specific affinity to GABA$_B$ receptor and Sepharose gels, and these gels were equilibrated with 50mM Tris-HCl buffer containing 0.2% cholic acid and 0.02% asolectin (buffer A). The solubilized fraction prepared by the treatment with various detergents was applied to the affinity column, and it was washed with buffer A. The receptor protein retained in the column was then eluted by a linear gradient of NaSCN (1 to 2M) or KCl (1M) in buffer A, and the eluted fraction were immediately dialyzed and used for GABA$_B$ receptor binding assay.

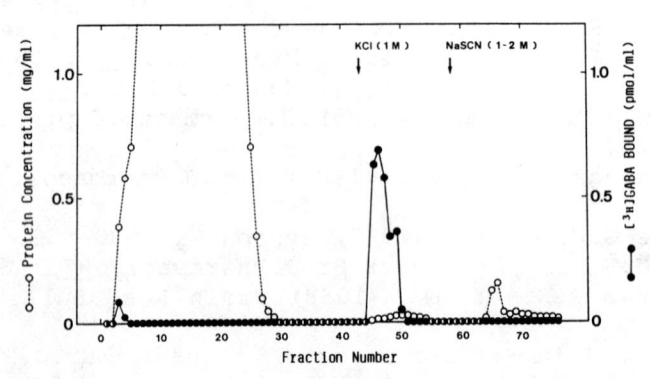

Fig.1 Affinity column chromatography using baclofen-epoxy-activated Sepharose 6B of solubilized fraction from bovine cerebral cortex.

Table 1 Summary on chromatographic separation of CHAPS-solubilized
        $GABA_B$ receptor from bovine cerebral cortex.

step	Total activity (pmol)	Specific activity (pmol/mg)	Purification (-fold)
Solubilized	0.71	0.006	1
Baclofen-Sepharose 6B	0.74	17.68	2828

RESULTS

The affinity column chromatography using baclofen-epoxy-activated Sepharose 6B of CHAPS-solubilized preparation resulted in a 2828-fold purification with no loss in total binding activity (Table 1). All of [^{3}H]GABA binding activity emerged from this column as a symmetrical peak following elution with 1M KCl (Fig.1). The specificity of partially purified $GABA_B$ receptor obtained was then examined by competition of the binding with various compounds. The binding was displaced by various compounds having specific affinity to $GABA_B$ receptor such as GABA, baclofen and 2-hydroxy saclofen in a concentration-dependent manner.

DISCUSSION

By the use of newly developed affinity column chromatographic procedures described here, substantial degree of purification of cerebral $GABA_B$ receptor has been achieved. The affinity matrix prepared by immobilized $GABA_B$ receptor agonist, baclofen, on Sepharose 6B demonstrated successful achievement with regard to both adsorption and elution of the soluble $GABA_B$ receptor. Binding capacity of the matrix was relatively high and most of the applied soluble $GABA_B$ receptor could be adsorbed on the affinity column, and all of the receptor protein retaining specificity as $GABA_B$ receptor could be eluted by KCl. Although SDS-polyacrylamide gel electrophoresis showed several protein band and thus the molecular weight of $GABA_B$ receptor could not be estimated, modification of this column chromatographic procedures may well become an useful tool for further purification and molecular characterization of $GABA_B$ receptor.

REFERENCES

1. Haga, K. and Haga, T. J. Biol. Chem. 260 (13) : 7927-7935, 1985.
2. Lomasney, J. W. et al. J. Biol. Chem. 261 (17) : 7710-7716, 1986.
3. Ohmori, Y. and Kuriyama, K. Neurochem. Int. 15 (3) : 359-363, 1989.
4. Wojcik, W. J. and Neff, N. H. Mol. Pharmacol. 25 : 24-28, 1983.

GABA$_B$-RECEPTORS IN THE HIPPOCAMPUS: ACTIONS ON PRE- AND POSTSYNAPTIC SITES

B.H. GÄHWILER*, D.A. BROWN**, T. KNÖPFEL* and S.M. THOMPSON*
*Brain Research Institute, University of Zürich, CH-8029 Zürich, Switzerland, and
**University College, London WC1E 6BT, United Kingdom

In the hippocampus, the inhibitory neurotransmitter GABA interacts with two unique types of receptors which have been designated GABA$_A$ and GABA$_B$ receptors (1). GABA$_A$ receptors are selectively activated by the GABA analogue muscimol and mediate an increased Cl$^-$ conductance. A selective agonist for the GABA$_B$ receptor is the antispastic agent baclofen (1). To identify the ionic mechanism of GABA$_B$ receptor-mediated inhibition, we have analyzed the postsynaptic permeability changes induced by baclofen in voltage-clamped hippocampal pyramidal cell somata under conditions in which actions on K$^+$ and Ca^{2+} can be discriminated (2). Furthermore, we have characterized the GABA$_B$ receptor-mediated presynaptic inhibition in hippocampal neurons (3).

METHODS

Experiments were performed on hippocampal slices prepared from 5 to 6-day-old Wistar rats and cultured organotypically for 3-5 weeks as described previously (4). Individual CA$_3$ pyramidal cells were impaled under visual control and single-electrode voltage-clamped. Synaptic potentials were evoked with 100 µs anodal current pulses using monopolar microelectrodes. For measurements of cytosolic Ca^{2+}-concentrations, the Ca^{2+} indicator fura-2 was injected intrasomatically, and epifluorescence excited either at 366 nm or 405 nm using a mercury arc lamp.

RESULTS

In CA$_3$ pyramidal cells, application of baclofen at a concentration of 10 µM induced an inwardly rectifying outward (hyperpolarizing) membrane current which reversed at -75 mV (with an external K$^+$ concentration of 5.8 mM). This current appeared to be a K$^+$ current since (i) its reversal potential showed the expected shift when extracellular K$^+$ was changed and (ii) it was blocked by external Ba^{2+} or internal Cs$^+$. This action of baclofen was closely imitated by GABA after GABA$_A$-mediated processes had been abolished with GABA-antagonist such as pitrazepin or bicuculline. The inward currents produced by baclofen and GABA at membrane potentials negative to their reversal potential were also blocked in a voltage-dependent manner by 1 mM external Cs$^+$.

When outward currents were blocked with internal Cs$^+$, the residual inward voltage-dependent Ca^{2+} current was not changed by baclofen. As a further test, we have examined the effect of baclofen on cytosolic Ca^{2+}-concentrations with fura-2. When CA3 pyramidal cells were voltage-clamped close to the resting potential, no change in cytosolic Ca^{2+}-concentrations was observed during application of 10 µM baclofen.

Negative feedback of synaptically released GABA onto presynaptic elements may result in a depression of evoked release. We have, therefore, examined the ability of GABA and its analogues to effect the IPSP under voltage clamp. Bath application of baclofen decreased the conductance underlying the IPSP without affecting the IPSP reversal potential, with an EC_{50} of about 5×10^{-7}M. A similar dose-dependent depression of IPSPs was observed with iontophoretic application of GABA. It appears likely that feedback of GABA onto presynaptic $GABA_B$ receptors is responsible for the activity-dependent reduction in the conductance underlying the IPSP following repetitive stimulation.

DISCUSSION

The present results indicate that activation of $GABA_B$ receptors in hippocampal pyramidal cells produces dual effects. At postsynaptic sites, GABA and the $GABA_B$ agonist baclofen hyperpolarize pyramidal cells by increasing K^+ permeability rather than by reducing Ca^{2+} permeability, as evidenced by voltage-clamp and optical recordings using the Ca^{2+} indicator fura-2. At presynaptic sites, GABA can decrease IPSPs by a $GABA_B$ receptor-mediated inhibition of release.

REFERENCES

1. Bowery, N.G. et al.: (-)Baclofen decreases neurotransmitter release in the mammalian CNS by an action at a novel GABA receptor. Nature (London) 283:92-94, 1980.

2. Gähwiler, B.H. and Brown, D.A.: $GABA_B$-receptor-activated K+ current in voltage-clamped CA_3 pyramidal cells in hippocampal cultures. Proc. Natl. Acad. Sci. USA 82:1558-1562, 1985.

3. Thompson, S.M. and Gähwiler, B.H.: Activity-dependent disinhibition. III. Desensitization and $GABA_B$ receptor-mediated presynaptic inhibition in the hippocampus in vitro. J. Neurophys. 61:524-533, 1989.

4. Gähwiler, B.H.: Organotypic monolayer cultures of nervous tissue. J. Neurosci. Meth. 4:329-342, 1981.

The role of GABA-B receptors in the control of neuronal excitability

H.-R. Olpe, G. Karlsson, M.W. Steinmann, C. Kolb*, F. Brugger, M.F. Pozza, A. Hausdorf
Research Department, Pharmaceuticals Division, CIBA-GEIGY Ltd., CH-4002 Basle, Switzerland
*University Clinic, Neurological Department, CH-4031 Basle, Switzerland

In view of the widespread distribution of $GABA_B$ receptors in the central nervous system, it is likely that they play important roles in the regulation of neuronal activity. Depending on the focus of analysis (synapse, neuron, neuronal network), the term function has to be defined separately. The analysis is hampered and complicated by the possible existence of multiple receptor types showing regional heterogeneity. $GABA_B$ receptors are localized both pre-and postsynaptically (Bowery, 1989). Presynaptic $GABA_B$ receptors have been shown to exert inhibitory actions on the release of various transmitters, including the release of GABA itself. Postsynaptically $GABA_B$ activation leads to reduced neuronal excitability through membrane hyperpolarization (Bowery, 1989). The present paper focusses on the role of $GABA_B$ receptors in the hippocampus and the sensorimotor cortex and deals with selected neurophysiological features of these neurons.

The importance of $GABA_B$ receptors in the regulation of neuronal activity is apparent from early in vivo studies. In these ionophoretic investigations the selective $GABA_B$ receptor agonist baclofen was shown to reduce the spontaneous activity of neurons in many brain areas. However, since there may be synaptic and extrasynaptic $GABA_B$ receptors, these early in vivo studies and subsequent in vitro studies were faced with interpretational problems. New opportunities to elucidate the role of $GABA_B$ receptors arose recently when selective $GABA_B$ receptor blockers became available. $GABA_B$ blockers are expected to reveal the actual role played by $GABA_B$ receptors in ongoing GABAergic transmission.

GABA acts postsynaptically on $GABA_A$ and $GABA_B$ receptors to elicit an early and late inhibitory postsynaptic potential (ipsp), respectively. The activation of $GABA_A$ receptors appears to have a more pronounced curtailing effect on postsynaptic activity than $GABA_B$ receptor activation. This may be due to the shorter latency, the larger change in conductance and the larger amplitude of the membrane hyperpolarization resulting from activation of $GABA_A$ receptors. It is therefore to be expected that selective blockade of the two receptors would reveal distinct effects on neuronal activity. In order to test this hypothesis we have performed experiments with the new $GABA_B$ receptor blocker CGP 35348. CGP 35348 binds to the $GABA_B$ receptor with an IC_{50} of 34 µM when ^{3}H-CGP 27492 is used as a ligand. In electrophysiological experiments performed in the neonate rat spinal cord and the hippocampal slice, CGP 35348 is ten to thirty times more potent than phaclofen.

The $GABA_A$ receptor blocker bicuculline and CGP 35348 were ionophoretically applied near to spontaneously active neurons in the CA1 area of the hippocampus and of the sensorimotor cortex of the anaesthetized rat. Bicuculline strongly excited all neurons tested including neurons of the hippocampus which fired no spontaneous action potentials prior to the application of bicuculline. Upon prolonged application of bicuculline, large epileptic-like field potentials were observed. The $GABA_B$ blocker CGP 35348 moderately increased the spontaneous firing of cortical and hippocampal neurons but epileptic-like discharges were not observed. In hippocampal coronal slices, bath-applied CGP 35348 blocked the late ipsp's evoked by stimulation of the Schaffer commissural/collaterals but did not affect the extra-and intracellularly recorded excitatory postsynaptic potentials. CGP 35348, in contrast to bicuculline, did not induce multiple population spikes. In slices made epileptic by bath-applied bicuculline, or penicillin or by lowered Mg^{2+}-levels (from 2 to 0.1 mM), CGP 35348 (100 µM) moderately increased the frequency of epileptic-like discharges. These in vitro studies were corroborated by in vivo investigations which showed that CGP 35348 did not have clearcut proconvulsive features in a number of classical convulsion tests in mice. Taken together, these data suggest that $GABA_B$ receptors have a less profound impact on neuronal activity than $GABA_A$ receptors. They may have, however, a subtle modulatory role. This idea is supported by intracellular investigations in rat and cat cortical slices which suggest that $GABA_B$ receptor-mediated late ipsp's may reduce the responsiveness to weak excitatory stimuli but leave the responses to strong stimuli unimpaired (Connors et al., 1988). The precise role of $GABA_B$ receptors in cortical function remains, however, to be elucidated.

Given the possibility of a moderate disinhibitory effect of CGP 35348, we investigated the influence of this compound on synaptic plasticity. Experiments were performed on rat hippocampal slices. Long-term potentiation (LTP) of population spikes recorded in the CA1 area was induced by tetanic stimulation of the Schaffer collateral/commissural fibers. CGP 35348 (100 µM) and phaclofen (1mM) both significantly facilitated LTP. These results point to a possible role of $GABA_B$ receptor in the control of synaptic plasticity.

Connors, B.W. et al., J. Physiol. **406** (1988) 443.
Bowery, N., TIPS **10**, (1989) 401.

GABA-B RECEPTORS: FROM NEUROTRANSMISSION TO BEHAVIOUR

H. BITTIGER, R. BERNASCONI, F.BRUGGER, W. FROESTL, R. HALL*,
G. KARLSSON, K. KLEBS, H.-R. OLPE, M.F. POZZA, M.W. STEINMANN
AND H. VAN RIEZEN
Research and Development Department, Pharmaceuticals
Division, CIBA-GEIGY AG, CH 4002 Basel and Central Research
Laboratories*, CIBA-GEIGY Ltd. Tennax Road, Trafford Park,
Manchester M17 1WT, England

INTRODUCTION

Studies on the possible physiological role of GABA-B receptors were recently intensified when the first GABA-B antagonists became available (3,4). These were weak and active only in vitro . As a consequence, current ideas about possible behavioural effects of GABA-B receptor blockade and the possible therapeutic applications of GABA-B antagonists derive exclusively from in vitro data. We discovered recently a novel, centrally active GABA-B antagonist, CGP 35 348, which crosses the blood-brain barrier after parenteral administration. This compound allowed the study of biochemical, electrophysiological and behavioural changes following the manipulation of the GABA transmission by blockade of the GABA-B receptors. One important question in these studies was, whether the effects of GABA-B receptor blockade would be opposite to those of the GABA-B agonist baclofen such as: inhibition of release of neurotransmitters (2,5), reduction of neuronal firing, sedation, analgesia, inhibition of spinal reflexes and muscle relaxation (1,2).

PROPERTIES AND ACTIVITIES OF CGP 35 348

CGP 35 348 is a substituted linear phosphoamino acid [P-(3-aminopropyl)-P-diethoxymethyl-phosphinic acid]. It interacted selectively with GABA-B receptors (IC50 = 34 µM) and showed no interactions with GABA-A, NMDA, quisqualate, kainate, muscarinic cholinergic, biogenic amine and histamine receptors at a concentration of 1 mM. CGP 35 348 antagonized a number of effects of the GABA-B agonist baclofen in vitro at concentrations of 10 - 100µM: the potentiation of the stimulation of adenylyl cyclase by noradrenaline in rat cortex slices, the inhibition of GABA-release induced by electrical stimulation in the same preparation, the suppression of spontaneous electrical activity of hippocampal CA1 neurons, the inhibition of mono- and polysynaptic reflexes in spinal cord preparations and the reduction of paired pulse inhibition in hippocampal slices. In some, but not all of these systems CGP 35 348 alone showed activity: it increased the GABA release of electrically stimulated slices and augmented the paired pulse inhibition in hippocampal slices, to some extent the activity of spontaneously active neurons in the hippocampus and spinal cord was increased and the amplitude of the monosynaptic reflex in spinal cord preparations. Antagonism against effects of baclofen was demonstrated also in vivo: 1.Suppression of neuronal activity in experiments where baclofen was ionophoretically applied near to rat cortical neurons and the antagonist was given parenterally,2.the inhibition of GABA - turnover,3.the increase in the power of the EEG at low frequencies (2 -4 Hz), 4. the impairment of rotarod behaviour and 5.the sedation. Active doses were 30 - 100mg/kg ip of CGP 35 348. The compound administered alone did not have obvious effects on the GABA turnover, the neuronal activity, the EEG and the rotarod behaviour even at high doses, which readily blocked the effects of baclofen. Grooming and stereotypies were observed in mice, but not in rats and at 1000mg/kg ip proconvulsive effects appeared.

CONCLUSIONS

CGP 35 348 interacts selectively with GABA-B receptors. Antagonism of effects of baclofen is seen in biochemical and electrophysiological experiments at concentrations of 10 - 100 µM and in vivo at doses of 30 - 100 mg/kg ip in the GABA turnover, ionophoretic experiments, the EEG and the rotarod model.Pronounced effects of CGP 35 348 alone can be demonstrated under conditions of electrical stimulation (GABA release from electrical stimulated slices, paired pulse inhibition) whereas slight increase in firing is found in spontaneously active hippocampal cells and and increased amplitudes of spinal reflexes in vitro.Mice are stimulated behaviourally. In conclusion, the GABA-B antagonist CGP 35 348 appears to be a "soft" positive modulator of neurotransmission. Possible therapeutic effects, as discussed by Bowery (this Symposium) may include improvement of cognitive processes and antidepressant activity. However, studies in a variety of complex animal models will be necessary to substantiate these speculations.

REFERENCES

1. Bein, H.J.(1972) In: Spasticity, a topical Survey,W.Birkmayer, pp 76-82, Hans Huber, Vienna
2. Bowery, N.G.(1989) Trends Pharmacol. Science 10: 401-407
3. Kerr, D.I.B. et al.(1987) Brain Res.405: 150-154
4. Kerr, D.I.B. et al.(1988) Neuroscience Lett.92: 92-96
5. Waldmeier, P.C. et al (1988) Naunyn-Schmiedeberg's Arch.Pharmacol. 337: 289-295

INTRATHECAL BACLOFEN IN THE TREATMENT OF SPINAL SPASTICITY

R.D. Penn, J.S. Kroin and J.M. Magolan
Department of Neurosurgery, Rush Medical College, Chicago, IL, USA

The $GABA_B$ agonist, baclofen, is extremely effective in reducing spasticity when administered intrathecally (2,3). We have treated 44 multiple sclerosis and spinal cord injury patients over the past 6 years using an implanted drug pump to chronically infuse baclofen. In most patients the dose to achieve a stable clinical result increases over the first 6 to 12 months and then stabilizes. In approximately ten percent of patients the dose continues to increase and tolerance becomes a problem for continued treatment. We have investigated baclofen tolerance in the laboratory and used drug holidays to deal with this clinical problem.

METHODS AND RESULTS

Five patients, whose increased muscle tone and spasms were well controlled by intrathecal baclofen, required dose escalations up to the high microgram/day range (mean 746 µg/d). Rather than risk side-effects by increasing the dose further in these long-term patients (mean duration 33 months), they were switched to intrathecal opiates

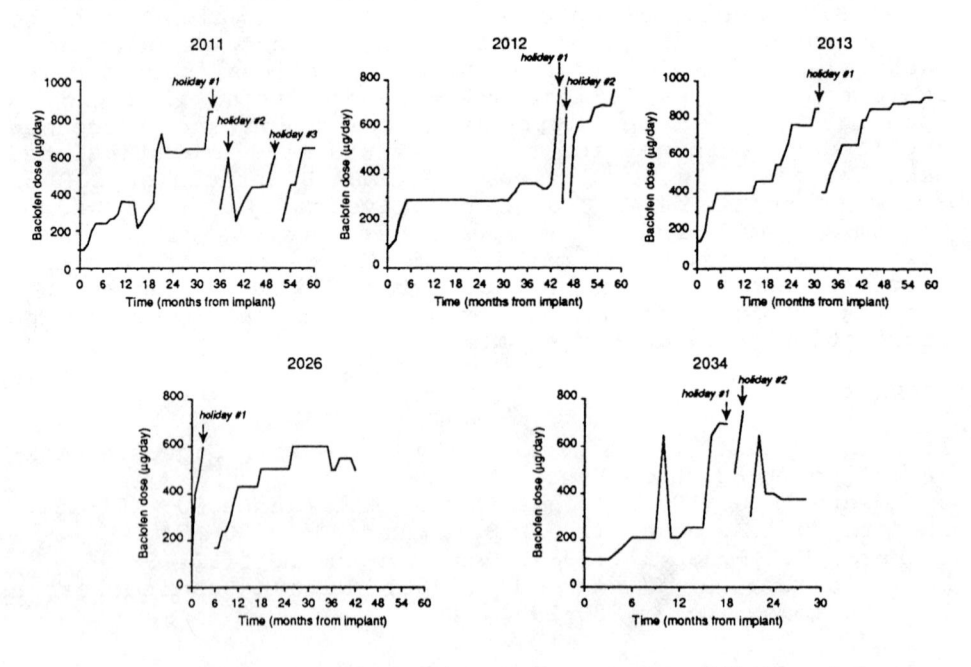

FIG.1.Dosage requirements for individual patients exhibiting tolerance

(usually morphine) for several weeks (mean duration 55 days). When these patients were then returned to intrathecal baclofen, their required dosage to control spasticity was approximately half of the value prior to this baclofen holiday (FIG. 1). Thus, sensitivity to baclofen is restored after a drug holiday.

Rats were implanted with Alzet osmotic minipumps to perfuse the lumbar spinal cord with baclofen or saline (1). Quantitative autoradiography was used to measure receptor levels. Chronic exposure of the cord for 28 days reduced spinal $GABA_B$ receptors in the dorsal grey by 36%. This is parallel to the decrease in sensitivity to baclofen in patients.

DISCUSSION

Continuous intrathecal baclofen controls spasticity at the spinal cord level at doses that do not effect sensation or descending motor performance. It is not clear yet whether following spinal lesions the $GABA_B$ receptor numbers or affinity change. However, patients appear to be exquisitely sensitive to a $GABA_B$ agonist. Tolerance in patients appears to be due to overstimulation of the $GABA_B$ receptors, since drug holidays allow treatment to resume with a smaller dosage.

REFERENCES

1. Kroin, J.S., Singh, R., Penn, R.D., et al: Chronic intrathecal baclofen reduces $GABA_B$ binding in rat substantia gelatinosa. Soc Neurosci Abstr 15:975, 1989.

2. Penn, R.D., Kroin, J,S: Continuous intrathecal baclofen for severe spasticity. Lancet, 2:125-127, 1985.

3. Penn, R.D., Savoy, S., Corcos, D., et al: Intrathecal baclofen for severe spinal spasticity: a double-blind crossover study. N Eng J Med 320:1517-1521, 1989.

GENE TRANSFER INTO NEURAL CREST DERIVED POST MITOTIC CELLS

A.L. BOUTILLIER[*], F. BARTHEL[*], B.A. DEMENEIX[°] and J.P. LOEFFLER[*+]
Institut de Physiologie[*+], Université Louis Pasteur, 21 rue René Descartes, 67084 STRASBOURG Cedex and Museum d'Histoire Naturelle[°], 57 rue Cuvier, 75231 PARIS Cedex 05, Correspondance to J.P. Loeffler[+]

DNA transfer studies are powerfull tools for studying gene expression or analyzing the role of given intracellular proteins. Despite steady progress in molecular biology techniques over the last decade, gene transfer studies have been restricted to investigation in established cell lines. Indeed, calcium phosphate/DNA coprecipitation and Dextran based transfection methods are too deleterious for very sensitive cells like primary neurons or endocrine cells. We have recently developped a gene transfer method based on the use of DNA binding lipids (1). Here we show that this method can be applied to primary chromaffin cells and central nervous system neurons.

METHODS

Chromaffin cells (3) and cerebellar granular neurons (6) were cultured as previously described. Transfection studies were carried out 3 days after plating. The appropriate plasmid/lipid complex (1) was obtained by freshly mixing 500 μl of DNA solution (2 μg/well) with 500 μl of lipid solution (final concentration, 6 μM of dioctadecylamidoglycylspermine: DOGS). The transfection step lasted 2 to 6 hours and chloramphenicol acetyl transferase (CAT) activity was measured after 24 hours according to Gormann et al. (5). Plasmids TRE/tk-CAT (6) and pENKAT-12 (2) have been described previously.

RESULTS

Proenkephalin gene expression control by neurotransmitters was studied in primary chromaffin cells after introduction of the human proenkephalin-CAT fusion gene (2). Transcription stimulation from this promoter by nicotine (5.10^{-6} M) and histamine (5.10^{-6} M), two membrane receptor agonists which also stimulate proenkephalin mRNA accumulation (3, 4) is depicted on Fig 1.

Fig 1. Chromaffin cells (10^5 cells) were plated in DMEM medium supplemented with 10 % fetal calf serum. After 3 days cell were transfected with 2 µg DNA (ENKAT-12) for 6 hours and treated with appropriate drugs for 48 hours in serum free medium (ct): no treatment, N: nicotine (5.10^{-6} M), H: histamine (5.10^{-6} M).

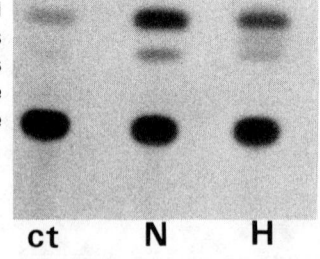

This strategy of gene transfer was further extended to central nervous system neurons (6). 48 hours after transfection with 2 µg TRE/tk-CAT plasmid, viability was evaluated by the trypan blue exclusion test (Fig 2A)

and CAT activity was determined (Fig 2B). No morphological differences or increased cell death was observed after transfection (a) as compared to untreated neurons (b).

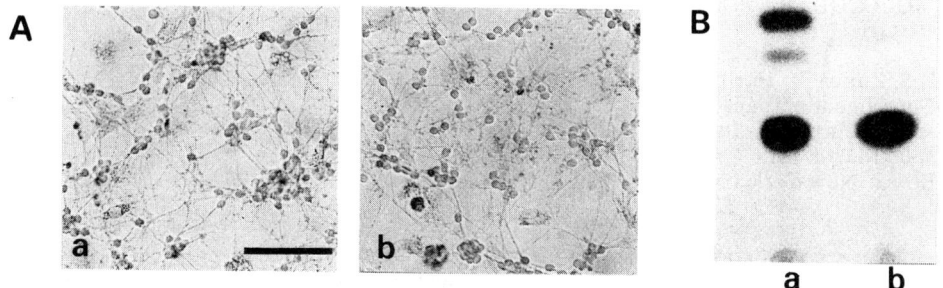

Fig 2. A: trypan blue exclusion test on transfected (a) and control neurons, (b: no lipid and no DNA added). Horizontal calibration bar represents 100 µm. B: autoradiogram represents a CAT analysis from transfected (a) and control neurons (b).

DISCUSSION

The present report illustrates that lipopolyamine mediated gene transfer can be used for studying gene expression in primary neuron and neural crest derived post-mitotic cells. Under standard transfection conditions, this method has no toxic side effects (Fig 2A) and the introduced fusion genes are responsive to recognized regulatory transmitters (Fig 1). Thus, this technique can be used to study tissue specific gene regulation in its physiological environment (primary cells as opposed to transformed or established cell lines), for example, during terminal neuronal differentiation in vitro.

ACKNOWLEDGEMENTS

We thank Dr P. Sassone-Corsi and M. Comb for the gift of TRE/tk-CAT and pENKAT-12. This work was supported by grant 6089 from ARC.

REFERENCES

1. Behr, J.P. et al. Efficient gene transfer into mammalian primary endocrine cells with lipopolyamine coated DNA. Proc. Natl. Acad. Sci. USA 86:6982-6986, 1989.
2. Comb, M. et al. A cyclic AMP-and phorbol ester-inducible DNA element. Nature 323:353-356, 1986.
3. Kley, N. et al. Proenkephalin A gene expression in bovine adrenal chromaffin cells is regulated by changes in electrical activity. EMBO J. 5:967-970, 1986.
4. Kley, N. et al. Histaminergic regulation of proenkephalin mRNA levels in culture adrenal chromaffin cells. Neuroendocrinology 46:89-92, 1987.
5. Gormann, C.M. et al. Recombinant genomes which express chloramphenical acetyl transferase in mammalian cells. Mol. Cell. Biol. 2:1044-1051, 1982.
6. Loeffler, J.P. et al. Lipopolyamine-mediated transfection allows gene expression studies in primary neuronal cells. J. Neurochem. (in press).

MOLECULAR STUDIES OF NMDA RECEPTORS

R.S. Zukin, R. Haring, L. Kushner, J. Lerma and M.V.L. Bennett
Department of Neuroscience
Albert Einstein College of Medicine
1300 Morris Park Avenue
Bronx, New York 10461 USA

The excitatory neurotransmitter glutamate activates multiple receptors defined by the actions of the selective agonists kainate, quisqualate and N-methyl-D-aspartate (NMDA). Recent evidence suggests that the N-methyl-D-aspartate (NMDA) receptor is functionally and structurally associated with the phencyclidine (PCP) receptor which mediates the psychotomimetic effects of PCP, σ opioids and dioxalanes (for a review see (5)). To investigate the relationship between NMDA and PCP receptors on a molecular level, the regulation of NMDA-activated channels by PCP was studied in *Xenopus* oocytes injected with rat brain mRNA (3). In oocytes injected with brain mRNA (50 ng/cell), NMDA application (with glycine) evoked a partially-desensitizing inward current that was potentiated by glycine and blocked by D-(-)-amino-5-phosphonovaleric acid (AP5), by Zn^{2+}, and, in a voltage-dependent manner, by Mg^{2+}. These results show that the distinguishing features of rat brain NMDA channels are reproduced in this translation system. In addition, kainic acid elicited a non-desensitizing inward current at short latency and quisqualate elicited both a short latency inward current and a delayed oscillatory inward current, presumably mediated by a second messenger system. Responses to glutamate had both short latency and delayed components.

The PCP derivative N-[1-(2-thienyl)cyclohexyl]piperidine(TCP) blocked the NMDA-evoked current, and its potency was comparable to its binding affinity in rat brain membranes. Onset of block required the presence of agonist. Antagonism was stereoselective in that the active ligand dexoxadrol was a more effective blocker than its relatively inactive stereoisomer levoxadrol. Other PCP receptor ligands, (+)SKF-10,047 and MK-801, also blocked. Potencies of compounds active at NMDA and PCP receptors in oocytes were comparable to those obtained previously in electrophysiological and binding assays on neural tissues. These results indicate the coexpression of neuronal PCP and NMDA receptors in *Xenopus* oocytes.

The mouse neuroblastoma-Chinese hamster brain hybrid cell line NCB-20 is the only cell line in which binding studies indicate the presence of phencyclidine (PCP) receptors. *Xenopus* oocytes injected with NCB-20 cell poly (A)$^+$ RNA express NMDA-activated channels (4). In injected oocytes, NMDA application evoked a partially desensitizing inward current that is potentiated by glycine, blocked by the competitive antagonist (AP5), blocked by Mg^{2+} and by Zn^{2+}, and blocked in a use-dependent manner by the PCP receptor ligands PCP and MK-801. There was no response to kainate or quisqualate. Thus, NMDA receptors expressed from NCB-20 cell mRNA exhibit properties similar to those of the neuronal receptors. The absence of expression of other excitatory amino acid receptors in this system makes it particularly useful for study of NMDA-evoked responses.

To characterize the polypeptide components of NCB-20 cell NMDA receptors, cell membranes were reacted with the photolabile PCP derivative [^{3}H]azido-PCP (1). SDS-

PAGE analysis of NCB-20 cell membranes reacted with [^{3}H]azido-PCP showed the presence of five major labelled bands (M_r90000, 68000, 49000, 40000 and 3300), a pattern similar to that observed for rat brain membranes. MK-801 and AP5 selectively inhibited the labelling of M_r68000 and 90000 polypeptides, indicating at least two different PCP binding proteins. The M_r68000 and 90000 components correspond to a high affinity site (20% of total [^{3}H]TCP sites) which exhibits the pharmacology expected for the NMDA receptor.

Reconstitution of functional, solubilized NMDA channels, followed by introduction into lipid bilayers, permits comparison of biochemical and functional properties. We have developed a methodology for the solubilization of NMDA receptors from rat forebrain membranes and reincorporation into lipid vesicles of active receptors (2). Recovery of [^{3}H]MK-801 binding activity is nearly 100% with about a 10-fold purification. Retention of pharmacological properties is indicated by the finding that PCP receptor ligands compete for [^{3}H]MK-801 binding in a rank order of potency that parallels their behavior potencies. Moreover, binding of [^{3}H]TCP is prevented by D(-)AP5 and potentiated by glutamate and glycine. Photoaffinity labelling of reconstituted receptor preparations with [^{3}H]azido-PCP resulted in two bands of radioactivity corresponding to polypeptides of M_r59000 and 98000, close in size to the two larger polypeptides labelling in rat forebrain membranes. Photoaffinity labelling of these bands was largely inhibited by both TCP and MK-801. Together, these results provide evidence for the reconstitution of NMDA receptors with binding activity in this liposome preparation.

The studies described demonstrate that rat brain mRNA directs the synthesis of at least four types of functional excitatory amino acid receptors in the *Xenopus* oocyte system, whereas in this system NCB-20 cell mRNA directs the synthesis of only the NMDA type of EAA receptor. The NMDA channel expressed in the oocyte, using either rat brain mRNA or NCB-20 cell mRNA, exhibits the pharmacological properties of the neuronal receptor, including the functional association with the PCP receptor located within the NMDA-gated channel. The demonstration that mRNA isolated from cells lacking functional NMDA-activated channels, but bearing PCP binding sites, can encode functional NMDA-activated channels in the oocyte indicates some defect or regulating step in posttranslational processing or insertion of the receptors into the plasma membrane in the cell of origin. The NCB-20 cell line is the only cell line known to have PCP receptors that appear to be associated with NMDA receptors. Development of a methodology for reconstitution of active NMDA receptors in artificial liposomes should be important for future electrophysiological characterization of this receptor class.

REFERENCES

1. Haring, R., Zukin, R.S., and Zukin, S.R. (1990) *Neurosci. Lett.* in press.
2. Haring, R., Zukin, R.S., Zukin, S.R., and Scheideler, M. Reconstitution and partial purification of brain NMDA receptors. Submitted for publication.
3. Kushner, L., Lerma, J., Zukin, R.S., and Bennett, M.V.L. (1988) *Proc. Natl. Acad. Sci. USA.* 85:3250-3254.
4. Lerma, J., Kushner, L., Spray, D.C., Bennett, V.L., and Zukin, R.S. (1989) *Proc. Natl. Acad. Sci. USA.* 86:1708-1711.
5. Zukin, R.S., and Zukin S.R. The σ Receptor. (1988) In *The Opiate Receptors*. G. Pasternak, ed. pp. 143-163. Human Press, New Jersey.

SPIDER TOXINS AS PROBES FOR GLUTAMATE RECEPTOR

N. Kawai,* T. Nakajima** and T. Takenawa***
*Tokyo Metropolitan Institute for Neurosciences, **Faculty of Pharmaceutical Sciences University of Tokyo and ***Tokyo Metropolitan Institute for Gerontology, Tokyo, Japan.

Animal toxins have served as important tools in the characterization of molecules involving neurotransmission. The venom of some orb-web spiders contain potent blockers of the glutamatergic neurotransmission. Joro spider toxin (JSTX) derived from Nephila clavata has been found to block excitatory postsynaptic potentials and glutamate-evoked responses in the neuromuscular synapse of crustacea, the squid giant synapse and the mammalian hippocampal synapse. Pharmacological studies using various agonists of glutamate indicated that JSTX preferentially blocked non-NMDA type receptors possibly quisqualate-sensitive subtype of the glutamate receptor (1).

So far, more than 15 compounds were isolated from the venom of Joro spiders and it was found that a unique 2,4-dihydroxyphenylacetyl asparaginyl cadaverine part was common to all toxins. By use of a range of synthesized analogs in studying the structure-activity relationship, we have concluded that 2,4-dihydroxyphenylacetyl asparaginyl part may be responsible for the suppressive action, while the remaining part containing the polyamine may enhance or promote the toxic activity (2).

Using JSTX we could separate the glutamate receptor in the presynaptic membrane from that in the postsynaptic membrane in the lobster neuromuscular synapse. While glutamate depolarized the postsynaptic membrane by eliciting Na^+ current, it hyperpolarized the presynaptic membrane by activation of K^+ channels. This K^+ current induced by the presynaptic glutamate receptor, "glutamate$_B$", was not sensitive to JSTX but was blocked by pertussis toxin (3).

Labeling of synthesized JSTX-3 was used for histological investigation of glutamate receptors. By use of autoradiography with ^{125}JSTX-3, radioactive spots were localized in the subsynaptic membrane of the lobster muscle(4). Histochemical study utilizing the interaction of biotinylated JSTX with avidin showed specific binding of the toxin in the rat brain. Strong binding of biotinyl JSTX was observed in pyramidal cells of hippocampus and Purkinje cells of cerebellum where main transmission are glutamatergic.

Isolation and purification of the JSTX-3 binding protein have been done using JSTX-3. Crude synaptic membrane fraction from rat hippocampus and cerebellum was solubilized by Triton X-100. Using various kinds of affinity chromatography JSTX-3 binding proteins were purified from rat hippocampus and cerebellum (5). SDS-PAGE of the affinity-purified JSTX-3 binding protein showed at least four bands migrating with Mr values of 90K to 40K, which suggests an oligomeric composition of the receptor. JSTX-binding proteins with similar Mr sizes were also isolated from bovine brain and crustacean muscles.

The affinity-purified protein was reconstituted into giant liposomes formed by lipid films. The functional activity of the reconstituted protein was studied by using the patch clamp recording. The liposomes with reconstituted protein induced discrete glutamate-sensitive conductance.

Antibodies obtained by immunization with the JSTX-3 binding protein in guinea-pig antiserum reacted with the polypeptide bands. Small amount of antiserum showed inhibition of the excitatory postsynaptic currents in lobster neuromuscular synapse and also in the synapse of hippocampal pyramidal neurons of rat.

REFERENCES

1. Abe, T. et al. Effects of a spider toxin on the glutaminergic synapse of lobster muscle. J. Physiol. 339:243-252, 1983.
2. Kawai, N. and Nakajima, T. Characterization of glutamate receptor by spider toxin. J. Toxicol. Toxin Reviews in press.
3. Miwa, A. et al. G protein is coupled to presynaptic glutamate and GABA receptors in lobster neuromuscular synapse. J. Neurophyiol. 63:173-180,1990.
4. Shimazaki, K. et al. An autoradiographic study of binding of iodinated spider toxin to lobster muscle. Neurosci. Lett. 84:173-177,1988.
5. Shimazaki, K. et al. A spider toxin (JSTX)-binding protein in rat hippocampus. Biomed. Res. 10:401-403,1989.

THE STRUCTURE AND FUNCTION OF Na^+ and Cl^--COUPLED GABA TRANSPORTER(S)

B.I. KANNER*, R. RADIAN*, A. BENDAHAN*, S. KEYNAN*, N. MABJEESH*,
A. SHOUFFANI*, J. GUASTELLA**, H.A. LESTER**, N. DAVIDSON**,
H. NELSON*** and N. NELSON***
*Department of Biochemistry, Hadassah Medical School, Hebrew University, Jerusalem; **Division of Biology, 156-29, California Institute of Technology, Pasadena, CA 91125; ***Roche Institute of Molecular Biology, Roche Research Center, Nutley, NJ 07110.

The plasma membranes of neurons and glial cells possess sodium-dependent neurotransmitter transporters. They are proposed to terminate synaptic activity (1) and are capable of releasing neurotransmitters from cytoplasmic stores in a calcium-independent fashion (11). The transporters are able to accumulate the transmitters against their concentration gradient by cotransport with sodium ions. The latter move down their electrochemical gradient and this provides the energy for the process. Interestingly, additional ions are co- or counter-transported as well. For instance, γ-aminobutyric acid (GABA) is cotransported with sodium and chloride (2-4,7) and l-glutamate is cotransported with sodium and countertransported with potassium (2-4). Here we describe some of our recent studies on the GABA system.

The (Na^+-Cl^-)-coupled GABA transporter has been purified to an apparent homogeneity and functionally reconstituted into liposomes (9). It is a glycoprotein consisting of one type of polypeptide of 80 kDa (9). Antibodies raised against this polypeptide are able to quantitatively precipitate this polypeptide and remove the reconstitutable GABA transport activity (9). This, together with the cloning and expression of the GABA transporter (Guastella et al., submitted, see below) conclusively demonstrates that one type of polypeptide is sufficient for the transport reaction. The anti-GABA transporter antibodies are directed against epitopes on the protein, since they still interact with the fully deglycosylated transporter (5). The latter runs as a 60 kDa polypeptide on SDS-PAGE (5). Upon limited proteolysis a 60-65 kDa polypeptide is generated which still contains the glycan moiety but has lost reactivity towards the transporter. This polypeptide is - upon reconstitution - still capable of catalyzing (Na^+-Cl^-)-coupled GABA transport activity (5). These observations indicate that the transporter contains exposed domains which are not important for function.

Reconstitution of the GABA transporter into asolectin liposomes requires the addition of brain lipids. The active component in the brain lipids was found to be cholesterol (12). Optimal activity can be reconstituted by a combination of any of a series of phospholipids and cholesterol. Cholesterol analogues are ineffective (12). Also, reconstitution of l-glutamate transport exhibits the requirement for cholesterol. This requirement is not due to effects on membrane fluidity, intactness of the liposomes or the incorporation of proteins into them, but is probably due to direct interactions with the co-transporters.

The polyclonal antibodies raised against the GABA transporter (GABA-Tp) have been used for the immunocytochemical localization of the antigen in several rat brain areas. It was found that GABA-Tp is localized in the same type of axons that contain endogeneous GABA. The GABA-Tp antiserum, in contrast to the GABA antiserum, did not produce detectable labelling of nerve cell bodies. It did however label GABA-Tp in glial processes (10).

In crude synaptosomal membrane vesicles we have identified two pharmacologically distinct sodium- and chloride-coupled high affinity GABA transporters. One is inhibited by cis-3-amino-cyclohexane carboxylic acid (ACHC), the other by β-alanine. Upon solubilization and fractionation, a protein fraction was obtained which upon reconstitution exhibited GABA transport which was exclusively sensitive to ACHC, whereas β-alanine sensitive activity was found in a different fraction (6). In addition to this diversity of high-affinity transporters, two low-affinity transporters were detected as well. One simply represents the cytosolic aspect(s) of the high affinity transporters, whereas the other is a different transporter (8).

Using protein sequence of the highly purified GABA transporter, degenerate anti-sense oligonucleotides were synthesized and used to probe a λ zapII rat brain library. One cDNA clone was found which upon transcription - in one direction only - yielded synthetic RNA which was able to give rise to expression of GABA transport when injected into oocytes (Guastella et al., submitted). Further details will be provided in the lecture.

REFERENCES

1. Iversen, L.L.: The Uptake and Storage of Noradrenaline in Sympathetic Neurons (Cambridge University Press, London, 1967).
2. Kanner, B.I. (1983) Biochim. Biophys. Acta 726, 293-316.
3. Kanner, B.I. (1989) Current Opinion in Cell Biology 1, 735-738.
4. Kanner, B.I. and Schuldiner, S. (1987) CRC Critical Reviews in Biochemistry 22, 1-38.
5. Kanner, B.I., Keynan, S. and Radian, R. (1989) Biochemistry 28, 3728-3737.
6. Kanner, B.I. and Bendahan, A. (1990) Proc. Natl. Acad. Sci. USA, in press.
7. Keynan, S. and Kanner, B.I. (1988) Biochemistry 27, 12-17.
8. Mabjeesh, N.J. and Kanner, B.I. (1989) Biochemistry 28, 7694-7699.
9. Radian, R., Bendahan, A. and Kanner, B.I. (1986) J. Biol. Chem. 261, 15437-15441.
10. Radian et al. (1990) J. Neurosci., in press.
11. Schwartz, E.A. (1987) Science 238, 350-355.
12. Shouffani, A. and Kanner, B.I. (1990) J. Biol. Chem., in press.

INTERMEDIARY METABOLISM DISTURBANCE IN AD/SDAT AND ITS RELATION TO MOLECULAR EVENTS

S. HOYER
Department of Pathochemistry & General Neurochemistry, University of Heidelberg, F.R.G.

The mature, healthy, non-starved mammalian brain uses glucose only as a source of energy in the form of ATP. Glucose breakdown contributes to the formation of the neurotransmitters acetylcholine, glutamate, aspartate, gamma-aminobutyrate, and glycine, too (1, 2, 3). The sufficient formation and turnover rate of energy as ATP guarantees the maintenance of intracellular ion homeostasis, axoplasmatic flux, synapse function and structural integrity of a neuron (4, 5). The glycolytic breakdown of glucose yields 20% of total ATP only, whereas 80% of total ATP are formed by glucose oxidation. Any perturbation of the neuronal glucose metabolism may thus give rise to a cellular energy deficit which subsequently induces abnormalities in neuronal homeostasis and thus neuronal stress.
In normoglycemic patients suffering from early-onset dementia of Alzheimer type (AD), an early and predominant disturbance was found in a 44% reduction in cerebral glucose utilization whereas cerebral blood flow and oxygen utilization were unaltered (6). Reduced neuronal glucose utilization is obviously substituted by means of endogenous glutamate utilization via the aspartate aminotransferase reaction (7). This condition generates both an energy deficit and changes in the amino acid composition at the cellular level. The latter includes a rise of the aspartic acid concentration which may change the neuronal calcium homeostasis via the N-methyl-D-aspartate receptor. Furthermore, ammonia increases to neurotoxic levels (7), being a potent factor for glial proliferation (8), and for the induction of heat shock protein (9). The latter are induced under stress conditions (10), bind specifically to heat shock control elements of the amyloid A4 precursor gene which is activated by its promotor (11). Thus, the damage in neuronal glucose homeostasis and related metabolism may play a pivotal role in the generation of amyloid in DAT brain, and may precede this morphological abnormality. The same cellular and molecular pathobiochemistry may be set into motion, too, in late-onset DAT (SDAT), when cerebral glucose utilization is likewise diminished, but cerebral blood flow and oxygen utilization are starting to fall (12).

References
1. Hoyer, S., (1970): Klin.Wschr., 48: 1239-1243
2. Siesjö, B.K., (1978): Brain Energy Metabolism. Wiley, Chichester, chapters 1 and 6
3. Erecinska, M., and Silver, I.A., (1989): J.Cereb. Blood Flow Metabol., 9: 2-19
4. Whittingham, T.S., and Lipton, P., (1984): J.Neurochem., 37: 1618-1621
5. Siesjö, B.K., (1981): J.Cereb.Blood Flow Metabol., 1: 155-185
6. Hoyer, S., Oesterreich, K., and Wagner, O., (1988): J.Neurol., 235: 143-148
7. Hoyer, S., and Nitsch, R., (1989): J.Neural Transm., 75: 227-232
8. Cavanagh, J.B., and Kyu, M.K., (1971): J.Neurol.Sci., 12: 63-75
9. Dienel, G.A., and Cruz, N.F., (1984): J.Neurochem., 42: 1053-1061
10. Lindquist, S., (1986): Ann.Rev.Biochem., 55: 1151-1191
11. Salbaum, J.M., et al., (1988): EMBO J., 7: 2807-2813
12. Hoyer, S., (1978): In Alzheimer's Disease: Senile Dementia and Related Disorders, R.Katzman, R.D.Terry, and K.L. Bick, eds., pp 219-226. Raven Press, New York

NEUROTRANSMITTER CHANGES IN EARLY- AND LATE-ONSET ALZHEIMER-TYPE DEMENTIA

H. ARAI and R. IIZUKA
Department of Psychiatry, Juntendo University School of Medicine, Tokyo 113, Japan.

Alzheimer-type dementia (ATD) is one representative disease which causes dementia. Recent biochemical studies have revealed transmitter deficits in the cholinergic and other systems. However, replacement therapy for such deficits has not been successful in the treatment of ATD patients.
According to neuropathological findings, Alzheimer's disease (early-onset ATD) and senile dementia of Alzheimer-type (late-onset ATD) are included in the one disease-category of ATD. In the present study, however, we focus on the differences of neurochemical findings between early- and late-onset ATD, and briefly discuss drug therapy for ATD.

SUBJECTS AND METHODS

Postmortem human brains obtained in ATD cases and age-matched controls with no neuropsychiatric disorders were examined in the present study. All of the brains used were verified neuropathologically. Detailed clinical and postmortem data, and methods for the determination of biochemical data have been already reported elsewhere (1).

RESULTS AND DISCUSSION
Neurotransmitter changes in ATD
Neurochemical investigations revealed the existence in ATD brains of depletion of cholinergic enzyme activities, of concentration of biogenic amines and their metabolites, of several neuropeptide immunoreactivities and of glutamate concentration. These findings suggest the involvement of not only the cholinergic system but of also many other neurotransmitter systems. ATD may be called a multi-neurotransmitter systems disorder.
Difference between early- and late-onset ATD
The ATD group was divided according to age at onset. Neurotransmitter changes in the early-onset ATD group (< 65 yrs) were compared to those in the late-onset group.
The activities of choline acetyltransferase and acetylcholinesterase were more severely depleted in the early-onset ATD group. Turnover rate in the serotonergic system was decreased more clearly in the early-onset ATD group than in the late-onset ATD group (Fig.). This data and other biochemical differences suggested that the ATD group was not homogenous.

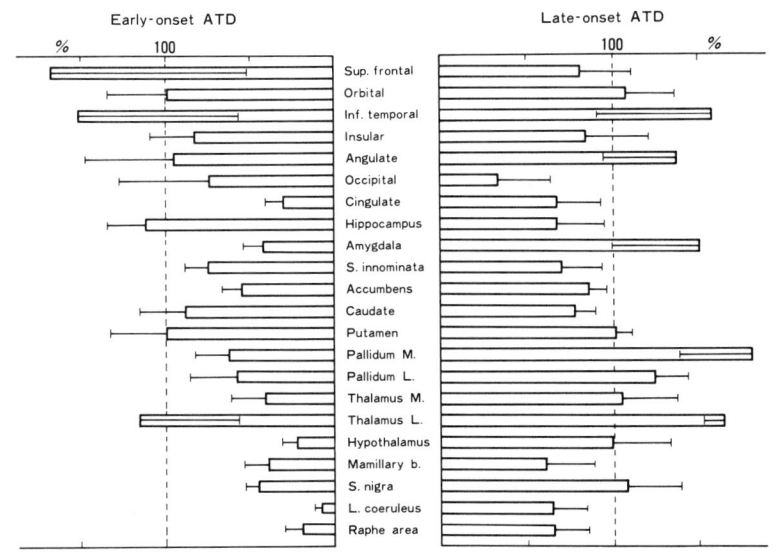

Fig. Turnover rate (5-HIAA/5-HT) in serotonergic system

Replacement therapy for transmitter deficits

The results revealed that neurotransmitter changes were more profound in the early-onset group. Replacement therapy for such deficits, therefore, might be more suitable and effective in the early-onset ATD group. On the other hand, since the late-onset ATD group displayed fewer changes, other pathogenetic factors as well as neurotransmitter changes might cause development of serious dementia symptoms in late-onset ATD. It seems of importance, therefore, to select early-onset ATD cases when replacement therapy for neurotransmitter deficits is examined.

Cholinergic deficit has received attention in ATD. However, out of the neurotransmitter changes we found in ATD brains, serotonergic deficit was the most marked. Accordingly, we here propose replacement therapy for the serotonergic deficit, or combined therapy of cholinergic and serotonergic drugs in the treatment of ATD.

How to evaluate an efficacy of drug therapy

When a new drug is clinically examined, what kind of scale should be used to evaluate its efficacy ? Demented patients show a lot of symptoms, therefore, a multi-discriminative scale like the GBS scale (2), with which we can evaluate even small changes in any symptom, is needed.

REFERENCES

1. Arai, H. et al. Changes of biogenic amines and their matabolites in postmortem brains from patients with Alzheimer-type dementia. J. Neurochem. 43:388-393, 1984.
2. Gottfries, C.G. et al. A new rating scale for dementia syndroms. Arch. Gerontol. Geriatr. 1:311-321, 1982.

NEUROCHEMICAL CHANGES IN GREY AND WHITE MATTER AND NEUROENDOCRINE DISTURBANCES IN DEMENTIA DISORDERS

C.G. GOTTFRIES
Department of Psychiatry and Neurochemistry, Gothenburg University, Gothenburg, Sweden

Several investigations have shown changes in the neurochemistry of the brain from patients with AD/SDAT. A severe disturbance of the acetylcholine (ACh) system has been reported by several authors, as marked by losses of acetylcholine esterase and choline acetyltransferase activity in biopsy and postmortal brain tissue. There is also evidence that the number of cell bodies is reduced in the nucleus basalis of Meynert in AD/SDAT (10). However, there are also disturbances in other neurotransmitter systems. In postmortem investigations it was shown as early as 1969 (2) that there was a dementia-related reduction of homovanillic acid (HVA) in the caudate nucleus of patients with AD/SDAT. Reduced concentrations of dopamine (DA), HVA, noradrenaline (NA), 5-hydroxytryptamine (5-HT) and 5-hydroxyindoleacetic acid (5-HIAA) have also been shown in several studies (for a review see 3,4). Reduced cell numbers in the substantia nigra, raphe nuclei and locus caerulus also support a disturbance of the monoaminergic systems in brains from patients with AD/SDAT.

Investigations have focused on neurotransmitter disturbances in grey matter, but changes in white matter have also been reported. Neurochemical investigations have shown that white matter components are reduced in AD/SDAT (8). White matter changes are described as incomplete infarctions, but the true nature of these disturbances is not fully known. Neither is it known to what extent they are related to the dementia syndrome. It is obvious, however, that white matter changes are not only a secondary phenomenon to the changes in grey matter.

Human brain monoamine oxidase activity can be divided into two forms, MAO-A and MAO-B. It has long been known that MAO-B activity in the human brain increases with age and that this activity is even more increased in brains from patients with AD/SDAT (1). Increased MAO-B activity has been found not only in grey, but also in white matter. Further investigations of MAO enzymes support the assumption that the increase is due to an increased concentration of otherwise unchanged MAO-B molecules. The most simple explanation of the MAO-B increase would be that the degenerative process, as a result of e.g. aging, AD/SDAT, or lesions in animal experiments, induces the growth of extra neuronal cells (e.g. glia) which are relatively rich in MAO-B activity compared with the original tissue. Thus, MAO-B activity can be considered to be a marker of gliosis. The faster rate of increase in MAO-B activity with age in white matter than in grey matter both in controls and in AD/SDAT patients indicates that the degenerative processes underlying MAO-B activity are more pronounced in white matter. It might even be speculated that they start in white matter and that the brain dysfunction is secondary to degenerative processes in the myelin-containing cells.

Neurohormonal changes have been reported in patients with AD/SDAT. 50-70% of patients have a pathological response to the dexamethasone test. Postmortem human brain investigations (9) have shown reduced concentrations of 5-HIAA and significantly increased concentrations of somatostatin, neurotensin, galanin and arginine vasopressin (AVP) in the hypothalamus of patients with AD/SDAT. Increased activity of AVP has been found in aged rats and in patients with SDAT (7). As AVP is considered of importance for the control of activity in the hypothalamus-pituitary-adrenal (HPA) axis, these postmortem findings are of pathogenetic interest. Whether the increased activity in the HPA axis is induced by incapacity to turn off stress reactions or is caused by disturbances in higher control systems for the hypothalamic function is at present not known. According to McEwen (5), the feedback system mediated by glucocorticoids via the hippocampus seems to be disturbed in AD/SDAT. It is of interest that treatment with citalopram, a 5-HT reuptake inhibitor, seems to suppress the activity in the HPA axis (6). Similar findings with tricyclic antidepressants have been made in rats.

In conclusion, it is evident that in brains from patients with AD/SDAT there are multiple changes in both grey and white matter. It is not possible, however, to single out any one of these changes as of special significance for the disease. The changes may well be secondary phenomena to a more fundamental change in the metabolism of the brain in these patients. Still, as the recorded changes may be of importance for the symptoms and possibly also for the neuroendocrine disturbances seen in AD/SDAT, they might be of use in the formulation of pharmacological treatment strategies.

REFERENCES

1. Adolfsson, et al., (1980): Life Sci., 27:1029-1034.
2. Gottfries, C.G., Gottfries, I. and Roos, B.E. (1969): J Neurochem., 16:1341-1345.
3. Gottfries, C.G. (1988): Compr. Gerontol., C 2:47-62.
4. Hardy, et al., (1985): Neurochem. Int., 7:545-563.
5. McEwen, B.S. (1987): Biochem. Pharmacol., 36:1755-1763.
6. Nyth, A.L. and Gottfries, C.G. (1990): Br. J. Psychiatry, (in press).
7. Swaab, D.F. Fliers E. and Partiman, T.S. (1985): Brain Res., 342:37-44.
8. Svennerholm, L., Gottfries, C.G. and Karlsson, I. (1988): In A multidisciplinary approach to myelin disease, G. Serlupi Crescenzi, ed., pp. 319-328. Plenum, New York.
9. Wallin, et al., (1990): Pharmacopsychiatry, (in press).
10. Whitehouse, et al., (1982): Science, 215:1237-1239.

CYTOSKELETAL ABERRATION IN ALZHEIMER'S DISEASE FIBROBLASTS

T.NISHIMURA and M.TAKEDA
Department of Neuropsychiatry, Osaka University Medical School, Fukushima, Osaka 553 JAPAN

Though the etiology of Alzheimer's disease is still unknown, recent findings suggest that Alzheimer's disease is associated with pathologic changes in cells outside the brain. There are papers reporting abnormalities in Alzheimer fibroblasts, including alteration of energy metabolism, increased sensitivity to x-rays, altered calcium binding, decreased adhesiveness, and altered protein phosphorylation. The change in cytoskeletal proteins of the cultured fibroblasts from Alzheimer's disease patients is reported.

MATERIALS AND METHODS

Fibroblasts were cultured from the cutaneous tissue of patients with clinically diagnosed Alzheimer's disease. The cells were maintained in Dulbecco's modified essential medium (DMEM) supplemented with 10 % fetal calf serum (FCS). The cells in the passage of 8-12 were used for the experiments. Fibroblasts grown to 80 % confluency on a polylysine-coated cover glass in DMEM supplemented with 10% FCS were fixed by 4% paraformaldehyde and immunostained. The antibodies used are anti-vimentin (Amersham), anti-actin (Transformation Res.), anti-fodrin (Amersham) and FITC-labeled anti-mouse IgG (Tago). Cells were harvested and the cell pellets were electrophoresed on a 7.5% acrylamide gel. The electrophoresed protein was transfered and immunostained with anti-vimentin and anti-fodrin antibodies. Peroxidase-labeled anti-mouse IgG were layered and developed with 0.07% H_2O_2/chloronaphthol.

RESULTS

After incubating the cells under serum-free medium for ten days, the fiobroblasts were immunostained with anti-actin, anti-tibulin, and anti-vimentin antibodies. The immunofluorescent staining with anti-actin and anti-tubulin antibodies showed no difference in the distribution of actin fibers and microtubules between control fibroblasts and Alzheimer fibroblasts. The staining with anti-vimentin antibody, however, revealed a significant difference in the distribution of vimentin fibers between control and Alzheimer fibroblasts. The control cells showed highly ordered arrangement of complex interconnecting networks, emanating from a perinuclear ring, from which vimentin fibers appear to connect to nuclear surface and extend throughout the cytoplasm terminating at the plasm membrane. Alzheimer fibroblasts showed a unique aberration of vimentin fibers arrangement. The even distribution of vimentin fibers were no more observed and vimentin fibers were stained strongly in some regions but weakin other regions. The continuity of

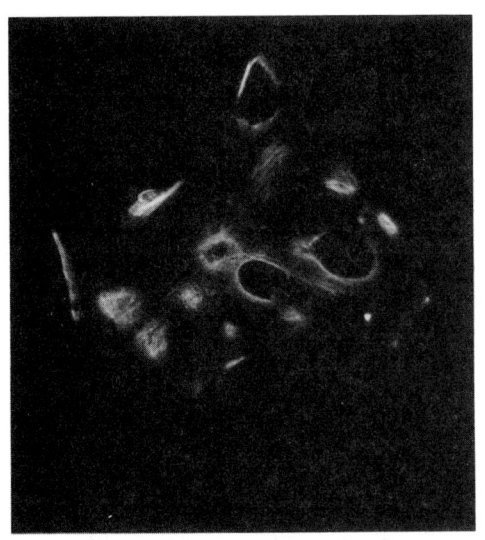

Fig.1 Anti-vimentin staining
of Alzheimer fibroblast

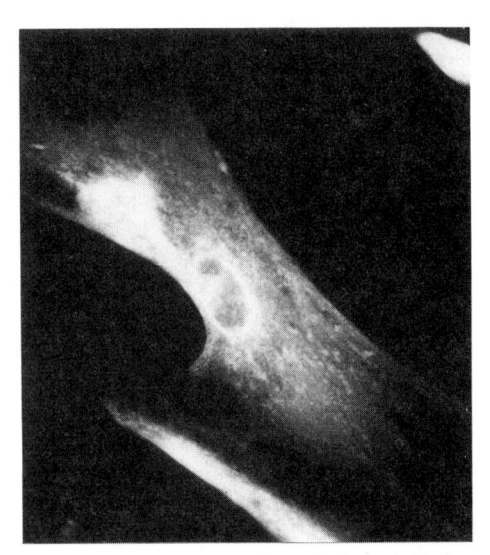

Fig.2 Anti-fodrin staining
of Alzheimer fibroblast

vimentin fibers seemed to be maintained. Patchy areas of intense vimentin immunostaining were observed in most of Alzheimer fibroblasts (Fig.1). Anti-fodrin staining of Alzheimer fibroblasts also showed different distribution of fodrin molecules from that of the control cells (Fig.2).

The fibroblast homogenate was studied by Western blotting using anti-vimentin and anti-fodrin antibodies. The anti-vimentin immunoblotting showed the six bands between 57k and 50k with control and Alzheimer cells. There was no difference in the molecular size of vimentin between Alzheimer and control cells. The immunoblotting with anti-fodrin antibody showed the higher molecular weight of fodrin bands with Alzheimer cells than the control cells.

DISCUSSION

Vimentin, a major intermediate filament in fibroblast, exists in meninges, ependyma, and subpopulation of glial cella in the central nervous system. The vimentin distribution in Alzheimer fibroblasts was shown to be quite different from that of the control cells. Though the molecular size and the quantity of Alzheimer vimentin is the same with that of control cells, the function of vimentin fibers may be changed in Alzheimer fibroblasts. The molecular size of fodrin is quite different in Alzheimer cells. Since fodrin is known to be located in submembrane area of cells, this finding indicates the change in membrane structure in Alzheimer's fibroblasts. It is possible that aberration of vimentin distribution is caused by the abnormal fodrin molecule in Alzheimer fibroblasts.

THE NEUROTRANSMITTER BASES FOR DEPRESSION AND DEMENTIA IN ALZHEIMER'S DISEASE

V. CHAN-PALAY
Neurology Clinic, University Hospital, 8091 Zürich, Switzerland

This paper summarises results on a quantitative study of catecholamine neurons in the locus coeruleus of controls, patients with senile dementia of the Alzheimer type and in chronic depression.

MATERIAL AND METHODS

All patients belonged to the Zurich study on dementia. Normal controls included the brains of 11 patients, 4 male and 7 female, ranging in age from 43 to 89 years, with no clinical history of neurological or psychiatric disease as confirmed by postmortem gross and microscopic neuropathological examination. Data assembled in three paradigm control cases in the age group of the patients in the Alzheimer's group served as control values for quantitative analysis (Table). Appropriate levels of normal mental function in patients was shown by results of between 22 and 26 from a possible 30 points in the last available mini-mental status tests. In the group of senile dementia of the Alzheimer's type (SDAT) cases the brains of 8 patients that had met the NINCDS-ADRDA criteria for the diagnosis of Alzheimer's disease were studied, 2 male and 6 female cases with ages ranging from 71 to 85 years. Cases of dementia due to other neurological disorders, such as ischemia, multiple infarcts, Pick's disease etc were excluded. Postmortem delays ranged from 3 to 16 hours: Seriously impaired mental function in these patients was indicated by a score of 0 to 5 points in the last available mini-mental status tests. The depressed patients had 18 or more years of history of major depressive episodes without cognitive defect.

RESULTS

Identification of norepinephrine (NE)-producing neurons in the locus coeruleus (Lc) is done by immunocytochemical demonstration of two NE biosynthetic enzymes, tyrosine hydroxylase (TH) and DBH, and immunoreactions are visualized by the peroxidase-antiperoxydase (PAP) and immunogold-silver-staining (IGSS) methods. It is demontrated that the reactions with antisera against TH and DBH yield equivalent results and that both immunocytochemical visualization methods allow detailed analysis of neuronal morphology. The neurons of the human LC fall into four distinct classes: large multipolar neurons with round or multiangular somata (LM), large elliptical "bipolar" neurons (LB), small multipolar neurons with round or multiangular somata (SM) and small ovoid "bipolar" (SB) neurons. In SDAT, the four basic LC neuron classes found in the normal human brain are recognizable in the remaining cells, but the cell somata are generally larger, the cell bodies are swollen and misshapen, and the dendrites are forshortened and thick and less branched than in neurons of control LCs. Quantitative analysis confirms the qualitative observations. The reduction of absolute numbers of LC-NE neurons in paradigm cases of SDAT and depression as compared to controls are shown in the table below.

Case	Age	Sex	Neuron number x 10^3
Control	79	m	47.5
Control	78	f	40.9
SDAT (mild)	78	m	34.0
SDAT (severe)	74	f	18.8
SDAT (severe)	77	f	5.7
Depression	86	f	29.08

A reduction of total neuron numbers of the LC of between 3.5% and 87.5% as compared to age-matched controls is found in SDAT. This neuron loss is topographically arranged: in the rostral part of the LC, the reduction is greatest, being more than 28% in the case least affected in this part, and 97% in the case most severely affected. The middle part is less, and the caudal part least affected by cell loss in all cases. The average rostrocaudal nuclear length in SDAT cases is reduced as compared to controls (13 mm and 14.9 mm respectively). The neuron loss is also extreme in the cases with major depression (-55%), with severe reduction of levels of TH within the remaining neurons.

REFERENCES

1. Chan-Palay V. and Asan E. Quantitation of catecholamine neurons in the locus coeruleus in human brains of young and older adults and in depression. J.Comp.Neurol.,287:357 (1989).

2. Chan-Palay V. and Asan E. Alterations in catecholamine neurons of the locus coeruleus in senile dementia of the Alzheimer's type, and in Parkinson's disease with and without dementia and depression. J. Comp. Neurol., 287:373 (1989).

3. Chan-Palay V., Jentsch B., Lang W., Höchli M., Asan E. Distribution of Neuropeptide Y, C-terminal flanking peptide of NPY, and Galanin coexistence with catecholamine in the locus coeruleus of normal human, Alzheimer's dementia and Parkinson's disease. Dementia, 18-31 1990.

THE USE OF A 5-HYDROXYTRYPTAMINE REUPTAKE BLOCKER (CITALOPRAM) AS AN EMOTIONAL STABILIZER IN DEMENTIA SYNDROMES

A.L. NYTH[*] and C.G. GOTTFRIES[*]
[*]Psychiatry and Neurochemistry, Gothenburg University, Gothenburg, Sweden

It is well known there are serious disturbances of the serotonergic (5-HT) metabolism in brains of patients with dementia of Alzheimer type (AD/SDAT). These findings implicate that drugs inhibiting the neuronal 5-HT reuptake might have a beneficial effect in patients with AD/SDAT. Hyttel (3) has shown that Citalopram blocks the entrance of 5-HT into serotonergic neurons, with no effect on the uptake of noradrenaline or dopamine. Harenko (2) and Nyth (5) have reported an improvement of emotional functions in patients with dementia after treatment with Citalopram.

SUBJECT AND METHOD

Recently we reported a study of the effects of Citalopram in patients with moderate AD/SDAT or vascular dementia (6). In this presentation the data from 73 patients with AD/SDAT will be given. The patients, ranging in age from 56 to 94 (mean=77.2) were studied in a combined placebo-controlled double-blind and open design. Treatment dose varied between 10 and 30 mg Citalopram or placebo. After four weeks of double-blind treatment, the patients were rated with a series of rating scales.

RESULTS

The GBS ratings (1) at baseline indicated moderate cognitive disturbances. In addition many patients also had depressed mood, reduced motivation, anxiety or confusion. The assessment after four weeks of double-blind treatment comprised 63 patients. Significant improvements were found in the GBS items: emotional bluntness, confusion, irritability, anxiety, fear-panic, depressed mood and restlessness in patients treated with Citalopram (FIG. 1). No significant improvements were recorded in the placebo treated patients. There was no improvement recorded on any of the intellectual items.

Eleven symptoms recorded on the UKU Side effect Scale (4) were rated as probably induced by test treatment. Four of these were recorded both during treatment with Citalopram and placebo. Concentration difficulties, depression, emotional indifference, orthostatic dizziness, diminished sexual desire, ejaculatory dysfunction and orgastic dysfunction were recorded only during treatment with Citalopram. Most symptoms were mild or moderate. Except bradycardia in three patients with an initial heart rate of 48, 52 and 60 respectively, no clinically significant cardiovascular reactions or blood pressure changes were recorded.

DISCUSSION

The results of the present double-blind study and our clinical impressions indicate that Citalopram is not only a mood stabilizer but also has effect on emotional bluntness, irritability, anxiety, fear-panic, and restlessness. Therefore the drug can be considered an emotional stabilizer. Emotional disturbances are common and are most troublesome for the demented patients themselves and for their relatives. Few side effects were recorded. The results of this study suggest that Citalopram may be particularly suitable for treatment of elderly patients with AD/SDAT.

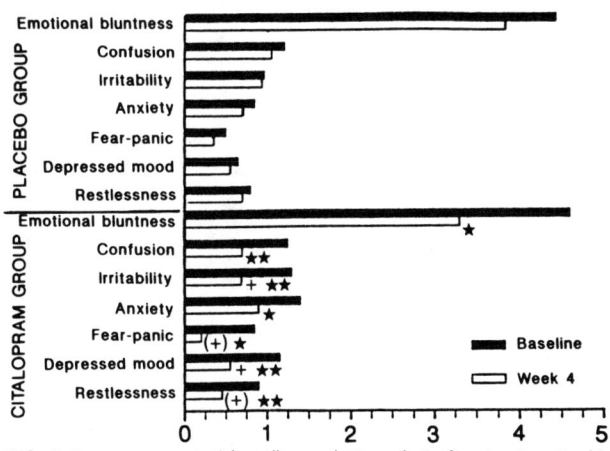

FIG. 1. Average scores at baseline and at week 4 after treatment with double-blind technique.
+ p<0.05, (+) p<0.10, unpaired t-test (between groups).
★ p<0.05, ★★p<0.01, paired t-test (within group).

REFERENCES

1. Gottfries, et al., (1982): Arch. Gerontol. Geriatr. 1: 311-330.
2. Harenko (1984) On a clinical phase II study of Citalopram in elderly depressed patients. H. Lundbeck A/S Report 19/831.
3. Hyttel, (1982): Prog. Neuro-psychopharmacol. Biol. Psychiatry 6: 277-295.
4. Lingjaerde, et al., (1987): Acta Psych. Scand. Suppl 334.
5. Nyth, et al., (1987): Nord. Psykiatr. Tidsskr. 41: 423-430.
6. Nyth, and Gottfries (1990): Br. J. Psychiatry (in press).

COURSE AND OUTCOME IN PANIC DISORDER

M.B. Keller*
*Department of Psychiatry & Human Behavior, Brown University,
Providence, RI, USA

Investigators have documented high rates of chronicity among patients suffering from anxiety disorders (1; 3 - 6). Longitudinal studies of patients with generalized anxiety disorder, agoraphobia, and panic disorder have indicated that patients with these disorders report having suffered from symptoms of anxiety/stress for one-sixth to one-half their lives. According to a number of published reports, high rates of comorbid affective disorders also complicate the course of anxiety disorders, leading to increased chronicity and severity of both anxiety and depression (2,6).

Subjects and Methods

450 subjects with a diagnosis of DSM-IIIR current or past panic disorder (with or without phobic avoidance or social phobia) or current or past agoraphobia were enrolled in a 12-site, longitudinal, naturalistic, prospective study of the clinical course of anxiety disorders. Since this is a naturalistic study, subjects received treatment (if any) by physician's choice, and were monitored by the investigators during the follow-up period.

Subjects were followed-up at six month intervals for one year and assessed for: current and lifetime (longitudinal) diagnosis and course of illness as obtained by structural interview (with the SCID and LIFE) at six and 12 months; assessment of psychosocial functioning, by patient questionnaire at intake, 6 months, and 12 months; and interim summaries of clinical status and treatment harvested from the treating physician/clinician over the 12-month period following intake.

Results

At this time preliminary, six month data has been analyzed for the first 150 patients enrolled in the study. This subsample includes 47 men (31%) and 103 women (69%). Average age of the subjects is 41; age range is 18 - 65.

Preliminary analyses indicated that 99 subjects, or 66%, had a lifetime episode of panic disorder with or without agoraphobia; 75 subjects (50%) were in an episode of panic disorder on intake. Further analyses showed that 24 subjects (16%) were in an episode of panic disorder only, while 51 (34%) were in an episode of panic disorder with agoraphobia.

A significant proportion of subjects with panic disorder were found to also have a comorbid affective disorder at intake. 14 of 75 panic disorder subjects (19%) had a comorbid major depression, and 8 (11%) had a diagnosis of intermittent depressive disorder.

Median age of onset of the panic disorder was 28. Median duration of the intake episode was 7.9 years; for those patients with a past panic disorder, median time since their last episode was 2.2 years.

Rates of recovery were calculated for 38 panic disorder subjects after six months of inclusion in the study. Ten, or 26% of this subsample, had recovered.

Discussion

These preliminary analyses confirm the findings of other investigators who have noted significant degrees of chronicity and comorbidity in panic disorder. The overall 28% comorbidity of depression in these subjects suggests that clinicians treating panic disorder patients should be aware of the need to vigorously treat the depression as well as the anxiety disorder. Further analyses are needed to provide a more complete understanding of the long-term course of this disorder.

References

1. Aronson T, Logue C: On the longitudinal course of panic disorder: Developmental history and predictors of phobic complications. Comprehensive Psychiatry, Vol. 28, No. 4 (July/August) 1987: pp. 344 - 355.

2. Coryell W, Noyes R, Clancy J: Panic disorder and primary unipolar depression. J Affective Disord 5: 311 - 317, 1983.

3. Errera P, Coleman JV: A long-term follow-up study of neurotic phobic patients in a psychiatry clinic. J Nerv Ment Dis 136: 267 - 271, 1963.

4. Katon W, Vitaliano P, Anderson K et al.: Panic disorder: Residual symptoms after acute attacks abate. Comprehensive Psychiatry, Vol. 28, No. 2 (March/April), 1987: pp. 151 - 158.

5. Marks I, Lader M: Anxiety states (anxiety neurosis): A review. J Ner Ment Dis 1973, Vol. 156 No. 1, pp. 1 - 18.

6. Reich J: The epidemiology of anxiety. J Nerv Ment Dis. Vol. 174 No. 3, March 1986, pp. 129 - 136.

THE PATHOPHYSIOLOGY OF SPONTANEOUS PANIC AS RELATED TO RESPIRATORY DYSCONTROL

Donald F. Klein, M.D.
Department of Psychiatry
Columbia University, College of Physicians & Surgeons
New York, NY, U.S.A.

That there is some relationship between hyperventilation and panic disorder seems plain. Although some believe that hyperventilation is both a necessary and sufficient condition for the occurrence of spontaneous panics, most now emphasize the need for a misconception of the physical symptoms as signs of immediate danger. Direct tests of room air hyperventilation in several laboratories have shown that although panic patients frequently develop more distress than normals, the actual precipitation of panics is not common. Further, the amount of distress is markedly affected by the instructional set.

The acute symptomatology of the spontaneous panic attack is predominantly cardiorespiratory with marked dyspnea and an urge to get out into fresh air. This must be accounted for.

Ernst Mayr has pointed out "need to distinguish two causations underlying all phenomena or processes in organisims. These have been referred to by earlier authors as proximate and ultimate causations. The proximate causes consists of answers to "how?" questions; they are responsible for all physiological and developmental processes in the living organism, and their domain is the phenotype. The ultimate or evolutionary causes consists of the answers to the "why?" questions, and provide the historical explanation for the occurrence of these phenomena. Their domain is the genotype..."

What we will address here is how a close evaluation of the "how?" mechanisms helps develop a hypothesis as to "why?". Several studies have shown that patients with panic disorder often display evidence of chronic compensated respiratory alkalosis, leading to the inference that they chronically hyperventilate. This normalizes, with treatment, which is usually interpreted as indicating that the chronic hyperventilation is secondary to the panic attacks. An alternative hypothesis is that an antecedent dysregulation causes both chronic hyperventilation and panics.

Respiratory studies of patients with spontaneous panic, in our laboratory, have shown that in the 1 or 2 minutes preceding the onset of the panic, there is the onset of marked hyperventilation. In panic precipitated by the dl-lactate infusion, respiratory hyperventilation is much decreased and is only evident as a small consistent change across many subjects. We hypothesize an unfolding of the panic process which includes a preliminary phase of hyperventilation, that does not serve as the basis for a cognitive misinterpretation. To attribute the panic to the hyperventilation is a post hoc fallacy. It is of particular interest that sodium lactate produces hyperventilation despite the concomitant metabolic alkalosis which should suppress respiration in a homeostatic attempt to stabilize the pH by retaining carbon dioxide. This, however, probably accounts for the fact that the degree of hyperventilation, produced by sodium lactate, is substantially less than that during the spontaneous panic.

That patients who panic with a particular challenge have an initial phase of hyperventilation is also supported by our sodium bicarbonate infusion work, which shows a drop in PCO_2 in those patients who go on to panic, whereas those who do not have the expectable rise in PCO_2.

Carbon dioxide, as a panicogen, also causes a greater increase in minute volume in panic patients than in controls, even in those patients who do not go on to panic.

We had also hypothesized that lactate and bicarbonate would result in a brain hypercapnia, which is consistent with the recent RCBF and PET findings that lactate increases brain hemic perfusion. Carbon dioxide is a particularly strong stimulus for this response.

To tie together the panic phenomenology, the antecedent hyperventilation, and the sensitivity to dl-lactate bicarbonate and CO_2, is possible if one hypothesizes that the derangement is in a specific detector for potential asphyxiation. Evidence is gathered, from a number of sources, as to whether one is in a state of potential asphyxiation. The initial response is hyperventilation and when a threshold is crossed, an emergency is declared with release of suffocation feelings. The panic attack is a false alarm, but not some sort of generic false alarm, but a specific false alarm that relates to asphyxiation detection.

INTERMITTENT VS MAINTENANCE MEDICATION IN SCHIZOPHRENIA
TWO YEAR RESULTS

M.I. HERZ*, W.M. GLAZER**, M.A. MOSTERT*, M.A. SHEARD**, H.V. SZYMANSKI*

*Department of Psychiatry, State University of New York at Buffalo, Buffalo, NY, U.S.A.; **Department of Psychiatry, Yale University, New Haven, CT, U.S.A.

It is common practice for aftercare clinics to treat chronic schizophrenic patients with maintenance neuroleptic medication on an indefinite basis. Despite the efficacy of these drugs in helping to prevent relapse (1), there is growing concern that prolonged administration of antipsychotic medication may have serious consequences, especially tardive dyskinesia, which is believed to increase with long-term use of the drugs. In the belief that reducing exposure to neuroleptic medication may decrease the side effects, we became interested in an intermittent treatment approach, that is, the use of antipsychotic drugs only when early signs of relapse appear.

This two-year study evaluates the relative efficacy of intermittent medication compared to maintenance medication for stable schizophrenic outpatients. Since it was a double-blind study, an early intervention strategy with active medication and crisis counseling was offered for all patients when prodromal symptoms appeared.

METHOD

One hundred and one patients were randomized after successfully completing a gradual drug withdrawal, 51 into the maintenance medication group and 50 into the intermittent medication group. The differential effectiveness of the two drug strategies was evaluated by comparing patients cross-sectionally on admission and at 12 and 24 months in terms of major dimensions of psychopathology, role functioning, family burden, and drug side effects, including abnormal involuntary movements. Patients were terminated from the study if they had three prodromal episodes in one year or if an episode lasted more than nine weeks.

RESULTS

Seventy-three percent of the maintenance patients and 38% of the intermittent patients completed the study, a statistically significant difference ($p < 0.001$). As expected, the intermittent group had more prodromal episodes, but the length and severity of the episodes showed no significant differences between groups. There were significantly ($p < 0.001$) more protocol terminations in the intermittent group (46%), compared with the maintenance group (14%). However, percentage of relapses after two years was 16% for the maintenance group versus 30% in the intermittent group, a nonsignificant difference. Relapse was defined as an increase in any Problem Appraisal Scale (3) psychotic symptom to moderate or severe, and a Global Assessment Scale (2) of 30 or less, and with more than two days' duration of the episode. Only 20% of all patients were hospitalized, 16% in the maintenance group, 24% in the intermittent group, a nonsignificant difference. The few differences in symptomatology and family burden ratings on cross-sectional evaluations generally favored the maintenance group. Measurements of side effects showed no differences between the groups.

DISCUSSION

Overall results favored the maintenance drug strategy. Therefore, there seems to be no advantage in using the intermittent approach for the majority of stable schizophrenic outpatients who are on moderate doses of antipsychotic medication. It appears that the low relapse and rehospitalization rates for intermittent patients resulted from the use of an early intervention strategy.

REFERENCES

1. Davis, J.M. and Andriukaitis, M.A. (1986): The natural course of schizophrenia and effective drug treatment. J. Clin. Psychopharmacol. 6 (1 suppl):2-10.
2. Endicott, J. et al. (1976): The Global Assessment Scale: a procedure for measuring overall severity of psychiatric disturbance. Arch. Gen. Psychiatry 33:766-771.
3. Spitzer, R.L., Endicott, J. (1971): An integrated group of forms for automated psychiatric case records; a progress report. Arch. Gen. Psychiatry 24:448-453.

Indication and informed consent for neuroleptic longterm treatment in schizophrenia.
H. HELMCHEN

Indications of neuroleptic longterm treatment are
- stabilization of remission
  after successful acute neuroleptic treatment, or
- suppression of persistent psychotic symptons, or
- prophylaxis of relapses.

The advantages aimed at by these indications must be weighed against the risks of neuroleptic longterm treatment. The most important risk is tardive dyskinesia because it may be, at least partly, in some patients and to some degree
- irreversible,
- untreatable, and
- frequent (ca. 20%, severe disabling tardive dyskinesia in ca. 1%).

Valid predictors for this risk are not known, but major supposed risk factors are
- longer duration of neuroleptic treatment for at least 3-6 months
  - perhaps higher dosage, both cumulative or daily
  - perhaps intermittent application
- old age
  - perhaps particularly in postmenopausal females
- brain lesions (atrophies?)
  - perhaps particularly around the 3 rd ventricle
  - perhaps subtypes of psychosis with cognitive dysfunctions and negative symptons.

Therefore, the cost-benefit-ratio of neuroleptic longterm treatment is acceptable individually only if there would be a high risk of subjective suffering or serious social consequences of nonmedication and the risk of tardive dyskinesia will be minimized by application of the lowest possible dose, perhaps continuously by a depot-neuroleptic and regularly screening for signs of beginning tardive dyskinesia. In that latter case a change to the atypical neuroleptic clozapine should be done as well as it should be considered in old people and those with a large 3rd ventricle. However, with clozapine regular and tight blood counts are unavoidable for control of the rare but serious risk of agranulocytosis.

When has the patient to be informed about these risks in order to get a valid consent? The time informing the patient is the moment of indicating and starting a longterm treatment. Although, of course, longterm treatment is another treatment with other indications and risks as an acute one, sometimes this seems to be forgotten if an initially neuroleptic treatment of an acute psychosis will be continued

without any interruption for more than 3-6 months.
At this time the patient should be informed on the expected benefits and possible risks of a neuroleptic treatment. If the competent patient refuses the medication then he should be trained to recognize first signs of a relapse and to be invited to repeat the treatment. He should be helped to evaluate his own experience of becoming ill again (and again) as well as that of side effects. In other, noncompliant patients their competence may be doubted and implementation of a legal guardianship be considered as a last chance for the patient.

References:
1. HAAG, H., GREIL, W., HAAG, M., BENDER, W., RÜTHER, E.: Tardive dyskniezia and medication history. Pharmacopsychiatry 18: 35-36 (1985)
2. HELMCHEN, H.: Clinical experience with clozapine in Germany. Psychopharmacol. 99: 80-83 (1989)
3. KANE, J.M.: The current status of neuroleptic therapy. J. Clin. Psychiatgry 50: 322-328 (1989)
4. MÖLLER, H.-J.: Indikation und Differentialindikation der neuroleptischen Langzeitmedikation. In Neuroleptika. Rückschau 1952-1986. Künftige Entwicklungen, P. PICHOT, H.-J. MÖLLER, eds. p.63-79, Springer, Berlin-Heidelberg-New York 1987

THE CLINICAL SIGNIFICANCE OF A PLASMA HALOPERIDOL AND FLUPHENAZINE LEVEL

T. VAN PUTTEN, S.R. MARDER, W.C. WIRSHING ET AL
Veterans Administration Medical Center, Los Angeles, U.S.A.

Two studies were conducted to investigate the relationships between plasma levels of neuroleptic (haloperidol and fluphenazine) and clinical response.

Study I:

SUBJECTS AND METHOD

Sixty-seven (67) newly re-admitted drug free schizophrenic men were randomly assigned to receive haloperidol (HPL) either 5, 10 or 20 mg daily for four weeks. Clinical response was measured at baseline, and weekly for the first four weeks, and at week 8 after the flexible dose period. Clinical ratings were made blind to plasma levels. Haloperidol was assayed by a radioimmunoassay[2].

RESULTS

We found a curvilinear relationship between clinical response and plasma HPL during fixed dose treatment. The therapeutic "window" appeared to be between 2 and 12 ng/ml. The "acid test", however, was whether patients with plasma levels greater than 12 ng/ml would improve as their plasma levels were lowered. When plasma levels above 12 ng/ml were lowered into the therapeutic window, all cases improved to varying degrees, and no patient deteriorated. When nonresponders within the therapeutic window had their plasma levels raised above 12 ng/ml (as in routine practice) they, on balance, deteriorated in that these patients became more dysphoric. Patients with plasma level below 2 ng/ml improved as their plasma levels were raised into the therapeutic window. On the 20 mg dose, half the patients had plasma levels above 12 ng/ml.

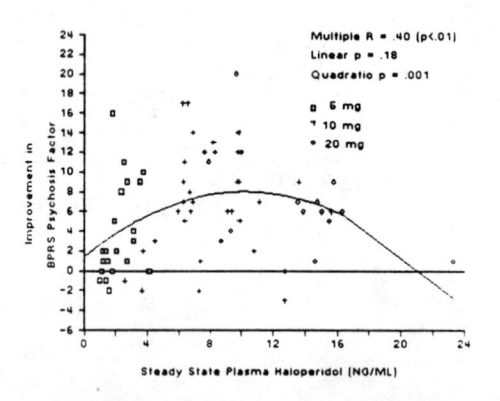

Study II:

SUBJECTS AND METHODS

Seventy-two (72) newly admitted schizophrenic (by DSM-III) patients who had not received neuroleptic for at least two months were randomly assigned to treatment with fixed doses of fluphenazine either 5, 10 or 20 mg daily for four weeks. Plasma levels were drawn weekly and analyzed for fluphenazine, fluphenazine sulfoxide, fluphenazine N-oxide and 7OH-fluphenazine by a sensitive radioimmunoassay[1]. Clinical response was measured weekly by a Global Impression Scale (which rates global improvement and side effects categorized into "none," "do not significantly interfere with patient's functioning," "significantly interfere with patient's functioning" and "outweighs therapeutic effect"), the Brief Psychiatric Rating Scale (BPRS) and an Extrapyramidal Side Effect scale.

RESULTS

A logistic regression indicated that Global Improvement was significantly related to plasma fluphenazine (p=.015). A logistic regression also indicated that disabling side effects (defined as side effects that "significantly interfere with patient's functioning" or side effects that "outweigh therapeutic effects") were significantly related to plasma fluphenazine (p=.0008). The figure shows both the improvement and disabling side effect curves and demonstrates that these curves are much closer together than is commonly appreciated. The therapeutic index for fluphenazine is much narrower than formerly thought. A multivariate analysis suggested that fluphenazine N-oxide is a toxic metabolite in that Flu N-oxide was significantly related to disabling side effects when analyzed in isolation (p=.003), and remained significant (p=.021) in a full model that included parent fluphenazine as well as the other two metabolites. Relationships between fluphenazine and its metabolites and BPRS scores will be available in time for the meeting.

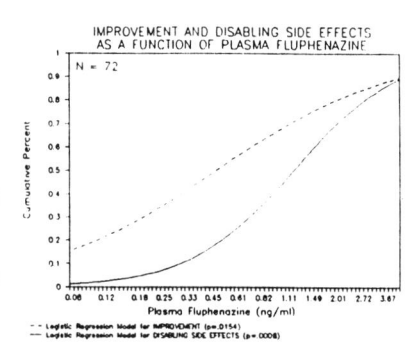

DISCUSSION

A plasma haloperidol or fluphenazine level may be useful in finding the minimal effective dose in maintenance treatment; to detect noncompliance; in drug interactions (e.g. with carbamazepine); and possibly in the refractory patient.

REFERENCES

1. McKay G., et al., (1990): Development and application of a radioimmunoassay for fluphenazine based on monoclonal antibodies and its comparison with alternate assay methods. J Pharm Sci., in press.

2. Poland R.E. and Rubin R.T. (1981): Radioimmunoassay of haloperidol in human serum: correlation of serum haloperidol with serum prolactin. Life Sciences, 29:1837-1845.

CLINICAL AND BIOLOGICAL PREDICTORS OF RELAPSE IN SCHIZOPHRENIA

S.R. MARDER, T. VAN PUTTEN, M. ARAVAGIRI, W.C. WIRSHING, K. JOHNSON-CRONK, M. LEBELL
Brentwood Division, West Los Angeles V.A. Medical Center and Department of Psychiatry and Biobehavioral Sciences, UCLA School of Medicine, Los Angeles, California, U.S.A.

Concerns about the toxicity of chronic neuroleptic treatment have led to a search for methods for treating schizophrenic patients with the lowest effective dose of medication. However, a number of studies indicate that dosage reduction is associated with an increased rate of relapse. This report will review our findings from a comparison of low and conventional doses of fluphenazine decanoate. In addition, we will also report on clinical and biological variables including prodromal symptoms and neuroleptic plasma levels which may be useful in predicting when patients are vulnerable for relapse.

SUBJECTS AND METHODS

The low dose study was a double-blind trial of either 5 mg or 25 mg of fluphenazine decanoate administered every two weeks for two years. The subjects were 66 male veterans who fulfilled DSM III criteria for schizophrenic disorder. Patients were followed for two years with regular ratings using the BPRS, SCL-90, and side effects scales at regular intervals. Blood was drawn for fluphenazine level at baseline, every month for the first three months, and then every 3 months. Samples were drawn 2 weeks following the previous injection or just before the next injection was administered. When subjects demonstrated an increase of 3 or more points on BPRS cluster scores for thought disturbance or paranoia they were considered to have had a "psychotic exacerbation". When patients demonstrated an exacerbation, the clinician was permitted to double their dose up to 10 mg in the low dose group or 50 mg in the conventional dose group. If patients could not be stabilized in a few days, they were considered to have had a relapse, our other measure of negative outcome.

Prodromal Symptoms. For this study, 50 stabilized schizophrenic patients, (diagnosed according to DSM IIIR), who received a low dose of fluphenazine decanoate (5 to 10 mg every 2 weeks) were monitored with weekly evaluations to determine whether they met criteria for nonpsychotic prodromal episodes. The following scales were evaluated: (1) the Anxious-Depression subscale of the Brief Psychiatric Rating Scale (BPRS); (2) a modification of the patient self-report Early Signs Questionnaire (Herz and Melville, 1980); and (3) the Idiosyncratic Prodromal Scale (IPS), ratings on a 100-point scale of three or more signs or symptoms that were selected after reviewing the onset of prior episodes with each individual patient and his or her family members. The three measures were compared with regard to their ability to correctly identify impending symptomatic exacerbation.

RESULTS

Fluphenazine plasma levels. Plasma levels of fluphenazine (FLU) were measured using a previously described radioimmunoassay (Midha et al, 1980). We studied the relationship between log transformed plasma levels at 6 and 9 months and rate of psychotic exacerbations with logistic regression during the year following the evaluation when the plasma level was drawn. Both analyses were statistically significant (at 6 months, chi square=4.38, df=1, p=.04; at 9 months, chi square=6.62, df=1, p=.003). The relationship between plasma level and the rate of psychotic exacerbations over the subsequent twelve month period was also studied by survival analysis using the log transformed FLU levels as a covariate (Cox Models). Using this method, we also found significant relationships between the log transformed FLU level and the risk of exacerbations at both time points (for 26 weeks, chi square = 3.77, df, 1, p=.052; for 38 weeks, global chi square = 11.25, df = 1, p =.0008).

Prodromal Symptoms. We used receiver operating characteristic (ROC) methods (Hsiao et al, 1989) for comparing the different instruments as methods for predicting whether patients would or would not demonstrate a psychotic exacerbation in the 4 weeks following the assessment. The area under the ROC curve (AUC) is an overall measure of a test's effectiveness. We calculated the AUC for each measure, and evaluated whether it indicated better than chance performance using a bootstrap method. Both the IPS and the BPRS cluster score were significantly better than chance at correctly identifying period of vulnerability to psychotic exacerbation (p <.01), but their sensitivity was modest at best. The ROC analyses suggest that relatively small changes in the signs and symptoms of chronic schizophrenic patients in maintenance treatment may be clinically meaningful.

CONCLUSIONS

Each of the clinical and biological measures provided useful information for clinicians who are treating chronic schizophrenic patients. Our results indicate that patients with low neuroleptic plasma levels or patients who are experiencing prodromal symptoms are at a greater risk for relapse.

REFERENCES

Herz MI, Melville C (1980) Relapse in schizophrenia. Amer J Psychiatry, 137:801-805.

Hsiao JK, Bartko JJ, Potter WZ (1989) Diagnosing diagnoses: Receiver Operating Characteristic Methods and Psychiatry. Arch Gen Psychiatry., 46:664-667.

Midha KK, Cooper JK, Hubbard JW. (1980) Radioimmunoassay for fluphenazine in human plasma. Commun Psychopharmacology, 4:107-114.

PREDICTION OF RELAPSE IN SCHIZOPHRENIA

J.LIEBERMAN*, J. KANE*, M. WOERNER*, J. ALVIR*, M. BORENSTEIN*, H. NOVACENKO**
*Hillside Hospital, division of Long Island Jewish Medical Center, Glen Oaks, NY, USA; **New York State Psychiatric Institute, New York, NY, USA.

Despite the proven efficacy of neuroleptic maintenance treatment in preventing relapse, the course of schizophrenia continues to be heterogeneous (1). There are no proven clinical predictors of outcome that can guide clinicians in determining optimal maintenance treatment strategies for individual patients (2). We evaluated the predictive validity of two provocative tests (behavioral response to methylphenidate and prolactin response to haloperidol) in two samples of stable outpatient chronic schizophrenics prior to undergoing neuroleptic withdrawal or dose reduction.

SUBJECT AND METHODS

1. 41 patients (71% schizophrenia, 29% schizoaffective disorder, mean ± SD age = 30 ± 6.1 years, 61% male) who were stable and receiving neuroleptic maintenance treatment for at least six months underwent provocative testing with methylphenidate (0.5mg/kg IV) and placebo in a randomized order under double blind conditions prior to and following neuroleptic withdrawal. Patients were then followed off medication for one year or until relapse.

2. 56 male patients (84% schizophrenic, 16% schizoaffective disorder, mean ± SD age = 26 ± 5.8 years) who were stable and receiving neuroleptic maintenance treatment for at least six months received a provocative test with haloperidol (2mg IM) prior to their random assignment to one of three doses of fluphenazine decanoate (12.5-50mg IM q2wks; 2.5-10mg IM q2wks; 1.25-5mg IM q2wks) and followed for one year or until relapse.

RESULTS

1. Patients who exhibited transient psychotic symptoms activation to methylphenidate were significantly more likely to relapse than nonactivating patients (Wilcoxon STAT = 8.03, df=1, p=.005 Figure 1).

2. Reduced PRL response to haloperidol was associated with the likelihood of relapse. In the low dose treatment group 75% of patients with PRL <50ng/ml relapsed compared to 33% of patients with PRL >50ng/ml (Figure 2).

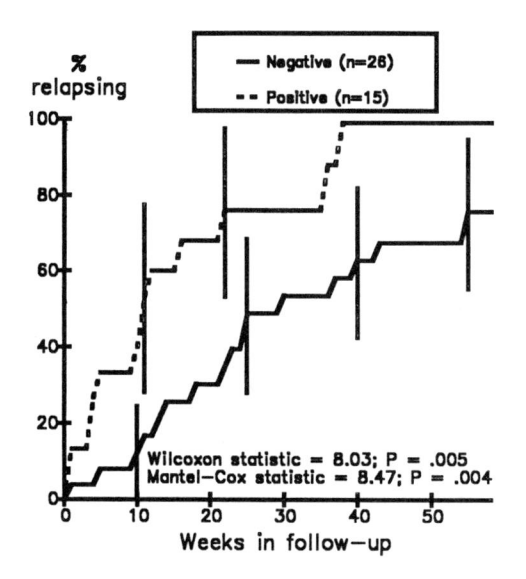

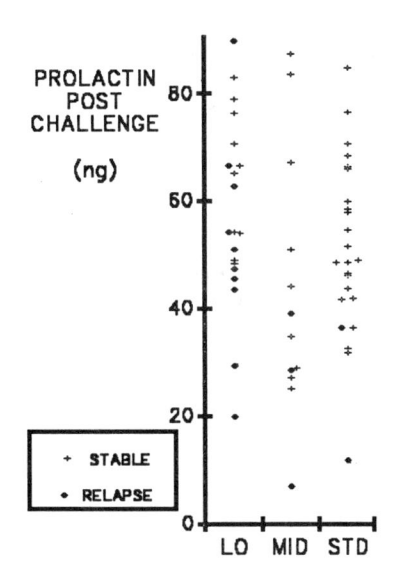

Fig. 1: Cumulative proportion (%) of schizophrenic patients relapsing by response to methylphenidate infusion.

Fig. 2: Relapse as a function of challenge response.

DISCUSSION

These results are consistent with prior reports in the literature (3,4,5,6) and suggest that pharmacologic probes of dopamine neural systems can elucidate pathophysiologic features of schizophrenia which have clinical utility.

REFERENCES

1. Angrist, et al. (1981): Relationship between responses to dopamine agonists, psychopathology, neuroleptic maintenance in schizophrenic subjects. In Recent Advances in Neuropsychopharmacology, Angrist, B, Burrows, GD (eds.), pp 49-51, Pergamon Press, New York.
2. Davidson, et al.: L-Dopa challenge and relapse in schizophrenia. Am. J. Psychiat. 144:934-938, 1987.
3. Kane, J. and Lieberman, J. (1987): Maintenance pharmacotherapy in schizophrenia. In Psychopharmacology Third Generation of Progress: The Energenic of Molecular Biology and Biological Psychiatry, Meltzer HY (ed.), pp. 1103-1110. Raven Press, New York.
4. Keks, et al.: Abnormal Prolactin Response to Haloperidol Challenge in Men with Schizophrenia. Am. J. Psychiat. 144:1335-1337, 1987.
5. Lieberman, J.A. and Kane, J.M. (eds.) (1986): Predictors of Relapse in Schizophrenia, American Psychiatric Press, Washington D.C.
6. VanKammen, et al.: d-Amphetamine induced heterogenous changes in psychotic behavior in schizophrenia. Am. J. Psychiat. 139:991-997, 1982.

PREDICTION OF RELAPSE FOLLOWING NEUROLEPTIC WITHDRAWAL: THE ROLE OF NORADRENALINE

D.P. van KAMMEN, J. PETERS, J. YAO, D. MC ADAM, A. MOUTON, W. BREEDING
VA Medical Center, Highland Drive, Pittsburgh, PA 15206, U.S.A.
Department of Psychiatry, Western Psychiatric Institute and Clinic, University of Pittsburgh, School of Medicine, Pittsburgh, PA, U.S.A.

In present day clinical practice schizophrenic patients are maintained on neuroleptics for up to 6 months after a psychotic episode. At present, there are no reliable clinical tests to assess whether schizophrenic patients can be safely withdrawn from neuroleptics, although patients may stop taking medication when their symptoms are under control. Amphetamine challenge test response during neuroleptic drug treatment has been reported to identify patients who are at risk to relapse soon after neuroleptic withdrawal (Angrist and van Kammen, 1985; van Kammen et al., 1982). Amphetamine releases both dopamine and noradrenaline (NA). The psychotogenic response to d-amphetamine, in spite of D_2-receptor blockade, in patients who relapsed after neuroleptic withdrawal suggested that NA activity could play a role in relapse.

METHODS

32 male DSM-IIIR schizophrenic patients (mean age: 34 ± 7.6 years) treated with oral maintenance haloperidol (mean dose: 12 mg/day) participated after signing informed consent. CSF NA, 3-methoxy-4-hydroxy phenolglycol (MHPG) and homovanillic acid (HVA) were determined with HPLC [van Kammen et al., 1989;1990]. The growth hormone (GH) response to a single dose of clonidine (0.005 mg/kg, po), i.e. the clonidine challenge test (CCT), were used to test the role of NA in relapse following haloperidol withdrawal in 29 patients. After double blind discontinuation of haloperidol, patients were placed on placebo for up to six weeks. Relapse was determined by an increase of 3 points in the 3-day-mean of the Bunney-Hamburg psychosis ratings [van Kammen et al., 1990]. Fourteen patients relapsed (22 ± 5 days drug-free) and 18 remained stable (45 days drug-free). After testing patients were put on antipsychotic drugs as clinically indicated.

RESULTS

a. CSF variables. CSF NA was significantly higher in the patients who relapsed subsequent to haloperidol withdrawal (0.79 ± 0.356 vs 0.52 ± 0.348 nmol/ml, p= 0.04, 2-tailed). None of the CSF monoamine metabolites were different between the two groups. b. Clonidine Challenge Test. At 90 min (7.2 ± 10.01 vs 1.6 ± 1.46 ng/ml, p<0.05) and 120 min (5.2 ± 6.3 vs 1.9 ± 2.09 ngm/ml, p<0.035) past the clonidine administration GH levels were significantly higher in the relapsers (p<0.05, 1-tailed). In the nonrelapsers no increases in GH levels were observed (FIG).

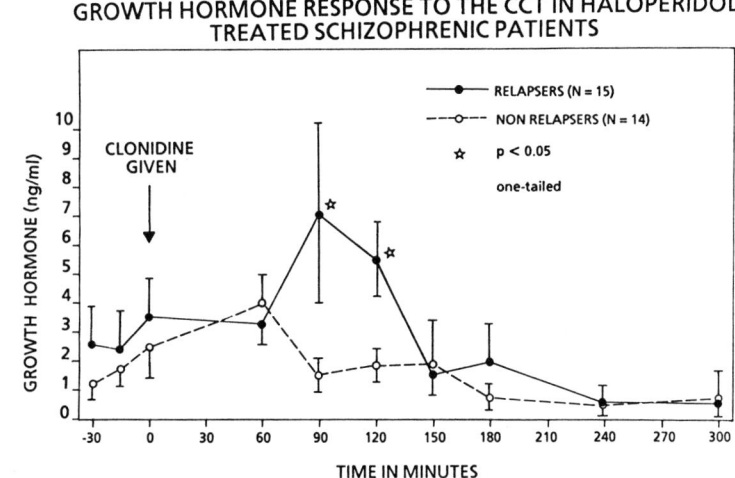

Figure 1
GROWTH HORMONE RESPONSE TO THE CCT IN HALOPERIDOL TREATED SCHIZOPHRENIC PATIENTS

DISCUSSION

The increases in CSF NE and the GH response to the CCT (functional α_2 receptor activity) suggest an overall relatively increased NE activity in the relapsers. GH peaks and CSF NE correlated significantly in the relapsers. The GH peaks were significantly lower than in our normal controls, while not all relapsers showed GH peaks at the expected time points. Our data indicate a potential dissociation between NE release and α_2 receptor activity (down regulation) in the nonrelapsers. **We propose that NA activity is relatively increased as a prodrome of psychotic relapse and that clinical stability is associated with decreased or normal CSF NA levels and subsensitive α_2-receptor activity.**

REFERENCES

1. Angrist, B., van Kammen, D.P. CNS stimulants as tools in the study of schizophrenia. TINS, 7:388-390, 1984.
2. van Kammen, D.P., Docherty J.P., Bunney W.E., Jr. Prediction of early relapse after pimozide discontinuation by response to d-amphetamine during pimozide treatment. Biol. Psychiat., 17:233-242, 1982.
3. van Kammen, D.P., Peters J., van Kammen, W.B., Nugent, A., Goetz, K.L., Yao, J., Linnoila, M. CSF norepinephrine in schizophrenia is elevated prior to relapse after haloperidol withdrawal. Biol. Psychiat., 26:176-188, 1989.
4. van Kammen, D.P., Peters, J., Yao, J., van Kammen, W.B., Neylan, T., Shaw, D, Linnoila, M. Norepinephrine in acute exacerbations of chronic schizophrenia: Negative symptoms revisited. Arch. Gen. Psychiat., 47:161-168, 1990.

NOVEL Ca^{2+} CURRENTS IN MAMMALIAN CNS NEURONS

N. AKAIKE and K. TAKAHASHI
Department of Neurophysiology, Tohoku University School of Medicine, Sendai 980, Japan

In the rat and mongolian gerbils models of vessel occlusion, the hippocampal CA1 pyramidal cells are highly sensitive to ischemia (4). Voltage-dependent Ca currents (I_{Ca}) classified into three groups (T-, N-, and L-types) on the basis of their kinetics, voltage-dependence, and unique pharmacologic sensitivities were observed in the hippocampal neurons (3, 7). Unexpectedly, we also found an additional tetrodotoxin (TTX)-sensitive transient Ca current (termed as TTX-I_{Ca}) in the pyramidal cells. Thus, in the present experiments, we have investigated the pharmacologic properties, the current kinetics, and the regional distribution of the TTX-I_{Ca}.

METHODS

Experiments were performed on the pyramidal neurons freshly isolated from rat CA1 region. Single neurons were isolated from 2-weeks-old-rats. Neurons were internally perfused with the use of suction pipette technique under the voltage-clamp (1), and the external solution surrounding a neuron was rapidly exchanged by 'concentration-clamp' technique (2). Membrane currents were recorded using amplifier EPC-7 L/M type.

RESULTS

The different regional distribution of TTX-I_{Ca} and T-type I_{Ca} in the hippocampal CA1 region was observed. The TTX-I_{Ca} was found dominantly at the dorsal portion of hippocampus whereas the T-type I_{Ca} at the ventral portion. The TTX-I_{Ca} developed linearly with increasing the extracellular Ca^{2+} concentration. On the other hand, T-type I_{Ca} showed a hyperbolic increase with the increase of external Ca^{2+} concentration. The ionic selectivity of TTX-sensitive channel for divalent cations was in the order of $Ca^{2+} \gg Sr^{2+} > Ba^{2+}$, which differed from that of T-, N, or L-type Ca^{2+} channels. The TTX-I_{Ca} was not affected by adding inorganic Ca^{2+} channel blockers such as La^{3+}, Ni^{2+}, and Cd^{2+}, but it was sensitive to TTX, scorpin toxin, and lidocaine, like voltage-dependent Na^+ channel did. The time constants of activation and inactivation of TTX-I_{Ca} were larger than those of Na^+ current (I_{Na}) but smaller than those of T-type I_{Ca}. The inactivation of TTX-I_{Ca} showed a double exponential decay as well as I_{Na}.

DISCUSSION

Histopathological studies showed that in brain area suffering a homogenous ischemic insult the hippocampal pyramidal neurons of CA1 region were damaged and disintegrate during the recovery phase. Moreover, the damage in percent of total cells in CA1 region was much serious in the dorsal portion than in the ventral portion (6). Interestingly, in the present experiments, there was different regional distribution of TTX-I_{Ca} along all hippocampal CA1 region, where TTX-I_{Ca} shared the dorsal portion. In CNS neurons, the T-type I_{Ca} plays an important role in functions by contributing to spontaneous depolarization waves and rebound excitation (5). Because, it can be effectively controlled by small membrane potential changes switched off even by slight depolarization or put into action again by membrane hyperpolarization. The threshold potential of TTX-I_{Ca} in the hippocampal pyramidal neurons was more negative than that of T-type I_{Ca}, and the inactivation time constant of former was smaller than that of latter. Thereby, in combination with Ca^{2+}-activated K^+ currents, TTX-I_{Ca} may created much effective mechanism for generation of membrane potential oscillations and autorhythmicity as compared with T-type I_{Ca}, suggesting that the excess excitation of TTX-sensitive channels might be associated with the cell death in the dorsal portion of CA1 region where TTX-sensitive channels exist.

REFERENCES

1. Akaike, N. et al. The calcium current of Helix neuron. J. Gen. Physiol. 71:509-531, 1978.
2. Akaike, N. et al. 'Concentration clamp' study of &C-aminobutyric-acid-induced chloride current kinetics of frog sensory neurones. J. Physiol. Lond. 379:171-185, 1986.
3. Akaike, N. et al. Dihydropyridine-sensitive low-threshold calcium channels in isolated rat hypothalamic neurones. J. Physiol. Lond. 412:181-195, 1989.
4. Alps, B. J. et al. The delayed post-ischemic treatment effects of nicardipine in a rat model of four vessel occlusion. Br. J. Pharmacol. 91: p312, 1987.
5. Llinás, R. and Yarom, Y. Properites and distribution of ionic conductance generating electro responsiveness of mammalian olivary neurones in vitro. J. Physiol. Lond. 315:569-584, 1981.
6. Smith, M.-L. et al. The density and distribution of ischemic brain injury in the rat following 2-10 min of forebrain ischemia. Acta Neuropathol. Berl. 64:319-332, 1984.
7. Takahashi, K. and Akaike, N. Nicergoline inhibits T-type Ca^{2+} channel in the isolated rat hippocampal CA1 pyramidal neurones. Br. J. Pharmacol. In press.

MUSCARINIC RECEPTORS, PHOSPHOINOSITIDE METABOLISM AND INTRACELLULAR CALCIUM IN NEURONAL CELLS

S.R. NAHORSKI, D.G. LAMBERT, R.J.H. WOJCIKIEWICZ, S. SAFRANY and E.M. WHITHAM.
Department of Pharmacology and Therapeutics, University of Leicester, P.O. Box 138, Medical Sciences Building, University Road, LEICESTER. LE1 9HN. U.K.

There is much evidence that implicates a central signalling role for Ca^{2+} in neurones and that a variety of neurotransmitter receptors are linked to phosphoinositide metabolism in the CNS (4,6). However, despite the fact that cerebral tissue can readily accumulate inositol-(1,4,5)trisphosphate $(Ins(1,4,5)P_3)$ and inositol$(1,3,4,5)$tetrakisphosphate $(Ins(1,3,4,5)P_4)$ (1,2) and possess a high density of Ins-$(1,4,5)P_3$ and $Ins(1,3,4,5)P_4$ receptor binding sites (8,3), the complexity of the CNS has prevented a clear indication of potential roles for inositol polyphosphates in neuronal Ca^{2+} homeostasis. We have recently used a human neuroblastoma (SH-SY5Y) cell and neonatal rat cerebellar granule cells to examine muscarinic receptor control of intracellular Ca^{2+} and potential regulation by $Ins(1,4,5)P_3$ and Ins-$(1,3,4,5)P_4$.

SH-SY5Y cells loaded with Fura-2 and stimulated with muscarinic agonists display changes in fluorescence indicative of a substantial release of intracellular Ca^{2+} stores and entry of this cation through the plasma membrane. These components can be studied individually by several experimental designs and suggest that they are both dependent on continued activation of the muscarinic receptor and may be regulated independently of each other. In particular, Ca^{2+} entry occurs at low concentrations of full muscarinic agonists and is the only component observed with partial agonists.

SH-SY5Y cells, in our hands (5) only express M_3 muscarinic receptors and stimulation of these sites leads to a large accumulation of the mass of $Ins(1,4,5)P_3$ in the first few seconds following agonist addition. This decays to a lower, but nevertheless elevated, steady-state that is maintained for at least 5 min. $Ins(1,3,4,5)P_4$, assayed by a mass radioreceptor assay, also accumulates and is maintained at a level 5-10 fold above basal for at least 5 min.

SH-SY5Y cells have been permeabilised by electroporation and still maintain muscarinic agonist and guanine nucleotide-dependent inositol polyphosphate accumulation. Permeabilised cells loaded with $^{45}Ca^{2+}$ or monitored with a Ca^{2+} sensitive electrode, display a large release of Ca^{2+} stores in response to $Ins(1,4,5)P_3$ and the nature of this intracellular receptor has been characterised by a variety of inositol polyphosphates including synthetic metabolically stable analogues (7). Furthermore, permeabilised cells respond to muscarinic agonists with a release of intracellular Ca^{2+} and GTPYS dramatically alters the relationship between muscarinic receptor occupation and Ca^{2+} release.

We have also examined the cerebellar granule cell using similar experimental approaches. This cell is relatively homogenous in culture and possesses several receptors (muscarinic, alpha$_1$ adrenoceptor, 5HT$_2$ and histamine H$_1$) linked to phosphoinositide metabolism. We have characterised the muscarinic receptor as M$_3$ pharmacologically and demonstrated that these primary neuronal cells accumulate Ins(1,4,5)P$_3$ mass in response to carbachol over the first 5-10 sec. Cerebellar granule cells permeabilised with saponin display intracellular stores of Ca^{2+} that can be loaded in an ATP-dependent manner and released by Ins(1,4,5)-P$_3$. The ability of these cells to release glutamate in response to depolarising stimuli may allow examination of modulatory roles for phosphoinositide-linked receptors in this release mechanism.

Overall, these simple neuronal cells have started to reveal the details of the relation between receptor stimulation, phosphoinositide metabolism and control of Ca^{2+} signalling. This may allow examination of potential Ca^{2+} effectors in neurones and their role in information storage and communication between neurones.

ACKNOWLEDGEMENTS:

The authors would like to thank The Wellcome Trust and SERC for financial support.

REFERENCES:

1. Batty, I. et al., (1985): Biochem. J. 232, 315-321.
2. Batty, I. and Nahorski, S.R. (1989): Biochem. J. 260, 237-241.
3. Challiss, R.A.J. and Nahorski, S.R. (1990): J. Neurochem. (in press)
4. Chuang, D. (1989): Ann. Rev. Pharmacol. 29, 71-110.
5. Lambert, D.G. et al., (1989): Eur. J. Pharmacol. 165, 71-77.
6. Nahorski, S.R. (1988): Trends. Neurosci. 11, 444-448.
7. Nahorski, S.R. and Potter, B.V.L. (1989): Trends. Pharmacol. 10, 139-144.
8. Willcocks A.L. et al., (1987): Biochem. Biophys. Res. Comm. 146, 1071-1078.

SPATIALLY ORGANIZED INTRACELLULAR Ca^{2+} SIGNALS IN RESPONSE TO DIFFERENT SECRETAGOGUES IN ADRENAL CHROMAFFIN CELLS.

T.R. CHEEK[*], T.R. JACKSON[**], R.B. MORETON[*], A.J. O'SULLIVAN[***], R.D. BURGOYNE[***] and M.J. BERRIDGE[*].
[*]AFRC Unit of Insect Neurophysiology and Pharmacology, Department of Zoology, Cambridge University, Downing Street, Cambridge CB2 3EJ UK.
[**]Medical Research Council Laboratory of Molecular Biology, Cambridge CB2 2QH UK. [***]Department of Physiology, Liverpool University, Brownlow Hill, Liverpool L69 3BX UK.

Bovine adrenal chromaffin cells secrete catecholamine *in vivo* in response to acetylcholine that is released from the splanchnic nerve terminal. The intracellular trigger for this process is the rise in $[Ca^{2+}]i$ that results from nicotinic receptor-induced Ca^{2+} entry.
  These cells also possess receptors for muscarinic agonists and peptides such as bradykinin and angiotensin II. Although these receptors activate phospholipase C, release $InsP_3$ and then subsequently mobilize internally stored Ca^{2+}, they trigger little or no secretion. In order to understand why entry of external Ca^{2+}, but not release of internally stored Ca^{2+}, is capable of triggering secretion from these cells, we have used fura-2 imaging techniques to study in detail the agonist-induced changes in $[Ca^{2+}]i$ that occurs in single cells. The results show that different classes of stimuli give rise to different spatial localizations of internal Ca^{2+}, and that only one specific pattern of internal Ca^{2+} is associated with a full secretory response.

METHODS
Chromaffin cells cultured on coverslips were incubated with 2uM fura-2/AM for 30min at room temperature and then imaged after equilibration to 37 C using an Imagine image processing system (Synoptics Ltd, Cambridge UK). The ratio image (340nm/380nm) was obtained at video rate and filtered with a time constant of 200ms. Full details are given in Cheek et al (1).
In order to simultaneously measure secretion from single cells, the chromaffin cells were co-cultured with fura-2-loaded NIH-3T3[t] fibroblasts. These cells do not respond to chromaffin cell secretagogues, but do respond with a rise in $[Ca^{2+}]i$ to ATP that is co-released with the catecholamine from the chromaffin cells. Full details are given in Cheek et al (1).

RESULTS AND DISCUSSION
The Ca^{2+} response to nicotine (and high K^+) is generated in two phases (Fig 1a). Initially Ca^{2+} is localized exclusively to the entire subplasmalemmal area, consistent with it entering the cell from the external medium; Ca^{2+} then rapidly infills until it is evenly distributed throughout the cell. The second phase consists of a further, large, increase in $[Ca^{2+}]i$ that is often confined to one pole of the cell. Using the co-culture technique it has been shown that this pattern of intracellular Ca^{2+} results in a 'full' secretory response that occurs over the entire cell surface.

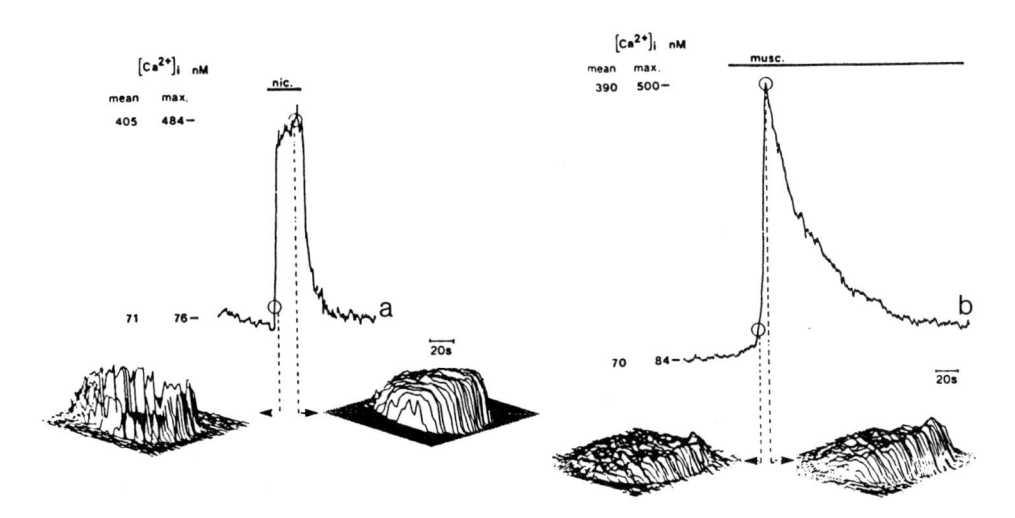

Fig 1. Time course and spatial distribution of changes in $[Ca^{2+}]i$ in single fura-2 loaded chromaffin cells in response to 10uM nicotine (a) and 0.3mM muscarine (b).

In contrast, the $InsP_3$-mobilizing agonists angiotensin II and muscarine result in a highly localized release of internal Ca^{2+} which, in the main, remains confined to the area of the cell from which it originated (Fig 1b). This pattern of internal Ca^{2+} is in marked contrast to the infilling effect seen in response to depolarizing stimuli, and was shown using the co-culture technique not to trigger secretion from 65% of chromaffin cells that gave a large (~160nM) rise in $[Ca^{2+}]i$ in response to angiotensin II. This data suggests that full exocytosis is triggered by initial Ca^{2+} activation of the entire subplasmalemmal area of the cell and not by Ca^{2+} that is spatially restricted. The restricted Ca^{2+} localization did however result, in the remaining 35% of cells, in a release of catecholamine that was polarized to the area of the plasma membrane that was activated by Ca^{2+}. Imaging studies on fura-2 quenching following Mn^{2+} entry suggest that this may have resulted from a localized Ca^{2+} influx that accompanies and/or follows Ca^{2+} mobilization. In contrast to angiotensin II, histamine which also mobilizes internal Ca^{2+} is a more effective secretagogue since it, in addition, activates Ca^{2+} entry over the entire plasma membrane.

All of these results strongly suggest that exocytosis from these cells is triggered by Ca^{2+} activation of the subplasmalemmal region of the cell, and that this is only achieved by the promotion of Ca^{2+} influx.

REFERENCE
1. Cheek, T.R. et al. Simultaneous measurements of cytosolic calcium and secretion in single bovine adrenal chromaffin cells by fluorescent imaging of fura-2 in co-cultured cells. J.Cell Biol. 109:1219-1227, 1989.

INTRACELLULAR Ca^{2+} STORES IN NON- MUSCLE CELLS: AN OVERVIEW

Susan Treves[1], Francesco Zorzato[1], Paola Chiozzi[1], Monica De Mattei[1], Francesco Michelangeli[2], Antonello Villa[3], Paola Podini[3], Tomohide Satoh[3], Jacopo Meldolesi[3] and Tullio Pozzan[1]

[1] Inst. of General Pathology, University of Ferrara, Ferrara, Italy.
[2] Inst. of General Pathology, University of Padova, Padova, Italy
[3] Dept. of Pharmacology, CNR Center of Cytopharmacology and Peripheral Neuropathology Center, University of Milano, Milano, Italy.

Great progress has been made on the molecular characterization of the various components of the Ca^{2+} homeostatic machinery: Ca^{2+} pumps and channels from plasma membrane and organelles, as well as a number of Ca^{2+} binding proteins have been purified and their primary sequence determined (8). However, at the cellular level, controversies concerning the identification of the intracellular Ca^{2+} stores and the interplay between second messengers in the regulation of $[Ca^{2+}]_i$ have yet to be clarified. In fact, general consensus has only been reached on the pivotal role of $Ins1,4,5P_3$ in receptor mediated Ca^{2+} mobilization from a non-mitochondrial store (2). The nature of this pool, the existence of other mechanisms for Ca^{2+} mobilization and the correlation between Ca^{2+} mobilization vs Ca^{2+} influx are still largely unknown.

In this contribution we discuss data from the recent literature concerning the identification of the $Ins1,4,5P_3$ sensitive Ca^{2+} store in different cell types, as well as discussing some of our recent results on the characterization of Ca^{2+} stores in non-muscle cells and in particular in the Purkinje cells of rat cerebelum.

RESULTS AND DISCUSSION

The observation that the microsomal fraction from non-muscle cells is endowed with an ATP dependent Ca^{2+} accumulation system goes back to the early 70's (7). Up to 1987 subcellular fractionation experiments simply confirmed the initial observations that microsomal fractions from a number of tissues contain most of the $Ins1,4,5P_3$ sensitive Ca^{2+} stores. Since ER is the most abundant component of microsomes, the idea that this organelle is the $Ins1,4,5P_3$ sensitive Ca^{2+} pool was taken for granted. More recent data suggest, instead, that the $Ins1,4,5P_3$ sensitive Ca^{2+} stores can be identified with a subfraction of microsomes; in some tissues this fraction copurified with plasma membrane markers, while in others with rough or smooth ER (4,5). In other studies no correlation with ER and plasma membrane markers was observed (1).

Our data obtained with rat liver microsomes offer some clues which may help solve this apparent contradiction. We found in fact that the correlation between $Ins1,4,5P_3$ binding and plasma membrane or ER markers simply depends on the purification procedure employed (Treves et al. in preparation). On the other hand we found that there is always an excellent quantitative correlation between the enrichment of the intralumenal Ca^{2+} binding protein calreticulin, CR, and that of $Ins1,4,5P_3$ binding, suggesting that these two markers belong to the same vesicle population.

The situation in intact cells is, by no means, clearer than that discussed above for subcellular fractions. Electron-microprobe analysis, in the absence of precipitating anions and under conditions minimizing diffusional artifacts suggest that ER, or a specialized part of it, represents the $Ins1,4,5P_3$ sensitive Ca^{2+} store (3). Another recently used approach is that of localizing the subcellular origin of the $[Ca^{2+}]_i$ rise following stimulus application and correlating it to the morphology and distribution of intracellular organelles. Summarizing a wealth of data, using this approach, a number of groups concluded that a subfraction of ER is endowed with $Ins1,4,5P_3$ sensitive Ca^{2+} release. A third type of approach was utilized by our group, i.e subcellular localization by immunocytochemistry at the electron microscope level of the protein markers of Ca^{2+} storage compartments (6,10). As basic markers of a Ca^{2+} store compartments we identified a Ca^{2+} ATPase, an intralumenal low affinity Ca^{2+} binding protein and a Ca^{2+} release channel or an $Ins1,4,5P_3$ receptor. In peripheral tissues only the first two markers could be studied, since, up to date, neither a Ca^{2+} release channel nor an $Ins1,4,5P_3$ receptor has been identified in molecular terms. The morphological data are not consistent with the identification of the bulk of ER as the organelle containing CR and a Ca^{2+} ATPase crossreactive with that of skeletal muscle, but rather appear consistent with the subfractionation data previously described, where CR and $Ins1,4,5P_3$ were mostly enriched in a unique subcellular fraction.

The cerebellar Purkinje cell has become very popular among students of signal transduction because it has been found to contain an extraordinary high level of $Ins1,4,5P_3$ receptors. The subcellular distribution of the $Ins1,4,5P_3$ receptor in Purkinje cells has been studied by three different groups and some apparent contradictions exist among them (8). We recently carried out a detailed quantitative study on cryosections of Purkinje cells using the immunogold technique (9). In particular: i) labelling of ER was found to be strikingly heterogeneous. The nuclear membrane and most of rough ER were poorly labelled by the anti $Ins1,4,5P_3$ receptor antibodies, while the highest density of labelling was found in smooth cysternae present on the cell body, on the dendrites and in the spines. We have also recently undertaken a kinetic characterization of the chicken cerebellum microsomal Ca^{2+} ATPase. Our data demonstrate that this protein (100 KDa MW) is distinct from both the cardiac and the skeletal isoform.

AKNOWLEDGMENTS

This work was supported in part by grants from Italian CNR, Special Projects "Biotechnology" and "Signal Transduction". We are indebted to Mr. M. Lanfredi for the excellent technical assistance . S.T. was supported by a grant from the "Banca Popolare di Padova e Rovigo".

REFERENCES

1) Alderson B. and Volpe P. (1989) Distribution of endoplsmic reticulum and calciosome markers in membrane fractions isolated from different regions of the canine brain Arch. Biochem. and Biophys. 272,162-174.

2) Berridge M.J. and Irvine R.F. (1989) Inositol phosphates and cell signalling Nature 341,197-205.

3) Bond M., Vadasz G. Somlyo A.V. and Somlyo A.P. (1987). Subcellular calcium and magnesium mobilization in rat liver stimulated in vivo with vasopressin and glucagon. J. Biol. Chem. 262,15639-15636.

4) Ghosh T.K., Mullaney J.M.,Taranzi F.I. and Gill D.L. (1989) GTP-activated communication between distinct inositol 1,4,5-trisphosphate-sensitive and -insensitive calcium pools Nature 340,236-239.

5) Guillemette G., Balla T., Bankal A.J., Spat A and Catt K.J. (1987). Intracellular receptors for inositol 1,4,5-triphosphate in angiotesin II target tissues. J. Biol. Chem. 262,1010-1015.

6) Hashimoto S., Bruno B.,Lew D.P.,Pozzan T.,Volpe P. and Meldolesi J. (1988) Immunocytochemistry of calciosomes in liver and pancreas J. Cell Biol. 107,2523-2531.

7) Moore L., Chen T., Knapp H.R.Jr and Landon E.J. (1975). Energy-dependent calcium homeostasis in isolated hepatocytes. J. Biol. Chem. 250,4562-4568.

8) Pietrobon D., Di Virgilio F. and Pozzan T. (1990) Functional and structural characteristics of the Ca^{2+} homeostatic machinery in eukariotic cells Europ. J. Biochem. in press.

9) Satoh T., Ross C.A., Supattapone S., Pozzan T., Snyder S.H. and Meldolesi J. (1990) Inositol 1,4,5-trisphosphate receptor in cerebellar Purkinje cells. Quantitative immunogold labeling reveals concentration in an endoplasmic reticulum subcompartment. J. Cell Biol. in press.

10) Volpe P., Krause K.H., Hashimoto S., Zorzato F., Pozzan T., Meldolesi J. and Lew D.P. (1988). Calciosome, a cytoplasmic organelle: the inositol 1,4,5-triphosphate-sensitive Ca^{2+} store of non muscle cells? Proc. Natl. Acad. Sci. USA 85,1091-1095.

PHARMACOLOGICAL ANALYSIS OF NEURONAL CALCIUM CHANNELS: INTERACTION WITH
G PROTEINS, SECOND MESSENGERS AND CALCIUM CHANNEL LIGANDS

A.C. Dolphin, E. Huston, R.H. Scott and J.F. Wootton[+]
Dept. Pharmacology St. George's Hospital Medical School, Cranmer
Terrace, London SW17 0RE U.K. and [+]Dept. Physiology, Cornell
University, Ithaca, N.Y. U.S.A.

CLASSES OF Ca CHANNELS IN NEURONES

The existence of the high threshold dihydropyridine sensitive L channel in neurones is now well documented (1). The presence of a small conductance low threshold, transient (T) channel was subsequently shown in peripheral and central neurones (2). It is suggested that there is another distinct subtype of channel which is present only in neurones. This channel was originally described in dorsal root ganglion (DRG) neurones and has been termed an N channel (1). It is not diydropyridine-sensitive and has a single channel conductance and kinetics of activation and inactivation intermediate between T and L channels. It has been suggested that activation of N channels underlies the transient component of the high threshold whole cell current. However it remains unclear whether N current results from activation of a single class of channel since its properties vary with cell type (1,3).

G PROTEIN MODULATION OF Ca CHANNELS

A class of neurotransmitter receptors (including α_2, $GABA_B$ and adenosine A_1) are coupled to inhibitory G proteins (G_i, G_o) and inhibit neuronal Ca currents. The response can be mimicked by internal GTP analogues, and is blocked by pertussis toxin (4,5,6). It is unclear whether the effect on Ca channels is direct (4) but in neurones it also involves G_o (7). In many cases, neurotransmitters inhibit the transient component of the whole cell current, which has been taken as an indication that N channels are selectively inhibited (3,8). It may also represent a marked slowing of the channel activation kinetics (5). It has recently been shown that this slowed activation of the calcium current in the presence of activated G protein represents a block of the channel which is slowly overcome upon depolarization (9,10). We have suggested that when the closed channel is complexed with activated G protein it is not available to open, and dissociation of this complex to the free closed state represents the rate limiting step (11).

INTERACTION OF G PROTEINS WITH LOW THRESHOLD T CHANNELS

Low threshold channels are also regulated by G proteins, whose activation can both increase and decrease T currents (12). A low concentration of GTP.S enhanced, whereas a high concentration inhibited T currents (12). It is possible that more than one type of G protein is involved, since the inhibition but not the enhancement was blocked by pertussis toxin, and neither effect was mimicked by cholera toxin. The $GABA_B$ agonist baclofen increased T current amplitude at $2\mu M$ and inhibited the current at $100\mu M$ (12).

INTERACTION BETWEEN Ca CHANNEL LIGAND BINDING SITES AND G PROTEIN ACTIVATION.

We have recently shown that there is an interaction between G protein activation and the effect of Ca channel ligands on L type Ca channels in cultured rat DRGs and sympathetic neurones (13,14,15). Ca channel antagonists including nifedipine, (-)202-791, diltiazem and D600 were observed to show only agonist properties on Ca channel currents in the presence of internal non-hydrolysable guanine nucleotide analogues. G protein activation reduces steady-state inactivation of calcium channels (5,15), stabilising the resting state of the channels. Further studies have now indicated that a phosphorylation step is involved (16). It is possible that G protein activation, by stabilising neuronal high threshold calcium channels in their resting state, prevents the antagonist action of calcium channel ligands, which results from their binding to the inactivated state of the channel (15,16). It is further possible that the enhancement occurs from binding of calcium channel ligands to an 'activator site' which is available on channels in their resting state and either promotes their phosphorylation, or reduces dephosphorylation of the channels.

Ca CHANNEL INVOLVEMENT IN NEUROTRANSMITTER RELEASE AND ITS MODULATION

Neurotransmitter release requires Ca^{2+} entry at the presynaptic terminal through voltage-sensitive Ca channels. The nature of the channels subserving transmitter release is unclear, as they do not show a unified pharmacology between different systems. Presynaptic inhibition by agents such as opiates and $GABA_B$ agonists may be due to the inhibition of presynaptic Ca channels, not necessarily those directly subserving release. The nature of these channels is also unclear (1,8,11,17).

REFERENCES
1. Tsien, R.W. et al. (1988) Trends in Neurosciences 11 431-437.
2. Carbone, E. & Lux, H.D. (1984) Nature, 310, 501-502.
3. Plummer et al (1989) Neuron 1 1453-1463.
4. Dolphin, A.C., McGuirk, S.M. & Scott, R.H. (1989) Brit. J. Pharmacol. 97 263-273.
5. Dolphin, A.C. & Scott, R.H. (1987). J. Physiol. 386, 1-17.
6. Holz, G.G., Rane, S.G. and Dunlap, K. (1986) Nature 319 670-672.
7. Hescheler, J. et al (1987) Nature 325 445-447.
8. Lipscombe, D., Kongsamut, S. & Tsien, R.W. (1989) Nature 340 639.
9. Grassi, F. and Lux, H.D. (1989) Neuroscience Letts. 105 113-117.
10. Scott, R.H. and Dolphin, A.C.(1990) Brit. J. Pharmacol.(in press).
11. Dolphin, A.C., Huston, E. and Scott, R.H.(1990) Biochemical Society Symposium 55.
12. Scott, R.H. & Wootton, J.F. and Dolphin, A.C. (1990) Neuroscience (in press).
13. Scott, R.H. & Dolphin, A.C. (1987). Nature 330, 760-762.
14. Scott, R.H. & Dolphin, A.C. (1988) Neurosci. Letts, 89, 170-175.
15. Dolphin, A.C. & Scott, R.H. (1989). J. Physiol. 413 271-288.
16. Dolphin, A.C. (1990) J. Physiol. (submitted).
17. Huston, E., Scott., R.H. and Dolphin, A.C. (1990) Neuroscience (submitted).

ROLE OF EXTRACELLULAR CALCIUM IN EXCITOTOXIC INJURY OF CULTURED CORTICAL NEURONS.

D.W. CHOI, J.H. WEISS, and D.M. HARTLEY
Department of Neurology, Stanford Medical School, Stanford, CA, U.S.A.

Cytotoxic overstimulation of neuronal glutamate receptors may contribute to the pathogenesis of certain neurological diseases. We have examined such excitotoxic injury in murine cortical cell cultures, and summarize here several arguments suggesting that it may be importantly mediated by an influx of extracellular Ca^{2+}. Controlled exposure to excitatory amino acids was carried out in defined buffer solutions; neuronal damage was assessed morphologically, and by the efflux of the cytosolic enzyme lactate dehydrogenase to the bathing medium.

Two main types of excitotoxic injury occur in our cultures: 1) a fast neurotoxicity induced by intense stimulation of N-methyl-D-aspartate (NMDA) type glutamate receptors; and 2) a slow neurotoxicity induced either by stimulation of non-NMDA type glutamate receptors, or by low level stimulation of NMDA receptors (1,2).

FAST GLUTAMATE RECEPTOR-MEDIATED NEUROTOXICITY

Only a few minutes of intense activation of NMDA receptors, either selectively, by agonists such as aspartate or homocysteate, or non-selectively, by glutamate, is followed over the next day by widespread neuronal degeneration. This injury can be separated into two components, distinguishable by differences in time course, ionic dependence, and receptor pharmacology. The first component, marked by immediate neuronal swelling, depends on the presence of extracellular Na^+. Most likely, there is Na^+ influx though ligand-gated and voltage-gated channels, accompanied by passive Cl^- and water influx. The second component, marked by delayed cell degeneration, depends on the presence of extracellular Ca^{2+} and the activation of NMDA receptors; it may thus be triggered by excessive Ca^{2+} influx through the NMDA receptor-gated channel. NMDA antagonists can substantially reduce glutamate-induced late neuronal degeneration even if added after glutamate washout, suggesting that the injury incurred during initial exposure to exogenous glutamate may be augmented by the subsequent activation of NMDA receptors by endogenously released agonists.

Three observations support the idea that the dependence of fast glutamate neurotoxicity on extracellular Ca^{2+} reflects a requirement for Ca^{2+} influx through the NMDA receptor-gated ionophore. First, delayed neuronal degeneration can be induced by the Ca^{2+} ionophore, A23187. Second, neuronal intracellular free Ca^{2+} rises during stimulation of NMDA receptors, although work in hippocampal neurons has suggested that this rise does not correlate in a simple fashion with resultant degeneration (3). Third, brief intense activation of NMDA receptors induces a neuronal accumulation of $^{45}Ca^{2+}$. This NMDA receptor-induced $^{45}Ca^{2+}$ accumulation correlates with subsequent degeneration; it is several-fold larger than the accumulation induced by either 90 mM K^+, or high concentrations of glutamate in the presence of an NMDA antagonist.

Excess entry of Ca^{2+} through NMDA receptor-gated ionophores is likely to be supplemented by Ca^{2+} entry through other routes, and the release of intracellular Ca^{2+} stores. These movements will produce localized elevations of intracellular free Ca^{2+}, which can trigger several cytotoxic cascades bearing direct responsibility for neuronal disintegration. Of particular importance may be the activation of proteases, lipases, and endonucleases; and the generation of free radicals through increased arachidonic acid metabolism (4).

SLOW GLUTAMATE RECEPTOR-MEDIATED NEUROTOXICITY

While high concentrations of potent NMDA agonists can trigger degeneration of cultured mouse cortical neurons after exposure times of only a few minutes, selective non-NMDA agonists or low levels of NMDA agonists require exposure times exceeding several hours to induce comparable damage. It is not possible to remove extracellular Ca^{2+} for such lengthy periods of time, but pharmacological studies have suggested that Ca^{2+} influx may also be important in this form of excitotoxicity.

100 μM nifedipine had only a small downward effect on the $^{45}Ca^{++}$ accumulation or widespread neuronal degeneration induced by brief exposure to high concentrations of NMDA; but 10 - 100 μM concentrations of either nifedipine or nimodipine substantially attenuated the comparable neurotoxicity produced by 24 hour exposure to submaximal concentrations of alpha-amino-3-hydroxy-5-methyl-4-isoxazole propionate (AMPA), kainate, or quinolinate (2). $^{45}Ca^{2+}$ accumulation induced by brief exposure to non-NMDA agonists was small and thus technically hard to work with, but preliminary experiments have suggested that it can be attenuated by high concentrations of dihydropyridines. Nifedipine was not a glutamate receptor antagonist as it did not reduce excitatory amino acid-induced inward currents in voltage-clamped neurons.

Thus slow glutamate receptor-mediated neurotoxicity may be substantially mediated by entry of extracellular Ca^{2+} through voltage-gated Ca^{2+} channels.

REFERENCES

1. Choi, D.W. (1988): Neuron, 1: 623-634.
2. Weiss, J.H. et al. (1990): Science, in press.
3. Michaels, R.L. and Rothman, S.M. (1990): J. Neurosci. 10: 283-292.
4. Choi, D.W. (1990): Cerebrovasc. Brain Metab. Rev., in press.

ENHANCEMENT OF REINFORCING EFFICACY BY DEVELOPMENT OF PHYSICAL DEPENDENCE

K. TAKADA*, Y. WAKASA* and T. YANAGITA
Department of Psychopharmacology*, Preclinical Research Laboratories,
Central Institute for Experimental Animals, Kawasaki, Japan

It is well-known that once physical dependence on heroin or morphine is developed in drug users, their drug-seeking becomes compulsive in order to avoid or escape from the withdrawal discomfort. However, it is not clear whether or to what extent such enhancement exists with prototypic dependence-producing drugs including morphine, codeine, and cocaine. To answer this, we examined changes in reinforcing efficacy before and after treating rhesus monkeys with repeated intravenous administration of test drugs.

General Methods
An intravenous catheter was implanted in 4-5 rhesus monkeys per group, and they were trained to self-administer drugs under a progressive ratio (PR) schedudule, which requires increasing number of lever-presses ($\sqrt[4]{2}$ times the previous ratio) in order to receive each injection. The lever-press ratio at the last obtained injection (final ratio) was then regarded as indicating the intensity of the drug-seeking behavior. After the training, the monkeys were pretreated with forced intravenous injections of a test drug or saline, after which testing under the PR schedule to self-administer the drug was started usually following a 1- or 2-days' withdrawal period.

Opioids
The pretreatment dosing schedule were: morphine, 0.25 mg/kg every 6 hrs (Low) or every 90 min (High) for 2 weeks; dihydrocodeine, 1 mg/kg hourly for 3 days (Short) or for 2 weeks (Long); and pentazocine, 1 mg/kg every 90 min for 3 days followed by hourly injections for 11 days. The unit doses of the test drugs during the PR period were: morphine, 0.25 mg/kg; dihydrocodeine, 1 mg/kg; pentazocine, 0.25mg/kg. Withdrawal observations were conducted during the withdrawal and PR periods. The severity of the withdrawal signs were quantified for each item by converting the observed values rated on a 2- or 4-level scale to a scale of 0 to 60. The values for each item were weighted according to the grade of morphine withdrawal signs after Seevers, 1936.[1] The mean maximum withdrawal scores during the withdrawal period, range of final ratios, and the percent increase infinal ratios against saline pretreatment value, are shown in Table 1. As can be seen, the withdrawal scores after pentazocine as well as the lower dose conditions of morphine and dihydrocodeine did not differ from those after saline, but the final ratios were increased 2- to 4-fold. After the higher dose conditions, the withdrawal scores were significantly higher than with saline, but the final ratios were not significantly increased compared to the lower dose conditions.

Stimulants
The pretreatment dosing schedule of nicotine was 0.25 mg/kg hourly for 28 days. As for cocaine, monkeys were given 24-hr access to 0.11 mg/kg/inj under a

FR100 schedule for 4 weeks instead of forced injections. Cocaine 0.11 mg/kg and nicotine 0.25 mg/kg were used as the unit doses during the PR period. With cocaine, the ratio was doubled after every 4th injection. No increase in the final ratio was observed in any of the monkeys, and the average percent increase against saline was 68.8 and 62.5, repectively, for cocaine and nicotine. No apparant withdrawal signs were observed with either drug.

Table 1. Maximum withdrawal score and ranges of final ratios obtained after each drug treatment, and percent increase in the final ratios against saline-pretreatment.

Drugs	Pretreatment	Maximum withdrawal score	Final ratio range	%Increase in final ratio
Saline	Saline	5.3 ± 1.1	140- 570	-
Morphine	Saline	-	340- 1600	
	Morphine Low	7.5 ± 2.1	2260- 3810	331.6 ± 114.9
	High	15.3 ± 2.1*@	2260- 6400	405.5 ± 103.7
DC[a]	Saline	-	950- 1600	-
	DC Short	7.5 ± 0.9	2690- 7610	441.3 ± 110.3
	Long	12.0 ± 1.4*@	4530-10760	549.8 ± 163.3
PZC[b]	Saline	-	1350- 3810	-
	PZC	8.3 ± 1.5	2260- 3810	166.3 ± 39.9

*: $p<0.05$ vs. saline   @: $p<0.05$ vs. lower dose condition
a) Dihydrocodeine   b) Pentazocine

Discussion

Marked enhancement of reinforcing efficacy was observed after the development of physical dependence on morphine and dihydrocodeine even when no grossly observable withdrawal signs were apparant, while only weak enhancement was observed with pentazocine. Previous experiments on ethanol,[2] pentobarbital, and diazepam conducted in our institute under similar conditions revealed that enhancement was weak with the former two drugs and equivocal with diazepam, although withdrawal signs of the barbital-type graded as mild to intermediate[3] were observed during the PR period following the period of forced drug injection or free-access condition. Thus it can be said that the manifestation of withdrawal signs does not necessarily result in enhancement of reinforcing efficacy. No enhancement was observed with cocaine or nicotine, and the final ratios tended to decrease after exposure to these drugs with no apparant withdrawal signs being observed.

References
1) Seevers, M.H. (1936): J. Pharmacol. Exp. Ther., 56:147-156.
2) Yanagita, T. (1976): Pharmacol. Rev., 27:503-509.
3) Yanagita, T. and Takahashi, S. (1970): J. Pharmacol. Exp. Ther., 172:163-169

GENETIC APPROACHES TO THE ANALYSIS OF ADDICTION PROCESSES

FRANK R. GEORGE, Ph.D.
National Institute on Drug Abuse, Addiction Research Center, Box 5180,
Baltimore, MD 21224, USA

Behavioral genetics is the study of both genetic and environmental influences upon behavior. Some behaviors are highly genetically determined, while others are primarily influenced by environmental factors. Behavioral responses to drugs, especially drug seeking behaviors, appear to lie somewhere between these two extremes, so that both genetic and environmental influences, and their interactions, are critical.

One powerful method for studying drug seeking behavior is the use of operant self-administration procedures, which combine several key criteria necessary for an effective animal model of drug abuse. However, until recently, these studies had focussed solely on environmental conditions important in drug-seeking behaviors. Individual differences found in these studies were generally attributed to differences in training and subject history, or often ignored. It is possible that genetic differences in sensitivity, metabolism or the reinforcing effects of drugs may have produced this variability.

The use of inbred strains in many drug preference studies has provided valuable information about the contribution of genetic factors to alcohol(1), opioid(2) and cocaine(3) taking. These findings provide foundation evidence that genetic factors play an important role in determining drug taking behaviors.

We first examined genetic factors in response to cocaine by studying acute cocaine administration in LEWIS (LEW) and F344 rats. We found that LEW rats were more sensitive to the locomotor stimulant effects of cocaine. Conversely, F344 rats were more sensitive to the lethal effects of cocaine(3). We next tested whether these rats would consume a cocaine solution in preference to water. Following adjunctive training procedures, intake of cocaine was higher in LEW relative to F344 rats (8.0 vs. 2.7 mg/kg per hour test session respectively), and exceeded intake of water only in LEW rats(3). Thus, cocaine appears to readily function as a reinforcer for LEW but not F344 rats, suggesting that significant genetic differences may exist in response to cocaine. In addition, the results of these initial studies suggest that the stimulant, reinforcing and lethal effects of cocaine are not highly correlated.

Operant drug self-administration studies indicate that genotype is a critical determinant of ethanol reinforced behavior(3), but little is known concerning genetic differences in operant self-administration of non-alcohol drugs. We recently studied operant self-administration of cocaine as well as the potent, orally active opiate agonist etonitazine (ETZ) in LEW and F344 rats, the same strains known to differ in both ethanol-seeking(4) and cocaine preference(3) behavior. Strategies used previously to establish oral intake of ethanol(4) were effective in establishing cocaine and ETZ as a reinforcer, but only for LEW rats. Responding for cocaine or ETZ was actually lower than vehicle intake for F344 rats.

It is unlikely that specific "addiction" genes exist. It seems more probable that the biological contributions to drug addiction result from the interactions among several genes, each of which regulates a common and necessary biological system. In the case of persons who would be at high risk for drug abuse, the specific versions of these genes are present in a combination which is most conducive to making a drug an effective reinforcer. Experimentally, the integration of behavioral genetic methods with those of operant conditioning has great potential for increasing our understanding of addiction processes. Genetic factors are being shown to play a critical role in addiction, and the use and study of genetic models in this area will not only improve our understanding of these genetic contributions to addiction, but, via the powerful approaches of behavior genetic methods, will ultimately aid in our overall understanding of the serious problem of drug addiction.

REFERENCES

1. Broadhurst, P.L. (1979): Drugs and the Inheritance of Behavior: A Survey of Comparative Pharmacogenetics. Plenum Press, New York.

2. George F.R. and Goldberg, S.R. (1989): Trends Pharmacological Sci, 10:78-83.

3. Rodgers, D.A. and McClearn G.E. (1962): Q. J. Stud. Alcohol, 23:26-33.

4. Suzuki, T., George, F.R. and Meisch, R.A. (1988): J Pharm. Exp. Ther., 245:164-170.

INDIVIDUAL DIFFERENCES IN DRUG PREFERENCE IN HUMANS

H. DE WIT

Department of Psychiatry, University of Chicago, Chicago IL 60637

It is not known why some individuals and not others develop problems with drug or alcohol abuse. Risk factors predisposing certain individuals to abuse drugs or alcohol may be studied by examining individual differences in subjective (mood-altering) and behavioral (reinforcing) effects of drugs under laboratory conditions. These effects, measured using standardized procedures, are good predictors of drug use outside the laboratory (9, 10).

Our laboratory has used a drug preference procedure to study individuals hypothesized to be at risk for drug or alcohol abuse (3). Subjects exhibiting certain characteristics are tested using a laboratory choice procedure, in which they first sample a drug and a placebo (PL) under double-blind conditions, and then choose the substance they prefer (i.e., drug or PL). The proportion of drug choices is the measure of preference. Several studies have been completed.

A. <u>Psychiatric symptomatology</u>. Individuals with psychiatric symptoms may be predisposed to use drugs that relieve their symptoms (2, 5). We tested the hypothesis that preference for the anxiolytic, diazepam (DZP; 10 mg vs PL), would be higher in volunteers exhibiting high levels of anxiety compared to non-anxious controls. We also tested the hypothesis that amphetamine (AMP) preference (10 mg vs PL) would be higher in volunteers with higher-than-normal levels of depression. In neither study did the symptomatic volunteers choose the drug more often: Both anxious subjects and controls chose DZP infrequently (22% vs 30% DZP choice), and both non-depressed and depressed volunteers preferred AMP over PL (70% vs 60% AMP choice). Thus, these data did not support the "self-medication" hypothesis of drug use.

B. <u>Genetic history.</u> Sons of male alcoholics are at high risk for developing alcoholism, but the mechanisms underlying this predisposition are not known. We assessed whether males with and without an alcoholic relative differed in their subjective and behavioral responses to an acute dose of ethanol (ETH; 8). The two groups did not differ: they exhibited similar subjective responses to ETH, and both groups chose ETH with about the same frequency (60% vs 63% ETH choice). Thus, a family history of alcoholism was not correlated with either subjective or behavioral effects of ETH.

Because use of benzodiazepines is known to be especially high among alcoholics, we conducted a similar study (in preparation) to compare preference for DZP (20 mg vs PL) in males with and without an alcoholic relative. Subjects with alcoholic relatives chose DZP slightly, but not significantly, more often than subjects without alcoholic relatives (52% vs 38% DZP choice), and the two groups exhibited similar subjective responses to the drug. Thus, family history of alcoholism also was not correlated with responses to a moderate dose of DZP.

C. <u>Drug use history</u>. Because of the apparent association between alcohol consumption and benzodiazepine use or abuse, we tested preference for DZP (20 mg vs PL) in two groups of normal social drinkers who differed in alcohol use (i.e., light [1-5 dks/wk] or moderate [7-15 dks/wk] (7). Moderate drinkers chose the DZP significantly more often than light drinkers (100% vs 66% DZP choice) suggesting that prior alcohol use may be a significant risk factor in use or abuse of benzodiazepines.

D. <u>Post-hoc analyses of heterogeneous subject groups.</u> We have also examined individual differences in subjective responses to drugs by conducting post-hoc analyses of data from several choice studies (1, 4, 6). In these analyses, subjects who chose a drug most frequently were compared to those who chose it least frequently, on a variety of intra- and extra-experimental variables. Subjective drug effects were found to be related to drug choice for several drugs. For example, in a study with ETH the most frequent choosers reported stimulant-like subjective effects from the drug whereas infrequent choosers reported only sedation after ETH.

E. <u>Summary.</u> Laboratory studies measuring the reinforcing and subjective effects of drugs in human subjects may help us understand why some individuals develop problems of excessive drug use or drug abuse. The studies completed to date indicate that, while psychiatric symptomatology and genetic factors were not related to drug preference, prior drug or alcohol use may predict the use of certain drugs. Individual variations in the subjective responses to drugs have also been found to be related to drug preferences.

REFERENCES
1. de Wit, H., Uhlenhuth, E.H. and Johanson, C.E. (1986a): <u>Drug Alcohol Dep</u> 16: 341-360.
2. de Wit, H. et al., (1986b): <u>Arch Gen Psychiatry</u> 43: 533-541.
3. de Wit, H. and Johanson, C.E. (1987a): In <u>Methods of Assessing Reinforcing Properties of Abused Drugs</u>. M. Bozarth, ed. pp. 559-572. Springer-Verlag, New York.
4. de Wit, H. et al., (1987b): <u>Alcoholism</u> 11: 52-59.
5. de Wit, H. et al., (1987c): <u>Clin Pharmacol Ther</u> 42: 127-136.
6. de Wit, H., Pierri, J. and Johanson, C.E. (1989a): <u>Psychopharmacology</u> 98: 113-119.
7. de Wit, H., Pierri, J. and Johanson, C.E. (1989b): <u>Pharmacol Biochem Beh</u> 33: 205-213.
8. de Wit, H. and McCracken, S.M. (1990): <u>Alcoholism</u> 14: 63-70.
9. Griffiths, R.R., Bigelow, G.E. and Henningfield, J.E. (1980): In <u>Advances in substance abuse: Behavioral and biological research</u> (Vol I). N.K. Mello, ed. pp. 1-90. JAI Press, Greenwich.
10. Johanson, C.E., Woolverton, W.L. and Schuster, C.R. (1987): In <u>Psychopharmacology: The Third Generation of Progress</u> H.Y. Meltzer, ed. pp. 1617-1626. Raven Press, New York.

BEHAVIORAL AND PHARMACOLOGICAL STRATEGIES FOR REDUCING DRUG ABUSE

M. E. CARROLL
Department of Psychiatry, University of Minnesota, Minneapolis, MN, U.S.A.

There are many parallels between drug self-administration in the animal laboratory and drug abuse in humans. The animal models have allowed for the identification of factors that control the initiation and maintenance of drug abuse, and these models have also been valuable in studies of tolerance, cross tolerance, dependence and screening drugs for abuse liability. The purpose of the research presented here was to test behavioral and pharmacological interventions on self-administration of cocaine and phencyclidine in rats and monkeys. The drugs were self-administered orally, intravenously or by smoking. The behavioral treatments consisted of presenting a nondrug alternative reinforcer concurrently with the drug, and the pharmacological treatments were injections of buprenorphine, an opioid mixed agonist-antagonist that has been reported to reduce cocaine use in humans (1) and i.v. cocaine self-administration in monkeys (2), and fluoxetine, a serotonin uptake blocker used clinically as an antidepressant.

SUBJECTS AND METHODS

Intravenous drug self-administration. Rats were implanted with chronic jugular catheters and trained to press a lever for a 5 sec infusion of cocaine (0.1, 0.2, or 0.4 mg/kg) or fentanyl (2.5, 5 or 10 µg/kg). Four lever presses were required for each infusion (fixed ratio or FR 4 schedule), and infusions were available continuously. Water and food intake were measured daily. After behavior stabilized, a non-drug reinforcer, a sweet drinking solution of glucose and saccharin (G+S), was presented to a group of 5 rats for 5 days, and the effect on cocaine self-administration was determined. In other experiments, groups of 5 rats were injected with buprenorphine (0.1, 0.2 or 0.4 mg/kg) or fluoxetine (2.5, 5 or 10 mg/kg) twice daily for 5 days. Control groups self-administered the orally-delivered G+S solution but not cocaine and received the same drug injections. These groups were included to examine the effect of the drug treatments on behavior rewarded by a nondrug substance. The buprenorphine experiment was replicated with rats self-administering fentanyl (2.5, 5 and 10 µg/kg).

Oral drug self-administration. Rhesus monkeys were trained to make lip-contact responses for deliveries (0.6 ml) of phencyclidine (0.25 mg/ml) and water under concurrent FR 16 schedules during daily 3 hr sessions. In one group of 5 monkeys, after behavior stabilized, a saccharin solution (0.03 % wt/vol) replaced water during the sessions to examine the effect of an alternative nondrug reinforcer on phencyclidine self-administration. The response requirements for phencyclidine and saccharin were varied independently and simultaneously (FR 4, 8, 16, 32, 64 and 128). Each condition was held constant until behavior stabilized for at least 5 days. In another experiment with 3 monkeys the effect of buprenorphine on phencyclidine self-administration was tested. The monkeys were injected i.m. with 5 doses of buprenorphine (0.1, 0.2, 0.4, 0.8 and 1.6 mg/kg) or saline (0) 30 min before session onset for 5 days. Control monkeys received the same buprenorphine treatment, but they self-administered orally-delivered saccharin or ethanol.

Smoking behavior. Four monkeys were trained to respond on a lever under a progressive ratio schedule, and then to make 5 inhalation responses on a tube to receive a fixed quantity of cocaine smoke (2 mg/kg). Ten smoking trials were available each day, and there was a 15 min timeout after each smoke delivery. When behavior had stabilized, buprenorphine (doses listed above) injections were administered i.m. 30 min before session onset for 5 consecutive days. The effect on number of smoke deliveries was determined.

RESULTS

The <u>behavioral interventions</u> reduced cocaine and phencyclidine self-administration behavior in rats and monkeys, respectively. Cocaine infusions decreased by a mean of 26% during the 5 days that the alternative reinforcer was added to the environment. Phencyclidine self-administration was decreased by 30 - 93% by the presence of a concurrent saccharin solution, and the percentage increased as the phencyclidine FR increased. Thus, saccharin interfered more with phencyclidine intake as the cost of phencyclidine increased. Similarly, when the cost of phencyclidine and saccharin changed simultaneously, saccharin reduced the phencyclidine deliveries from 18 to 65.5 % as the FRs increased from 4 to 128.

The <u>pharmacological interventions</u> (buprenorphine and fluoxetine) reduced i.v. cocaine self-administration in rats in a dose-dependent manner. Food and water intake were not similarly affected. Control groups responding for a G+S solution also showed dose-related decrements in responding. They were more effective as cocaine dose decreased. At the highest cocaine dose (0.4 mg/kg) fluoxetine had almost no effect. Fluoxetine reduced fentanyl self-administration with similar dose effect relationships. Figure 1 shows that all doses of buprenorphine amost completely reduced self-administration of orally-delivered phencyclidine in 2 monkeys and by 50% in a third monkey. Figure 2 shows that buprenorphine markedly reduced cocaine smoking in 2 of 3 monkeys. Tests with control monkeys receiving orally-delivered saccharin and ethanol showed that behavior maintained by these substances was also greatly reduced by buprenorphine administration.

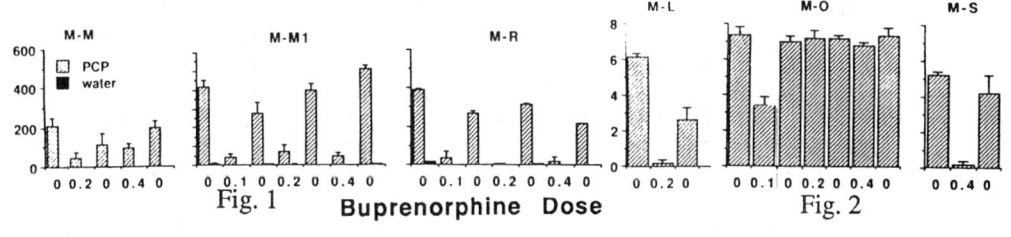

Phencyclidine liq. (Fig. 1) and cocaine-base smoke (Fig. 2) deliveries X buprenorphine dose.

DISCUSSION

These results indicate that nondrug alternative reinforcer are effective in reducing drug self-administration, especially if the cost of drug is high and the cost of the alternative reinforcer is moderate. It was also demonstrated that potential treatment drugs such as buprenorphine and fluoxetine effectively reduce drug self-administration, but their action is not specific across drugs or classes of reinforcers (e.g., drug, palatable substance). An explanation of the reduction in drug self-administration due to pretreatment with drugs could be based on the ability of the treatment drug to block reinforcing effects of the self-administered drug, to substitute as a reinforcer, to produce a generalized decrement in behavior, to punish drug-taking behavior or to a combination of factors. Food and water intake and saline infusions were not substantially reduced by buprenorphine or fluoxetine, arguing against a general suppression of behavior. Thus, collectively, the present results suggest that buprenorphine and fluoxetine alter the reinforcing effects of drug and nondrug substances.

REFERENCES

1. Kosten, T.R., Kleber, H.D. and Morgan, C. Role of opioid antagonists in treating intravenous cocaine abuse. Life Sci. 44:887-892, 1989.
2. Mello, N.K., Mendelson, J.H., Bree, M.P. et al. Buprenorphine suppresses cocaine self-administration by rhesus monkeys. Science, 245:859-862.

BRAIN CIRCUITRY COMPUTER RECONSTRUCTION: HUMAN BRAIN PROJECT

STEPHEN H. KOSLOW AND ALAN I. LESHNER
National Institute of Mental Health, Rockville, MD, U.S.A.

The time is now propitious for the bringing together of modern computer science with modern neuroscience through the development of the "human brain project." A recent report from the National Academy of Sciences (1), "Models for Biomedical Research: A New Perspective" says, "We seem to be at a point in the history of biology at which new generalizations and higher order biological laws are being approached, but may be obscured by the simple mass of data." The two communities, neuro and computer scientists, are currently in the process of planning and developing the approach for the human brain project, which will promote innovative and cutting edge science.

The human brain project will be a comprehensive interactive computer database of information in brain anatomy, physiology, neuronal biochemistry, neuronal systems, and behavioral and cognitive functions. As we envision this system, the human brain project will receive input from both experimental and clinical researchers. This 3-dimensional human brain project will have the capability of acquisition, storage, analysis and display of anatomical and physiological data on rodent, primate and human brain structures and their functions.

There are a number of driving forces which have been set in motion which now demand that the neuroscience community address this problem. Paramount is the sheer amount of, and growth of, data related to the brain, its neurochemicals and its function. For the last decade we have been in a period of accelerated experimentation with data being accumulated at a rate which makes it impossible for any one individual to completely assimilate and integrate the information. Retrieval of the information in its current context is fragmented and difficult to handle in any synthetic format. However, the computer industry, has developed, and is developing further, both hardware and software which can address these needs. For example, we now have the capacity for 3-dimensional graphic display of animal and human brain information.

The number of neuroscientists working on problems related to nervous system function has increased exponentially in the last two decades to the point where the annual Society for Neuroscience meeting has an attendance of approximately 13,000 scientists. There has been a logarithmic increase in information on nervous system neurotransmitters, including the classical neurotransmitters and newer neuropeptides. In addition, there has been discovery of a number of trophic factors and genomic approaches to studying the brain. Newer methods of approaching brain function include not only the direct chemical measures but also the now common noninvasive imaging techniques such as Magnetic Resonance Imaging (MRI), Positron Emission Topography (PET), and Single Photon Emission Computer Tomography (SPECT), as well as mapping of brain electrical activity.

The human brain project would allow for the synthesis and greater understanding of how the multitude of parts of the brain act in concert to yield healthy or pathological behavior. Such an approach should lead to major conceptual and medical breakthroughs. On the simplest level, the human brain project will speed the progress of neuroscience research. This project has the ability to gather, reduce duplication of effort and permit more open sharing of new data among colleagues. From a practical perspective, it will also provide current information to clinicians and educators. As it presently exists, the database is far too complex and fragmented, and as previously stated the expansion rate of information makes the unaided and unstructured search for such information a virtual impossibility. The human brain project will allow anyone to search the knowledge base in a short period of time, integrate information which may appear to be only tangential to the original question. The ultimate goal of the human brain project will allow for the integration of an unlimited range of information, the design of new categories of experiments, and the development of new theories.

REFERENCES

1. National Academy of Science. (1985): <u>Models for Biomedical Research: A New Perspective</u>. National Academy Press, Washington, D.C.

STRUCTURE-FUNCTION CORRELATION OF THE LIVING HUMAN BRAIN WITH MRI AND PET: A MEANS OF ANATOMICAL AND FUNCTIONAL LOCALIZATION

J.C. MAZZIOTTA*, D. VALENTINO*, C.A. PELIZZARI**, G.T. CHEN**, AND F. BOOKSTEIN***
*Department of Radiology, UCLA, Los Angeles; **Department of Radiology/Oncology, University of Chicago, Chicago, Illinois; ***University of Michigan, Ann Arbor, MI, U.S.A.

The integration of structural images, from MRI or CT, with functional images from PET or SPECT, provides the opportunity to analyze functional data based on anatomical landmarks. The most reliable approach to this process has been the subject of debate (2,3) for the last six years. We have proposed a system that integrates images, first, within a subject ("Merger One") and then between subjects ("Merger Two") (Fig. 1) so as to optimize the solution to this data analysis and display problem. The resulting images can be displayed as multi-dimensional maps of structure-function superimpositions and provide a comprehensive view of this integrated data in a format familiar to anyone with knowledge of brain anatomy.

Merger One: A system has been developed (4) which produces aligned, registered, scaled, and resliced image sets within a given subject and, either, between (e.g., MRI-PET) or within (e.g., MRI-MRI) imaging modalities. This approach fits the 3D surface of a common boundary between data sets. For example, the outer surface of the skull or skin, which can be found in MRI and transmission PET images can serve as the appropriate surface. Once fit, the resulting match can be expressed as a function of the degree of misalignment, which typically has an error that is comparable in magnitude to the voxel size of the imaging device with the poorest spatial resolution. Once an appropriate structure-function match has been produced (Fig. 2), regions of interest (ROIs) can be manually drawn on the anatomical image using structural landmarks and transferred automatically to the functional PET image for quantification of the variable of interest. Such regionalization can be performed in 3D with volumes of interest (VOIs).

Merger Two: A more difficult problem is the distortion of one brain data set from a given individual to that of another individual, a population, or an idealized model. Because of the anatomical variations in normal brains, it has largely been impossible to provide a 3D distortion system with reproducible accuracy that works for all brain regions. Through the use of morphometrics (1), it may be possible to achieve this type of 3D distortion. Such an approach has been successful in two dimensions and is being extended to 3D for the purpose of this study. By selecting landmarks distributed throughout the 3D volume of brain anatomy, we are currently testing the morphometric approach to determine its reliability and accuracy. Landmarks are chosen at points in the brain because of their geometric site or for their inherent stability (e.g., growth centers, vascular bifurcations, or points of tissue curvature).

If successful, Merger Two provides the opportunity to compare individual studies of structure and function with studies of other individuals, groups, or an idealized brain model. In the latter case, one could have preassigned VOIs drawn to identify all cerebral structures. When a given patient study is merged with the idealized model, automated regionalization of the functional data would occur. These data could then, in turn, be compared with values from normal individuals or subjects with specific disorders. Such an approach would have both practical clinical as well as investigational value. For the former, it would provide an automated method of determining normality or similarity to specific disease entities. For the latter, it could be used to identify the distribution of a functional response to a specific task or drug stimulus, to study the variations and natural history of a disease process or the effects of interventions such as drug therapy, surgery, or rehabilitation.

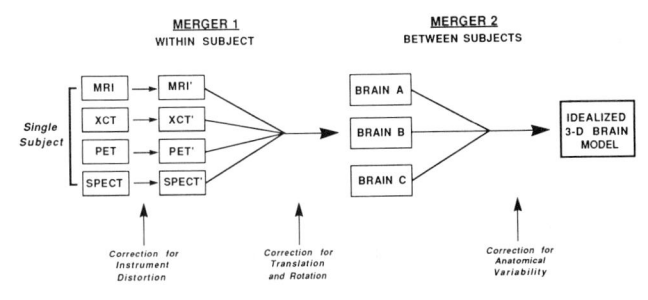

Fig. 1.   Merger Scheme

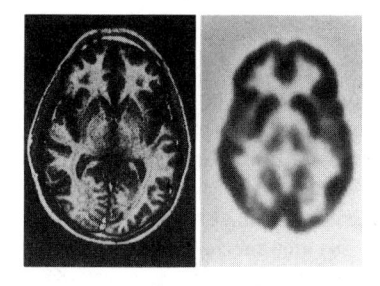

Fig. 2.   PET and MRI images displayed after Merger One (3) matching.

REFERENCES

1. Bookstein F.L. IEEE Tran Pat Anal Mach Intell, (1989): PMA I-11, S67-S85.
2. Mazziotta J.C. J Cereb Bld Flow Met (1984): 4:481-483.
3. Mazziotta J.C., Koslow SH. J Cereb Bld Flow Met (1987): 7:S1-S31.
4. Pelizzari C.A., Chen GT, et al. J Comput Assist Tomo (1989): 13:20-26.

VISUALIZING THE 3-D STRUCTURE, FUNCTION OF BRAIN

ARTHUR W. TOGA
The Laboratory of Neuro Imaging
Department of Neurology, UCLA School of Medicine
710 Westwood Plaza, Los Angeles, California 90024

ABSTRACT

Autoradiographic and histologic preparations are two of many methods which have provided neuroscientists with a more comprehensive understanding of brain structure and function.

This paper describes methods for displaying functional and anatomic data on arbitrary collections of surfaces on or within the brain. The resulting displays provide quantitative information on the magnitude of functional activity as well as accurate perception of surface form.

INTRODUCTION

Many basic science experiments (animal models) require the physical sectioning of tissue to examine anatomy (structure) or function (physiology) deep to the surface at acceptable resolutions. Recent efforts at 3D reconstruction have concentrated on systems that model structure **or** function. Volume rendering techniques have displayed the volume of data directly, without constructing an intermediate surface representation. This approach alone cannot be used for displaying and analyzing structures which are not definable by densitometric criteria. Other methods are surface based techniques, which generate a complete surface model before viewing. Surface models have a dual role, in that they can be used for modelling, partitioning space and delineating particular structures, as well as for viewing.

Techniques have been developed for mapping biological function on 3D structure. Surface based methods include direct mapping of function (pseudocoloring) without surface shading and solid texturing. A volume of quantitative data in the brain can be thought of as a solid texture where color variations correspond to degrees of functional activity. Our goal is to permit functional mapping on arbitrary surfaces within or on the brain, within a flexible graphics environment.

In this paper, we present a system for mapping functional data upon arbitrary surfaces within or on the brain. The resulting models have applications in neurobiology because they provide an alternative to cutaways for viewing patterns of internal functional activity.

METHODS

Surfaces of structures (e.g. cortex) were constructed using a technique which triangulates between the outlines (contours) of successive sections. Images were aligned with respect to each other and Z-values calculated.

A solid texture function was constructed from quantitative data for surface mapping. The original sections provided the density data. A trilinear interpolant was useds for points not lying on the sampled lattice. The data used here was a set of 50 slices (512x512x8 bits) using quantitative autoradiographic techniques for measuring glucose metabolism in an epileptic monkey.

Surface viewing required the designation of various parameters such as color, transparency, hardness, and priority. Next, **geometric transformations** were applied for rotation, translation, scaling, and perspective. The final **rendering** process displayed surfaces of the triangular models with an A-buffer method, and applied solid texturing where appropriate.

RESULTS AND DISCUSSION

These methods for the functional mapping of brain were applied to the cortical surface, the surface of internal nuclear structures, and arbitrary cutting planes. Because the surfaces are natural and complex, special consideration was necessary to provide realistic displays without sacrificing quantitation.

The comprehensibility of solid-textured views of complicated surfaces requires the viewer to be able to extract several independent features including object orientation in space and quantitative magnitude of the functional data over the object surface. The pseudocoloring scheme for the solid texture function must be selected with care if these components are to be kept independent. We used a simple spectral sequence, from high activity red through low activity violet, with 16 categories. Displaying the data with transparencies, and solid textured cutting planes can provide very informative displays.

CONCLUSIONS

We have shown a system for displaying neurobiological surface models with reference to structure and function. We combined quantitative data with surface rendering and shading algorithms in a defined way. The functional mapping allows both form and function to be appreciated in a three dimensional context. This approach has several desirable features. Complex, convoluted surfaces can be shown with the shading cues necessary to understand their shapes. Viewpoint, object position, illumination and perspective can all be varied as needed. Multiple objects can be shown in one view, with or without transparency to allow internal surfaces and intersecting objects to be shown in relation to each other. Quantitative information can be superposed on biological or otherwise defined surfaces anywhere within the volume. As a result, both quantitative and positional information can be understood in its global context.

MULTIMODAL 3D IMAGING OF EEG AND MRI

MICHAEL W. TORELLO
Department of Psychiatry and Psychology, Ohio State University, Columbus, Ohio, 43210, U.S.A.

Both EEG imaging and MR imaging represent relatively new and separate neuroimaging technologies. EEG imaging techniques have been developed to deal with the problem of data reduction and interpretation. This methodology can condense, summarize, and display spectral, spatial, and temporal information of brain activity from multiple scalp locations and produces a topographic map of electrical activity across the entire scalp. MR data are typically displayed as multiple 2D slices. The clinician must mentally visualize these slices as 3D images in order to comprehend relationships between structures. The 3D visualization of these 2D images is now possible due to improvements in computer graphics technology. In addition, we felt that the development of techniques to integrate images from multiple modalities (functional and structural) would provide new insight into the relationships of scalp electrode placement, scalp-recorded electrical activity and the underlying brain anatomy.

Our overlapping imaging techniques have produced combinational images showing brain structure, brain electrical activity and scalp electrode placements in one visualization (4,5). Our first subject was a healthy 37 year-old male righthander. Eyes closed resting EEG was recorded using a Biologic Brain Atlas III and artifact-free data were analyzed using a Fast Fourier Transform and converted to color-coded spectral maps. In order to subsequently visualize placements of scalp EEG electrodes, oil-filled capsules pasted to the scalp acted as electrode markers according to a system of electrode placement (3). Next, the subject was given an MR scan (General Electric 1.5 Tesla) and serial, sagittal slices (256 X 256 pixels), 5mm thick using a partial saturation sequence were obtained. The electrode markers were visualized as high intensity circular areas on the scalp. The MR data was converted to RGB format and displayed on a high resolution graphics monitor (SUN 3/160 workstation and Pixar II image computer). MR sections showing cerebral cortex were manually traced using a computer cursor and mouse. The cortical surface of the brain was then reconstructed from these tracings as a 3D perspective image constructed from thousands of polygons. These polygons described the surface of the brain. A color-coded map of alpha eyes-closed electrical activity scalp distribution was recomputed after its overlay onto the 3D MR image. Since the original color-coded EEG image was an equal area projection 2D map, and since the reconstructed multi-slice MR image is a perspective image, we first overlayed a translucent "skull cap" onto the MR image. Then, we used the original EEG microvolt values measured from the electrodes and did a four-point weighted linear interpolation to determine the microvolt values of each pixel that made up the "skull cap". Color codes of microvolt values were assigned to each pixel. The EEG image was made translucent to allow the viewing of the underlying brain and perpendiculars were extended from the scalp electrode markers to the underlying cortex to preserve their relationship to the brain's surface. The final image could be rotated in any axis to facilitate viewing.

Presently, we have dramatically improved the 3D reconstruction algorithms and visualizations of the brain. In addition, our reconstructed 3D MR image no longer represents just cortical surface of the brain but the entire brain volume can now be displayed and manipulated. We have also reduced slice thickness to 3mm with an interslice interval of .5mm (total slices 50-60). This results in a striking improvement of anatomical detail upon reconstruction. Initially, image reconstructions required 2 1/2 hours using a SUN 3/160 workstation with 8 Mb of memory. For rapid image processing, utilizing a Cray Y-MP 8/864 we have reduced this time to 80 seconds and further optimization is expected.

It was noted that electrodes were not placed over brain areas predicted by the International 10/20 System (3). This system does not guarantee systematic electrode placement with respect to underlying brain areas, but it does provide a standardized placement with respect to skull landmarks (2). The relationship between specific cortical structures and standard electrode placements is only approximate, since the brain and skull size and shape vary widely from individual to individual (1). We suspect that electrode placement inaccuracy, with respect to underlying brain anatomy, can contribute artifactually to the spatial variations in scalp-recorded brain potentials which have been documented in patients. It is critical to the understanding of various neurodiseases to know whether functional asymmetries are in whole or part artifactual or represent a valid neurophysiological difference.

The strength of this integrated imaging technique is that, a) if specific regional correlations do exist between brain anatomical abnormalities and EEG abnormalities within a given individual, they will now be easily visualized; b) the visualization of brain anatomy in 3D will provide easier appreciation of the boundaries of tumors and other anatomical irregularities that are observed from multiple 2D MR slices; and c) the visualization of the precise locations of scalp electrodes with respect to the underlying cortical tissue within a given subject is now possible. Further, this technique could lead to an improved system of scalp electrode placement, through the development of a correction procedure which should provide better scalp electrode correlations with underlying brain landmarks between subjects. This approach of combining imaging modalities into a unified visualization represents a significant advance in brain research.

REFERENCES

1. Galaburda, A.M. and Sanides, F. Cytoarchitectonic organization of the human auditory cortex, J. Comp. Neurol., 190:597, 1980.

2. Homan, R.W., Herman, J. and Purdy, P. Cerebral location of international 10-20 electrode placement. Electroencept. Clin. Neurophysiol. 66: 376-382, 1987.

3. Jasper, H.H. The ten-twenty electrode system of the International Federation. Electroenceph. Clin. Neurophysiol. 10: 371, 1958.

4. Torello, M.W., Garabis, J.M., Hunter, W.W. and Csuri, C.A. Combinational imaging: structure and function of the brain displayed simultaneously: Proceedings of the Society Magnetic Resonance in Medicine, 1986.

5. Torello, M.W., Phillips, T. Hunter, W.W., and Csuri, C.A. Combinational imaging: magnetic resonance imaging and EEG displayed simultaneously. J. Clin. Neurophysiol. 4 (3): 274, 1987.

Approach to benzodiazepine dependence studies through ligand receptor binding in vivo

Osamu Inoue and Toshiro Yamasaki

Division of Clinical Research, National Institute of Radiological Sciences, 4-9-1 Anagawa, Chiba-shi 260, Japan.

In vivo measurement of neuroreceptors in the living human brain by PET would be of great value for drug dependence studies. The binding potentials of receptors and the receptor occupancy by various types of drugs can be directly measured(1). However it has been reported that there are significant discrepancies between in vitro and in vivo receptor binding. For example, in vivo binding of benzodiazepine(BZ) receptors was altered by stress(2) or treatment with drugs which did not interact with BZ receptors in vitro(3). Although the mechanism for such discrepancies is yet unclear, the in vivo binding technique is valuable for the investigation of neural interaction , such as GABA and dopaminergic neuron. Even though the functional roles of dopamine in benzodiazepine dependence is unknown,the reward pathway might be related to drug dependency.In this study,the effect of sedative and hypnotic drugs (ethanol, pentobarbital and clonazepam) on the in vivo binding of dopamine D1 and D2 receptors were investigated.

Method

Male ddY mice weighing about 35-40 g (8-9 weeks old) were used. Mice were treated with varying doses of ethanol, pentobarbital and 2 mg/kg of clonazepam 30 min prior to the tracer injection. Mice were intravenously injected with 0.2 ml of 3H-SCH 23390 or 3H-NMSP, and decapitated at 45 min after the tracer injection. Radioactivity in the striatum, cerebral cortex and cerebellum was measured and the ratio of radioactivity in the striatum or cerebral cortex to that in the cerebellum was used as index of the binding potential(BP) of dopamine D1 and D2 receptors.

Results

Acute treatment with ethanol significantly reduced BP of dopamine D1 receptors in the striatum in a dose-dependent manner, while BP of dopamine D2 receptors in the same region was not changed by 1 g/kg of ethanol. In vivo binding of 3H-SCH 23390 and 3H-NMSP in the cerebral cortex which might contain a serotonergic component, was not altered by ethanol. Pentobarbital also affected the in vivo binding of both 3H-SCH 23390 and 3H-NMSP in the striatum. A significant decrease in binding of both 3H-SCH 23390 and 3H-NMSP was also seen in clonazepam-treated mouse striatum. These results are summarized in Fig 1.

Discussion

In vivo binding of 3H-SCH 23390 and 3H-NMSP was significantly affected by sedative and hypnotic drugs. These changes in binding might be caused by an alteration in the rates of association or dissociation in vivo probably through GABA-mediated process. One possible explanation for such changes in receptor binding is that the diffusion barrier to the synapse is changed by sedative and hypnotic drugs. Membrane fluidity seems to be a critical factor in the diffusion barrier. As membrane fluidity has been reported to be changed by drug tolerance and drug addiction(4), it is of interest to examine whether in vivo binding of dopamine receptors is altered by repeated treatment with such sedative and hypnotic drugs or not. The neural interaction study through receptor binding in vivo seems to be a valuable method for drug dependence studies including benzodiazepines.

Fig 1. Relative binding potential (BP) of dopamine D1 and D2 receptors in vivo.

Mice were treated with ethanol, clonazepam and pentobarbital 30 min prior to the tracer injection.

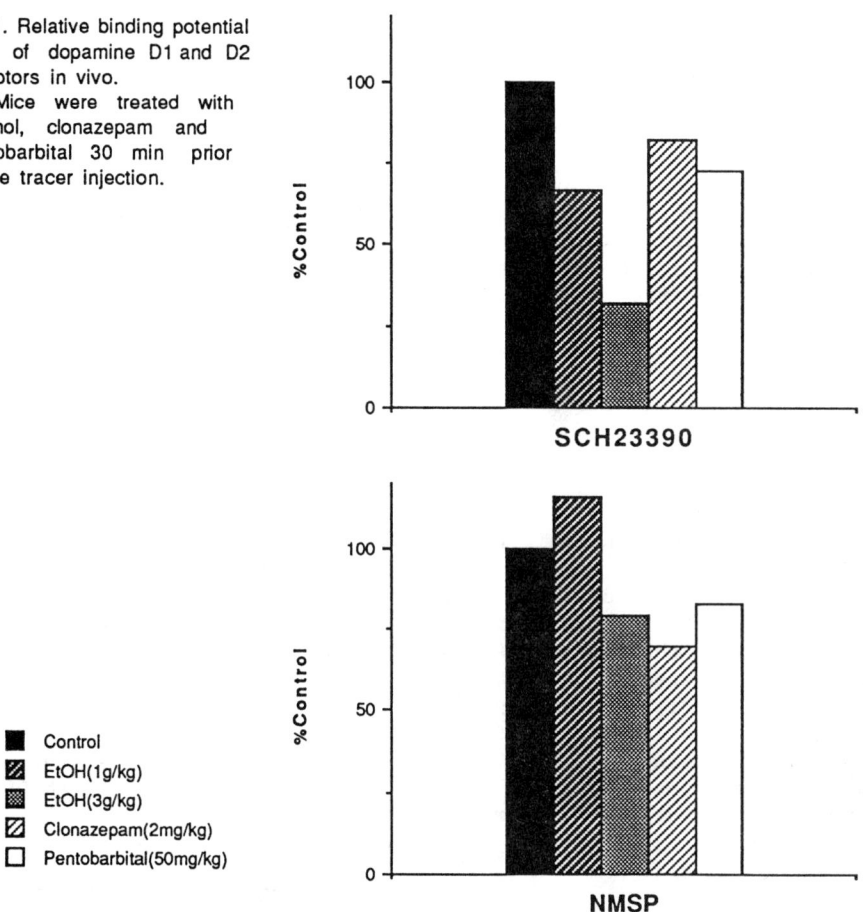

- ■ Control
- EtOH(1g/kg)
- EtOH(3g/kg)
- Clonazepam(2mg/kg)
- □ Pentobarbital(50mg/kg)

References

(1) Shinotho,H.et al. Detection of benzodiazepine receptor occupancy in the human brain by positron emission tomography.Psychopharmacol.99:202-207,1989
(2) Weizman,R.et al. Repeated swim stress alters brain benzodiazepine receptors measured in vivo.J.Pharmacol.Exp.Ther.249(3):701-707,1989
(3) Jeevangee,F.et al. Enhancement of [3H]flunitrazepam binding by mianserine in vivo.Neuroscience Letters.46:305-309,1984
(4) Heron,D.S. et al. Adaptive modulation of brain membrane lipid fluidity in drug addiction and denervation supersensitivity. Biochem.Pharmacol.31(14):2435-2438,1982

EFFECTS OF BENZODIAZEPINE AND NONBENZODIAZEPINE HYPNOTICS ON THE
HIPPOCAMPAL RHYTHMIC ACTIVITY IN CATS

N. YAMAGUCHI, Y. KIYOTA, Y. KUBOTA, H. KIDO, H. SAKAMOTO*
and N. AKIYAMA**
Department of Neuropsychiatry, Kanazawa University School of Medicine,
Kanazawa 920* and Awazu Nervous Sanatorium, Komatsu 923-03**, Japan

In 1954, Green and Arduini (2) have reported that the hippocampal electrical activity on rabbits showed the rhythmic slow activity (RSA) during wakefulness. Afterwards, Jouvet et al. (5) observed the hippocampal RSA during the paradoxical sleep in cats and Shimazono et al. (6) also observed the same phenomenon in dogs. We discovered in 1968 (7) that the frequency of hippocampal RSA decreased after the application of nitrazepam on cats. The present paper is concerned with the effects of hypnotics of benzodiazepine (triazolam) and nonbenzodiazepine cyclopyrrolone derivatives (zopiclone) on the hippocampal RSA during wakefulness and paradoxical sleep in cats.

SUBJECT AND METHOD

Adult cats were used in this study. As surgical procedures of implantation of electrodes were previously described (8), the particulars have been omitted here. Stainless steel screws were placed bilaterally on the cranial dura mater for recording electrical activities from the anterior (motor area) and posterior sigmoid gyri (somatosensory area). Concentric electrodes were implanted into the thalamus, the dorsal hippocampus and the mesencephalic reticular formation. Chronic experiments usually started not earlier than 2 weeks after the surgery. Polygraphic recordings of the EEG, ECG, EOG and respiration curve were carried out continuosly for two hours before and for 6 hours after the intravenous injection of drugs. The frequency of dorsal hippocampal activity was analyzed by using an automatic frequency analyzer.

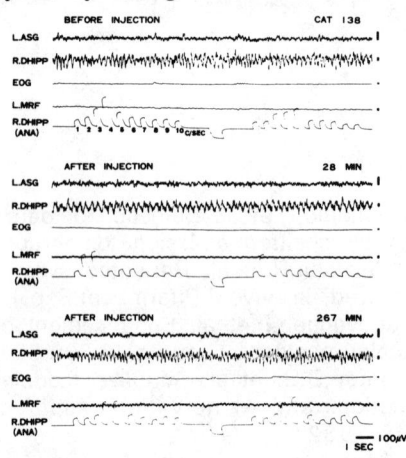

Fig. 1: The hippocampal rhythmic activity during the paradoxical sleep stage before and after the intravenous application of triazolam of 0.02 mg/kg. Abbreviations for this and following illustrations : L, left ; R, right ; ASG, anterior sigmoid gyrus ; DHIPP, dorsal hippocampus ; EOG, electrooculogram ; MRF, midbrain reticular formation ; ANA, frequency analysis by an automatic frequency analyzer.

Fig. 2: The hippocampal rhythmic activity during the paradoxical sleep stage before and after the intravenous application of zopiclone of 0.4 mg/kg.

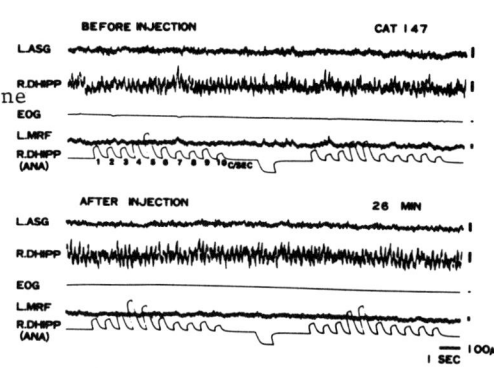

RESULTS

The frequency of hippocampal rhythmic activity during the paradoxical sleep diminished from 5 Hz to 3 Hz after the application of triazolam (0.01-0.02 mg/kg) and returned gradually to the original frequency (Fig. 1). The frequency of hippocampal rhythmic activity during wakefulness also diminished from 3 Hz to 2 Hz after the administration of triazolam. The slowing of the hippocampal rhythmic activity following the application of triazolam was prolonged by the simultaneous injection of ethylalcohol (100 mg/kg). On the other hand, there were no changes to the frequency of hippocampal rhythmic activity in the paradoxical sleep and in the wakefulness after the application of nonbenzodiazepine zopiclone (0.2-0.8 mg/kg) (Fig. 2).

DISCUSSION

Certain facts are already established concerning anterograde amnesic effect of diazepam (3). Hazama and Kawahara (4) reported a case suffered from impairment of short term memory induced by triazolam. Adey et al. (1) observed that regular theta rhythm becomes restricted in its representation to the dorsal hippocampus and entorhinal cortex with development of an approach learning. In our present experiments, the frequency of hippocampal rhythmic activity diminished after the application of triazolam. It is assumed that the slowing of the hippocampal activity may be attributed to the cause of the impairment of memory processing after the application of benzodiazepine derivatives.

REFERENCES

1. Adey, W.R. et al.: A.M.A. Arch. Neurol. 3:74-90, 1960.
2. Green, J.D. & Arduini, A.A.: J. Neruophysiol. 17:533-557, 1954.
3. Gregg, J.M. et al.: J. Oral Surg. 32:651-664, 1974.
4. Hazama, H. & Kawahara, R.: Seishin Igaku (Tokyo). 23:361-365, 1981.
5. Jouvet, M. et al.: C.R. Soc. Biol. (Paris). 153:1024-1028, 1959.
6. Shimazono, Y. et al.: Neurol. medico-chir. (Tokyo). 2:82-88, 1960.
7. Takeshima, T., Yamaguchi, N. et al.: Brain and Nerve (Tokyo). 20: 209-216, 1968.
8. Yamaguchi, N. et al.: Electroenceph. clin. Neurophysiol. 17: 246-254, 1964.

DISCRIMINATIVE STIMULUS AND REINFORCING EFFECTS OF BENZODIAZEPINES IN NORMAL HUMAN VOLUNTTERS

C.E. JOHANSON
Psychiatry, Uniformed Services University of the Health Sciences, Bethesda, MD, U.S.A.

The experimental evaluation of the dependence potential of drugs in animal models has included studies of discriminative stimulus and reinforcing effects. It has been shown that drugs which share discriminative stimulus properties with a known drug of abuse are also likely to have dependence potential. Furthermore, drugs which function as positive reinforcers in animals, i.e., are self-administered, are drugs which are abused by humans. This concordance has led to the use of these two procedures in the prediction of dependence potential and self-administration methods have also been used to evaluate behavioral and pharmacological factors which modify reinforcing properties. While most studies of this type have been carried out in animals, studies are also being conducted in humans. In the present series of studies, the discriminative stimulus and reinforcing effects of diazepam (DZ) and other benzodiazepines were evaluated in normal volunteers.

SUBJECTS

All experimental subjects were normal volunteers between 21 and 35. Candidates with a previous history of drug abuse or dependence, a history of Axis I disorders according to DSM-IIIR criteria, or any significant present or past medical or psychiatric problem were excluded. The protocol was approved by the local institutional human use committee and informed consent was obtained. Subjects were paid for their participation.

PROCEDURE AND RESULTS OF DRUG DISCRIMINATION EXPERIMENTS

Subjects were instructed that their job was to learn to discriminate between two different drugs, 10 mg DZ and placebo. On each session, participants filled out mood questionnaires, ingested a capsule, and then were free to leave. One, 3 and 6 hrs later, subjects filled out additional questionnaires. During phase 1 (4 sessions), 10 mg DZ and placebo were administered on separate sessions and identified prior to ingestion using letter codes. During phase 2, subjects were not told which capsule they received and were asked to telephone 6 hrs after ingestion to report their discrimination. If they were correct, they received bonus money. If a subject correctly identified the capsules on 5 of the 7 sessions, they participated in a third phase of 12 sessions. Six of these sessions were additional training sessions. Randomly intermixed with training were 6 test sessions when subjects received other drugs. Subjects were not aware that a test session was scheduled until they telephoned and they received bonus money regardless of their response.

In the first experiment, sixteen of 19 subjects learned the discrimination with overall accuracy of 90% during phase 2 which was maintained at a level of 85% during phase 3. When 2 and 5 mg DZ were administered during test sessions, drug-appropriate responding was 7% and 64%, respectively. Drug-appropriate responding increased from 29% when 1 mg lorazepam was tested to 86% at 2 mg. Sixty-four percent of the subjects called 50 mg pentobarbital drug whereas only 21% discriminated amphetamine as DZ. The subjective effects of DZ were typical of benzodiazepines. These results indicate that it is possible to train humans to discriminate DZ and this discrimination is sensitive to differences in dose and appears specific to sedative-like drugs. In a second study which is presently ongoing, two additional anxiolytics, triazolam and buspirone, and the antihistamine tripelennamine are being evaluated.

PROCEDURE AND RESULTS OF SELF-ADMINISTRATION STUDIES

Outpatient Procedure. The reinforcing properties of benzodiazepines were evaluated using a choice procedure consisting of 9 experimental sessions. During the first 4 sessions, subjects received either drug or placebo which were identified using letter codes. On the last 5 sessions subjects were given a choice of which capsule they preferred to take. The measure of self-administration was the number of drug choices versus the number of placebo choices. On all experimental sessions, participants filled out mood questionnaires, ingested a capsule, and then were free to leave, i.e., they returned to their daily activities. One, 3 and 6 hrs later, subjects filled out additional questionnaires.

Laboratory-Based Procedure. Similar studies with DZ were also conducted under controlled laboratory conditions with subjects participating in groups of 4. Each experiment consisted of 7 sessions, 4 sampling and 3 choice. In the first study, subjects received (sampling) or choose (choice) a single dose of DZ (20 mg) or placebo at the beginning of the 4-hr session. In the second study, the protocol was similar except that DZ was administered in divided doses of 4 mg. During the drug sampling sessions, each subject received a total of 5 divided doses over the 1st 2 hrs of the session and during placebo sessions, these 4 capsules all contained placebo. During choice trials, subjects first chose which type of capsule they wished to take throughout the session (DZ or placebo). They then had the opportunity to choose an additional 6 capsules (total of 28 mg for DZ) distributed over the 1st 3 hrs of the session.

Several different studies were conducted with between 9 and 18 subjects participating in each study. In the first study using the outpatient procedure, 2, 5, and 10 mg DZ were compared to placebo in 3 separate experiments. As dose was increased, drug choice decreased from 58% to 27%, i.e., subjects preferred placebo. These results were in contrast to a previous study using an identical procedure which showed that normal volunteers preferred amphetamine and other psychomotor stimulants to placebo. Additional studies were conducted with lorazepam and flurazepam which yielded similar results, i.e., these benzodiazepines were not self-administered and choice decreased as dose was increased. For all three benzodiazepines, the subjective effects were typical of sedative-like drugs. Because the drugs were administered in the morning hours and subjects were returning to work-related activities, it was possible that the administration of sedative drugs was interfering with performance. Therefore an additional study was conducted in the evening with subjects returning home after capsule administration. Despite this time-change, placebo was still preferred to 5 and 10 mg DZ.

In the laboratory study with the administration of a single dose of 20 mg, subjects still preferred placebo over DZ. However, DZ choice increased dramatically when subjects were administered the drug in divided doses. Under these conditions, over 60% of choices were DZ although the subjective effects produced by the drug were similar to those obtained in previous studies where DZ did not maintain drug-taking behavior.

SUMMARY

The present studies demonstrated that DZ and other benzodiazepines share discriminative stimulus properties in humans and the results obtained correspond to results obtained in other animals species. Likewise, these drugs do not have strong reinforcing effects which has also been shown in animal studies. However, the results obtained with the divided dose procedure with subjects participating under controlled laboratory conditions with a group of friends indicates that there are conditions which can augment the reinforcing effects of DZ. Further studies are needed to determine the factors responsible for this increase in reinforcing effects and whether they are additional risk factors that increase the likelihood that humans will self-administer DZ.

PRECLINICAL AND CLINICAL STUDIES OF THE ABUSE AND DEPENDENCE
POTENTIAL OF BENZODIAZEPINES AND OTHER SEDATIVES

ROLAND R. GRIFFITHS
Departments of Psychiatry and Neuroscience, The Johns Hopkins
University School of Medicine, Baltimore, MD, U.S.A.

The benzodiazepine anxiolytics and hypnotics are among the most widely prescribed of all compounds. Two significant problems with these compounds are: 1. they are abused by people with histories of drug abuse (i.e. they are used at high doses for non-therapeutic purposes and they are bought and sold illegally); and 2. they produce physical dependence at both high and therapeutic dose levels. In addition to being an adverse effect of drug use, physical dependence represents a mechanism for maintaining inappropriate chronic use of these compounds by both drug abusers and by patients. This paper will review data from human and infrahuman studies that provide information about the abuse and physical dependence potential of benzodiazepines and other sedatives.

Reinforcing effects in animals: Drug self-administration procedures in laboratory animals permit assessment of the relative efficacy with which different drugs maintain drug self-administration. The validity of this approach for providing information relevant to human drug abuse is supported by the good correspondence between those drugs that are self-administered by laboratory animals and those that are self-administered and abused by humans. Various sedative compounds were evaluated for self-injection in baboons using a standard substitution paradigm in which each drug was substituted for cocaine for 12 or more days under a continuously available fixed-ratio 160 schedule with a 3-h timeout following each injection. These studies showed that abecarnil (a benzodiazepine receptor mediated ß-carboline anxiolytic), buspirone, chlorpromazine and phenobarbital either did not maintain self-injection behavior above vehicle control levels or maintained only very low rates. A series of benzodiazepines (alprazolam, bromazepam, chlordiazepoxide, clonazepam, clorazepate, diazepam, flurazepam, lorazepam, medazepam, midazolam and triazolam) maintained low to intermediate rates of self-injection, with triazolam and midazolam maintaining the highest rates among the benzodiazepines. Amobarbital, methohexital, pentobarbital and secobarbital maintained the highest rates of self-injection which approximated those maintained by cocaine.

Physical dependence-producing effects in animals:

Physical dependence on sedatives can be evaluated by characterizing spontaneous withdrawal or flumazenil (a benzodiazepine antagonist) precipitated withdrawal after a period of chronic administration of a test drug. Withdrawal severity is an increasing function of dose and duration of sedative administration and, with benzodiazepines, an increasing function of flumazenil dose. Spontaneous withdrawal from lorazepam and diazepam have shown increases in abnormal postures, twitch jerks, limb and body tremor, and disruption of food intake. Flumazenil precipitated withdrawal from diazepam and lorazepam showed increases in bruxism, retching vomiting, tremor and abnormal postures. Spontaneous and precipitated withdrawal studies with tandospirone (a $5-HT_{1A}$ receptor mediated anxiolytic) and abecarnil indicated less severe physical dependence than with diazepam and lorazepam.

Reinforcing effects in humans:

The reinforcing effects of drugs in humans can be studied directly by using drug self-administration and choice procedures, or can be studied indirectly by having subjects rate subjective effects believed to be correlated with reinforcing effects (e.g. drug liking or positive mood states). The best validated approach for providing information predictive of the abuse liability of sedative drugs is to evaluate compounds under placebo-controlled, double-blind conditions in subjects with histories of sedative drug abuse. Studies showed that a various benzodiazepines (alprazolam, diazepam, lorazepam, oxazepam and triazolam) have some abuse liability. Related studies suggest that the abuse liabilities of pentobarbital and meprobamate are greater than benzodiazepines while the abuse liabilities of chlorpromazine and diphenhydramine are less than benzodiazepines.

Physical dependence in humans:

The withdrawal syndrome following termination of both high and therapeutic doses of benzodiazepines in humans has been well characterized. The profile, intensity, and time-course of signs and symptoms that emerge upon termination of drug administration has permitted differentiation of true pharmacological withdrawal from a simple re-emergence of pre-existing anxiety or insomnia. Although the most severe withdrawal signs (seizures and delirium) are generally absent in therapeutic dose dependence, a variety of disturbing signs and symptoms remain, including anxiety, insomnia, irritability, tremor, muscle twitching, headache, GI disturbance, depersonalization perceptual changes). A recent study has provided evidence for a mild flumazenil precipitated withdrawal syndrome after short-term treatment (3 to 14 days) with lorazepam (3.0 mg/day) in normal humans. As with the preclinical research, it may be possible to use flumazenil as a tool for developing safe and effective procedures for assaying the physical dependence potential of new compounds with activity at the benzodiazepine receptor.

BENZODIAZEPINE DEPENDENCE AND THE MANAGEMENT OF WITHDRAWAL

J. Guy EDWARDS, Timothy CANTOPHER and Stefano OLIVIERI,
Department of Psychiatry, Royal South Hants Hospital, Southampton,
SO9 4PE, U.K.

Benzodiazepine (BDZ) dependence has stimulated an enormous amount of medical and legal interest during the last decade, but although much has been learnt about the problem there are more unanswered than answered questions. More time and energy has been spent in identifying the BDZ withdrawal syndrome and describing its features than in its management. Of the treatments that have been used propranolol has produced encouraging results, while most authorities recommend gradual withdrawal. We report a study comparing abrupt withdrawal under propranolol cover (PW group) with a gradual step-like withdrawal over 10 weeks (SW group).

PATIENTS AND PROCEDURE

Thirty-four patients who had taken BDZs for a mean of nine years and were thought to be dependent gave their informed consent for inclusion in the study which was carried out under double-blind conditions. No patient had a concomitant psychiatric or relevant physical illness or was receiving another psychotropic drug. Patients taking BDZs other than diazepam at the time of entry into the trial were changed to equivalent doses of diazepam. At baseline the existing tablets were changed to active diazepam plus propranolol placebo and patients were randomly allocated to one of the two treatment groups. In both groups active treatment was stopped at week 10 and placebo stopped at week 12. Patients were followed up for six months. During the study patients received general support and advice but no specific psychological or other pharmacological treatment.

RESULTS

There were three drop-outs prior to random allocation to the withdrawal groups, leaving 15 patients in the PW group and 16 in the SW group. Eleven of the patients in the latter group were successfully withdrawn compared with only four in the PW group. Twelve out of the 16 patients who failed to withdraw dropped out during the first four weeks of withdrawal. All subjects who completed withdrawal remained drug free at six months follow-up. Withdrawal symptoms in the SW group were mild, while those in the PW group ranged from mild to severe. All of the alleged withdrawal symptoms were similar to those encountered in abnormal emotional states and we did not observe bizarre perceptual disturbances, psychotic phenomena or convulsive seizures.

Temporary but significant worsening on the following scales occurred between week 0 and 2 in the PW group but not in the SW group: Hamilton Rating Scale for Anxiety (2), Hospital Anxiety and Depression Scale (3), visual analogue and global assessment scales.

By week 14 and at six months follow-up both groups had improved on all scales compared with baseline, although this trend reached significance only in the Hamilton anxiety scale and global severity scales in the SW group. The PW group showed larger mean changes in each scale between baseline and week 2 compared with the SW group, although the difference between groups only reached significance in the Hamilton anxiety scale. When data from only those who successfully completed the withdrawal phase was analysed, the differences between the groups disappeared. However, the non-significant trend towards improvement from the start to the end of the trial remained.

No significant changes in alcohol or nicotine consumption occurred in either groups. The plasma diazepam and desmethyldiazepam estimations confirmed that compliance with treatment was good in both groups.

Contrary to expectations, older patients were more often successful in withdrawing from benzodiazepines than young ones. A possible explanation for this is that an older liver metabolises diazepam more slowly than a younger one, thereby producing a more gradual removal of the benzodiazepine and its active metabolites from the body. Those who were more severely anxious at the start of the trial had more difficulty in withdrawing than less anxious patients.

Full details of the study have been reported elsewhere (1).

CONCLUSIONS

Gradual withdrawal of diazepam from patients with chronic benzodiazepine dependence is more successful than abrupt withdrawal under propranolol cover. Younger subjects and those who are more severely anxious have more difficulty in withdrawing than older and less anxious patients, respectively. Most patients can be successfuly withdrawn from their benzodiazepines by gradual withdrawal combined with non-specific counselling, simple support and advice.

REFERENCES

1. Cantopher, T. et al. Chronic benzodiazepine dependence. A comparative study of abrupt withdrawal under propranolol cover versus gradual withdrawal. Brit. J. Psyciat. 156: 406-411, 1990.

2. Hamilton, M. A rating scale for anxiety. Brit. J. Med. Psychol. 32: 50-55, 1959.

3. Zigmond, A. and Snaith, R. The Hospital Anxiety and Depression Scale. Acta Psychiat. Scand. 86: 1-7, 1983.

INTERNATIONAL REGULATION OF BENZODIAZEPINES

Dr Inayat Khan, Chief Medical Officer, Psychotropic and Narcotic Drugs Unit, World Health Organization, Geneva

With the coming into force of the 1971 convention WHO set in motion a critical examination of procedures and methods used by WHO, Commission on Narcotic Drugs (CND) and experts who participated in the evaluations which was resulted in more formalized and explicit process. The process began when WHO Expert Committee on Drug Dependence met and wrote a report that specified laboratory procedures that were acceptable for assessing dependence and CNS alternations (TRS 618, 1978). This group stated that because the reinforcing effect on drug seeking and drug taking behaviour is a property common in all types of psychotropic substances that produces and/or perpetuate the repeated use of drugs in humans, the evaluation of reinforcing properties using drug self-administration methods is essential for predicting dependence. Another important pharmacological property of a drug of abuse is its ability to produce physical dependence. Assessing physical dependence is particularly important to determine whether withdrawal manifestations are life threatening.

In 1980, another expert committee met and deliberated specifically defining the types of data useful for determining public health and social problems, produce by a drug being considered for control as well as possible means for obtaining these types of data. The report covered methods for estimating extent of use, drug related health problems and drug related social problems (TRS 656, 1981).

Beginning in 1984, the WHO new procedures were used by WHO in the review of drugs for scheduling recommendations under the Single and 1971 Conventions. The document entitled "Guidelines for the WHO Review of Dependence-Producing Psychoactive Substance for International Control" (MNH/PAD/86.5, 1986) summarizes the approved changes and their underlying principle. The WHO Executive Board in its eighty-fifth session held in January 1990 have approved some modifications to those guidelines as were proposed to them in the light of the experiences gained by WHO.

During the plenipotentiary conference for the creation of the 1971 Convention on Psychotropic Substances, as early as in January/February 1971, a discussion took place to control four benzodiazepines, which were widely available at that time, under the new convention. These were diazepam, chlordiazepoxide, oxazepam andnitrazepam. These recommendations from WHO was based on the report of the 17th Expert Committee on Drug Dependence (TRS 437). The recommendations were not accepted. The WHO's eight review of psychoactive drugs was convened in response to a resolution 4 (xxx) of the United Nations Commission on Narcotic Drugs in February 1983, which requested WHO to urgently review and assess all benzodiazepines on the market for international control. In February 1984, the UN Commission on Narcotic Drugs decided to place 33 commercially available benzodiazepines under Schedule IV of the 1971 Convention based on the recommendations of WHO as contained in a document MNH/83.28.

In April 1989, the 26th Expert Committee on Drug Dependence met and reviewed the status of 4 benzodiazepines, which were not reviewed earlier. These were brotizolam, etizolam, midazolam and quazepam. The data was reviewed under the following headings:

- i) substance identification
- ii) similarity to already known substances and effects on the central nervous system
- iii) dependence potential
- iv) abuse liability (likelihood of abuse)
- v) therapeutic usefulness

The group recommended control only for midazolam. Their recommendations for such a control was, "On the basis of the available data concerning the pharmacological profile, dependence potential and actual abuse, the Committee rated the abuse liability of midazolam as moderate and the therapeutic usefulness as moderate to high. Some public health and social problems are currently associated with the use of midazolam. As with all benzodiazepine agonists studied to date, it can be inferred from the preclinical studies that midazolam is capable of producing a state of dependence in humans subjects similar to that observed with diazepam.

In addition, the Committee noted that the availability of the substance in an injectable form enhances the likelihood of abuse. The Committee therefore considered that midazolam is likely to be abused so as to constitute a public health and social problem warranting the placing of the substance under international control in Schedule IV of the 1971 Convention.

MOLECULAR GENETICS OF AFFECTIVE DISORDERS

J. MENDLEWICZ[*], D. HIRSCH[*], C. VAN BROECKHOVEN[**]

[*] University Clinics of Brussels, Erasme Hospital - Free University of Brussels - Department of Psychiatry, Route de Lennik 808 - 1070 Brussels - Belgium
[**] Neurogenetics Lab. Dept. of Biochemistry, U.I.A. Universiteitsplein 1, 2610 Antwerpen - Belgium

Recently, linkage studies with classical genetic markers have provided consistant evidence of the presence of a major single gene located on the distal end of the long arm of the X chromosme, in bipolar manic- depression (1,2) but this type of inheritance has not been observed in all families studied (1). In addition, using the DNA recombinant method in molecular genetic studies of manic depression, a close linkage has been demonstrated between manic depression and Factor 9 (Hemophylia B) on the distal end of the long arm of chromosome X in a new set of pedigrees (3). Some families show possible linkage between affective illness and the ST14 probe (close to G6PD and CB suggesting the presence of a major locus for manic-depression between ST 14 and factor IX genes. Conversely, the localisation of a gene situated on the distal part of the short arm of chromosome 11 has also been reported in one family originating from the old Amish community (4), but this chromosomal linkage has not yet been confirmed in other pedigrees (5-7), using the same chromosomal markers in informative families selected in different geographical areas. Furthermore, a recent reevaluation of the old order Amish (8) on a newly extended family showed lod scores to be considerably weakened, indicating that a single locus linked to INS and HRAS1 was unlikely to be the sole causal factor for affective disorder. Thus these new chromosomal linkage findings reveal the existence of several distinct genetic forms of bipolar illness, with at least two potential different chromosomal locations, one on the tip of the long arm of the X chromosome and the other (if confirmed) by other groups on the short arm of chromosome 11. Other pedigrees of bipolars have been reported not to show linkage with the above genetic markers (1). These results provide strong support for the hypothesis of molecular heterogeneity in the genetic etiology of bipolar manic-depressive illness. The application of molecular genetics such as the use of various RFLP and polymerase chain reaction (PCR) for gene amplification will provide new powerfull tools for data banking of genetic material.

Chromosomal rearrangements are also to be studied in psychiatric disorders, because these observations could help targeting new chromosomal probes in specific chromosomal regions of interest.

REFERENCES

1. J. Mendlewicz. Population and family studies in depression and mania. British Journal of Psychiatry, 153 (suppl. 3) 16-25, 1988.
2. J. Mendlewicz. X-linked transmission of affective illness : current status and new evidence. Biological Psychiatry. Eds. C. Shagass, R. Josiassen, W. Bridger, K. Weiss, D. Stoff, G. Simpson, Elsevier, vol. 7, 46-48, 1986.
3. J. Mendlewicz, P. Simon, F. Charon, H. Brocas, S. Legros, G. Vassart. A polymorphic DNA marker on X chromosome and manic-depression. The Lancet, 1230-1232, 1987.
4. J.A. Egeland, D.S. Gerhard, D.L. Pauls, J.S. Sussex, K.K. Kidd, C.R. Allen, A.M. Hostetter, D.E. Housman. Bipolar affective disorders linked to DNA markers on chromosome 11. Nature, 325, 783-787, 1987.
5. S.D. Detera-Wadleigh, W.H. Berretini, L.R. Goldin, D. Boorman S.B. Anderson, E.S. Gershon. Close linkage of C-Harvey-ras-1 and the insulin gene to affective disorder is ruled out in three North American pedigrees. Nature, 325, 806-808, 1987.
6. S. Hodgkinson, R. Sherrington, H. Gurling, R. Marchbanks, S. Reeders, J. Mallet, M. McInnes, H. Petursson, J. Brynjolfson. Molecular genetic evidence of heterogeneity in manic-depression. Nature, 325, 805-806, 1987.
7. G. Michael, P. McKeon, P. Humphries. Linkage analysis of manic-depression in an Irish family using H-ras 1 and INS DNA markers. Journal of Medical Genetics, 25, 634-637, 1988.
8. J.R. Kelsoe, E.I. Gings, J.A. Egeland, D.S. Gerhard, A.M. Goldstein, S.J. Bale, D.L. Pauls, R.T. Long, K.K. Kidd, G. Conte, D.E. Housman, S.M. Paul. Re-evaluation of the linkage relationship between chromosome 11 p loci and the gene for bipolar affective disorder in the old order Amish. Nature, vol 342, 238-243, 1989.

LINKAGE STUDIES ON CHROMOSOME 11q IN SCHIZOPHRENIA

D.H.R. BLACKWOOD, W.J. MUIR, D.M. ST CLAIR, A.HUBBARD, D.BAILLIE, M. WALKER.
Department of Psychiatry, University of Edinburgh, Royal Edinburgh Hospital and MRC Human Genetics Unit, Western General Hospital, Edinburgh, Scotland.

Attempts to find linkage between DNA polymorphisms and schizophrenia in families are hampered by uncertainties about the mode of inheritance, the clinical definition of the phenotype and the probable heterogeneity of the disease. The neuropathological basis of schizophrenia is completely unknown so there are no clear cut candidate regions which could be the starting point for linkage studies. Cytogenetic studies however may provide important clues if mental illness can be shown to segregate with a particular chromosomal rearrangement. We have previously described a balanced translocation t(1,11) (q43,q21) associated with schizophrenia and other psychiatric illnesses over four generations in a large extended Scottish pedigree (1). In this family, psychiatric illness was diagnosed in 16 out of the 34 subjects who carried the translocation. Diagnoses were schizophrenia (3), schizoaffective disorder (2), major depressive disorder (6), generalized anxiety (2) and adolescent conduct and emotional disorder (3). Among the 43 family members with a normal karyotype, only five received a psychiatric diagnosis: generalized anxiety (1), minor depression (1), alcoholism (3). The likelihood that the chromosome 1:11 translocation was linked to mental illness in this family was analysed using the Linkage programmes. A maximum LOD score of 3.3 was obtained when the phenotype was defined to include cases of schizophrenia, schizoaffective disorder and major depressive disorder, and a LOD score of 4.3 was obtained when the phenotype was defined to include the cases of severe adolescent mood and conduct disorder. However, when the phenotype was very broadly defined to include minor depression, anxiety and alcoholism, the LOD score was diminished to less than 2.

This single family provided some evidence to support the view that a gene implicated in the pathogenesis of schizophrenia and other psychiatric illnesses is located in the region of the translocation breakpoints on chromosome 11 or chromosome 1. Mapped to this region on the long arm of chromosome 11 are several genes of possible relevance to schizophrenia, including the Dopamine D2 receptor. Two other groups have also reported families in which a translocation involving the long arm of chromosome 11 is found together with mental illness (2), Holland et al, Personal communication). Therefore linkage studies using seven markers (including one for D2 receptor) mapped to the region of the translocation on 11q were carried out in 17 multiply affected schizophrenic pedigrees. Data were analyzed with the LINKAGE programmes using both broad and narrow definitions of the schizophrenia phenotype. Even when schizophrenia was strictly defined (only cases with schizophrenia, schizoaffective illness and unspecified functional psychosis) the results of two point analysis did not support linkage of illness with these chromosome 11 polymorphisms. Heterogeneity of LOD scores from our 17 families could not be detected using the HOMOG programmes. However the size of families studied make it unlikely that heterogeneity if it existed would be detected in a sample of this size.

We conclude that in these schizophrenic families there is no linkage between illness and polymorphisms mapped to the region of the chromosome 11 breakpoint. It is possible that the difference in linkage findings between the large karyotypically abnormal family and the other 17 schizophrenic pedigrees is due to genetic heterogeneity in schizophrenia, and this was not detectable in our group of medium sized families. Alternatively a connection between the chromosome translocation and schizophrenia may be an indirect one and psychiatric illness could be a result of a number of abnormal karyotypes.

1. St Clair, et al 1990 Lancet (In Press).
2. Smith et al 1989 A.M.J. Human Genet. 45: A220.

MOLECULAR GENETICS OF FAMILIAL ALZHEIMER's DISEASE

C. VAN BROECKHOVEN[*], H. BACKHOVENS[*,**], G. VAN CAMP[*], P. STINISSEN[*], W. VAN HUL[*], A. LOFGREN[*], M. CRUTS[*], A. WEHNERT[*,**], G. DE WINTER[*,**], A. VANDENBERGHE[*], M. BRUYLAND[***], J. GHEUENS[****] and J-J. MARTIN[****].
Department of Biochemistry[*] and Department of Medicine[****], University of Antwerp (UIA), Born-Bunge Foundation, Antwerpen; Innogenetics[**], Gent; Department of Medicine[***], University of Brussels (VUB), Brussel, Belgium.

The involvement of genetic factors in the etiology of Alzheimer's disease (AD), an age-related disorder of the central nervous system, has been recognized for several years. At present several AD families are known in which the disease is inherited as an autosomal dominant trait. Genetic linkage analysis indicated the existence in some AD families of a gene predisposing to the disease located in the pericentromeric region of chromosome 21 (1,4,7). The implication of chromosome 21 in AD had previously been suggested by the consistent finding of similar pathological hallmarks in the brains of aged Down Syndrome (trisomy 21) patients. However, in several other AD families the chromosome 21 linkage could not be confirmed suggesting that AD is genetically and/or etiologically heterogeneous (2,3).

SUBJECT AND METHOD

We analyzed two extended Belgian pedigrees AD/A and AD/B, with early onset, autosomal dominant AD, for linkage with the chromosome 21q21 DNA markers D21S1/S11, D21S16 and D21S13. Both families have been used previously in the exclusion analysis of the gene coding for the amyloid precursor protein (APP), the major component of the senile plaques, located in band 21q21 near the obligate Down Syndrome phenotype region (6). Since then the clinical and pathological characteristics of the patients in families AD/A and AD/B were re-evaluated. Furthermore additional family members have been sampled, new AD patients identified and paternity and family relationships analyzed using hypervariable DNA markers. Current information on both AD pedigrees is summarized in table 1.

RESULTS AND DISCUSSION

Initial results suggested linkage of the families AD/A and AD/B to the marker locus D21S13 located close to the centromere (7). However, linkage to chromosome 21 could not

TABLE 1: THE BELGIAN AD PEDIGREES

	AD/A	AD/B
NUMBER OF GENERATIONS	6	5
NUMBER OF AD PATIENTS	39	24
NUMBER OF PATHOLOGICAL CONFIRMED AD CASES	11	6
MEAN AGE AT ONSET (years ± SD)	35.1 ± 4.8	34.7 ± 3.0
MEAN AGE AT DEATH (years ± SD)	41.1 ± 4.2	42.2 ± 2.2

be proved due to lack of sufficient informative meioses in the AD pedigrees, a common problem inherent to the adult onset and short duration of the disease. Three approaches are currently followed in our lab to overcome this problem. First, we searched for additional polymorphisms for the presently linked DNA markers. New polymorphisms were detected for D21S13 and D21S16 (5,8,10). Second, we selected new DNA markers from a chromosome 21 phage library and localized them in relation to the existing marker loci (9,11). Third, we extracted DNA of pathological specimens of deceased AD patients belonging to the elder generations of both pedigrees. The DNA is severely degraded but the genetic information can be reconstructed after amplification of the sequence of interest with the Polymerase Chain Reaction (PCR) technique.

REFERENCES

1. Goate, A. et al. (1989): The Lancet, i:352-355.
2. Pericak-Vance, M. et al. (1988): Exp. Neurol., 102:271-279.
3. Schellenberg, G. et al. (1988): Science, 241:1507-1510.
4. St. George-Hyslop, P. et al. (1987): Science, 235:885-890.
5. Stinissen, P., Vandenberghe, A., Van Broeckhoven, C. (1990): Nucl. Acids. Res., in press.
6. Van Broeckhoven, C. et al. (1987): Nature, 329:153-155.
7. Van Broeckhoven, C. et al. (1988): In Genetics and Alzheimer's disease, P.M. Sinet, Y. Lamour, Y. Christen eds., pp. 124-129. Springer-Verlag.
8. Van Broeckhoven, C. et al. (1989): Cytogenet. Cell Genet., 51:1096.
9. Van Camp, G. et al. (1989): Hum. Genet., 83: 58-60.
10. Van Camp, G. et al. (1990): Hum. Genet., in press.
11. Van Camp, G. et al. (1990): Somatic. Cell Molec. Genet., in press.

MOLECULAR GENETIC RESEARCH IN NEURODEGENERATIVE DISEASE

Katsuhiko MIKOSHIBA
Institute for Protein Research, Osaka University, 3-2 Yamadaoka,
Suita, Osaka 565, Japan

Recently many neurodegenerative mutant animals have been reported which have abnormality in the development of the nervous system. The analysis of these mutants comparing with the control animals offers great information on the cellular and molecular mechanism of the development of the nervous system. I present the data on myelin deficient and cerebellar mutants.

MYELIN DEFICIENT MUTANTS

Myelin is mainly composed of two major proteins, myelin basic protein (MBP) and proteolipid protein (PLP). MBP and PLP account for 30 and 50 % of the total myelin protein respectively. Shiverer and mld mutant have abnormality in the MBP gene resulting in the absence or very poor production of MBP. MBP gene contains 7 exons. Shiverer mutant is a deletion mutant of MBP gene where large portion including exon 3 to 7 are deleted. The mutant mld is an allelic mutant to shiverer, and, therefore, is symboled as shi^{mld}. It is not a deletion mutant contrary to shiverer. The MBP gene in mld is duplicated and the upstream gene has large inversion (from exon 3 to 7) causing antisense RNA production (1,2). Down stream gene is an intact gene, but its expression is suppressed presumably by the antisense RNA which would be synthesized from the inverted MBP gene in upstream region, by forming RNA-RNA duplex with the RNA formed from the normal down stream gene. We have succeeded to detect RNA-RNA duplex only in mld mutant brain.

Jimpy mutant has abnormality in the PLP gene. Only one base is changed to another base causing the splicing abnormality in the PLP gene expression, resulting in abnormal expression of PLP (3,4). In these myelin deficient mutants, due to the genetic abnormalities, the protein synthesis is greatly reduced causing the abnormal myelin formation.

Cerebellar mutants: Cerebellar cortex is composed of only five types of neurons and the neural network is well studied. There are only two inputs and single output. Besides, we can easily identify each neuron from morphological criteria. Cerebellum is an important center for controlling motor movement. Advantage of analysing the cerebellum is that we have many cerebellar mutants. Nervous, pcd are the mutants which lack Purkinje cell neuron. Weaver is characterized by the absence of granule cells. Staggerer is a mutant which have abnormality in the morphogenesis of Purkinje cell. The dendritic arborization of the Purkinje cell in the staggerer is so poor and the spines which should be formed on the dendrites for the formation of synaptic contact with the outer inputs are absent. The mutant shows also absence of calcium spikes in the Purkinje cells. Staggerer mutant cerebellum lacks high molecular weight protein, named P_{400} (5). The protein is also greatly decreased in the Purkinje cell deficient mutants. Biochemical and molecular genetic studies have revealed that P_{400} protein is an inositol trisphosphate (InsP3) receptor which is essential to calcium moblization from the calcium store site in the cell after receiving signals from outside the cell (9). P_{400} protein was localized in the dendrites as well as soma of the Purkinje cell(6,7). We succeeded to clone and sequence the cDNA of P_{400}. The length of cDNA was about 10 kbp having two polyA additional signals (8). Transfection of the cDNA to L-cell showed the expression of enhanced InsP3 binding activity and also the calcium release activity in the presence of InsP3. It is presumed that calcium metabolism including InsP3 receptor is neccessary for the normal development of the Purkinje cells in the cerebellum.

Analysis of neuropathological mutant animals comparing with that of the control animals at cellular and molecular level offers a great infomation on the development, growth and differentiation of the nervous system which are not usually obtained from the analysis of the normal animals.

REFERENCES

1. Okano et al. Gene organization and transcription of duplicated MBP genes of myelin deficient (shi^{mld}) mutant mouse. EMBO J. 7: 77-83, 1988
2. Okano, H. et al. Recombination within the upstream gene of duplicated myelin basic protein genes of myelin deficient shi^{mld} mouse results in the production of antisense RNA. EMBO J. 7: 3407-3412, 1988
3. Moriguchi, A. et al. The fifth exon of the myelin proteolipid protein-coding gene is not utilized in the brain of jimpy mutant mice. Gene 55: 333-337, 1987
4. Ikenaka, K. et al. Myelin proteolipid protein gene structure and its regulation of expression in normal and jimpy mutant mice. J. Mol. Biol. 199, 587-596, 1988
5. Mikoshaiba, K. et al. Biochemical and immunological studies on the P_{400} proatein, a protein characteristic of the Purkinje cell from mouse and rat cerebellum. Dev. Neurosci. 2: 254-275
6. Maeda, N. et al. Purification and characterization of P_{400} protein, a glycoprotein characteristic of Purkinje cell, from mouse cerebellum. J. Neurochem. 51, 1724-1730, 1988
7. Maeda, N. et al. Developmental expression and intracellular location of P_{400} protein characteristic of Purkinje cells in the mouse cerebellum. Dev. Biol. 133: 67-76, 1989
8. Furuichi, T. et al. Primary structure and functional expression of the inositol 1,4,5-trisphosphate-binding protein P_{400}. Nature 342: 32-38, 1989
9. Maeda, N. et al. A cerebellar Purkinje cell marker P_{400} protein is an inositol 1,4,5-trisphospate (InsP3) receptor protein. Purification and characterization of InsP3 receptor complex. EMBO J. 9: 61-67, 1990

NEUROPATHOLOGICAL AND BEHAVIORAL CHANGES IN ALZHEIMER'S DISEASE

PETER J. WHITEHOUSE, M.D., Ph.D.
Associate Professor of Neurology and Chief, Division of Behavioral Neurology, Case Western Reserve University and Director, Alzheimer Center, University Hospitals of Cleveland, Cleveland, Ohio

Alzheimer's Disease (AD) is characterized clinically by both cognitive and behavioral abnormalities. Considerable attention has been paid to characterizing the memory, language, perceptual, and praxis problems that occur in this disorder. Only recently has attention been paid to the prominent behavioral abnormalities which are a major source of caregiver stress. Studies of both lay and professional caregivers have demonstrated that disruptive behaviors are more predictive of stress on the health care system than the primary cognitive abnormalities.

In our recent studies of the behavioral abnormalities in AD, we have examined both our clinical charts retrospectively as well as prospectively evaluated patients using two new instruments specifically designed to assess psychiatric symptoms in dementia. We have employed the Behav-AD to survey of psychiatric symptoms and the Cornell Scale for Depression in Dementia to assess specific affective symptoms. A large number of AD subjects suffer from hallucinations, delusions, and affective disorders. In addition, other behaviors, such as agitation and wandering, which are harder to assign to formal psychiatric diagnostic categories, are also common. In our clinical management programs, we are investigating both behavioral and biological approaches to treating these behavioral disturbances. New medications developed for the treatment of primary psychiatric illnesses may be helpful in better managing these psychiatric conditions in dementia.

We have learned a considerable amount about the neuropathological basis of cognitive symptoms in AD over the last several years. Pathology in hippocampus, amygdala, cortex, as well as subcortical regions such as the cholinergic basal forebrain undoubtedly play a role in underlying memory and other cognitive disturbances. The pathology in the cholinergic basal forebrain is particularly interesting because of their short- and long-term pharmacological treatment implications. Considerable investment is being made to the development of both cholinesterases and muscarinic agonists to substitute for the missing cholinergic cells. Our long-term treatment strategy for this condition will focus on the mechanisms of cell death and neuroplasticity. We are currently focusing on nerve growth factor, fibroblast growth factor and other related trophic factors that may preserve the viability of cholinergic basal forebrain neurons and other affected populations.

Our neuropathological investigations are also exploring the biological basis of the behavioral disturbances in AD. Biological psychiatrists have for some time been hypothesizing that abnormalities in brain bioamines underlie depression and psychosis. Preliminary evidence has been provided by groups at Hopkins and Pittsburgh that alterations in noradrenergic locus coeruleus and serotonergic raphe nucleii may lead to some predisposition for depression in AD. Our own research programs are designed to understand more of the mechanisms and consequences of the loss of cells in these brainstem bioaminergic nucleii. In the future, we hope that understanding the mechanisms of cell death in these structures may lead to developing more effective therapies that will not only palliate the symptoms of the disease--both cognitive and behavioral--but also to reverse the progression of the disease.

NGF AND ALZHEIMER'S DISEASE. PERSPECTIVES FROM BASIC RESEARCH

G. VANTINI, M. FUSCO, L. CAVICCHIOLI, G. TOFFANO and A. LEON
Fidia Research Laboratories, Abano Terme, Italy

Recent investigations on newborn and adult rats have shown that forebrain cholinergic neurons respond to exogenous NGF with a selective and prominent increase of choline acetyltransferase (ChAT) activity, the enzyme involved in the synthesis of acetylcholine. In addition, measurable levels of NGF, mRNA coding for NGF, NGF receptors and mRNA coding for NGF receptors are present in rat brain and their regional distribution suggests that NGF may regulate the functions of the above-mentioned cholinergic neurons (for a review see 4,7).

Studies conducted in our laboratory aiming to further elucidate the physiological role of NGF in the CNS have indicated that:

1. Anti-NGF antibodies administered intracerebroventricularly (i.c.v.) to either neonatal or adult rats are capable of decreasing ChAT activity in brain regions shown to be sensitive to endogenous NGF. This observation directly supports the notion that endogenous NGF plays a physiological role in CNS (8).

2. Continuous i.c.v. infusion of murine NGF (mNGF) in adult rat brain produces a significant increase of ChAT activity in forebrain cholinergic neurons with or without a prior lesion. These results suggest that a prior lesion is not an essential prerequisite for responsiveness to exogenous NGF in adult brain (2). In addition, the effect elicited by NGF is dose-dependent and lasts several weeks upon discontinuation of NGF administration.

3. I.c.v. administration of mNGF amplifies the expression of NGF receptor mRNA and corresponding protein levels in basal forebrain of newborn, adult (1) and aged (24-month-old) rats. These findings are suggestive of a self-cooperativity between NGF and its CNS target structures. Self-cooperativity may play an important role in regulating forebrain cholinergic function and suggests that deficits in NGF function may also occur as a consequence of alterations in the autoregulation of the synthesis of NGF receptors.

4. Recombinant human NGF (rhNGF) is able to affect in vivo forebrain cholinergic neurons. Like mNGF, rhNGF

was effective in increasing ChAT activity in both neonatal and adult rats.

Since morphofunctional alterations of forebrain cholinergic neurons appear to be one of the most consistent features of Alzheimer's disease, NGF deficits have been implicated and a potential therapeutical utility of NGF has been proposed in this disease (3,5,6). All together, our results are consistent with the rationale for the use of NGF or agents capable of facilitating or mimicking its action in the treatment of Alzheimer's disease and point to a need for recombinant DNA technology to identify a reliable source of "well-characterized" human NGF in sufficient quantity for continuing comprehensive research programs.

REFERENCES

1. Cavicchioli, L. et al., (1989): Eur. J. Neurosci., 1: 258-262.
2. Fusco, M. et al., (1989): Neuroscience, 33(1):47-52.
3. Hefti, F. and Weiner, W. (1989): Ann. Neurol., 20:275-281, 1989.
4. Hefti, F., Hartikka J. and Knusel, B. (1989): Neurobiol. Aging, 10:515-533.
5. Marx, J. (1990): Science, 247:408-410.
6. Phelps, C.H. et al., (1989): Science, 243:11.
7. Thoenen, H., Bandtlow, C. and Heumann, R. (1987): Rev. Physiol. Biochem. Pharmacol., 109:145-178.
8. Vantini, G. et al., (1989): Neuron, 3:267-273.

TETRAHYDROAMINOACRIDINE IN ALZHEIMER'S DISEASE

LEON J. THAL, M.D.
Department of Neurology, San Diego VA Medical Center and Department of Neurosciences, University of California at San Diego, San Diego, CA, U.S.A.

Tetrahydroaminoacridine (THA) is an intermediate length cholinesterase inhibitor with good oral absorption and distribution. In animal studies, THA has been reported to improve performance in: adult mice in a t-maze active avoidance task, middle aged monkeys in a color discrimination task, memory impaired aged monkeys in automated tests of recent memory, NBM-lesioned rats in acquisition of ultrasound passive avoidance, hippocampally deficient mice in a water maze, scopolamine-impaired passive avoidance learning in mice, and rats with scopolamine-induced amnesia in a t-maze.

Several human clinical trials with THA in Alzheimer's disease (AD) have now been completed. A small pilot intravenous THA study was reported to result in improvement in severely advanced AD patients. An oral study using low dose (30 mg/day) plus lecithin was reported to improve verbal memory only when THA was combined with lecithin (4). The report of dramatic improvement in 16 out of 17 patients (6) prompted renewed interest in this compound. A small double-blind (2) and three larger double-blind crossover studies, using oral doses of 100-125 mg of THA plus lecithin have recently been reported (1,3,5). All of these studies failed to demonstrate cognitive improvement. Carry-over effect between periods was detected in one study (3).

A large multicenter trial to test the efficacy of THA in AD was initiated in the United States in 1987. This study was designed to be carried out in several phases. In phase I, a dose-titration phase, subjects are exposed to a series of THA doses in order to determine if a best dose response occurs. Patients failing to demonstrate a best dose response are dropped from the study. Individuals demonstrating a best dose response are randomized to treatment with drug at their best dose or to placebo. As of March 16, 1990, 567 patients have entered this study; 184 have entered the double-blind phase, and 167 have completed the double-blind phase.
Approximately 40% of patients exposed to the drug show a best dose response during the titration phase. Approximately 35% exposed to drug demonstrated elevated transaminase levels. After 100 patients completed the study, an interim analysis was carried out which indicated that continuation of the study was warranted. Whether THA will prove to be useful, effective, and safe in the treatment of AD remains to be demonstrated.

REFERENCES

1. Chatellier G, Lacomblez L (1990): Tacrine (tetrahydroaminoacridine; THA) and lecithin in senile dementia of the Alzheimer type: a multicentre trial. Br. Med. J. 300:495-499.
2. Fitten LJ, Perryman KM, Gross P, Steinberg A (1988): Chronic oral THA

administration in mice, monkeys and man. In: Current Research in Alzheimer Therapy. Giacobini E and Becker R (Eds) pp 211-216. Taylor & Francis, New York, and personal communication.

3. Gauthier S, Bouchard R, Lamontagne A, Bailey P, Bergman H, Ratner J, Tesfaye Y, Saint-Martin M, Bacher Y, Carrier L, Charbonneau R, Clarfield AM, Collier B, Dastoor D, Gauthier L, Germain M, Kissel C, Krieger M, Kushnir S, Masson H, Morin J, Nair V, Neirinck L, Suissa S (1990): Tetrahydroaminoacridine - lecithin combination treatment in intermediate stage Alzheimer's disease: results of a Canadian double-blind cross-over multicentre study. N. Eng. J. Med., in press.

4. Kaye WH, Stiaram N, Weingartner H, Ebert MH, Smallberg S, Gillin JC (1982): Modest facilitation of memory in dementia with combined lecithin and anticholinesterase treatment. Biol. Psychiatry 17:275-280.

5. Molloy DW (1990): Effect of tetrahydroaminoacridine on cognition, function, and behavior in Alzheimer disease. Lancet, in press.

6. Summers WK, Majowski LV, Marsh GM, Tachiki K, Kling A (1986): Oral tetrahydroaminoacridine in long term treatment of senile dementia, Alzheimer type. N. Engl. J. Med. 315:1241-1245.

TABLE

TETRAHYDROAMINOACRIDINE IN ALZHEIMER'S DISEASE

Study	Daily dose (mg)	Type of Study	Duration	Subj.	Results
Kaye (1982)	30 + lecithin	double-blind	3 doses	10	+
Summers (1986)	to 200 + lecithin	double-blind	3 weeks	17	+
Fitten (1988)	to 250	double-blind	7 days	10	-
Chatellier (1990)	to 125 + lecithin	double-blind	4 weeks	60	-
Gauthier (1990)	to 100 + lecithin	double-blind	8 weeks	39	-
Molloy (1990)	100 + lecithin	double-blind	3 weeks	22	-

All of the above studies are cross-over designs.

PRECLINICAL PHARMACOLOGY OF PHOSPHATIDYLSERINE

G. PEPEU, M.G. VANNUCCHI AND F. CASAMENTI
Department of Pharmacology, University of Florence, Italy.

Phosphatidylserine (Ptdser) is the most effective phospholipid for protein kinase C activation (6). According to Bruni (2) it plays a role in cell communication and enhances evoked histamine release from mastcells. Ptdser (75-150 mg/kg i.p.) in adult rats, increases ACh release from the cerebral cortex in adult rats in vivo (3), and antagonizes the amnesic effects of scopolamine (9). In aging rats, Ptdser (25-50 mg/Kg i.p.) significantly ameliorates the age-associated deficit in a passive avoidance conditioned response (4).

The age-related cognitive dysfunctions which occur in animals and man have been attributed to an impairment of brain cholinergic mechanisms (1). An impairment of brain cholinergic mechanisms has been repeatedly described in aging rodents. A 50% decrease in the electrically stimulated acetylcholine (ACh) release was observed in cortical slices prepared from old rats in comparison with young rats (7), and a significant decline in ACh release from the cerebral cortex, hippocampus and caudate was detected in freely moving old rats by intracerebral microdialysis technique (12). The decrease in ACh release from electrically stimulated cortical slices can be prevented by pretreating the aging rats with Ptdser (8). It was demonstrated that a 7 days pretreatment with 15 mg/kg i.p. of Ptdser is sufficient to restore ACh release in aging rats, and that the effect lasts for 5 days after interruption of the treatment (10). By investigating the mechanism of Ptdser action it was shown that, in the aging rats, Ptdser is able to increase the avaibility of endogenous Ch for de novo ACh synthesis and release (11).

In this work we investigated the effects of Ptdser on ACh release from the cerebral cortex in freely moving unanaesthetized aging rats by the microdialysis technique.

MATERIALS AND METHODS

Four, 19 and 25 month-old male Wistar Charles River rats were used. Transverse dialysis tubes were implanted according to the procedure of Wu et al. (12). The tubes were perfused with Ringer's solution containing physostigmine 7 um at the constant rate of 2.0 ul/min.

Samples were collected every 20 min and ACh and Ch content of the dialysates was quantified using a HPLC method (11). Purified Ptdser from bovine brain was administered by i.p injection, as a sonicated suspension in 0.05 M Tris buffer, or orally in drinking water.

RESULTS AND DISCUSSION

ACh and Ch release from the cerebral cortex in 4 month-old rats was 247±16 fmol/min and 7.6±0.5 pmol/min (n=15), respectively.
In 19 month-old rats it was 35±4 and 25±3% (n=8, P<0.01) lower, respectively, than in 4 month-old rats. However, in 19 month-old rats treated for 8 days with Ptdser 15 mg/kg i.p. ACh and Ch releases were not statistically different from those in young rats (n=8). In 25 month-old rats ACh and Ch release were 66 and 33% (n=7, P<0.01) lower, respectively, than in 4 month-old rats. In 25 month-old rats treated orally with 50 mg/kg of Ptdser for 9 months a 39% decrease in ACh release only was found, in comparison with the young rats, while Ch decrease was not modified. Oral administration of Ptdser for 15 and 30 days was ineffective.
Our results demonstrate that the age-associated impairment of the cholinergic system in the rat can be corrected by i.p. and oral Ptdser administration. However, the oral route requires a much longer treatment than the parenteral route, raising the question of Ptdser fate in the body. Recovery of cholinergic deficit in aging rats has been also obtained (5) by intracerebral long-term infusion of NGF.

REFERENCES

1) Bartus et al. (1982): Science 217:408-417.
2) Bruni A. (1988): Pharmacol. Res. Comm. 20: 529-544.
3) Casamenti,F. et al., (1979): J. Neurochem., 32:529-533.
4) Corwin,J. et al.,(1985): Neurobiol. Aging 6:11-15.
5) Fisher,W. et al. (1987): Nature 329:65-68.
6) Hirisawa,K. and Nishizuka,Y. (1985): Ann. Rev. Pharmacol. Toxicol. 25: 147-170.
7) Pedata,F. et al. (1983): Neurobiol. Aging 4:31-35.
8) Pedata,F. et al. (1985): Neurobiol. Aging 6:337-339.
9) Pepeu,G., Gori,G. and Bartolini,L. (1980): In Phospholipids in the nervous system, N.G. Bazan, L.A. Horrocks, and G. Toffano, eds., pp.271-274. Raven Press, New York.
10) Vannucchi,M.G. et al. (1987): Neurobiol. Aging 8:403-407.
11) Vannucchi,M.G. et al. (1990): J. Neurochem. (in press).
12) Wu,C.F. et al. (1988): Neurobiol. Aging 9:357-361.

CLINICAL TRIALS WITH PHOSPHATIDYLSERINE (PS)

Amaducci L., Bracco L., and Lippi A.
Department of Neurology, University of Florence, Italy.

The evaluation of the real activity of a drug requires numerous and extensive investigations. Great care should be payed to check blindness of investigators and patients, definition of objectives and characteristics of the studied population, methods of data collection and analysis, identification of specific endpoints and outcomes. Clinical trials on dementia present some further difficulties. The possibility of obtaining valid results from clinical trials on dementia depends upon two principal factors: the correct diagnosis of the disease underlying the dementia syndrome; and the detection of specific cognitive and behavioral disturbances using neuropsychological measures minimally influenced by age, sex and educational level, inter-rater variability and repeated administrations. Finally, an important aspect of clinical trials on dementia, mainly Alzheimer's Disease (AD), is the identification of specific outcomes of the treatment. Infact, the course of the disease is variable and the real meaning of cognitive and behavioural disturbances in patients' daily living activities is not completely clarified. The evaluation of drug effects on these parameters is quite complicated. According to these considerations, we present a short review of the most significant double blind, randomized, controlled clinical trials on treatment with PS. Delwaide et al. (2) carried out a clinical trial on 42 patients affected by mild-moderate dementia. PS 300mg/d or placebo were administered for 6 weeks. Patients were evaluated basally, after 1, 6 and 9 weeks using two behavioural scales (Crichton and Peri Scale) and one psychometric test (Circle Crossing Test). After 6 weeks of treatment, the patients treated with PS showed an improvement of several Peri Scale items in comparison to the placebo group. After 3 weeks of wash-out the effect was significantly reduced. In a study conducted on 87 patients suffering from "organic dementia" (3) the administration of PS 300mg/d for two months induced some improvements in long term memory, as evaluated by the Five Words Test, and in some items of the Geriatric Rating Scale that explores inhibition, self-sufficiency overall decline, sleep disturbances, socialization and maladaptive behaviour. This effect was present even after one month of wash-out. The trial carried out by Villardita et al. (4) is characterized by: a great number of patients (313) suggering from mild mental impairment and selected according to several exclusion criteria even if no definite clinical diagnosis was made; an extensive neuropsychological examination investigating attention, memory, language, constructive and categorical abilities. Patients taking PS experienced improvement of memory, attention and verbal fluency after 45 and 90 days of treatment. The effect was still present after one month of wash-out. On the other hand, the placebo group showed a progressive impairment of all the explored cognitive functions. Amaducci and the SMID Group carried out a trial on 142 patients suffering from clinically diagnosed AD (1). The subjects were selected according to rigorous inclusion and exclusion criteria and the clinical diagnosis of probable AD was based on a specific branching decision procedure. This study was designed as a multicentric, parallel, randomized, double-blind clinical trial. These patients were evaluated basally, after 3 months of treatment with PS 200mg/d or placebo and after 3 subsequent months of wash-out. The assessment was carried out by means of an extensive neuropsychological battery evaluating the daily-living activity, orientation, information, concentration, short and long term memory, language and visuospatial ability. After 3 months of treatment no significant difference between treated and placebo group was found. However, in the patient subgroup with severe impairment, three out of twenty neuropsychological tests were performed better by the patients on PS that those on placebo. The same differences in favour of the treated group were observed 3 months after ending of treatment. Daily living performance as evaluated by the Blessed Dementia Scale showed a moderate, but statistically significant improvement in the treated group. The same trend was noticed using the Blessed, Roth Information-Memory-Concentration test. According to the Set Test, a significant improvement in verbal fluency was observed in the treated patients. As a whole, the data obtained in these studies indicate a moderate, although statistically significant improvement in some out of numerous explored neuropsychological functions. These effects appear to persist and sometimes to increase after a period of wash-out and are more evident in the seriously impaired subgroup of AD patients.

REFERENCES

1. Amaducci, L., and the Smid Group (1988): Psychofarm Bull, 24:130-134.

2. Delwaide, P.J., et al. (1986): Acta Neurol Scand, 73:136-140.

3. Palmieri, G., et al. (1987): Clin Trials J 24:73-83.

4. Villardita, C., et al. (1987):. Satellite Symposyum of the ISN-ASN Joint Meeting "Phospholipids in the nervous system: biochemical and molecular pathology", Puerto La cruz (Venuezuela), June 6-9, 1987.

WHAT'S TREATABLE IN DEMENTIA?
THE TREATMENT OF DEPRESSION IN DEMENTIA

R.J. ANCILL
Division of Geriatric Psychiatry, Department of Psychiatry, University of British Columbia, Canada.

Depression is a common problem in the elderly especially those with dementia. It is unclear what the exact prevalence of depression in demented patients is, and it is even unclear in elderly populations with estimates varying from 3.7% when strict DSM-III criteria are used to 34.5% when all types of presenting syndromes are included. It appears that only a small proportion of the elderly who are depressed, whether they are demented or not, appear to meet the criteria for Major Depression as found in DSM-III or DSM-IIIR, but this does not necessarily mean that only this small number are depressed. There are many studies that have suggested that around 10% of the elderly have a range of symptoms that would be diagnosed as depression although again this is somewhat difficult to determine in patients who also have cognitive impairment.

The most important feature of depression in the elderly has been the concurrent presentation of dementia and depression. Although much has been published on depressive pseudodementia since it was first described in 1961 by Kiloh (3), much attention has been paid to discriminating between depression and dementia rather than the recognition of the two syndromes occurring together. Reifler described the concept of a cognitive-affective disorder which recognises the co-presentation of a mood disorder and cognitive impairment in the same patient (4). Reifler further classifies these disorders into two types: Type 1, which would be loosely equivalent to depressive pseudodementia where the cognitive impairment improves when the depression resolves, and Type 2 where although the depressive symptoms may resolve there is little improvement in overall cognitive function.

As biological factors appear to be more relevant in the aetiology of depression in the elderly, particularly those who have a demented disorder, it can be assumed that biological interventions should be successful. ECT is an effective and well tolerated treatment for severe depression in the elderly including those with dementia, but pharmacotherapy still remains the mainstay of treatment, with tricyclic antidepressants still forming the most common drugs prescribed for depression in the impaired elderly. However the elderly are especially prone to drug toxicity and unpredictable effects due to changes in kinetics, physiology, changes in compliance, multiple drug interactions with multiple pathologies, as well as poor prescribing practice and a failure to recognise side effects when they occur. The tertiary amine tricyclics, such as amitriptyline, imipramine, doxepin, trimipramine and clomipramine are still widely prescribed for the elderly even though these compounds are poorly tolerated in this age group. They are significantly anticholinergic and cause postural hypotension. They are also cardiotoxic. There are data to suggest that tertiary amine tricyclics are not well absorbed in the elderly especially when compared to the less anticholinergic secondary amines such as desipramine (2). In one study in the elderly (mean age 74), patients were randomly assigned to receive doxepin (n=18), trimipramine (n=8), desipramine (n=19) or trazodone (n=12), and steady-state plasma drug levels were determined. For doxepin and trimipramine, there was no significant relationship between the oral dose of the tricyclic and the plasma level obtained (r=+0.20 and r=-0.15 respectively). There was a significant correlation for desipramine (r=+0.60, p<0.01) and trazodone (r=0.91, p<0.001). Thus it seems that the more anticholinergic the antidepressant, the lower or more variable the plasma levels obtained, and this appears to reflect muscarinic receptor blockade in the gut with resulting delayed gastric emptying and disruption of normal motility.

In a retrospective study of 100 consecutive patients admitted to a Geriatric Psychiatry In-patient Programme with a diagnosis of dementia, 41% were also diagnosed after assessment as having a depression. This depression was characterised by fitful sleep, poor appetite with weight loss and diurnal variation of dysfunctional behaviour which was commonly worse in the morning. The high score on the Mini Mental State Examination (MMSE) (1) was 23 points. 86% of the 41 patients with both dementia and depression responded to antidepressant treatment of which 26% responded to ECT. Of the 86% who responded, 4 out of 5 showed improvement in cognitive function as measured by improvement in the MMSE of between 3 and 9 points.

Depression in the demented elderly is a common problem and may well present with features atypical of those expected in younger patients or described in DSM-IIIR. The concept of Cognitive-Affective disorder is a clinically useful one and treating depression in these patients is highly successful resulting in improvement of the depressive symptoms, but often also in improvements in cognitive function.

References

1. Folstein, M.F., Folstein, S.E. and McHugh, P.R. (1975): J. Psychiat. Res., 12: 189-198.
2. Gosselin, C. and Ancill, R.J. (1989): Can. J. Psychiat., 34: 921-924.
3. Kiloh, L.G. (1961): Acta Psychiat. Scand., 37: 336-351.
4. Reifler, B.V. (1986): J. Clin. Psychiat., 47: 354-356.

WHATS TREATABLE IN DEMENTIA?
AGGRESSION IN DEMENTIA

P.V. Rabins
Department of Psychiatry, John Hopkins University School Of Medicine, Baltimore, USA

There is little research, even of a descriptive nature, on the treatment of aggression in patients with dementia. Thus, clinical impressions serve the basis for both classification and intervention. Aggression is best approached as a behaviour which occurs more commonly in brain injured individuals than in comparison populations. Most commonly, the behaviour is intermittent and its frequency related to an environmental circumstance.

Aggression is defined as a behaviour with physical an/or verbal concomitants in which actual physical harm to others or self would result if the behaviour was carried to its completion.

Because underlying brain injuries increase the prevalence of cognitive and behavioural complications of drug therapy, the first intervention for aggression should be environmental. Frequently, however, the potential harm which could result from the behaviour necessitates pharmacologic intervention. Several classes of drugs are available to treat aggression.

1. Neuroleptics - Several controlled studies demonstrate the effectiveness of neuroleptics in decreasing aggression in the demented (4). Improvement is reported in approximately one-third of patients. Significant side effects occur with a similar frequency (5).

2. Antidepressants - Serotonin uptake blockers may have a unique role in the treatment of aggression e.g. Wilcox et al(7) reported that 4 of 6 cases of dementia and aggression responded to a combination of trazadone and tryptophan.

   Aggression can also be a symptom of major depression which occurs in approximately 20% of the demented. Although (3) was not able to show a benefit of imipramine compared to placebo in the treatment of depressive symptoms in Alzheimer's disease patients, clinical experience suggests that antidepressants can be of significant benefit in treating both mood and aggressive symptoms. Highly anticholinergic agents, such as amitriptyline, should be avoided since Alzheimer's disease has an associated cholinergic deficit.

3. <u>Anti-anxiety agents</u> - While benzodiazepines have long been used to treat aggression in demented patients, there are no controlled trials demonstrating their efficacy. Clinical experience suggests that paradoxical worsening of behaviour and agitation occurs in 15-20% of cases. Shorter acting agents such as oxazepam might be preferable to longer half-life agents, but again this has not been studied in aggressive individuals.

   Case reports suggest that buspirone might be a specific treatment for aggression (1,6). Few cases have been reported and it is unclear at what dosage patients respond.

4. <u>Anticonvulsants</u> - Carbamazepine has been touted as a useful agent in treating aggressive behaviour in head injured patients, but most studies have not included elderly individuals with dementia. The therapeutic/toxic range is narrow and the demented appear to be particularly prone to developing ataxia.

5. <u>Lithium</u> - Case reports suggest that lithium carbonate is effective in diminishing aggression in the brain injured (8), but there are few reports of its use in the demented elderly. Target blood levels in the cognitively normal elderly are 0.5-0.8 ng/dl and a similar or lower blood level range should be the target in the demented.

6. <u>Beta-blockers</u> - Open and controlled trials of several beta-blockers have been carried out (9). One double-blind study of pindolol demonstrated effectiveness in 11 subjects, all of whom were demented (2).

References

1. Colenda C.C., 1988: Lancet, 1:1169.
2. Greendyke R.M. and Kanter R.D., 1986: J Clin Psychiatry, 47: 423-426.
3. Reiffler B.V., Teri L. and Taskind M. et al, 1989: Am J Psychiatry, 146: 45-49.
4. Risse S.C. and Barnes R., 1986: JAGS, 34: 368-376.
5. Steele C, Lucas M.D. and Tune L., 1986: J Clin Psychiatry, 47: 310-312.
6. Tiller J.W.G., Dakis J.A. and Shaw J.M., 1988: Lancet, Aug 27: 510.
7. Wilcox G.K., Stevens J. and Perkins A., 1987: Lancet, April 18: 929-930.
8. Williams K.H. and Goldstein G., 1979: Am J Psychiatry, 136: 800-803.
9. Yudofsky S.C., Silver J.M. and Schneider S.E., 1987: Psychiatric Annals, 17: 397-407.

WHAT'S TREATABLE IN DEMENTIA?
THE PHARMACOLOGICAL MANAGEMENT OF COGNITIVE IMPAIRMENT IN THE DEMENTED PATIENT

M.S.J. PATHY.
University Department of Geriatric Medicine, University of Wales College of Medicine, Wales, UK.

Therapeutic intervention in Alzheimer's disease (AD) is influenced by three cardinal issues:
a) early diagnosis,
b) pharmacological development based on neurochemical brain research and
c) practical and internationally standardised neuropsychometric assessment.

NINCDS-ADRDA standards (2) for Alzheimer's Disease and DSM III(R) criteria for dementia are only fulfilled when AD is neuropathologically advanced. Memory impairment is a non-specific, but clinically simple and useful screening marker for dementia. The development of a hospital-based Memory Clinic in 1983, and additional community-based Memory Clinics in 1988 confirmed that clinical screening strategies can identify early cognitive impairment, but diagnostic differentiation will be uncertain as patient groups will be heterogeneous. AD itself is clinically and neuropathologically heterogeneous and a variable response to therapeutic agents is likely. Classification of the first 250 of 2,100 patients showed that 50% had Alzheimer's Disease, 10% multi-infarct dementia, 4% mixed Alzheimer's and multi-infarct dementia. Depression and memory impairment due to drugs were the commonest reversible presenting conditions. Treatment of chronic dementia is largely palliative at present. Advances in neuropathology and neurochemistry of dementia indicate that therapeutic models might be based on defined neurotransmitter deficiencies or on specific neuronal loss. Cognitive function is likely to involve multiple synapses and transmitters (1). Major therapeutic strategies are directed towards agents that modify cerebral cholinergic, serotonergic, GABAergic, dopaminergic and peptiderigic systems. Despite the link between SDAT and multiple neurotransmitter and neuropeptide systems deficits, the pivotal role of the cholinergic system is unarguable.

Cholinergic enhancement might be achieved by:
a) attempts to increase synthesis of acetylcholine by precursor administration. Choline and lecithin have failed to produce obvious clinical benefit.
b) reducing acetylcholine breakdown by acetylcholinesterase inhibitors (anti-AChE). Problems with these compounds are that

some are very short acting (physostigmine) or are poorly absorbed and poorly transmitted across the blood brain barrier (quaternary anti-AChE) or they may produce severe affective side-effects due to being tonic rather than phasic receptor agonists (oxotremorine) or other centrally-related symptoms.

Not withstanding the difficulties encountered in designing effective anti-AChE compounds, a long acting formulation of physostigmine is under study; Tacrine has given conflicting results in SDAT, but a closely related but less hepatotoxic compound HPO29 is under extensive clinical studies.

L-dopa and dopaminergic agonists have failed to show clinical benefit in SDAT. Although there is no evidence that experimental noradrenergic neuronal lesions affect cognition, mnemonic physostigmine effects do not occur in experimental combined noradrenergic and cholinergic lesions. Controlled systematic trials of noradrenergic therapies in dementia are lacking. Decreased serotonin concentrations in the brain in dementia suggests that potentiation of serotonergic transmission may be a useful strategy. Scopolamine-induced amnesia may be possibly reversed by GABAergic antagonists and inhibitory GABAergic neurones may influence basal forebrain cholinergic neuronal activity.

Consistent reduction in somatostatin and corticotrophin-releasing factor have been reported in AD, but no evidence has been reported to show that somatostatin deficiency affects cognition. The ability of neurotrophic nerve growth factor to reverse partially cholinergic neuronal atrophy holds out a potentially exciting breakthrough in the therapy of AD.

Assessment of multiple components of cognitive dysfunction require neuropsychometric instruments which are validated and practical for age and the progressive nature of dementia (3), and need to be tailored to identify those areas of cognition likely to be influenced by trial drugs.

References

1. Black, I.A. et al (1987): Science, 236: 1263 - 1268.
2. McKhann, G. et al (1984): Neurology, 34: 939 - 944.
3. Rosen W.G. et al (1984): Am. J. Psychiat., 141: 1356 - 1364.

WHAT'S TREATABLE IN DEMENTIA?
METHODOLOGICAL PROBLEMS IN CLINICAL RESEARCH IN DEMENTIA

A. CLARKE.
SmithKline Beecham Pharmaceuticals, Brentford, UK.

Clinical studies in dementia are bedevilled by fundamental difficulties. Despite recent advances, the reliable diagnosis of dementia requires detailed, time-consuming and expensive clinical work-up, and the differential diagnosis of dementia is hard to achieve. The tools available to assess the effects of therapeutic intervention are crude and not necessarily of clear clinical relevance.

Nonetheless, a focus on such fundamental problems can enable meaningful trials to be conducted. By use of investigations that are widely available, patients with secondary causes for cognitive impairment can be identified. For example, carefully taken medical and psychiatric histories, preferably with corroboration from a close relative, can help to chart the time-course of presenting symptomatology. Recent onset may indicate acute confusional states. Standard diagnostics, including physical and neurological examinations, haematology and clinical chemistry, chest X-ray, serum vitamin B_{12}, serum folate and serology for syphilis, may help to identify possible medical causes for the patients symptoms (1). CT scans or Magnetic Resonance Imaging can reveal space occupying lesions. Although dementia can co-present with other psychiatric disorders such as depression, a thorough psychiatric interview can exclude patients with other primary psychiatric diagnoses. Structured diagnostic interviews, such as the CAMDEX (4), can be useful in standardising the approach to diagnosis. However, their use with patients with attentional difficulties may be limited. By a serious search for secondary causes, a diagnosis of primary dementia can be arrived at by exclusion.

Differential diagnosis into vascular and non-vascular dementias is difficult. However, use of scales such as the Hachinski (3) attempt to categorise patients with differing pathologies. This may be important, since a differential response to a pharmacological agent may be seen in patients with dementias with differing aetiologies.
It is possible to use clear and clinically-meaningful endpoints with sample sizes adequate to enable drug-induced changes to be detected. Many trials have been reported, where unusual non-validated scales have been used to assess drug effects, or where the number of patients treated was too small to detect clinically-meaningful changes. Although the results of such trials may be interesting, a little more care in the choice of scales and an increase in patient numbers may have yielded results of

fundamentally greater reliability. It is naive to expect any drug to produce dramatic clinical improvements. However, common sense dictates that even small improvements in global scales such as the Mini-Mental State Examination (2) are of greater overall clinical relevance than large improvements in some neuro-psychological ratings that are not global and often not validated for use in the demented elderly. Expert statistical advice at the trial design stage, can not only ensure adequate sample size calculations, but also aid in the appropriate handling of confounding factors such as baseline mental state, co-presenting psychiatric and non-psychiatric disorders and concomitant medication.

Finally, the management of the patient and the surroundings in which they are assessed can minimise problems caused by anxiety, by lapses in attention and by the feeling of failure inherent in many assessment schedules. It is well recognised that patients perform better in their home environment and in familiar surroundings. Consequently, failure to take account of this, for example by transporting patients to out-patient clinics and assessing them as though they were attending a busy routine clinic, is liable to hinder reliable assessment.

Clinical trials are by their very nature a compromise, but nonetheless represent the science of the possible in a real clinical world. By adequately addressing the achievable, rather than highlighting the impossible, there are methods available today to enable high standards of clinical research in dementia to be undertaken, despite the methodological problems.

References

1. Byrne, E.J. (1987): Int. J. Ger. Psychiat., 2: 73-81.
2. Folstein, M.F., Folstein, S.E. and McHugh, P.R. (1975): J. Psychiat. Res., 12: 189-198.
3. Hachinski, et al (1975), Arch. Neurol., 32: 632-637.
4. Roth, et al (1986), Br. J. Psychiat., 149: 698-709.

ALCOHOL AND ANXIETY

R.G. LISTER
Laboratory of Clinical Studies, National Institute on Alcohol Abuse and Alcoholism, DICBR, Building 10 Room 3C218, 9000 Rockville Pike, Bethesda, MD 20892, U.S.A.

The relationship between alcohol and anxiety is complex (3,6). While it is clear that alcohol can reduce anxiety, the effect depends on a number of factors including the dose, the subject population and the context in which the alcohol is consumed (16).

The high incidence of alcohol abuse amongst phobic subjects may be due in part to self-medication of alcohol as an anxiolytic (1,11,12). However, experimental studies have found conflicting effects of alcohol on phobic anxiety and avoidance behavior in simple phobics (16). It has been suggested that the anxiety disorders that produce the greatest response to alcohol may be those in which the anxiety has a large cognitive component (16), e.g. agoraphobia. While alcohol may be used to self-medicate anxiety disorders, alcohol dependence may cause or exacerbate such disorders (14).

Animal studies generally support the notion that alcohol has anxiolytic or stress-reducing effects. In laboratory rodents the effects of alcohol resemble those of clinically effective anxiolytics in animal models of anxiety (7,9). In rat colonies, the alcohol consumption of subordinate males is higher than that of dominants (2,4). This increased consumption may be related to the stress of low position in the dominance hierarchy. Ethanol also appears capable of preventing a number of neurochemical changes caused by stress (8).

The mechanisms mediating ethanol's anxiolytic effects remain unclear. Behavioral pharmacological studies using animal models suggest that the mechanisms underlying alcohol's anxiolytic action differ from those involved in its other behavioral effects. For example, specific alpha-2 adrenoceptor antagonists are able to reduce ethanol-induced hypothermia and ataxia but fail to modify ethanol's anxiolytic effect (10). While the interaction of alcohol with GABAergic mechanisms has been well documented (15), the role of GABA in alcohol's anxiolytic effect remains unclear. Drugs that are capable of reducing ethanol's anxiolytic effect via an action at the benzodiazepine/GABA receptor complex all have intrinsic anxiogenic actions (7,10). The exact nature of the antagonism is, therefore, unclear. A recent study suggests that the benzodiazepine-

GABA receptor complex may be important in mediating anxiety associated with alcohol withdrawal (5).

REFERENCES

1. Bibb, J.L. and Chambless, D.L. Alcohol use and abuse among diagnosed agoraphobics. Behav. Res. Ther. 24:49-58, 1986.
2. Blanchard, R.J. et al. Social structure and ethanol consumption in the laboratory rat. Pharmacol. Biochem. Behav. 28:437-442, 1987.
3. Cappell, H. and Herman, P. Alcohol and tension reduction. Q. J. Stud. Alcohol 33: 33-64, 1972.
4. Ellison, G.D. A novel animal model of alcohol consumption based on the development of extremes of ethanol preference in colony housed but not isolated rats. Behav. Neurosci. 31:324-433, 1981.
5. File, S.E., Baldwin, H.A. and Hitchcott, P.K. Flumazenil but not nitrendipine reverses the increased anxiety during ethanol withdrawal in the rat. Psychopharmacology 98:262-264, 1989.
6. Hodgson, R.J., Stockwell, T.R. and Rankin, H.J. Can alcohol reduce tension? Behav. Res. Ther. 17:459-466, 1979.
7. Koob, G.F., Percy, L. and Britton, K.T. The effects of Ro 15-4513 on the behavioral actions of ethanol in an operant reaction time and a conflict test. Pharm. Biochem. Behav. 31:757-760, 1988.
8. Kuriyama, K., Kanmori, K. and Yoneda, Y. Preventive effects of alcohol against stress-induced alteration in control of monoamines in brain and adrenal gland. Neuropharmacology 23:649-653, 1984.
9. Lister, R.G. Ethologically-based animal models of anxiety disorders. Pharmac. Ther., in press.
10. Lister, R.G. Antagonizing the behavioral effects of drugs. J. Psychopharmacology 3:21-28, 1989.
11. Mullaney, J.A. and Trippett, C.J. Alcohol dependence and phobias: clinical description and relevance. Br. J. Psychiat. 135:565-573, 1979.
12. Schneier, F.R. et al. Alcohol abuse in social phobia. J. Anxiety Disorders 3:15-23, 1989.
13. Smail, P. et al. Alcohol dependence and phobic anxiety states: I. A prevalence study. Br. J. Psychiat. 144: 53-57, 1984.
14. Stockwell, T. et al. Alcohol dependence and phobic anxiety states. A retrospective study. Br. J. Psychiat. 144:58-63, 1984.
15. Ticku, M.K., Burch, T.P. and Davis, W.C. The interactions of ethanol with the benzodiazepine-GABA receptor ionophore complex. Pharmacol. Biochem. Behav. 18(Suppl. 1):15-18, 1983.
16. Wilson, G.T. Alcohol and anxiety. Behav. Res. Ther. 26:369-382, 1988.

ALCOHOL-INDUCED ALTERATIONS IN THE FUNCTION OF CEREBRAL GABA$_A$ RECEPTOR COMPLEX

T.Hashimoto, T.Ueha, H.Mizutani and K.Kuriyama. Department of Pharmacology, Kyoto Prefectural Univercity of Medicine, Kyoto 602, Japan

Although various studies dealing with the central actions of alcohol are present, exact molecular mechanisms underlying these actions as well as the establishment of alcohol dependence have not been clealy elucidated. In this study, we have investigated the effects of alcohol and alcohol dependence on the function of cerebral GABA$_A$ receptor, benzodiazepine(BZP) receptor and Cl ion channel complex.

METHOD

Alcohol dependent mice(ddy male mice,20-25g) were made by the inhalation of ethanol vapour for 1 week. These animals exhibited typical withdrawal symptoms at 8 hours after the termination of inhalation. The specific bindings of [^{3}H]muscimol([^{3}H]MUS 5.0nM : GABA$_A$ receptor, [^{3}H]flunitrazepam([^{3}H]FLU 0.5nM : BZP receptor) and t-butyl-bicycloorthobenzoate([^{3}H]TBOB 2.0nM : Cl ion channel) were measured using synaptic membrane, membrane vesicles (synaptoneurosomes) and reconstituted phospholipid vesicles with purified GABA$_A$ receptor complex. Purified GABA$_A$ receptor complex was obtained using 1012-S affinity gel column chromatography (1) following the solubilization of abovine cerebral synaptic membrane with CHAPS. The purified receptor

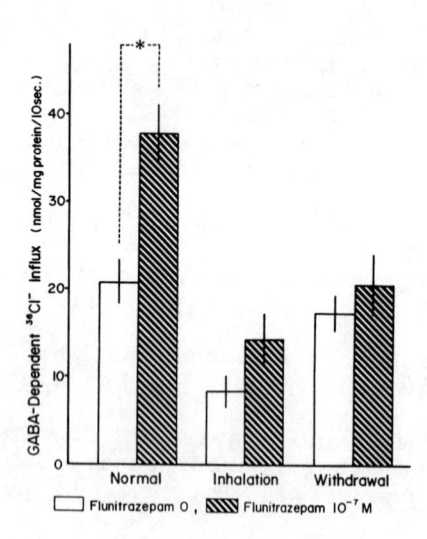

Fig 1. Effects of ethanol inhalation and its withdrawal on flunitrazepam-induced stimulation of GABA-dependent ^{36}Cl$^-$ influx into synaptoneurosomes from mouse brain. Each value represents the mean ± S.E.M. obtained from 3 to 4 separate experiments. *p<0.05, as compared with the value as indicated.

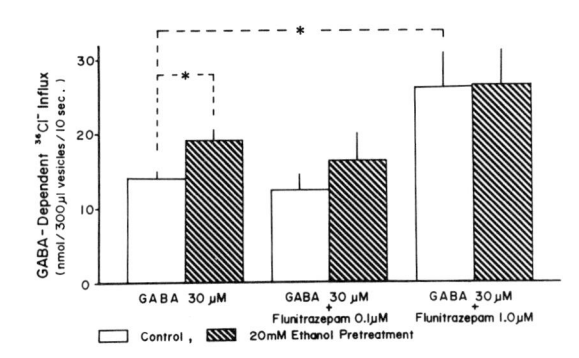

Fig 2. Effect of ethanol pretreatment on flunitrazepam induced GABA-dependent $^{36}Cl^-$ influx into reconstituted vesicles with purified GABA$_A$ receptor. Each value represents the mean ± S.E.M. obtained from 3 to 4 separate experiments. *$p<0.05$, as compared with the value as indicated.

was reconstituted into phospholipid vesicles according to the method of Haga et al. (2). The influxes of $^{36}Cl^-$ into reconstituted vesicles with purified GABA$_A$ receptor and membrane vesicles were measured at 30°C for 10 sec using $^{36}Cl^-$ (1.0 nCi) in the presence of GABA (3).

RESULTS

The specific bindings of [^{3}H]MUS, [^{3}H]FLU and [^{3}H]TBOB to cerebral synaptic membrane were not significantly altered in animals having alcohol dependence as well as exhibiting alcohol withdrawal syndrome. In contrast, GABA-dependent $^{36}Cl^-$ influx into cerebral membrane vesicles obtained from alcohol-dependent animals exhibited a significant decline, and this decrease was recovered following the withdrawal of alcohol inhalation. Furthermore, the accentuating effect of FLU on GABA-dependent $^{36}Cl^-$ influx was found to be eliminated under alcohol-dependent and alcohol withdrawal conditions (Fig 1). In reconstituted vesicles with purified GABA$_A$ rceptor, it was found that ethanol dose-dependently accelerated $^{36}Cl^-$ influx but eliminated the accentuating effect of FLU on GABA-dependent $^{36}Cl^-$ influx(Fig 2).

DISCUSSION AND CONCLUSION

The present results clearly indicate that alcohol has direct deteriorating effects on the functional coupling of GABA$_A$ receptor and BZP receptor as well as that with Cl ion channel without altering the receptor bindings. Furthermore, the present data suggest that these changes in GABA$_A$ receptor complex may be involved in the establishment of alcohol dependence as well as the exhibition of alcohol withdrawal syndrome in alcohol dependent subjects.

REFERENCES

1. Kuriyama K. and Taguchi J. (1987) : Neurochem. Int., 10 : 253-263.
2. Haga K. et al. (1985) : Nature, 316 : 731-733.
3. Hirouchi M. et al. (1987) : Biochem. Biophys. Res. Commun., 146 : 1471-1477.

ALCOHOL AND ANXIETY: ETHOPHARMACOLOGICAL APPROACHES

R. J. Blanchard[1,2] and D. C. Blanchard[2]
Department of Psychology[1] and Bekesy Laboratory of Neurobiology[2], University of Hawaii, Honolulu, HI U.S.A.

A possible anxiolytic effect of alcohol has long been regarded as important in the etiology of alcohol abuse. We are using an ethoexperimental approach to evaluate the effects of alcohol on anxiety through analysis of patterns of natural defensive behaviors.

Defensive Behaviors

For most vertebrate species, danger from attacking conspecifics, from environmental features, and from predators is a potent behavior-determining factor. Defensive behaviors may comprise the single most time-and effort-consuming behavioral component of the average vertebrate's life span, and one in which mistakes are extraordinarily damaging to the individual's extended fitness. The success of particular defensive reactions is strongly dependent on the situation as well as the type of threat source, suggesting that both situational and threat stimuli control the form of defensive behaviors.

Ethoexperimental Analysis.

Ethoexperimental analysis analyzes and investigates such natural behavior patterns in an experimental laboratory context. Its goal is to investigate evolved neurobehavioral systems not arbitrarily-selected behaviors. We have now created several test situations designed to elicit and measure a wide range of natural defensive behaviors, for use as dependent variables in studies of alcohol and other drug effects.

Alcohol effects on reactions to a present, discrete, threat stimulus.

When wild Rattus norvegicus confront an approaching human experimenter in an oval runway where escape is possible, the subject flees. When escape is not possible, it freezes, with both behaviors increasing in intensity as the experimenter-subject distance is reduced from 5 m to 1 m. At very short defensive distances (1.0 to 0.5 m), either freezing or flight tends to give way abruptly to a species-typical defensive threat/attack pattern, with the subject orienting to the oncoming threat, baring its teeth and audibly vocalizing, followed by a jump attack and bites.

Alcohol (0.3, 0.6, 1.2 and 1.8 g/kg, i.p.) did not alter the distance at which avoidance occurred, the proportion of animals avoiding, or the time required to run 25 m while being chased, until high dose levels (1.8 or 1.2 g/kg) were given. At these levels sharply increased times required to run 25 m suggested sedative or motoric effects of the drug. In contrast, jump attacks to an anesthetized conspecific showed a reliable increase at low alcohol doses, apparently declining at the highest doses given (1).

Alcohol effects on defense to situations associated with threat.

In contrast to flight, freezing, and defensive threat/attack to discrete threat stimuli, situations in which a threat stimulus has been presented, or, containing a nondiscrete threat stimulus (c.f. cat odor) tend to elicit a risk assessment pattern of proxemic spatial relationships, orientation, scanning and exploration with particular associated gait and postural characteristics; plus interference with ongoing nondefensive behaviors. On the basis of both similarities in eliciting situations and behavioral isomorphisms, we have suggested that the risk assessment pattern may provide a better model of anxiety than do other defensive behaviors (2,3).

In two situations involving previous exposure to a cat, 15 measures were taken for laboratory rats given 0, 0.6 or 1.2 g/kg of alcohol. On an initial test day two risk assessment measures, location near the cat area and transits to/from this area increased, along with increased general locomotion and a high magnitude but nonsignificant decrease in crouching. On the retest day two additional risk assessment measures increased, for a total of four altered risk assessment measures out of five. Three of the ten nondefensive behaviors increased with alcohol during the retest session as well (3). It is notable that increases in risk assessment from a baseline of crouching or freezing (as here) is interpretable as indicating anxiolytic action: Diazepam consistently increased risk assessment measures in these tasks with minimal impact on nondefensive behaviors (2).

In a straight alley containing a cloth stimulus saturated with the odor of a cat, controls showed high levels of risk assessment, including specific orientation/posture/movement such as "stretch attend" and "stretch approach". Alcohol (0.6 and 1.2 g/kg) did not alter nondefensive locomotion (curved back approach) but the higher dose reliably reduced stretched attend/approach behaviors (4).

The view that risk assessment may be altered by alcohol was confirmed in digitized locomotion/location data for rats exposed to a cat presented at one end of a rectangular test chamber. Alcohol (1.2 g/kg) reduced time immobile, with stereotypic time, but not duration of uprights, increasing proportionately. This effect was reliable only during the initial 10-min. period, notable because alcohol particularly alters initial reactions to potential threat sources (5). The location of the animal, near, rather than away from the area where the threat source had been presented, was also altered by the 1.2 g/kg alcohol dose (Fig. 1). This effect was reliable for both time periods.

Discussion

These results strongly suggest that alcohol, at 0.6 and 1.2 g/kg, produces a relatively consistent effect on risk assessment behaviors to partial threat stimuli and situations associated with threat. It is notable that the pattern of increases in risk assessment in the three situations in which an actual cat was used, against a freezing background, but, decreased risk assessment to the cat odor stimulus, a situation in which risk assessment was a more dominant reaction, was identical to that seen with diazepam (2,4). While the diazepam effect was stronger and more selective than that of alcohol, these studies support a view that alcohol also has a relatively selective effect on those components of defense most isomorphic to anxiety, while additionally producing a release in defensive threat/attack behaviors to discrete threat stimuli.

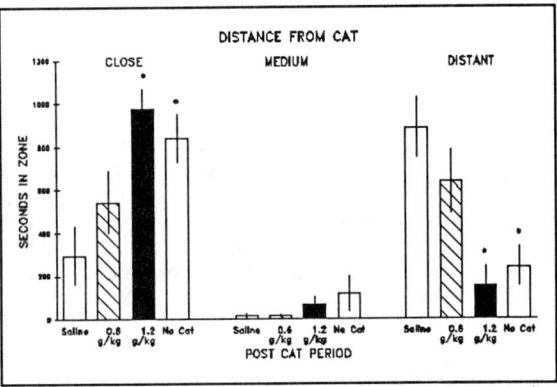

Figure 1: Location of rats injected with 0, 0.6, or 1.2 g/kg alcohol in areas "close", "medium", or "distant" from where a cat was encountered. The no-cat group received a saline injection.

1. Blanchard, R. J., Blanchard, D. C., Flannelly, K. J. and Hori, K. (1986): Ethanol changes patterns of defensive behavior in wild rats. Physiol. Behav., 38:645-650.

2. Blanchard, D. C., Blanchard, R. J., Tom, P. and Rodgers, R. J. Diazepam reduces risk assessment in an anxiety/defense test battery. Psychopharmacology, In Press.

3. Blanchard, R. J., Blanchard, D. C. and Weiss, S. M. Ethanol effects in an Anxiety/Defense Test Battery. Alcohol. In press.

4. Blanchard, R. J. and Blanchard, D. C., Rodgers, R. J., and Weiss, S. M. Effects of ethanol and diazepam on reactivity to predatory odors. Pharmacol. Biochem. Behav. In press.

5. Blanchard, R. J., Flannelly, K. J., Hori, K., Blanchard, D. C. and Hall, J. (1987): Ethanol effects on female agg. vary with opp. size and time within session. Pharmacol. Biochem. Behav. 27:645-648.

DRUG TREATMENT OF ANXIETY IN ALCOHOL WITHDRAWAL

S.E. FILE, A. ZHARKOVSKY and P.K. HITCHCOTT
Psychopharmacology Research Unit, UMDS Division of Pharmacology, University of London, Guy's Hospital, London, SE1 9RT, UK.

There has been considerable evidence for a role of calcium channels in the ethanol withdrawal syndrome and nitrendipine has been reported to reduce the incidence of tremor and seizures on withdrawal from chronic exposure to ethanol (1). We had previously found that nitrendipine (50 mg/kg) did not reduce increased anxiety that can be detected on withdrawal from 4 weeks of ethanol administration (2). The purpose of experiment 1 was to investigate a wider range of nitrendipine doses (25-100 mg/kg) and several different withdrawal responses.

Chronic ethanol treatment has also been found to reduce GABA concentrations and binding sites (3,4) and $GABA_A$ receptor agonists suppress some ethanol withdrawal symptoms (4). We have also found that flumazenil (4 mg/kg), a benzodiazepine receptor antagonist, reverses the increased anxiety that can be detected on withdrawal from chronic benzodiazepine or ethanol treatment (2,5). In experiment 2 we investigated whether the $GABA_B$ receptor agonist baclofen (1.25 - 5 mg/kg) could reverse ethanol withdrawal responses.

METHODS

Male hooded Lister rats were fed a liquid diet to which increasing concentrations of absolute ethanol were added to reach 10%. This was then maintained for a further 4-5 weeks (experiments 1 & 2, respectively) and the final daily intake was 14.5 ± 0.9 g/kg/day. The animals were tested 7.5 h after withdrawal of ethanol from the diet and 30 min after i.p. administration of nitrendipine or baclofen.

RESULTS

Nitrendipine (25-100 mg/kg) had no specific effect on the increased anxiety that was detected on withdrawal from ethanol in both the social social interaction and elevated plus-maze tests. However, nitrendipine (100 mg/kg) did reduce withdrawal tremor. Baclofen (1.25 & 2.5 mg/kg) significantly reversed the anxiogenic withdrawal responses in both tests. Baclofen (1.25 - 5 mg/kg) dose dependently reversed the increase in aggression, the incidence of tremor and muscle rigidity that occured on withdrawal from ethanol. Table 1 summarises the effects of the two drugs on the various withdrawal responses. The failure to find a reversal of withdrawal anxiety with nitrendipine suggests that this withdrawal response may be differently controlled from the withdrawal tremor responses and seizures.

TABLE 1: EFFECTS OF NITRENDIPINE AND BACLOFEN ON ETHANOL WITHDRAWAL
+ INHIBITION OF THE SIGN;   - NO EFFECT

WITHDRAWAL SIGNS	NITRENDIPINE	BACLOFEN
INCREASED ANXIETY	-	+
INCREASED AGGRESSION	-	+
TREMOR	+	+
MUSCLE RIGIDITY	-	+

DISCUSSION

The drug treatments of the increased anxiety seen on withdrawal from chronic ethanol administration will be compared with the treatments that both reverse (flumazenil) and prevent (flumazenil and verapamil) the increased anxiety seen on the withdrawal from chronic benzodiazepine treatment. The possible changes in neurotransmitter release will be discussed.

REFERENCES

1. Little, H.J. et al. Calcium channel antagonists decrease the ethanol withdrawal syndrome. Life Sci., 39:2054-2065, 1986.
2. File, S.E. et al. Flumazenil but not nitrendipine reverses the increased anxiety during ethanol withdrawal in the rat. Psychopharmacology, 98:262-264, 1989.
3. Sytinski, I.A. et al. The gamma-aminobutyric acid (GABA) system in brain during acute and chronic ethanol intoxication. J. Neurochem., 25:43-48, 1975.
4. Ticku, M.K. Ethanol and the benzodiazepine-GABA receptor-ionophore complex. Experientia, 45:413-417, 1989.
5. Baldwin H.A. and File S.E. Reversal of increased anxiety during benzodiazepine withdrawal: evidence for an anxiogenic endogenous ligand for the benzodiazepine receptor. Brain Research Bull., 20:603-606, 1988.

ALCOHOL AND ANXIETY: A CLINICAL PERSPECTIVE

DAVID T. GEORGE AND MARKKU LINNOILA
NATIONAL INSTITUTE ON ALCOHOL ABUSE AND ALCOHOLISM
BETHESDA, MARYLAND, U.S.A.

Studies on patients with alcoholism have found a higher than expected prevalence of panic disorder and suggest a positive correlation between the level of alcohol consumption and severity of anxiety (1). Conversely, there is an increased prevalence of alcoholism among patients with panic disorder and their blood relatives. A comparison of symptoms, physiological and neurochemical changes known to occur in both alcohol withdrawal and panic disorder reveals a degree of similarity between the two conditions (2). To explore possible biological determinants that might explain the comorbidity of alcoholism and panic disorder, we performed a number of studies.

Selection Criteria

1. Alcoholics fulfilled DSM III-R criteria for alcohol dependence and RDC criteria for alcoholism. Alcoholics with panic disorder fulfilled the additional DSM III R criteria for panic disorder.

2. Subjects had no somatic illness or mental disorder other than those being studied.

3. All subjects were medication-free for three weeks and were maintained on a low-monoamine diet for at least 72 hours prior to the study.

4. The alcoholic groups were hospitalized and abstinent for three weeks prior to the study.

Cerebrospinal Fluid

To assess brain neurotransmitter functions, we analyzed cerebrospinal fluid samples from alcoholics, alcoholics with panic disorder and controls. Of interest, alcoholics with panic disorder showed higher levels of B-endorphin (when covaried for height and weight) compared to the other two groups. Comparisons of CSF monoamine metabolite concentrations showed no significant differences between the groups. Our findings suggest that the proopiomelanocortin system may have a role in the etiology of panic disorder in alcoholics perhaps through its regulatory effect on the firing of presynaptic sympathetic and parasympathetic neurones.

Lactate Infusions

Since lactate has been shown to be an effective probe to elicit a panic attack in patients with panic disorder (but not controls), we elected to infuse 0.5M sodium lactate in alcoholics with panic disorder and compare the results to alcoholics and patients with panic disorder without alcoholism. We found alcoholics with panic disorder to be hyporesponsive to lactate with only 17% having a panic attack compared to 70% of patients with panic disorder without alcoholism having a panic attack (3). This finding suggests that alcoholics with panic disorder may represent a subgroup which differs biochemically from patients with panic disorder without alcoholism.

Clomipramine Infusion:

Clomipramine is a relatively specific serotonin reuptake inhibitor which has been thoroughly evaluated as a behavioral and neuroendocrine challenge in humans. Controls, alcoholics and alcoholics with panic disorder were infused with placebo and 12.5 mg of clomipramine on separate days. All subjects showed a significant increase in plasma prolactin, cortisol and ACTH concentrations following the clomipramine infusion. There were no significant differences between the groups. Behaviorally, clomipramine gave rise to a number of affective changes. During the infusion, patients with panic disorder showed significantly higher levels of anxiety and measures of depression. No subject expressed a desire to consume alcohol during or after the infusion.

Mechanism of Panic Attacks

Most studies to date have focused on the sympathetic nervous system to explain the etiology of panic attacks. They have, however failed to show clear overactivity of the sympathetic nervous system in patients with panic disorder either at baseline or during a panic attack. Preliminary procaine data show that alcoholics with panic disorder have a greater increase in heart rate per unit reduction of vagal tone compared to alcoholics without panic attacks or controls. These results suggest a dysregulation in the balance between the sympathetic and parasympathetic nervous systems and raises the question of whether prior alcohol abuse has contributed to this alteration.

REFERENCES

1. Stockwell T. et al. Alcohol dependence and phobic anxiety states II. A retrospective study. Brit. J. Psychiat. 144:58-63, 1984.

2. George D.T. et al. Panic attacks and alcohol withdrawal: Can subjects differentiate the symptoms? Biol. Psychiatry. 24:240-243, 1988.

3. George D.T. et al. Panic response to lactate administration in alcoholic and nonalcoholic patients with panic disorder. Am. J. Psychiatry, 146:1161-1165, 1989.

ACTIONS OF SEX HORMONES ON THE BRAIN

C. HIEMKE and M. BANGER
Department of Psychiatry, University of Mainz, Mainz, F.R.G.

Various central nervous functions are modulated by the gonadal steroid hormones progesterone, estradiol, and testosterone (Fig. 1). This view is based on animal studies and observations of human behavior. The sex steroid dependent functions seem to be linked closely and thus form a complex network in the brain.

Animal studies have given evidence that sex steroids interfere with brain differentiation during the perinatal phase especially in preoptic hypothalamic areas. This is well documented for the so-called sex dimorphic nucleus in rodents (1). The differentiating effects are visible in adulthood and indicated by sex-specific hormone respones of gonadotropin release or behavior.

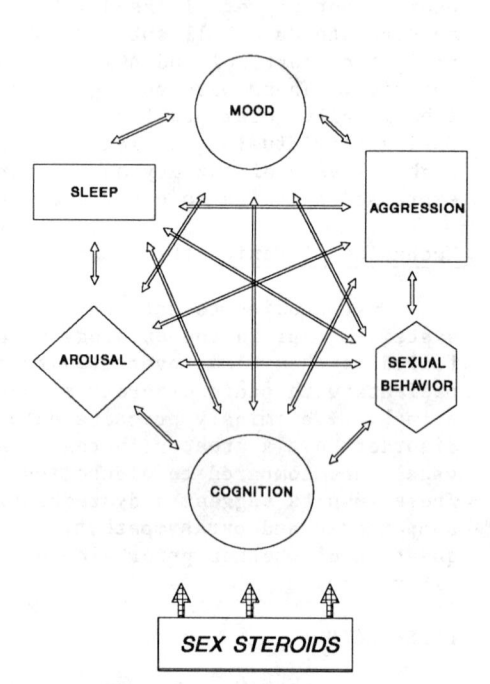

FIG.1. Central nervous functions that are under the modulatory control of sex steroid hormones.

The adult brain is also sensitive towards sex steroid hormones. Alterations in sexual behavior (2), secretion of gonadotropins, basal body temperature (3) or sleep architecture (4) occur after withdrawal from steroid hormone production by gonadectomy or administration of sex steroids. The alterations are accompanied by specific biochemical changes (5) such as the formation of metabolic energy, the synthesis, degradation or release of neurotransmitters, especially of monoamines or opioid peptides, or changes in the properties of neurotransmitter receptors. At least some of the biochemical changes are closely related to the behavoiral alterations which indicate that specific biochemical effects on distinct neurotransmitter systems might be the neural substrate that bring about the multiple changes of complex central nervous functions (Fig.1). The sex steroid induced actions on the central nervous system, however, are not unidirectional. They are highly dependent on the functional state of the target neurons. For example, estrogens can both, inhibit **or** enhance the release of hypothalamic luteinizing hormone releasing hormone depending on the endocrine state.

With regard to the mechanisms that bring about the varoius effects of sexual steroids on the brain genomic actions are certainly involved (6). They are mediated via intracellular sex steroid hormone receptors which subsequently change the synthesis or degradation of specific proteins. Classical intracellular estrogen, progestin, and androgen receptors are present in the brain (5) and estrogen induced alterations of catecholaminergic neurotransmission can be antagonized by the specific estrogen receptor antagonist hydroxytamoxifen (7). On the other hand, electrophysiological investigations and recent biochemical studies have shown direct short term effects on membrane associated receptors especially the $GABA_A$ receptor complex by gonadal steroids and some of their metabolites (8).

From observations of human behavior and feelings it was concluded that the human brain is a target for sex steroid hormones similar to that of animals. There are disorders of sexual differentiation that are often related with psychosexual disturbances. Moreover, it is well known that alterations of gonadal steroid production are frequently accompanied by disturbances of functions that are indicated in Fig. 1. The alterations include slight behavioral deviations up to psychotic disorders, e.g. the premenstrual syndrome or post partum psychosis (9). Moreover, our own recent investigations give evidence for specific changes in the formation and metabolism of estrogens in depressed patients.

The numerous reports in the literature taken together thus indicate that sex steroid hormones and some of their metabolites must be regarded as highly potent endogenous psychotropics.

REFERENCES

1. Raisman, G. and Field P.M. (1985): Brain Res., 54:1-29.
2. Meyerson, B. (1984): Prog. Brain Res., 61:271-281.
3. Hinckel, P. et al. (1989): In Thermoregulation: Research and Clinical Applications, P. Lomax and E. Schönbaum, eds., pp.49-53. Karger, Basel.
4. Block, A.J. et al. (1981): Am. J. Med., 70:506-510.
5. Pfaff, D. (1980): Estrogens and Brain Function, Springer Press, New York
6. McEwen, B.S. (1988): Neurochem. Res., 13:663-669.
7. Hiemke, C. et al. (1985): J.Endocrinol. 106: 37-42
8. Peters, J.A. et al. (1988): Br. J. Pharmacol. 94:1257-1269.
9. Halbreich, U. et al. (1983): Arch. Gen. Psychiatry 40:535-542.

SENSITIVITY OF HYPOTHALAMIC NEURONS TO OXYTOCIN IN VITRO: RELEVANCE TO ESTROGEN INDUCTION OF LORDOSIS BEHAVIOR

L.-M. KOW and D. W. PFAFF
Neurobiology and Behavior, The Rockefeller University, New York, NY, U.S.A.

In the induction of reproductive behaviors, estrogen can regulate gene expression and thereby modulate gene products (5). In some systems estrogen can even modulate more than one gene product. For example, estrogen appears to have a two-pronged effect on an oxytocin system. It not only enhances the synthesis of oxytocin mRNA (1) but also increases oxytocin binding (2), apparently by increasing oxytocin receptors. The question for this, as well as other, molecular biological actions is whether the modulation of gene products is physiologically significant and functionally relevant. To investigate this, we used in vitro hypothalamic slices to study neuronal responses to oxytocin and to see whether these responses were affected by estrogen in accordance to its molecular biological action. These responses were also compared with those to norepinephrine (NE) and acetylcholine (ACh), which are lordosis relevant (3), to assess the involvement of the estrogen-oxytocin relationship in the regulation of lordosis.

METHODS Hypothalamic slices were prepared from ovariectomized rats either treated with estrogen (OVX+E) or not (OVX). Extracellular single-unit activity was recorded from slices submerged in a perfusion chamber. Units were recorded exclusively from ventro-lateral ventromedial nucleus (VMN), where neurons can concentrate estrogen (see 4) and also show increase in oxytocin binding in response to estrogen treatment (2). After being classified according to their firing patterns and responses to electrical stimulation, recorded units were subjected to perfusion with oxytocin solutions. Some units were also tested with NE, ACh, and other agents.

RESULTS Many neurons responded to oxytocin, and the responses were predominantly excitation. The responsiveness, as summarized in Table 1, is both dose-dependent and estrogen-sensitive. When perfused with LO OXT, only OVX+E units responded, indicating that estrogen increased neuronal sensitivity to the peptide. The responsiveness is also dependent on unit types. It was highest in units firing intermittently or phasically, lower in units firing continuously, and lowest in silent units. For example, in OVX+E preparations perfused with LO OXT, 7 out of 9 intermittent and phasic units and 3 out of 28 continuous units responded, but none of the 10 silent or the 10 antidromically activated (AD) units tested were responsive. Results for AD units were not included in Table 1, because all of them were recorded from OVX+E preparations. This interesting result suggests that estrogen can also increase neuronal sensitivity to antidromic activation.

TABLE 1: NUMBER OF UNITS RESPONSIVE (RESP) OR NON-RESPONSIVE (NR) TO PERFUSION WITH A LOW (LO, 2×10^{-10} M) OR A HIGH (HI, 10^{-8} M) CONCENTRATION OF OXYTOCIN (OXT) SOLUTIONS.

PREPARATION TYPES	LO OXT RESP	LO OXT NR	HI OXT RESP	HI OXT NR	LO vs HI p(2-tailed)[*]
OVX+E	10	37	24	20	<0.01
OVX	0	54	14	34	<0.001
OVX+E vs OVX	p<0.001		p<0.05		

[*] Chi-square or Fisher exact probability test.

Comparison of responses showed that, in OVX+E but not OVX preparations, responses to oxytocin correlated with both of those to NE and ACh. Of the OVX+E units tested with oxytocin and ACh, 10 responded to both, 5 to either, and 9 to neither (Chi-square test, $p<0.02$, two-tailed). Of those tested with oxytocin and NE, the corresponding numbers are 16, 11 and 7 ($p<0.05$, one-tailed). In contrast, there was no such correlation for OVX units. The corresponding sets of numbers are 5, 23, and 8 for oxytocin and ACh; and 15, 24, and 6 for oxytocin and NE.

DISCUSSION The major findings of the present study are: A, oxytocin acted on many VMN neurons and its predominant action was excitation; B, estrogen enhanced the effectiveness of oxytocin actions; and C, under estrogen influence oxytocin tended to act on the same population of VMN neurons affected by NE and ACh.

Many lines of evidence indicate that estrogen induction of lordosis is correlated with the excitation of VMN neurons, especially those firing at low rate (see 3, 4). In the present study, we found that oxytocin had a predominantly excitatory action on VMN neurons, especially intermittent and phasic units, the types of units that have low firing rate. This oxytocin action is consistent with the lordosis-inducing action of estrogen, indicating that oxytocin, a gene product modulated by estrogen, can mediate the estrogen action.

The above indication is further supported by present findings that oxytocin action was potentiated by estrogen in a lordosis-relevant way. Corresponding to the demonstration of increased bindings (2), we found estrogen potentiated oxytocin action. Since this is an estrogen priming effect with a time frame appropriate for genomic action, the potentiation is probably due to an increase of oxytocin receptors induced by estrogen. This potentiation, or the increase in receptors, appeared to be specific to one population of VMN neurons, because estrogen was found to render oxytocin action better correlated with those of NE and ACh. This finding can be interpreted as estrogen acting specifically on NE- and ACh-responsive neurons. Since central actions of NE and ACh, particularly those on VMN neurons, can regulate lordosis (3), this population of VMN neurons are lordosis-relevant. By the same token, the correlation between oxytocin action and actions of NE and ACh indicates that oxytocin action is lordosis-relevant under estrogen influence. Putting these findings together, it seems that the ovarian hormone can, on one hand, enhance the synthesis of oxytocin and, on the other hand, induce the synthesis of oxytocin receptors in the lordosis-relevant neurons (ie, neurons acted on by lordosis-relevant NE and ACh) to allow oxytocin to act in a functionally relevant way. Thus, our study of the electrophysiological action of a gene product modulated by estrogen has shown that its two-pronged molecular biological action is physiologically significant and functionally relevant.

Portions of the study were conducted in collaboration with Dr. A.E. Johnson.

REFERENCES
1. Chung, S.K. et al., (1990): Estrogen influences on oxytocin mRNA in the forebrain and hypothalamus of the rat. Manuscript in preparation.
2. Johnson, A.E. et al., (1989): Anatomical localization of the effects of 17B-estradiol on oxytocin receptor binding in the ventromedial hypothalamic nucleus. Endocrinology 124:207-211.
3. Kow, L.-M. and Pfaff, D.W. (1988): Transmitter and peptide actions on hypothalamic neurons in vitro: implications for lordosis. Brain Res. Bull. 20:857-861.
4. Pfaff, D.W. (1980): Estrogen and Brain Function: Neural Analysis of a Hormone-Controlled Mammalian Reproductive Behavior. Springer-Verlag, New York.
5. Pfaff, D.W. (1989): Patterns of steroid hormone effects on electrical and molecular events in hypothalamic neurons. Molecular Neurobiology 3:135-154.

HORMONAL CONTROL OF SOCIO-SEXUAL APPROACH BEHAVIOR

B.J. MEYERSON
Department of Medical Pharmacology, University of Uppsala, Sweden.

The concept "sexual motivation" describes the condition that makes an individual willing to engage in sexual activity. The processes responsible for sexual motivation are a result of an interaction between sensory stimuli and hormonal influences both acting on inherent and acquired central nervous integrative processes. To investigate the various factors that organizes and activates sexual motivation, we need for animal experimental purposes, motor expressions that reflect such a condition. One form of behavior which reflect motivation is the approach (orientation) towards a partner. The neuropsychoendocrine and biochemical basis for this particular element of sexuality was investigated.

METHODS (3, 4, Fig. 1, 2)

Methods are established to measure the orientation in the laboratory rat towards a potential sexual partner. The experimental protocol includes measures of partner preference, sociability and visits to the incentive partner. To assure a sexual aim v. other social basis for the approach, various combinations of the sex and endocrine condition of the incentive subjects were used.

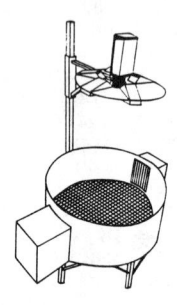

Fig. 1

HORMONES AND SEXUAL APPROACH IN THE FEMALE RAT (2, 4)

The female in estrous increases its contacts with a male. The urge to seek male contact declines after ovariectomy (ovx). Estradiol benzoate treatment restors the behavior. There is a consistent finding that a sexually active male is a more effective incentive than a female or castrated male during spontaneous or induced estrous. Also testosterone (T) is effective to stimulate the preference for a vigorous male in ovx female rats. Results with a non-aromatizable androgen indicate that T need not to be converted to estrogen in order to facilitate a male directed orientation in ovx females. Progesterone did not enhance estrogen induced partner preference unless the goal situation involved a sexual reward in terms of copulatory interactions.

HORMONES AND SEXUAL APPROACH IN THE MALE RAT (3, Fig. 2)

In an experimental situation in which the male does not have direct access to the female, the approach towards the female is dependent on gonadal hormones in the male. In the castrated male T not only increases the social performance but also the preference for the estrous v. anestrous female.

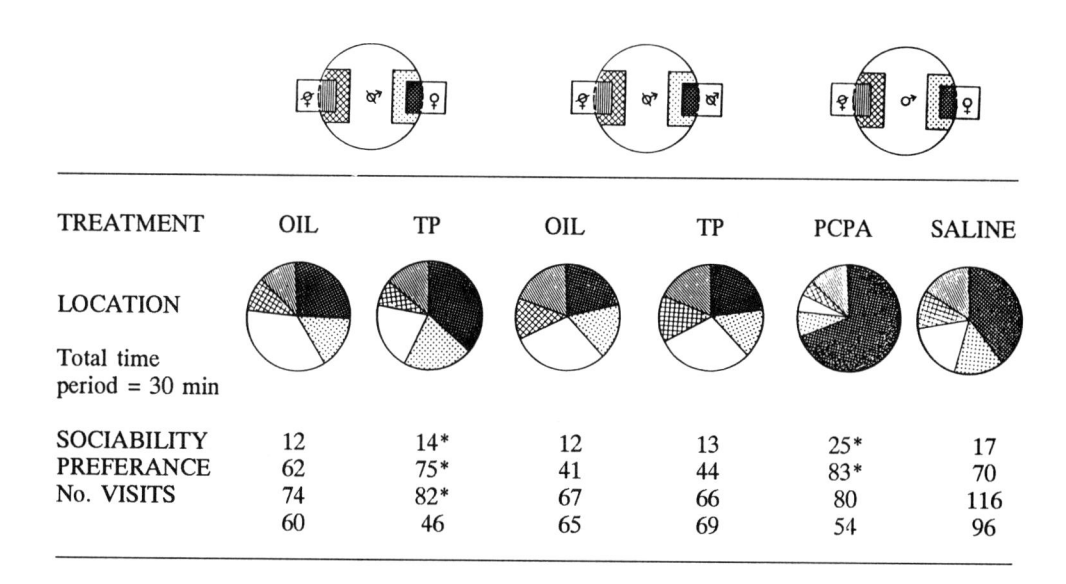

TREATMENT	OIL	TP	OIL	TP	PCPA	SALINE
LOCATION Total time period = 30 min						
SOCIABILITY	12	14*	12	13	25*	17
PREFERANCE	62	75*	41	44	83*	70
No. VISITS	74	82*	67	66	80	116
	60	46	65	69	54	96

FIG. 2. Socio-sexual approach behavior in castrated male rats treated with testosterone propionate 0.5 mg/kg, week (TP), oil vehicle (OIL) or intact males given PCPA 150 mg/kg s.c. N = 12 per group. * <0.05.

ONTOGENY AND PSYCHOSEXUAL DIFFERENTIATION (1, 5)

Before puberty females as well as males had a clear preference for a female v. male partner of the same age. The socio-sexual approach behavior adopts the adult pattern at or just after puberty. Female rats neonatally treated with T orients as adults more towards a female partner v. a male. Androgenized females are less incentive to males that normal females.

PSYCHOPHARMACOLOGY (fig. 2)

Various psychopharmacological agents are tested, mainly with an action associated to monoaminergic mechanisms. PCPA (p-chlorophenylalanine) increased social performance and preference for the receptive female v. not receptive female.

REFERENCES

1. De Jonge, F.H., and Meyerson, B.J. (1982): Horm. Behav., 16:1-12.
2. De Jonge, F.H., et al., (1986): Pharmacol. Biochem. Behav., 24:285-289.
3. Hetta, J., and Meyerson, B.J. (1978): Acta Physiol. Scand., Suppl. 453:1-68.
4. Meyerson, B.J., and Lindström, L. (1973): Acta Physiol. Scand., Suppl. 389:1-80.
5. Meyerson, B.J., et al., (1980): In Advances in the Bioscience, Vol. 25: The development of responsiveness to steroid hormones, A.M. Kaye and M. Kaye, eds., pp. 451-460. Pergamon Press, Oxford.

GONADAL HORMONES, OVULATION AND SYMPTOM FORMATION

T. BÄCKSTRÖM   Departments of Obstetrics and Gynecology, University of Uppsala, Sweden.

The menstrual cycle is characterized by changes of the ovarian hormones. The central nervous system (CNS) is also affected as can be noticed in the cyclical changes in epileptic seizures in many fertile women with epilepsy (2). Many symptoms, in the Pre Menstrual Syndrome (PMS), show cyclical pattern (7). The most common are mental symptoms with depression, irritability, lack of energy, tension and somatic symptoms of bloatedness, breast tenderness, changes in appetite and sexual interest (1,7,12,13,15,17). If one is not aware of the cyclical nature of the symptoms, the premenstrual state is impossible to distinguish from an ordinary anxiety or depressive state. An association exists between PMS and affective illness (8). The presence of psychological problems and a neurotic personality might obscure the relation to the menstrual cycle. Therefore the diagnosis is very important. Earlier the diagnosis was based on only the case history. Today it is generally accepted that the diagnosis and subclassification of the patients should be based on daily prospective symptom ratings (12).

The whole etiology of PMS is still unknown. A temporal relationship to the luteal phase of the menstrual cycle is however clear and many facts suggesting one or several provoking factors produced by the corpus luteum exists. The symptoms start to develop in parallel with the initial development of corpus luteum and disappear when the luteal phase end (3). During the preovulatory estradiol (E2) peak there are very few negative symptoms, instead, there is a period of well-being (3).

In anovulatory cycles induced by treatment with GnRH analogues administered nasally or subcutaneously, the GnRH analogues seem to diminish the cyclical mood changes as compared to placebo (5,9,16). E2 implants giving anovulation are also effective in abolishing cyclical mood changes (14). Danazol also inhibits ovulation and is reported effective (18), but have severe side effects.

Further support to the hypothesis of a factor from corpus luteum are in treatment of postmenopausal women. The estrogen/gestagen sequential replacement therapy (E/G) reassembles the hormonal variations during an ovulatory menstrual cycle, the E2-only treatment an anovulatory cycle. The women with E/G showed cyclicity in their mood and physical signs related to the addition of the gestagen, whereas those receiving E2 did not show any deterioration of mood at the end of the treatment cycle (10).

In PMS women studied during two menstrual cycles with daily prospective symptom ratings and daily blood samples for E2 and Progesterone (P) measurements, the cycle with higher luteal phase concentrations of both E2 and P, had more severe premenstrual symptoms than the cycle with lower concentration (11). The results were more clear for luteal phase E2 with higher degree of significance than for any of the other studied hormones (11). These results contradict the "lack of progesterone theory" (7) for the etiology of PMS.

Not all women have cyclical mood changes and the difference between women with and without PMS is unclear. One suggestion is that women with PMS are more sensitive to hormonal provocation than women without, as the hypothalamo-pituitary unit seem more sensitive to ovarian hormones in women with PMS compared to controls (4). Women who suffer from PMS are also the one who react badly on oral contraceptives (6).

REFERENCES

1. Andersch, B., et al. (1986). J. Psychosom. Obst. Gynaec., **5**: 39-49.
2. Bäckström, T.(1976) Acta Neurol. Scand., **54**: 321-347.
3. Bäckström, T., (1983): Psychosom. Med., **45**: 503-507.
4. Bäckström, T., et al. (1985): Clin. Endocrinol., **22**: 723-732.
5. Bancroft, J., et al. (1987): Clin Endocrinol., **27**: 171-182.
6. Cullberg, J. (1972): Acta Psychiat. Scand., Suppl 236.
7. Dalton, K. (1984). The premenstrual syndrome and progesterone therapy, William Heineman, London.
8. Endicott, J, et al. (1981): Psychosom. Med., **43**: 519-29
9. Hammarbäck, S. and Bäckström, T. (1988): Acta Obstet. et Gynec. Scand., **67**: 159-166.
10. Hammarbäck, S, et al. (1985): Acta Obstet. Gynecol. Scand., **64**: 515-518.
11. Hammarbäck, S, et al. (1989): J. Clin. Endocr. Metab., **68**: 125-130
12. Hammarbäck, S,. (1989): Acta Obstet. Gynecol. Scand. Suppl. 151.,
13. Halbreich, U. and Endicott, J. (1982). In: Behaviour and the Menstrual Cycle, R.C. Friedman (eds). pp 243-265. Marcel Dekker, New York
14. Magos, AL, et al.(1986): Br. Med. J., **292**: 1629-33.
15. Moos, R.H. (1969). Am. J. Obstet. Gynec., **103**: 390-402.
16. Muse, K.N., et al. N. Engl. J. Med., **311**: 1345-1349.
17. Sanders, D, et al. (1983). Psychosom. Med., **45**: 487-501.
18. Watts, JF, et al. (1985): J. Int. Med. Res., **13**: 127-8.

INFLUENCE OF GONADAL HORMONES ON COGNITIVE FUNCTION IN WOMEN

E. HAMPSON

Department of Psychology, University of Western Ontario, London, Canada

Very little is known about the influence of sex hormones on human brain function, and the possible behavioral consequences of such effects. In several recent studies, we have shown that certain cognitive and motor abilities may be among the human behaviors subject to modulation by gonadal steroids (1-3). Over the normal menstrual cycle, for example, we have found that variations in estrogen levels are accompanied by subtle variations in women's spatial, articulatory, and manual motor skills (1). In another study, women tested at the menstrual phase of the cycle showed superior performance on tests of spatial ability and inferential reasoning, compared with women tested at the midluteal phase (2). The midluteal phase, however, was associated with superior fine motor skills, verbal fluency, and perceptual speed & accuracy, skills that typically show sex differences in favor of women. This pattern is consistent with the higher levels of gonadal steroids typical of that phase.

In this paper, we examine whether oral contraceptive (OC) usage in young women is associated with any of the same cognitive and motor effects. Because most contraceptive agents are combinations of synthetic estrogens and progestins, a provisional hypothesis was that OC users would differ significantly from women tested during menses, when serum concentrations of endogenous sex hormones are low. To the extent that OCs mimic the hormonal environment of the midluteal phase of the cycle, OC users should show a similar pattern to that described above, i.e. poorer performance on tests known to favor men, and better performance on tests known to favor women, compared with subjects tested at the menstrual phase of the cycle.

SUBJECTS AND METHOD

Twenty-nine medically healthy young women, ranging in age from 20 to 30 yrs (mean = 22.2), who had been on low-dose OCs (35 mcg or less ethinyl estradiol) for a mean of 29.7 months, took part in the study. Each woman was administered a standard battery of cognitive and motor tests, described elsewhere (2), and was naive as to the purpose of the study. Mean number of pills left in the current pack at time of testing was 6.5 out of a possible 21 (range 17 to 0, i.e. had just taken last pill). Composite scores representing each unique cognitive and motor ability were derived, as in (2). The performance of OC-users was then compared statistically with published data from 45 spontaneously-cycling women tested on the same battery of tests (23 at the menstrual, 22 at the midluteal phase of the cycle)(2).

RESULTS

Differences between women at the menstrual phase and OC users were evaluated by one-tailed a priori contrasts. Fig 1 shows that the difference in mean performance was in the expected direction on all five composites, and was significant for manual speed/co-ordination [$t(71) = 2.55$, $p < .006$], speeded articulation [$t(71) = 1.67$, $p < .05$], and perceptual speed and accuracy [$t(71) = 1.69$, $p < .05$], where OC users performed somewhat better than menstruating women. Differences were not significant for the spatial composite or for the Inference Test, although the latter showed a trend in the expected direction [t (70) = 1.53, p < .065]. Performance of OC users in relation to women tested at the midluteal phase of the cycle was variable.

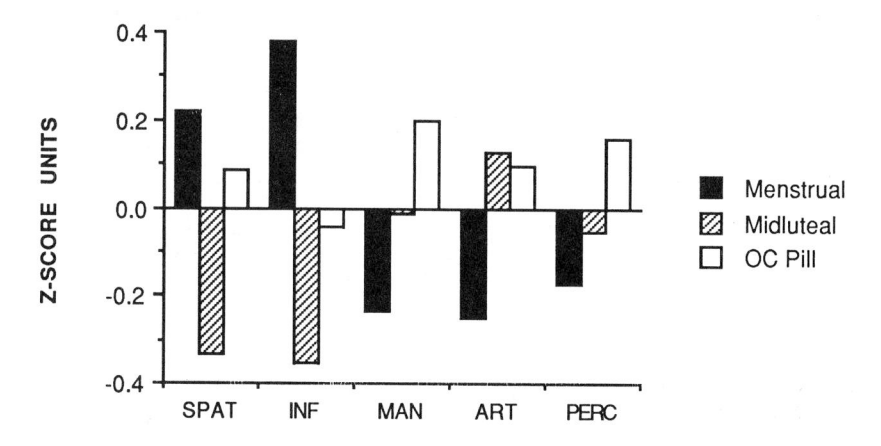

FIG. 1. Mean scores on the spatial, inference, manual speed/coordination, articulatory, and perceptual speed composites, for women in the three hormone conditions.

DISCUSSION

These preliminary results are compatible with the notion that the functionally high levels of sex hormones in OC users may have predictable implications for restricted aspects of cognitive and motor performance. Although the pattern of results was in the predicted direction relative to the menstrual phase of the cycle, the effects were not always the same as those seen in spontaneously-cycling women, particularly for spatial ability where the very slight diminution relative to menstrual phase performance was not statistically significant. Results further support the possibility that certain human abilities may be sensitive to sex hormones, and raise a host of questions for future research.

REFERENCES

1. Hampson, E. Estrogen-related variations in human spatial and articulatory-motor skills. Psychoneuroendocrinology 15(2): in press.
2. Hampson, E. Variations in sex-related cognitive abilities across the menstrual cycle. Brain Cog., in press.
3. Hampson, E. & Kimura, D. Reciprocal effects of hormonal fluctuations on human motor and perceptual-spatial skills. Behav. Neurosci. 102(3): 456-459, 1988.

Gonadal Hormones, Serotonin, Noradrenaline and Mood

U. HALBREICH,* N. ROJANSKY,* S. CARSON*, J. PILETZ,** AND A. HALARIS**

Departments of Psychiatry and Ob/Gyn, State University of New York at Buffalo, N.Y., U.S.A.* and Department of Psychiatry, Case Western Reserve School of Medicine, Cleveland, Ohio, U.S.A.**

It has been shown that gonadal hormones influence activity of several monoaminergic neurotransmitters (4) and this might be one of the mechanisms by which they are involved in modulation of behavior(2). levels of gonadal hormones as well as mood, fluctuate along the normal menstrual cycle (3) and therefore premenstrual dysphoric changes (PMC) might provide a model for the study of the interaction between hormones, mood and other biochemical variables. Here we report on a series of studies on several aspects of the serotonergic system as well as α_2 adrenoreceptor (α_2-AR) binding in platelets.

Clinical methods

All subjects were evaluated with the Premenstrual Assessment form - PAF, and the menstrually-related changes were prospectively confirmed with a Daily Rating Form (DRF). They were confirmed as being "Not Currently Mentally Ill" with a structured interview using the Schedule for Affective Disorders and Schizophrenia - SADS, and Research Diagnostic Criteria (RDC). The clinical evaluations were described in detail elsewhere (1).

Menstrually-related changes in hormonal response to tryptophan It has been hypothesized that menstrually-related changes in serotonergic activity and mood might be due to changes in availability of the 5-HT precursor tryptophan. Ten women with dysphoric PMC were given an oral dose of 8 grams twice - during the mid follicular phase and in the late luteal phase-when they had actual PMC. Cortisol and prolactin responses were higher during the follicular phase than the late luteal phase. Cortisol: Δ max ($\bar{\chi}$ $\pm$S.D.) = Follicular: 7.0$\pm$6.9, late luteal: 3.4$\pm$6.0 ug/dl, t = 4.15, p = 0.0004. Prolactin: Fol: 6.8$\pm$7.0, L.L.: -2.7$\pm$5.0 ng/ml, t = 3.17, p = 0.0044. These results are despite no phase-related changes in pharmacokinetics of tryptophan and might point to menstrually related changes in responsivity of the 5-HT system and not a change in the availability of the precursor-stimulus.

Imipramine receptor binding and serotonin uptake in platelets. 28 women were studied during the early luteal phase (non-symptomatic) and late luteal-symptomatic phase. IMI binding of women with PMC differed (was decreased) from women with no PMC during the early luteal phase, before formation of symptoms (t=2.59; p <0.02) but both groups had low IMI binding during the late luteal phase. there was no group difference or phase effect in 5-HT uptake. Therefore, some serotonergic mechanisms might be trait factors contributing to vulnerability to PMC, or they might change already sometime before symptom-formation.

Studies with the serotonergic agonist m-CPP:
Women with dysphoric PMC were studied in the mid-follicular and late luteal phases of the menstrual cycle. 0.5 mg/kg m-CPP was orally administered. Cortisol response to m-CPP was blunted during the late luteal phase; Δmax cortisol: 6.1 ± 6.8 vs 12.2 ± 8.0 ugr/dl; F = 9.32, p -0.008. There was no phase effect on the prolactin response: Δmax PRL: 11.6 ± 8.6 vs 13.6 ± 13.0 ng/ml, F = 0.26, N.S. This supports the notion on selected decreaed late luteal 5-HT responsivity in PMC.

α_2-AR Binding in Platelets of Women with Dysphoric PMC
Binding at the relative selectivity to high affinity α_2 site (site 2, 1.5nM) of women with dysphoric PMC was significantly higher than that of women with no PMC, during the mid follicular phase (98.2 ± 66.5 fmol ^{3}H-PAC/mg protein vs. 44.9 ± 13.4 fmol/mgpr, t = 2.68, p = 0.019). That difference became even larger during the symptomatic late luteal-premenstrual period (156.9 ± 100.9 vs 62.8 ± 23.4 fmol/mgpr, t = 3.32, p = 0.004).

The difference between the two groups was marginal for the relative selectivity to super high affinity α_2 site (sites 1, 0.06 nM) - (t = 2.17, p = 0.047). The site 2/site 1 ratios of the 2 groups did not differ during both menstrual cycle periods. Comparison of binding at site-2 of patients who were non-symptomatic during mid-follicular phase and symptomatic during the late luteal phase showed significantly higher late luteal binding (183.3 ± 114.0 vs 88.7 ± 74.2, t = 2.67, p = 0.032). There was only a tendency towards phase difference in binding in the site-1 (t=1.87, p=0.088) and no difference in the site 2/site 1 ratio (t = 0.23, p = 0.825). Binding at site-2 during the late luteal phase was highly correlated with severity of dysphoric PMC: r = 0.7812, p< 0.0001), and negatively correlated with plasma levels of progesterone: r = -0.6351, p = 0.048. There was no such correlation with E_2: r = -0.0137, n.s.

Comment
The data indicate that several functions of the serotonergic system might be selectively involved in the pathophysiology of menstrually-related mood changes. The increased α_2-AR in women with dysphoric PMC is suggestive of involvement of the Noradrenergic system. Furthermore, this finding might point to a biological association between dysphoric PMC and affective disorders. These data should be viewed in the context of a multidimensional homeostatic field involving gonadal hormones, neurotransmitters and other biological factors as well as individual vulnerability, environmental and psychological inputs(3).

References
1. Halbreich U, Endicott J, Nee J. (1983): Arch. Gen. Psychiat., 40: 535-542.
2. Halbreich U, (1987). Hormones and Depression, Raven Press, New York.
3. Halbreich U, Alt T, Paul L. (1988): Endocrin. Metab. Clin. N.Amer. 17: 173-194.
4. McEwen BS (1987), In, Hormones and Depression, U Halbreich, Ed. pp. 239-254. Raven Press, New York.

NEUROENDOCRINE AND PSYCHOSOCIAL MECHANISMS IN POST-PARTUM PSYCHOSIS

R. Kumar, A. Wieck, M. Marks, I.C. Campbell and S.A. Checkley, Institute of Psychiatry, De Crespigny Park, London SE5 8AF, U.K.

Psychosis after childbirth regularly occurs in about one in every thousand mothers and the relative risk of psychotic breakdown in a first time mother in the first month after delivery has been estimated as being 35 times higher than in a comparable month before conception (1). The risk of recurrence after a subsequent confinement or of relapse in a woman with a history of bipolar manic depressive illness that preceded childbearing is about 200 times higher than the overall rate of post-partum psychosis. The short delay between parturition and typical onset of illness, the apparent independence of rates of illness from cultural and social factors and some genetic evidence linking post-partum psychosis with manic-depressive illness provide further support for the hypothesis that the primary aetiology is in the physiological rather than in the social or environmental domain.

METHODS

We have been prospectively investigating aetiological mechanisms in women selected as being at high risk of experiencing a post-partum psychotic illness. The subjects so far investigated are 46 women with a previous history of affective illness and 46 control mothers without a prior history of psychiatric disorder. The subjects are studied repeatedly through pregnancy and up to six months post-partum and comparisons can thus be made between women who relapse and those who do not, and with controls. In this report we present preliminary data on two of the measures from this continuing study - first, the relationship between subsequent relapse and the functional status of hypothalamic dopaminergic (D_2) receptors on the 4th day post-partum and second, the possible contribution of adverse life events in the year preceding delivery to the onset (recurrence) of psychosis. Cerebral dopamine receptor activity is assayed by means of the growth hormone secretory response to a small dose of apomorphine (0.005 mg/kg s.c.) on the 4th day after delivery, i.e. before the onset of illness. This neuroendocrine test has been extensively applied in studies of schizophrenic patients and those with affective disorders (2) and the findings are largely inconclusive possibly because of persistent effects of psychotropic medication or other consequences of the illness itself. There is greater variation in patient populations and a suggestion of enhanced activity in a few schizophrenic subjects off medication for 3 months or more (3). The evidence which implicates stressful life events in the causation of post-partum psychosis is derived from large scale epidemiological studies and from investigations of case notes but the only direct investigation so far reported (4) failed to find an excess of such events. We have recorded the occurrence of life events by the method of Paykel et al. (5) and because the interviews were conducted prior to the likely onset of illness the data are relatively free from the bias that can arise in post hoc studies.

RESULTS

Figure 1 shows the growth hormone response of 14 subjects with a history of bipolar or schizo-manic illness, 8 of whom relapsed and six who remained well; also shown are 15 controls, none of whom developed a psychosis after delivery. The "base-line" GH levels in all groups were similar and the responses of the relapsed group were significantly elevated above the controls both in terms of the peaks and the areas under the curve ($p < 0.005$ and $p < 0.01$ respectively). The women who subsequently relapsed also had significantly higher peak GH responses than those who remained well ($p < 0.05$). These differences in GH response were not related to subjects' age or body weight or any medication after delivery. All the 'high risk' subjects had been free from drugs such as neuroleptics, antidepressants or lithium for a minimum of two months (range 2 months - 9 years). Relapse was also associated with the prior occurrence of severe life events; of the 16 'high risk' mothers who became severely ill again 7 (44%) had had at least one such event as compared with 5 of the 30 (17%) who remained well ($p < 0.05$).

DISCUSSION

These preliminary findings show that enhanced cerebral dopaminergic activity precedes the onset of an episode of bipolar or schizo-affective psychosis and later follow-up tests will clarify whether this abnormality persists after recovery. Further studies will examine the mechanisms underlying the enhanced response to the dopamine agonist. As more subjects are recruited we shall also be in a position to test for interactions between stressful life events and other psychosocial as well as physiological variables.

REFERENCES

1. Kendell, R.E. et al. Br. J. Psychiat. 150:662-673, 1987.
2. Matussek, N. Current Trends in Neuroendocrinology 8:141-182, 1988.
3. Cleghorn, J.M. et al. Biol. Psychiat. 18:875-885, 1983.
4. Martin, C.J. et al. J. Affect. Dis. 16:283-293, 1989.
5. Paykel, E.S. et al. Br. J. Psychiat. 136:339-346, 1980.

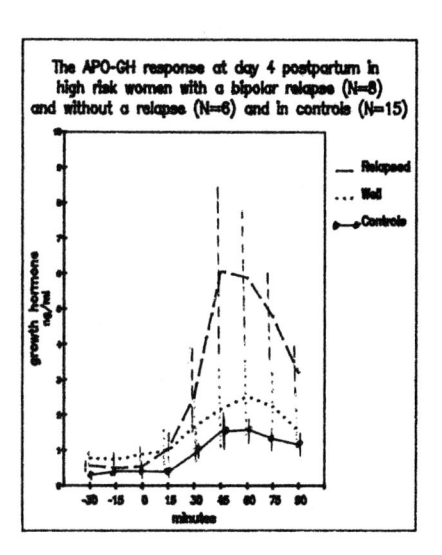

CLINICAL CLUES TO THE AETIOLOGY OF PUERPERAL PSYCHOSIS

IAN BROCKINGTON
Dept. of Psychiatry, University of Birmingham, England.

Puerperal or postpartum psychosis has been recognised for almost 200 years because of the very close temporal association between childbirth and severe mental disorders. This association has been demonstrated best by the epidemiological studies of Paffenbarger (1961-4) and Kendell (1976-1987). About 1 in 500 pregnancies are followed by a psychosis severe enough to lead to hospital admission. In spite of the often extreme severity of these illnesses, recovery is the rule, but 40% have relapses unrelated to childbirth, and recurrences after subsequent pregnancies are common (1/5 for each pregnancy).

There is much to suggest a neurochemical cause in view of the striking premorbid normality of most sufferers, their strong family history of mental disorder, the frequency of manic and confusional features and the response to electroconvulsive therapy. However the neurochemistry of the brain is so complex and obscure that we need more clues from clinical case lore to indicate the systems worthy of close study. In recent years some new clues have emerged, including the following:

(1) There is a close relationship between puerperal psychosis and manic depressive (bipolar) disease. This is clearly seen in patients with two episodes, one of which has taken the form of severe depression and another of mania.

(2) A minority of patients recover quickly but enter a phase of short-lived relapses which have some relationship to the menstrual cycle (1).

(3) Occasional patients have been encountered with multiple episodes of pregnancy-related mental illness, some of which have started after delivery and others in the 9th month of pregnancy, providing prima facie evidence of the prenatal onset of 'puerperal psychosis' (2).

(4) One patient who developed a typical puerperal psychosis after both her pregnancies developed a similar illness after evacuation of a hydatidiform mole (3).

(5) There have been several case reports of puerperal psychosis following bromocriptine treatment given to stop lactation, including two in which the psychosis cleared up rapidly without any treatment except stopping bromocriptine (4).

(6) Although a role for progesterone in the causation of this illness has been suggested, treatment with large doses of intramuscular progesterone, building up a blood level similar to that of late pregnancy, has no effect on the psychosis, even when treatment is started within 2 weeks of delivery.

REFERENCES

1) Brockington I F et al. Premenstrual relapse of puerperal pyschosis. J.Aff.Dis. 14: 287-292, 1988
2) Brockington I F et al. Prepartum psychosis. J.Aff.Dis. (In press)
3) Hopker S W & Brockington I F. Psychosis following hydatidiform mole. B.J.Psych. (In press)
4) Canterbury R J et al. Postpartum psychosis induced by bromocriptine. Sth. Med J. 80: 1463-4, 1987

DO BIOCHEMICAL FACTORS PLAY A PART IN POSTNATAL DEPRESSION?

Vivette Glover, Patricia Hannah, Merton Sandler
Department of Chemical Pathology, Queen Charlotte's and Chelsea Hospital,
Goldhawk Road, London W6 OXG, UK

Three types of postpartum mental disturbance are recognised, the "blues", puerperal psychosis and postnatal depression (4). While it is generally accepted that the profound hormonal changes associated with parturition are likely to play an important role in the first two, the connexion is less clear with postnatal depression. This may be because both the blues and psychosis occur in the first two weeks after birth but the definition of the term postnatal depression is less clear. It has been used for any depressive episode occurring within three or sometimes six months of giving birth. As thus defined, it seems likely to be a heterogeneous condition having multifactorial causation, with biological and social factors playing a varying role in different individuals.

It is not implausible that a sharp fall in circulating oestrogen and progesterone concentrations, hormones which a succession of animal studies have shown to have a pronounced effect on brain monoamine and GABA systems, might give rise to a disturbance of affect. In our recent studies, we have tried to investigate the time course of development of postnatal depression, to see whether it can be triggered by the biochemical events of parturition, to study its biochemical correlates, and determine whether subjects with a known biochemical vulnerability to depressive illness are particularly susceptible to this variant of the disorder.

It is clearly relevant to trace out the pattern of development of postnatal depression in different individuals, and to determine the progression of clinical features in these patients from the first postpartum week onwards. To this end, we have used the Edinburgh Postnatal Depression Scale (EPDS) (1) in a group of 217 patients both at 5 days and 6 weeks postpartum. There was a high overall correlation of score, and also a similar distribution of symptom pattern on each occasion. Two-thirds of the patients who suffered from depression at 6 weeks (EPDS score 13+) were showing dysphoria at 5 days (EPDS score 10+).

In a group of 71 multiparous women, we found that both a recollection of depression following a previous birth and a high 5-day EPDS score were risk factors: a 5-days EPDS score of 13+, together with this recollection increased the likelihood of depression at 6 weeks 85-fold.

In another study in which 39 women suffering from postnatal depression were interviewed using the SADS-L questionnaire, it emerged that about one-quarter had shown euphoric symptoms in the latter part of the first week postpartum. This raises the possibility of a continum of symptoms with postpartum psychosis, in which a substantial proportion of sufferers show features of manic depression.

A reduced Vmax of 5-hydroxytryptamine (5-HT) platelet uptake has been noted in several independent studies of major depression (5). We investigated this in 63 patients at 5-days postpartum and related the findings to individual EPDS scores obtained at the same time. Although no abnormality in Vmax could be detected, there was a significant reduction in Km for 5-HT uptake in women scoring 10+ (n=19), compared with those scoring below 10 on the EPDS (n=44, $p<0.01$). This finding suggests that, in the first week postpartum, there might be biochemical differences in the 5-HT system, correlating with mental state, of a kind distinct from those identified in other types of depression.

Although there are no definitively established biological trait markers for vulnerability to depression, the tyramine test continues to look promising. Patients with a lifetime history of endogenous unipolar depression, although not necessarily depressed at the time of examination, excrete less tyramine sulphate after an oral load of free tyramine than controls. This finding, has now been replicated by a number of different groups and appears to distinguish endogenous from neurotic depression of the same severity (2). It also appears to predict response to antidepressant medication (3). We are currently assessing its value as a marker for vulnerability to postnatal depression, and the results will be presented at the meeting.

REFERENCES

1. Cox, J.L., Holden, J.M., Sagovsky, R. (1987): Br. J. Psychiat., 150:782-786.

2. Hale, et al., (1986): Br. J. Psychiat., 20:251-261.

3. Hale, et al., (1989): Lancet, i:234-236.

4. Kumar, R., Brockington, I.F. (1988) (eds): Motherhood and Mental Illness 2, Butterworth, Cambridge.

5. Tuomisto, J., Tukiainen, E. (1976): Nature, 262:596-598.

ENDOCRINE STUDIES OF THE MATERNITY BLUES

T.OKANO and J.NOMURA
Department of Psychiatry, Mie University School of Medicine, Tsu, Mie, JAPAN

Transient weeping or mild depression which occurs in some women after childbirth has been called the maternity blues, but the cause of this syndrome is yet unknown. The syndrome offers a good opportunity to study the relationship between endocrine and mental changes. The present study is to investigate mood changes and adrenocortical as well as thyroid function in the maternity blues and in the postpartum depression in a prospective manner.

SUBJECT AND METHOD

Forty-seven subjects had normal deliveries without instrumentation or epidural anaesthesia. Women with any history of endocrine or psychiatric illnesses were excluded. Measurements of serum cortisol, psychiatric interview and assessment using the Schedule for Affective Disorders and Schizophrenia (SADS) and the Research Diagnostic Criteria (RDC), and self-rating by the Zung Self-Rating Depression Scale (SRDS) were carried out three times; the first in late pregnancy (36 weeks), the second on the 3rd or 4th day postpartum, the third at one month after delivery. The blood samples were taken at 10 a.m., but at 7 a.m. on the 3rd or 4th day postpartum. For the first five days postpartum, symptoms of the blues were rated by the Stein scale (3). One month after delivery, the 10-item Edinburgh Postnatal Depression Scale (EPDS) (1) was administered to all subjects. Serum levels of triiodothyronine, free-thyroxine, thyroid-stimulating hormone, microsomal and thyroglobulin antibodies were also measured at this time.

RESULTS

Using the above-mentioned criteria, twelve subjects (25.5%) were diagnosed as the maternity blues. At one month after delivery, two subjects were diagnosed as major depressive disorder and two were minor depressive disorder. Two of these subjects had experienced the blues. The scores of SRDS at any period did not show any difference between the blues group and the normal group. However, the scores of EPDS in the blues group were significantly higher than those in the normal group. The results show that the experience of

TABLE : SERUM LEVELS OF CORTISOL DURING PREGNANCY AND POSTPARTUM PERIOD

	LATE PREGNANCY 36 WEEKS	POSTPARTUM PERIOD 3-4 DAYS	POSTPARTUM PERIOD 1 MONTH
CORTISOL (μg/dl) NORMAL GROUP	26.9±4.9 (N=35)	22.2±5.9 (N=35) ⎤	8.6±2.3 (N=35)
BLUES GROUP	27.3±4.7 (N=12)	28.9±7.1 (N=12) ⎦ *	10.9±4.2 (N=12)

* $P < 0.005$

the blues may have an influence even after one month.

Table shows the serum levels of cortisol in late pregnancy and postpartum period. During pregnancy and one month after delivery, there was no difference of cortisol levels between the blues group and the normal group. However, 3rd or 4th day postpartum, serum levels of cortisol in the blues were significantly higher than those in the normal group.

At one month after delivery, there was no difference of the thyroid function between the depression group and the normal group. Four subjects showed positive microsomal antibodies and one showed positive thyroglobulin antibodies, but these results had no relation to the occurrence of postpartum depression.

DISCUSSION

The most important endocrine finding in this study is the high levels of serum cortisol in subjects with the maternity blues. The result confirms our preliminary study (2). There is a possibility that the hyperadrenocorticalism may play a part in the biological basis of the maternity blues. This study also indicates a possible relationship between maternity blues and postpartum depression.

REFERENCES

1. Cox,J.L., et al. (1987): Br.J.Psychiatry., 150:782-786.
2. Okano,T.(1989): Mie Medical.J., 39 (2):189-200.
3. Stein,G.(1980): J.Psychosom.Res., 24:165-167.

PHARMACOANTHROPOLOGY IN PSYCHIATRY

W. KALOW and T. INABA
Department of Pharmacology, University of Toronto,
Toronto, Canada, M5S 1A8

Pharmacogenetics has been called the study of the interrelation of hereditary constitution and response to drugs. All elements of pharmacogenetics are or may be parts of pharmaco-anthropology. Anthropology is a science of populations; it includes the study of their origins, their distinctions, their social and cultural features, and their biology as affected by heredity and environment. It is a science without political or nationalistic overtones. The term "transcultural" has been used when dealing with regional differences in psychiatric drug use or response, and all factors implied by this term are parts of pharmacoanthropology. Thus, PHARMACOANTHROPOLOGY IS THE MEDICAL SCIENCE WHICH DEALS WITH INTERETHNIC DIFFERENCES OF PHARMACOLOGICAL OR TOXICOLOGICAL CONCERN (2). It is concerned with both genetic and non-genetic factors that may affect the response to drugs.

Interethnic differences come in two varieties (3). First, there are countable, discrete differences, such as differences in the incidence of therapeutic failures, or in the frequency with which a particular toxicity occurs, or in the prevalence of subjects who have an inborn deficiency of a drug-metabolizing enzyme. Second, there are differences of continuous variables, as, for instance, different average dose requirements for a given drug, or different average activities of a drug-metabolizing enzyme, or the tendency for a shorter or longer halflife of a drug in two populations.

There are many examples to illustrate the countable differences (3). All monogenetic enzyme deficiencies tend to occur with different frequencies in the human races. In this context, one can cite debrisoquine hydroxylase, mephenytoin hydroxylase, aldehyde dehydrogenase, N-acetyltransferase, glutathione-S-transferase, cholinesterase, paraoxonase, or glucose-6-phosphate dehydrogenase. All except the last are drug-metabolizing enzymes. All deficiencies are genetic, and frequency distributions in any one population tend to be bimodal. A well established clinical consequence of psychiatric concern is the reduced incidence of alcoholism among persons with a deficiency of aldehyde dehydrogenase.

Differences of continuous variables between populations are more difficult to assess than are differences based on gene frequencies, and there are far fewer case reports. For example, the usual dose of diazepam or of halothane tends to be lower in Orientals than in

Caucasians. Other examples are the differences of average activity of aspirin esterase and other esterases between British and Nigerian populations, and the different metabolic ratios of debrisoquine between extensive metabolizers in Europe, in China, and in black Africa. These differences could be genetic or environmental; the distinction may have to await progress in molecular biology.

A lesson from pharmacogenetics may be the relative abundance of variants of drug-metabolizing enzymes, in comparison with the rarity of established receptor variants. This could be a matter of different discovery rates based on research technology, but it could also be that there are biological constraints upon receptor variation; by contrast, biological adaptation of our enzymatic defence systems against the ever-changing variety of chemical intruders may be expected to promote the variability of drug-metabolizing enzymes. If so, variability in the metabolism of psychiatric drugs deserves increasing attention.

Recent progress in pharmacogenetics brought to the fore the problems of drug metabolism in brain. For instance, we confirmed that the genetically variable debrisoquine hydroxylase occurs in brain, and we found it to be identical with the piperazine acceptor site, a molecule with similarities to the dopamine transporter (Niznik et al.) (4). Bertilsson et al. (1). found epidemiological evidence for some particular personality traits in poor metabolizers of debrisoquine. We expect that such exciting new insights of pharmacogenetics will not be long neglected in psychiatry, and will eventually enter pharmacoanthropology.

REFERENCES

1. Bertilsson, L. et al. Debrisoquine Hydroxylation Polymorphism and Personality. Lancet I: 555, 1989.
2. Kalow, W. Pharmacoanthropology: Outline, Problems, and the Nature of Case Histories. Fed. Proceed. 43: 2314-2318, 1984.
3. Kalow, W., Goedde, H.W., and Agarwal, D.P. (1986) Ethnic Differences in Reactions to Drugs and Xenobiotics, Alan R. Liss, New York.
4. Niznik, H.B. et al., The Dopamine Transporter and Cytochrome P450IID1 (Debrisoquine Hydroxylase) in Brain: Resolution and Identification of two Distinct [^{3}H]GBR-12935 Binding Proteins, Arch. Biochem. Biophys. 276: In press, 1990.

MEASUREMENT OF HALOPERIDOL REDUCTASE ACTIVITY IN RED BLOOD CELLS FROM THE JAPANESE PSYCHIATRIC PATIENTS

S. TAKAHASHI, T. SOMEYA, M. SHIBASAKI, N. ISHIDA, T. KATO and T. NOGUCHI
Department of Psychiatry, Shiga University of Medical Science, Otsu, Japan

Previous reports suggested interethnic difference to be present in reduced haloperidol (RHAL)/haloperidol (HAL) ratios in plasma from patients on HAL. The ratios reported were lower in Orientals than Caucasians. The ratios we measured in 45 Japanese patients had a dose-dependent relationship, while their distribution was skewed, likely to be bimodal (4). HAL reductase was found to be a type of ketone reductase in human liver (1), and was expected to be determined in tissues other than liver. We established a method for measuring HAL reductase activity in human red blood cells (2), and analyzed this enzyme activity in blood samples from patients treated with HAL.

SUBJECT AND METHOD

Blood samples were collected from 50 patients, 25 men and 25 women, 18-64 years old, hospitalized and treated with HAL for their active psychotic symptoms. Other neuroleptics or barbiturates were not given, but low doses of antiparkinson drugs and benzodiazepines as sleep inducers were allowed as needed. All met DSM-III-R criteria for schizophrenia (n=45) or schizophreniform disorder (n=5). Doses were titrated according to clinicians' treatment purposes in the range of 15-80 mg/day (mean=15.6 mg). Eighty-seven blood samples were collected at the steady state, after 12 hours of the last dose. Analytical method for HAL reductase activity in red blood cells was described elsewhere (2). Briefly, lysed RBC (0.1 ml) was diluted in 200 mM pH 7.4 phosphate buffer, to which 5 mM NADPH and HAL as substrate to make up the final concentration of 0.1 mM were added in the final volume of 2 ml, and incubated at 37°C for 30 min. Formed RHAL was determined according to Korpi (3). Red blood cell counts were used for calculation.

RESULTS

We examined characteristics of the HAL reductase in red blood cells. The optimum pH for this enzyme was found at 8.2-8.9. Vmax and Km were calculated as 1,600-5,800 pmol/hr/10^6 RBC and 30-330 respectively. This enzyme reaction was NADPH dependent. These values were identical to those we obtained previously in human liver experiments (1).
HAL reductase activities in patients samples were in the range of 5.5-23.1 pmol/hr/10^6 RBC (mean=13.4 $\pm$ 3.6, S.D.). Interindividual variability was as large as 32.5% (CVs), while intraindividual CVs were 11.7 % in 33 individuals examined repeatedly two weeks apart. No significant correlations were found between HAL reductase activity in RBC vs dose of HAL per body weight, or plasma RHAL/HAL ratios.

DISCUSSION

To date we have not noticed any previous report on HAL reductase activity measured in patient materials. Concentrations of HAL 0.1 mM as substrate and RHAL formed were more than 100 times higher than those in plasma, so that it is not likely for in vitro enzymatic reaction to be interfered in the medium. There is a possibility, however, that HAL reductase activity might be affected if pharmacotherapy with HAL and other neuroleptics lasted long, eventhough their doses were pretty low. In order to answer this possibility we should collect samples from new patients not ever treated. As far as the data we obtained from normal volunteers without HAL treatment, HAL reductase activity appeared to have no significant change between patients and normal volunteers (Fig.). Distribution of HAL reductase activity in patients appeared to be shifted slightly to the left.

REFERENCES

1. Inaba, T. and Kovacs, J.: Haloperidol reductase in human and guinea pig livers. Drug Metab. Disp. 17:330-333, 1989.
2. Inaba, T., Kalow, W., Someya, T., Takahashi,S. et al: Haloperidol reduction can be assayed in human red blood cells. Can. J. Physiol. Pharmacol. 67:1468-1469, 1989.
3. Korpi, E.R., Phelps, B.H., Granger, H. et al.: Simultaneous determination of haloperidol and its reduced metabolite in serum and plasma by liquid chromatography. Clin. Chem. 29:624-628, 1983.
4. Someya, T., Takahshi,S., Shibasaki, M. et al.: Reduced haloperidol/haloperidol ratios in plasma: polymorphism in Japanese psychiatric patients. Psychiat. Res. 31:111-120, 1990

FIG. Distribution of haloperidol reductase activity in red blood cells from patients on haloperidol and normal volunteers

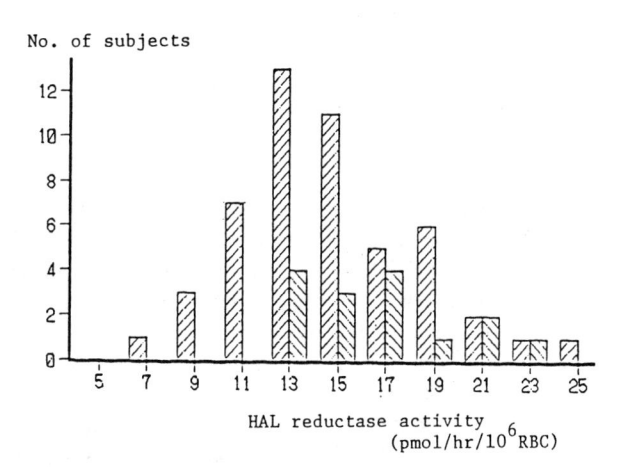

: patients (n=50, mean $\pm$ S.D.= 13.4 $\pm$ 3.6)
: normal volunteers (n=15, mean $\pm$ S.D.= 15.6 $\pm$ 3.2)

ETHNIC COMPARISON OF HALOPERIDOL AND REDUCED HALOPERIDOL PLASMA LEVELS:
CHINESE VERSUS NON-CHINESE

W. H. CHANG*, M. W. JANN***, H. G. HWU**, T. Y. CHEN*, E. K. YEH*, C. P. CHIEN*,
L. ERESHEFSKY****, S. R. SAKLAD**** and A. L. RICHARDS****
*Taipei City Psychiatric Center, **National Taiwan University, Taipei, Taiwan, ROC
***Mercer University, Atlanta, GA and ****The University of Texas at Austin, TX, USA

Haloperidol (HL) plasma levels (Cp) have been investigated by many researchers. A therapeutic range of 3-26 ng/ml has been suggested for HL Cp. HL is metabolized to an inactive compound, reduced HL (RH). However, RH is oxidized back to HL. Ethnic populations could metabolize HL and RH at different rates (1, 2).

METHODS

HL and RH Cp were measured in age- and dose-matched Chinese (C) and non-Chinese (NC) psychiatric patients (N=38). Concentrations were obtained at steady-state and 10-12 hours post-bedtime dose and prior to morning dose. HL and RH Cp were assayed by liquid chromatography and radioimmunoassay. The inter and intraassay coefficient of variation was less than 10% at 2-10 ng/ml for both assays. Patients were matched according to age (± 1 yr) and by HL dose that ranged between 10-60 mg/day. Accordingly, six study groups were formed: 10 mg (N=6); 20 mg (N=11); 30 mg (N=11); 40 mg (N=4); 50 mg (N=3); and 60 mg (N=3). Comparative analysis was completed with each group with paired Student's t-test.

RESULTS

No significant differences were calculated in each group in age, weight except in the 30 mg dose group and dose/weight as shown in Table 1. In each dose group, HL Cp were generally higher in C patients than the NC patients, though significance was only detected in the 30 mg group (26.1 ± 7.0 ng/ml vs. 18.8 ± 5.1 ng/ml, p= .035) and a slight trend in the 40 mg group (36.0 ± 15.0 ng/ml vs. 23.5 ± 10.4 ng/ml, p= .074). RH Cp were generally lower in C subjects in the HL dose groups 10 to 40 mg. However, at 50 mg and 60 mg, RH Cp were higher in C patients than the NC groups. A significant difference was noted only in the 60 mg group (61.6 ± 20.1 ng/ml vs. 48.0 ± 22.4 ng/ml, p= .028). RH/HL ratios were higher in the NC group in the 10 to 30 mg with a strong trend in the 20 mg and 30 mg groups (p= .06). At higher dosages, no difference in RH/HL ratios were noted. Whereas, in C patients, the ratio changed dramatically at higher dosage range (from .56 ± .28 of 40 mg group to 1.41 ± .52 of 50 mg group). In NC patients, a similar but less increase was noted (.74 ± .72 to 1.63 ± .71).

TABLE 1: SUMMARY OF HL AND RH CP IN C AND NC PSYCHIATRIC PATIENTS

DOSE (MG/DAY)	N	GROUP	AGE (YR)	WEIGHT (KG)	DOSE/WEIGHT (MG/KG)	HL CP (NG/ML)	RH CP (NG/ML)	RH/HL RATIO
10	6	C	34.2 ± 11.7	56.8 ± 8.8	.18 ± .04	8.6 ± 3.4	3.0 ± 2.5	.36 ± .18
		NC	33.8 ± 11.5	58.7 ± 16.5	.18 ± .05	6.6 ± 4.5	4.6 ± 4.4	.70 ± .31[a]
20	11	C	31.5 ± 11.3	54.3 ± 7.7	.37 ± .05	13.4 ± 5.6	3.1 ± 2.4	.22 ± .13
		NC	32.0 ± 11.5	64.7 ± 30.8	.36 ± .13	11.3 ± 7.0	5.6 ± 5.1	.58 ± .57[b]
30	11	C	28.4 ± 6.1	57.9 ± 7.6	.54 ± .15	26.1 ± 7.0	10.9 ± 6.9	.43 ± .26
		NC	28.6 ± 6.1	70.2 ± 13.6[c]	.44 ± .08	18.8 ± 5.1[d]	13.2 ± 6.2	.71 ± .34[e]
40	4	C	28.2 ± 8.1	54.5 ± 13.5	.77 ± .19	36.0 ± 15.0	19.9 ± 11.6	.56 ± .28
		NC	29.0 ± 7.8	67.1 ± 6.3[f]	.59 ± .06	23.5 ± 10.4[g]	23.0 ± 30.1	.74 ± .72
50	3	C	30.6 ± 4.7	55.0 ± 3.4	.91 ± .06	40.1 ± 10.8	59.4 ± 33.2	1.41 ± .52
		NC	31.3 ± 4.1	63.1 ± 8.7	.80 ± .11	33.0 ± 5.3	50.3 ± 13.1	1.63 ± .71
60	3	C	31.3 ± 5.5	61.7 ± 1.5	.97 ± .02	48.3 ± 17.8	61.6 ± 20.1	1.29 ± .07
		NC	32.3 ± 5.5	74.9 ± 11.9	.81 ± .11	29.7 ± 7.0	48.0 ± 22.4[h]	1.69 ± .94

[a]t=2.051, d.f.=5, p= .095; [b]t=2.068, d.f.=10, p= .066; [c]t=2.396, d.f.=10, p= .038; [d]t=2.442, d.f.=10, p= .035; [e]t=2.098, d.f.=10, p= .062; [f]t=2.715, d.f.=10, p= .073; [g]t=2.740, d.f.=3, p= .074; [h]t=5.863, d.f.=2, p= .028

DISCUSSION

In essence, this preliminary analysis further suggests the possibility of different metabolic rates between C and NC patients. Larger subject numbers at the higher dose are needed to fully investigate the shift in RH/HL ratios. The increase in RH/HL ratios at high dosages could suggest a saturation phenomenon.

REFERENCES

1. Chang, W.H. et al. Low plasma reduced haloperidol/haloperidol ratios in Chinese patients. Biol. Psychiatry 22:1406-1408, 1987.
2. Jann, M.W. et al. Haloperidol and reduced haloperidol plasma levels in Chinese vs. non-Chinese psychiatric patients. Psychiatry Res. 30:45-52, 1989.

CLOMIPRAMINE PLASMA LEVELS IN MAGHREBIAN AND FRENCH DEPRESSED PATIENTS

D. MOUSSAOUI*, H. LOO**, G. FERREY°, M.F. POIRIER**, N. AYMARD°°, N. KADRI*, A. SQUALLI†.
* University Psychiatric Center Ibn Rushd, Bd Tarik Ibn Ziad, Casablanca, Morocco.
** SHU de Santé Mentale et de Thérapeutique, Hôpital Ste Anne, Paris, France.
° Service de Psychiatrie, Hôpital Emile Roux, Eaubonne, France.
°° Service de Biologie, Hôpital Sainte Anne, 1, rue Cabanis, 75014 Paris, France.
† Department of Pharmacology, Faculty of Medicine, Casablanca, Morocco.

There is almost no study on pharmacokinetics of psychotropic medications between Caucasians and African subjects (north Africans or sub-saharian Africans), whereas many studies have been conducted between Caucasians and Asians on antidepressants and neuroleptics To our knowledge, there is only one team (Cuche et al.,1987), which studied incidentally tricyclic antidepressant plasma levels in French and in Algerians, showing a tendency to less desmethylate tricyclics in Algerians when compared to French patients. A collaborative study is at the present time conducted in order to measure clomipramine plasma levels in Moroccan depressed patients living in Morocco, in White French patients living in France and in Maghrebian (Algerian, Moroccan or Tunisian) patients living in France. The preliminary results from this study will be presented and discussed.

PROBLEMS IN LABORATORY EXPERIMENTATION IN NEUROBEHAVIORAL TOXICOLOGY AND TERATOLOGY

HUGH A. TILSON
Neurotoxicology Division, U.S. Environmental Protection Agency, Research Triangle Park, NC, U.S.A.

Neurotoxicology studies the immediate, persistent and delayed effects of chemical, biological and physical agents on the peripheral and central nervous system. Because the nervous system is highly plastic, certain changes in chemistry, structure and/or function are regarded as normal. However, some exposure-related changes in the nervous system can make it less able to function fully or forces it to compensate to function normally.

The effects of a potential neurotoxicant on the nervous system can be identified and characterized at multiple levels of organization, including molecular, subcellular, physiological and behavioral. One major problem in neurotoxicology concerns the interpretation of data collected at one level of neural organization as it relates to changes occurring elsewhere in the nervous system. This is particularly true in the case of neurobehavioral endpoints where the meaning of exposure-induced changes is sometimes unclear. The purpose of this presentation is to provide specific examples where chemical-induced changes in behavior have been used to study questions at the cellular or molecular levels.

p,p'-DDT is a chlorinated insecticide that produces tremor and hyperexcitability in vivo. At the cellular level, p,p'-DDT has been shown to interfere with neuronal function by holding sodium channels open once they are open, leading to repetitive firing of nerve cells. A spectral analysis procedure was used to characterize the tremorigenic effects of DDT in vivo. Pharmacological manipulations were used to study the possible relationship between DDT-induced tremorigenic activity and its cellular effects. Of the agents studied, phenytoin, which is thought to bind to the inactivation state of the sodium channel, counteracted the tremorigenic effects of DDT. Phenytoin also blocked DDT-induced hyperreactivity and changes in neurotransmitter levels in the brain, as well as blocking the tremor and hyperexcitability produced by another insecticide thought to act by the same mechanism of action. These experiments demonstrate the utility of behavioral procedures in studies of neurotoxic mechanism of action.

Polychlorinated biphenyls (PCB) are environmental agents having little specific neurotoxicity in adults. However, developmental exposure to PCB has been shown to produce a neurological syndrome consisting of abnormal motor movements and hyperactivity. Because of the known involvement of central dopaminergic systems in mediating motor function, behavioral data were used to focus subsequent neurochemical studies on PCB-induced changes in dopamine. Hyperactive PCB-exposed mice were found to have significantly reduced levels of dopamine in the corpus striatum. Litter mates of PCB-exposed mice that were less hyperactive and not showing the neurological syndrome were less affected. These studies demonstrate how behavioral observations can be used to direct additional research at the cellular level.

In adult animals, triethyl tin (TET) is a myelinopathic agent. Short-term exposure to TET postnatally in the rat produces persistent behavioral changes, including hyperactivity and learning deficits. Depending upon the device used, the hyperactivity produced by developmental exposure to TET can dissipate with time. One interpretation of these data is that there is a compensation in the nervous system of TET-exposed animals leading to apparent normal function. However, if these TET-exposed animals are exposed to a pharmacological challenge such as apomorphine, latent or silent neurotoxicity is evident. These data demonstrate how behavioral techniques can be used in combination with pharmacological manipulations to identify and help characterize compensatory changes occurring in the nervous system following developmental insult.

These and other studies illustrate the utility of behavioral techniques to identify and characterize the effects of neurotoxicant exposure. In addition, such studies underscore the need to conduct multidisciplinary research in which changes that occur at one level of analysis can be interpreted within the context of changes occurring at some other level of neural organization.

FUNCTIONAL BEHAVIOURAL ASSESSMENT OF CHANGES IN CNS REGULATORY SYSTEMS AFTER EARLY DRUG OR CHEMICAL EXPOSURE

G. BIGNAMI and E. ALLEVA
Laboratory of Organ and System Pathophysiology, Istituto Superiore di Sanità, Viale Regina Elena 299, I-00161 Roma, Italy.

Over the past years, behavioural toxicologists and teratologists have been confronted with a variety of problems which are partly similar to, and partly different from, those encountered in studies of lesion and drug effects. As concerns differences, the judgements on the relevance of the effects produced by various types of treatments cannot always rely on the same criteria. In pharmacological analyses, for example, a change of average locomotor activity deserves per se to be given appropriate consideration. The same does not necessarily apply when such an effect is found in a toxicological or teratological analysis, unless (i) a substantial proportion of the individual activity scores of treated animals are outside the normal range and/or (ii) other measurable effects are also present.

ASSESSMENT OF LEARNING AND MEMORY CHANGES

From other viewpoints, quite similar evaluation criteria are valid independently of the type of treatment. This is illustrated by studies which are aimed at assessing whether or not associative and/or cognitive processes are affected. In fact, behavioural neuroscientists and pharmacologists have long known that changes in response or error rates in a learning or performance paradigm cannot be directly taken as evidence for an impairment, or vice versa an improvement, of general learning capacities or memory capacities. For example, two-way (shuttle-box) avoidance acquisition and performance can be strikingly facilitated, rather than impaired, by extensive limbic lesions (4) and by antimuscarinics such as atropine and scopolamine (6). This obviously requires an explanation other than that of an improvement of learning or memory capacities.

Such messages have not yet been clearly received in the realms of behavioural toxicology and teratology, not to speak of the fact that they tend to be shelved and forgotten in the realms of behavioural neuroscience and pharmacology. This is shown, for example, by the extensive use of a variety of mazes -- particularly the radial maze -- to study lesion and drug effects on "working memory" and "reference memory". In fact, several such studies do not use the burdensome control procedures which are necessary to exclude a role of non-associative and non-cognitive effects of the treatment, such as subtle sensory, motor, or sensorimotor changes [see e.g. the critique in (3)].

In our early work on the effects in mice of prenatal benzodiazepine (oxazepam) exposure, an impairment of two-way active avoidance acquisition was observed at the young adult stage (2). Such a change might have been interpreted as a learning deficit if the test used (a go-no go avoidance discrimination task) had not required that the animals give both active and passive avoidance responses to different signals. Passive avoidance was learned and performed normally, which excluded not only a general learning or memory deficit, but also some other types of effects (e.g., sensory or motivational changes). The data rather pointed to a subtle and selective effect on the mechanisms involved in motor response activation, which was also supported by other changes seen at earlier developmental stages (see below).

ASSESSMENT OF CHANGES IN REGULATORY MECHANISMS

Another problem, particularly in behavioural teratology, is that of the functional evaluation of the changes recorded at various levels (physiological, biochemical, and behavioural) and at various time intervals after discontinuation of an early treatment. Short of devastating damages that can be identified by the microscope (or even by the naked eye and by the scales), powerful homoeostatic mechanisms can blur the picture to the point of making any interpretation quite difficult. On the one hand, behaviour can be apparently normal in a variety of tests in spite of substantial physiological-biochemical changes. On the other hand, there are no firm criteria to decide which one (or which ones) of several physiological and biochemical changes is (or are) responsible for the modification of one or the other behavioural function.

A partial solution of this problem has been offered by the ontogenetic study of appropriate combinations of behavioural tests and drug challenges (also called drug probes), such as agonists and antagonists which affect the functioning of neurotrasmission and neuromodulation systems. In the case of the prenatal benzodiazepine syndrome, for example, locomotor activity and the hyperactivity response to amphetamine were reduced at two weeks of age, but scopolamine hyperactivity, which normally appears at about three weeks of age, was not significantly affected (2). In addition, some of the morphine effects on activity were modified (although only during limited periods of development), while pain reactivity and morphine analgesia were not modified at any developmental stage (1).

OPEN PROBLEMS

The limited examples so far given should not create the illusion that we are now able to define the most effective strategies in functional-behavioural assessments. A final example can serve as a caveat, although it is taken from a study not aimed at teratological evaluations. In this study, the development of open field activity and habituation varied in rats in a complex fashion depending on whether the animals were given a single 30-min test or three 10-min tests at 24-hr intervals. Moreover, at the end of the second postnatal week amphetamine hyperactivity was much less in the former than in the latter condition, while the profile of drug effects was just the opposite at four weeks (5).

These data suggest that, depending on the organism's experience, there are differences in the way in which various mechanisms serving the modulation of motor activity (including habituation phenomena) are brought into play at successive developmental stages. For good and for bad, such complex test protocols have not yet been adopted for the purpose of behavioural-teratological assessments. In fact, we might be unable to understand the nature of the higher-order interactions that undoubtedly would emerge if the effects of an early treatment were evaluated by the use of a wide range of combinations of challenges, response end-points, and different test schedules.

REFERENCES

1. Alleva, E., Laviola, G., and Bignami, G. (1987): Psychopharmacology, 92:438-440.
2. Alleva, E., et al. (1985): Psychopharmacology, 87:434-441.
3. Godding, P.R., Rush, J.R., and Beatty, W.W. (1982): Pharmac. Biochem. Behav., 16:919-923.
4. Isaacson, R.L. (1974): The Lymbic System. Plenum, New York
5. Laviola, G., et al. (1988): Int. J. Devl. Neuroscience, 6:431-438.
6. Suits, E., and Isaacson, R.L. (1968): Int. J. Neuropharmacol., 7:441-446.

NEUROBEHAVIORAL TOXICITY OF IMMUNOACTIVE DRUGS

J. ELSNER and G. ZBINDEN
Institute of Toxicology, Swiss Federal Institute of Technology and University of Zurich, CH-8603 Schwerzenbach, Switzerland.

Recent studies have shown that cells from both the immune and the nervous systems possess receptors specific to humoral substances formerly attributed to one system only (11). Furthermore, cells from either system are able to produce molecules primarily associated with the other system (8,9). These properties result in a bidirectional information exchange network between the nervous and the immune systems able to cross-tune each other's functions. It is, therefore, not surprising that the prominent treatment-limiting side-effects in humans of immunomodulating drugs (natural or recombinant cytokines and immunosuppressants) are of neurobehavioral nature. Most cytokines (e.g. interleukins and interferons) are pyrogenic and induce a syndrome characterized by malaise, anorexia, increased threshold for thirst, sleepiness, depression (6), and other specific behavior which are believed to be part of a well organized life-saving mechanism (7). Other, more serious effects are cognitive, affective, and personality changes which, at moderate doses, remain limited, but which, at higher doses, may consist of disabling fatigue, numbness and paresthesias, confusion and stupor or coma (13). Immunosuppressants such as cyclosporine A have also been reported to induce severe neurotoxicity including seizures, encephalopathy and coma in humans (1) and rats (5). Whereas most of these manifestations are transitory, there are indications that in certain situations cytokines may produce permanent CNS lesions. E.g. IFN has been shown to permanently alter the behavior of mice treated in the neonatal period (10).

Preclinical toxicology is faced with the new challenge of assessing cognitive aspects of the neurobehavioral toxicity of immunoactive substances. With the aim to investigate the possibility for reproducing effects in laboratory animals which are comparative to the ones observed in humans, we used two experimental paradigms for the analysis of behavioral alterations induced by interleukine-2 (IL-2) and interferons (IFN): the wheel-shaped activity monitor and discrete trial spatial alternation operant conditioning.

MATERIAL, METHODS AND RESULTS

The wheel-shaped activity monitor (3) is a hexagonal structure of spoke, circular and blind alleys, in which the locomotor activity of rats is recorded in detail. In a first study, male Wistar rats (n=6) were injected intraperitoneally (ip) with a dose of 5×10^5 IU of human recombinant (hr) IFN-α-2a or 5×10^5 NU hrIL-2 per rat. This was followed by 2 injections of 10^5 IU or NU spaced 1 week apart. Locomotion activity registered for 90 min, 30 min after dosing, did not differ in magnitude from control rats receiving vehicle treatment. However, the selections of the paths in the monitor by the IL-2 treated rats were more stereotyped, as expressed by increased path iteration frequencies (PIF, $p<0.05$) In a second study, male Wistar rats (n=8) received single i.p. injections of 2 mg per rat of polyinosinic:polycytidylic acid (poly I:C, known to induce IFN-production (12)) or the vehicle in a cross-over design one week apart. The locomotion recorded 5 h after dosing was strongly reduced ($p=0.0002$) and the PIF were somewhat increased ($p<0.05$). 24 h after dosing, the locomotor activity was still moderately reduced ($p<0.05$) but PIF had completely recovered. In a third experiment, groups of 9 rats received on 3 consecutive days injections of 0.5 mg poly I:C per rat or the vehicle in a cross-over design one week apart. Some sedation (p<0.05) was seen 3 h after the last dose, but PIF was unchanged.

The indications of cognitive disturbances on the sequential-spatial perception in the activity monitor induced by acute IL-2 ask for further analysis. Therefore, this effect is investigated in the operant conditioning paradigm of discrete trial spatial alternation. In operant conditioning chambers (containing 2 glass-levers which can be illuminated from behind and which are located on each side of a central water-drop delivering spout) 12 male Wistar rats are trained daily to lever-press in discrete trials signalled by the lever-lights. The rats are reinforced if, on subsequent trials, they press alternate levers. After stable performance in this schedule, the rats will be injected i.p. on alternate days with a dose of 10^4 NU hrIL-2. With this procedure it will be possible to analyse in detail the effects on several variables which are indicative for short-time spatial memory, attention, perseveration, and performance speed (4). Results of this study will be presented at the 17th C.I.N.P. Congress in Kioto.

DISCUSSION

The experiments with the IFN-inducing poly I:C showed as prominent effect a marked and long-lasting sedation which is probably mediated by IFN release. A direct CNS action of poly I:C is highly unlikely since its penetration into the brain is improbable due to the large molecular weight. Moreover, the time course of the sedative effect closely parallels that known to exist in relation to IFN plasma concentrations. The fact that hrIFN-α-2a by itself was not sedating even after repeated administration may be due to the species specificity of this cytokine (a major problem for cytokine preclinical testing in general).

The major effect of IL-2 on locomotor structuring (PIF) and much less on activity magnitude may reflect the sometimes severe behavioral and cognitive disturbances (desorientation, delusions, delirium) observed in humans after administration of cytokines and in particular of IL-2 (2). We hope to be able to characterize these neurobehavioral changes in more detail in the operant conditioning experiment.

The complexity of the immune system probably exceeds by far the one of the nervous system. The interaction between these two systems may be even more complex. The analysis of behavioral modulations by cytokines will help in understanding the significances of this interplay.

REFERENCES
1. Appleton, R.E. et al. (1989): J. Neurol. Neurosurg. Psychiatry, 52:1068-1071.
2. Denicoff, K.D. et al., (1987): Ann. Intern. Med., 107: 293-300.
3. Elsner, J. (1986): Neurobehav. Toxicol. Teratol., 8: 573-584.
4. Elsner, J., et al. (1988): Psychopharmacology, 96: 194-205.
5. Famiglio, L. et al. (1989): Transplantation, 48: 316-321.
6. Fent, K. and Zbinden, G. (1987): TIPS, 8: 100-105.
7. Hart, B.L. (1988): Neurosci. Biobehav. Rev., 12: 123-137.
8. Kavelaars, A. et al., (1990): Endocrinology, 126: 759-764.
9. Ljungdahl, A. et al. (1989): J. Neurosci. Res., 24: 451-456.
10. Myers-Kazimer, R. et al., (1989): J. Interferon Res., 9: 11-21.
11. Plata Salaman,C.R., (1989): Brain Behav. Immun., 3: 193-213.
12. Rotondo, D. et al., (1987): Europ. J. Pharmacol., 137: 257-260.
13. Scott, G.M., (1983): Interferon, 5: 85-114.

FUNCTIONAL ALTERATIONS PRODUCED BY DEVELOPMENTAL EXPOSURE TO HORMONES

T.FUJII and M.HORINAKA
Department of Pharmacology, Teikyo University School of Medicine, Kaga, Itabashi-ku, Tokyo 173, Japan.

Behavioral endpoint has been considered as very sensitive parameters for the functional changes of the brain. The hippocampus plays a role in behavioral maturation (1) and has been recognized as a principal neural target tissue for glucocorticoids, with high concentrations of glucocorticoid receptors. Furthermore, numerous experimental results have indicated significant effects of thyroid hormones on neuronal differentiation and growth; thyroid hormone receptors also exist in the hippocampus (7). We have assessed the functional effects on the offspring after maternal exposure to drugs in a therapeutic dose and found alterations in the behavioral development, thermal regulation or responses to drugs (2-4). In this experiment, we studied the functional effects of developmental exposure to hormones, hydrocortisone and thyroxine, during the critical period of cerebral and hippocampal neurogenesis in the rat.

MATERIALS AND METHODS

Wistar-Imamichi pregnant rats were injected s.c with 10 mg/kg hydrocortisone-Na succinate (Hc, Solu-Cortef®), 5 µg/kg ℓ-thyroxine (T_4) or vehicle between 11:00-11:30 on days 13-15 of gestation. The day of birth was designated as day 1. All litters were culled to 14 per litter and pups were weaned on 21 days of age. The rats were kept in a temperature-controlled room (22±3°C) with a lighting schedule of 14 hr light (0600-2000) and 10 hr darkness and supplied a stock diet and tap water ad libitum. All pups were examined for the body growth and the age of eye opening. The open-field behavior and play fighting behavior were observed from day 13-21 and at 4-5 weeks of age, respectively. In addition the following pharmacological endpoints were used; 1)Muscle relaxation time by baclofen (5 mg/kg,i.p.) at 6 weeks of age; 2)Sniffing down frequency after administration of apomorphine (1 mg/kg, s.c.) at 8-9 weeks of age; 3)Response to kainic acid (12 mg/kg, i.p.) by counting the frequency of wet dog shakes and limbic seizures at 3 and 6 months of age. Only one pharmacological test was applied to each rat.

RESULTS

Growth Rate: Growth rate of the T_4-F_1 rats was accelerated till 15 days of age in males and till 17 days of age in females, and suppressed thereafter in males. Growth rate of the Hc-F_1 rats showed a tendency of decrease from 15 days of age in both sexes. The time of eye-opening in

the T_4-F_1 and Hc-F_1 rats did not differ significantly from the controls.
Open-field Test: Development of locomotor activities in the infantile T_4-F_1 rats showed a delay, particularly in males. There were no significant changes in the locomotor activities in the infantile Hc-F_1 rats. Rearing activities in the control rats were highest at 19 days of age in both sexes, whereas the frequency of rearing was significantly low in the Hc-F_1 male and female rats.
Baclofen Test: Muscle relaxation time in the T_4-F_1 and Hc-F_1 rats did not differ from that in the controls.
Apomorphine Test: Sniffing down frequency after apomorphine administration increased in the T_4-F_1 male and female rats as compared with that in the controls. However, no change was shown in the Hc-F_1 rats.
Kainic Acid Test: A marked reduction in the responsiveness to kainic acid was observed in the T_4-F_1 male rats as examined for wet dog shakes at 3 and 6 months of age. A significant reduction in the frequencies of wet dog shakes was also noted in the 3-month-old Hc-F_1 male rats. Response to kainic acid in the T_4-F_1 and Hc-F_1 female rats was lower than in the controls but statistically insignificant.

DISCUSSION

The results demonstrated that prenatal exposure to thyroxine or hydrocortisone during the period of neurogenesis in the hippocampal pyramidal neurons, cerebral cortex (6) in the rat induced a marked reduction in the response to kainic acid when examined at adulthood, suggesting alterations in the binding site of kainic acid and/or in the developmental integration of the hippocampal formation and related brain regions which involved in the manifestation of wet dog shakes after kainic acid treatment. The hippocampal formation contains one of the highest densities of kainic acid binding site in the brain (5). Besides their own action, thyroid hormones and glucocorticoids might possess a modulating activity via own receptors in the central nervous system. It has been indicated that pharmacological dose of glucocorticoids damage hippocampal neurons (8). Perinatal hypothyroidism has been observed to decrease hippocampal kainic acid binding in rats (7). The present results suggest that short-term exposure at the middle of gestation to excess amounts of glucocorticoid or thyroid hormone in the rat affect the functional development of the brain.

REFERENCES

1. Altman,J., Brunner, R.L. and Bayer, S.A.,(1973): Behavioral Biology, 8:557-596.
2. Fujii,T. and Ohtaki,Y.(1985): Develop. Pharmacol. Therap., 8:364-373.
3. Fujii,T. et al.,(1986): Neuropharmacology, 25:845-851.
4. Fujii,T. et al. (1987): In Functional Teratogenesis-Functional Effects on the Offspring after Parental Drug Exposure, T.Fujii and P.M.Adams, eds., pp.159-173. Teikyo Univ. Press, Tokyo.
5. Monaghan,D.T. and Cotman,C.W.,(1982): Brain Res., 252:91-100.
6. Rodier,P.M. (1988): Progr. Brain Res., 73:335-348.
7. Savage,D.D. et al.,(1990): Neuroendocrinology, 51:38-44.
8. Sapolsky,R.M. (1987): TINS, 10:346-349.

NEUROBEHAVIORAL CHANGES PRODUCED BY DEVELOPMENTAL EXPOSURE TO PSYCHOTROPIC DRUGS

V. CUOMO, R. CAGIANO, M.A. DE SALVIA, C. LACOMBA and G. RENNA
Institute of Pharmacology, University of Bari, Piazza G. Cesare, Policlinico, 70124 Bari, Italy.

The timing of developmental treatments with psychotropic drugs may be crucial for the induction of short- and long-term behavioral changes in rodents.
In particular, prenatal administration of some psychoactive drugs produces behavioral effects which differ significantly from those elicited by their administration during early postnatal life. Moreover, prenatal and/or early postnatal treatment with various psychotropic drugs induces behavioral changes which are markedly different from those occurring in response to drug administration to mature animals.
Most of the behavioral alterations produced by developmental exposure to some psychoactive compounds are still present at an age at which these drugs are no longer detectable in the CNS, indicating that their administration during periods of division or differentiation of cells in the brain will permanently alter the course of neural development.
These findings may have implications for the exposure of the human fetus or neonate to psychotropic drugs.
In the present paper, behavioral changes produced in rats by the developmental administration of some psychotropic drugs affecting central GABAergic and dopaminergic neurotransmission are reported.
In particular, we investigated the effects of prenatal exposure to an anxiolytic compound, like diazepam, and to a neuroleptic agent, like haloperidol, on emotional and motivational patterns in which both the benzodiazepine-GABA-receptor-chloride channel complex and the dopaminergic system seem to be involved.
Thus, the influence of prenatal treatment with diazepam (0.1 - 1 mg/kg s.c. from day 14 to day 20 of gestation) and haloperidol (0.5 mg/kg s.c. from day 4 to day 15 of gestation) on the following behavioral parameters in Sprague-Dawley rats was evaluated: (i) Ultrasonic emission in rat pups removed from their nest; this response represents an accurate test in which the development of emotionality of infant rats can be assessed. (ii) Ultrasonic vocalization during copulation in male rats; this behavioral pattern is a sensitive indicator of subtle changes in sexual motivation.

Prenatal exposure to diazepam

Rat pups treated with diazepam (0.1 - 1 mg/kg) during prenatal life exhibited significant alterations of the length pattern of ultrasonic calls during the first two weeks of postnatal life. These changes were paralleled by a significant decrease in activity in the open field, possibly suggesting increased emotionality (3).

Moreover, the results of the present study show that prenatal exposure to diazepam affected some parameters of sexual activity in adult male rats (120 day old); in particular, a significant increase in the latency of emission of the first precopulatory 50 kHz ultrasound as well as a significant increase in the latency of the first mount-intromission were found in diazepam (0.1 - 1 mg/kg)-treated animals.

Prenatal exposure to haloperidol

Prenatal treatment with haloperidol (0.5 mg/kg) did not affect the ultrasonic vocalization of rat pups removed from their nest. Conversely, our recent findings have shown that the neonatal administration of this dopamine receptor antagonist produced profound and long lasting alterations in several parameters of ultrasonic emission (1).

The comparative evaluation of changes in ultrasonic calling induced by prenatal and early postnatal exposure to haloperidol could shed light on other findings, e.g. that this neuroleptic produced different behavioral alterations in adult rats depending upon the period of its administration.

Furthermore, our results have shown that even though prenatal administration of haloperidol did not influence the typical parameters of sexual activity of male rats, the latency of emission of the first precopulatory 50 kHz ultrasound was significantly increased in haloperidol (0.5 mg/kg)-exposed rats. These data parallel our previous findings showing that the duration of the period of the 22 kHz post-ejaculatory call emission was also increased by prenatal treatment with haloperidol (2).

Thus, the present data together with our previous findings (4) indicate that the gestational exposure to drugs affecting GABAergic and dopaminergic system induces in rat offspring both short- and long-term behavioral changes characterized by altered emotional and motivational responsiveness to environmental challenges.

REFERENCES

1. Cagiano, R. et al.,(1986): Life Sci., 38:1417-1423.
2. Cagiano, R. et al.,(1988): Eur. J. Pharmacol., 157:45-50.
3. Cagiano, R. et al.,(1990): Eur. J. Pharmacol.,(in press).
4. Cuomo, V., (1987): Trends in Pharmacol. Sci., 8:346-350.

MOLECULAR PHARMACOLOGY OF THE GABA/BENZODIAZEPINE RECEPTOR COMPLEX

H. MOHLER, P. MALHERBE*, G.J. RICHARDS*
Institute of Pharmacology, University of Zurich, Switzerland; *Pharma Research, Hoffmann-La Roche, Basle, Switzerland.

Ligands of the benzodiazepine receptor
The complexity of the brain frequently prevents the identification of molecular control elements for higher brain functions. The identification of the benzodiazepine receptor (BZR ref.6,12), brought to light a molecular and synaptic mechanism for the regulation of anxiety, vigilance, muscle tension and epileptiform activity. The BZR is an allosteric control element of the $GABA_A$-receptor through which the GABA-gated chloride flux can be modulated. The BZR is unique in that it mediates two opposite effects, facilitation as well as reduction of $GABA_A$-receptor function. While potentiating ligands, termed agonists, reduce the level of anxiety, vigilance, muscle tension and epileptiform activity, ligands with negative intrinsic activity, termed inverse agonists, intensify these CNS states. The effects of both types of BZR ligands are most likely mediated via a common drug binding domain since flumazenil, a benzodiazepine antagonist, inhibits the effects of agonists as well as inverse agonists. Presently, partial agonists are being developed which promise to be useful tranquilizing agents with reduced sedative properties and less dependence liability than full agonists (1).

Recombinant receptors
Despite its functional prominence the structure of the $GABA_A$-receptor has remained unclear. Cloning of subunit-cDNAs revealed an unexpected subunit heterogeneity comprising at least six α-subunits, three β-subunits, one γ- and δ-subunit (2-4,9-11). When the $\alpha1$- and $\beta1$-subunits were co-expressed GABA-gated chloride channels were formed. Varying the α-subunit isoforms gave rise to receptors with different sensitivities to GABA (2,4,5,10). While the α/β-subunit combination either lacked a response to BZR ligands (bovine subunits, ref. 2) or displayed a functionally impaired BZR (rat subunits, ref. 4), a bi-directional modulation of the $GABA_A$-receptor function by BZR ligands was achieved when a $\gamma2$-subunit was co-expressed with the α- and β-subunits (3,9). However, the α, β, $\gamma2$-receptor isoform lacks the cooperativity of GABA in gating the channel, a key property of the receptor in vivo. Furthermore, the $\gamma2$-subunit does not

appear to be co-expressed in all neurons displaying α- and β-subunits. Thus, the structure of $GABA_A$-receptors in the brain is still elusive.

Mapping of signalling pathways
The types of neurons which respond to ligands of the BZR are largely unknown. Since they are characterized by the expression of $GABA_A$-receptor genes they can now be identified using in situ hybridization histochemistry of receptor subunit mRNA in brain sections. For instance, co-expression of α1-, β1- and γ2-subunits was apparent in mitral cells of olfactory bulb, pyramidal and granule cells of hippocampal formation and granule cells of cerebellum. In other brain regions a differential expression of subunits was found. Thus, those neurons which are sensitive to ligands of BZR can now be mapped and identified. They may represent useful targets for the development of novel drugs.

The final therapeutic response to ligands of the BZR involves the activation of numerous yet unidentified populations of neurons. Therefore, an attempt was made to visualize the pattern of trans-synaptic signalling triggered by GABA-receptor activation. Using the induction of certain protooncogenes such as c-fos and c-jun as marker for neuronal activity (8) the pattern of signalling pathways for inverse agonists of the BZR has been mapped in the brain (7).

REFERENCES

1) Haefely, W. (1989) in: E.A. Barnard and E. Costa, eds., Allosteric modulation of amino acid receptors: therapeutic implications. Raven press, pp.47-70.
2) Levitan, E.S. et al. (1988) Nature 335, 76-79.
3) Malherbe, P. et al. (1990) J. Neuroscience (in press)
4) Malherbe, P. et al. (1990) Mol.Brain Res. (in press)
5) Malherbe, P. et al. (1990) FEBS Lett (in press)
6) Mohler, H. and Okada, T. (1977) Science 198, 849-851.
7) Mohler, H. et al. (1989) in: E.A. Barnard and E. Costa, eds., Allosteric modulation of amino acid receptors: therapeutic implications, Raven press, pp 31-46.
8) Morgan, J.T. and Curran, T. (1989) Trends Neurosci. 12, 459-462.
9) Pritchett, D.B. et al. (1989) Nature, 338, 1582-1585.
10) Schofield, P.R. et al. (1987) Nature 328, 221-227
11) Shivers, B.D. et al. (1989) Neuron 3, 327-337.
12) Squires, R.F. and Braestup, C. (1977) Nature 266, 732-734.

ALLOSTERIC MODULATION OF GABA$_A$ RECEPTORS: PARTICIPATION OF MULTIPLE SIGNALS

A. GUIDOTTI
FIDIA Georgetown Institute for the Neurosciences, Georgetown University Medical School, Washington, D.C. 20007 U.S.A.

GABA Receptor Heterogeneity

A host of evidence supports the existence of at least two major subclasses of GABA receptors: GABA$_A$ and GABA$_B$.

GABA$_B$ receptors are selectively activated by baclofen (p-chlorophenyl GABA) and are insensitive to muscimol, bicuculline, and benzodiazepines (BZ). Transmembrane signaling at GABA$_B$ receptors involves gating of K^+ or CA^{2+} channels by indirect mechanisms requiring an inhibition of adenylate cyclase or a modulation by a guanine nucleotide binding protein (G-protein) (10). In contrast, GABA$_A$ receptors fail to bind baclofen and to be modulated by G-proteins. The activation of GABA$_A$ binding sites with GABA or muscimol results in generation of a Cl^- current across the neuronal membrane (1). This effect is inhibited competitively by bicuculline and can be modulated positively or negatively by drugs acting at: a) the channel gating mechanisms (barbiturates and steroids) and b) the allosteric modulatory BZ binding sites (anxiolytic and anticonvulsant BZs or anxiogenic and proconvulsant β-carboline esters).

BZ ligands, in addition to a direct action on GABAergic transmission via BZ binding sites associated with the allosteric modulatory center of GABA$_A$ receptors, may influence GABA$_A$ receptor function indirectly acting on BZ binding sites located on the outer layer of the mitochondrial membranes (9). These mitochondrial BZ sites participate in the regulation of cholesterol availability to enzymes situated at the inner mitochondrial membranes and regulate the formation of pregnenolone (4), the rate limiting step in the biosynthesis of neurosteroids (3). Neurosteroids, in turn may regulate GABA$_A$ receptor function binding to allosteric sites associated with the receptorial channel domain (7).

Heterogeneity of BZ Binding Sites Associated with GABA$_A$ Receptors

Pharmacological, electrophysiological, and molecular biological studies support the concept that the BZ binding sites associated with the allosteric modulatory center of the GABA$_A$ receptors show heterogeneity. For example, clonazepam and zolpidem (differently from diazepam) bind with high affinity to cerebellar membranes but fail to bind to rat and cow spinal cord membranes.

Recent experiments in our laboratory (Memo's personal communication) have suggested that the subunit composition of GABA$_A$ receptors in rat and cow spinal cord are quite different form that of cerebellum. In fact, while in the cerebellum there is a predominance of α_1 subunits over the other α subunits, in the spinal cord there is a predominant expression of the α_4 subunit (α_5, according to P. Seeburg classification). Interestingly, reconstituted GABA$_A$ receptors obtained by transfecting α_5, β_1, and γ_2 cDNAs in kidney tumor cell lines fail to bind zolpidem with high affinity, whereas transfecting α_1, β_1, and γ_2 cDNAs, the GABA$_A$ receptors, like the cerebellar GABA$_A$ receptors, bind zolpidem with high affinity (6).

The different pharmacological properties of clonazepam, diazepam, and zolpidem (i.e., regarding their ability to enhance bicuculline seizure threshold, to decrease locomotion, to induce ataxia, or to elicit anticonflict action) further support the concept that in the rat CNS the preferential occupancy of heterogeneous $GABA_A$ receptors by drugs can be related to the effect on behavior (Massotti, personal communication).

Modulation of $GABA_A$ Receptors by Endocoids

If there are various subclasses of $GABA_A$ receptors that differ in their capacity of express binding sites for positive and negative allosteric modulator drugs, an obvious question then is: Are the functional aspects of these allosteric modulatory sites regulated by a variety of specific endogenous ligands (endocoids)? The existence of at least 3 groups of endocoids for the modulation of $GABA_A$ receptors is now documented. These groups are 1) A 10 kDa diazepam binding inhibitor (DBI) peptide and its processing products which include ODN, an octadecaneuropeptide (DBI 33-50) and TTN, a triakontetraneuropeptide (DBI 17-50). These peptides are present in neurones and in some glial cells and act on both the BZ binding sites coupled to $GABA_A$ receptors (ODN and DBI) or the BZ binding sites present on the mitochondria (TTN and DBI) (8), thus stimulating steroidogenesis (Papadopoulos, personal communication).
2) Natural BZ like substances, here called endozepines, which include diazepam, desmethyl diazepam, and other yet unidentified BZs. There are at least six different types of endozepines that can be identified in rat and human brain after reverse phase HPLC separation, flunitrazepam binding, and radioimmunoassay techniques. The endozepine levels in human brain can be as high as 150 pmol/g of tissue. Endozepines increase 5- to 6-fold in the CSF of hepatic encephalopathic patients (9) and this observation agrees with the clinical report that flumazenil (an inert BZ ligand) rapidly improves the symptoms of HE (2).
3) The pioneering work of Baulieu and collaborators (3), and more recent work on the role of steroids on transmitter receptor function (1,4), have indicated that neurosteroids exist, which having lost their hormonal action, act at GABAergic synapses as neuromodulators of $GABA_A$ receptor function. Relevant to this neuronal action, it has been observed that BZ ligands which bind to the mitochondrial BZ recognition sites regulate the conversion of cholesterol to pregnenolone, the rate limiting step in the biosynthesis of steroids (4). In brain, the mitochondrial BZ binding sites are predominantly present in the glial cells. It has been reported that glial cells synthesize and release neurosteroids (3). Therefore, we are now working on the hypothesis that some of the pharmacological actions of so called peripheral BZ ligands such as Ro 5-4864 (4-Cl diazepam), PK-11195 (an isoquinoline carboxamide derivative), alpidem (an imidazopyridine derivative), and even diazepam (a 1-4 benzodiazepine), can be mediated by production and accumulation of neurosteroids in the proximity of the GABAergic synapses.

REFERENCES

1. Bormann, (1988): J. *TINS*, **11**: 112-116.
2. Grimm, G. et al., (1988): *Lancet*, **1**: 1392-1394.
3. Hu, Z.Y. et al., (1987): *Proc. Natl. Acad. Sci.*, **84**: 8215-8219.
4. Mukhin, A.G. et al., (1989): *PNAS*, **86**: 9813-9816.
5. Olasmaa, M. et al., (1989): *Lancet*, **1**: 491-492.
6. Pritchett, D.B. and Seeburg, P.H., (1990): *J. Neurochem.*, **54**: 1802-1804.
7. Puia, G. et al.: *Neurons*, (in press).
8. Slobodiansky, E. et al., (1989): *J. Neurochem.*, **53**: 1276-1284.
9. Sprengel, R. et al., (1989): *J. Biol. Chem.*, **264**: 20415-20421.
10. Wojcik, W.J., Paez, X., and Ulivi, M. (1989): In *The Allosteric Modulation of Amino Acid Receptors and Its Therapeutic Implications*, E. Barnard and E. Costa, eds., pp. 173-193. Raven Press, New York.

PHARMACOLOGICAL PROFILES OF NON-BENZODIAZEPINE LIGANDS FOR CENTRAL BENZODIAZEPINE RECEPTORS

C.R. GARDNER
Roussel Laboratories, Kingfisher Drive, Covingham, Swindon, U.K.

There are several non-benzodiazepine (BDZ) chemical series which selectively interact with central BDZ receptors and contain molecules with a range of agonist-antagonist-inverse agonist efficacies. Perhaps the best known series is substituted ß-carboline-3-carboxylate esters with examples of full agonism (ZK 93423) equivalent to classical BDZs such as diazepam, differing degrees of partial agonism (ZK 91296>ZK 112119), virtual antagonism with little efficacy (ZK 93426), partial inverse agonism (ßCM>FG 7142>ßCE) and full inverse agonism (DMCM) (2,5). We have utilised the cyclopropyl ketone moiety as a stable ester replacement on position 3 (RU 33873, Fig.1). This compound is a long-lasting inverse agonist in vivo. RU 33873 potentiated leptazol seizures in mice (ED_{50} = 0.45 mg/kg i.p.), enhanced suprahyoid muscle twitching in urethane-anaesthetised rats (as do other strong inverse agonists) and induced some overt seizures alone at 10-20 mg/kg i.p. which were prevented by the BDZ antagonist flumazenil.

A series of imidazo(2,1-b)benzothiazoles (Fig.1) show high affinity for BDZ receptors and the 2-cyclopropyl ketone compound (RU 33782) also showed similar inverse agonist properties but did not induce seizures. Substitution of the benzene ring induced efficacy changes similar to those induced by the equivalent substitutions on ß-carbolines. For example, the 7-benzyloxy compound (RU 33894) did not potentiate leptazol seizures but weakly antagonised them (ED_{50} = 26 mg/kg i.p.), suggestive of partial agonism.

A large series of imidazoquinolines and imidazopyrimidines (Fig.1) has shown specific affinity for BDZ receptors and has yielded examples of near-full agonism (RU 31719), degrees of partial agonism (RU 33203>RU 32698>RU 32514), antagonism (RU 33094) and weak (RU 33697) or strong (RU 34000) partial inverse agonism (3,4). Some of these molecules show relatively low affinity for BDZ receptors in vitro (≥0.5 µM) but retain potency in a wide range of rodent tests in vivo. Kinetics studies with selected compounds suggest that the low affinity is compensated for by increased bioavailability.

Several other chemical series have high affinity for BDZ receptors but cover more restricted ranges of efficacy (see 2). Pyrazoloquinolines have examples of weak partial agonism (CGS 9896), weak partial inverse agonism (CGS 8216) and stronger partial inverse agonism (S-135). Two different series of quinoline derivatives show antagonism (RU 40410) and partial agonism (PK 8165, RU 39419). There are now cyclopyrrolones with partial agonist (RP 60503) as well as full agonist (zopiclone) properties (1). The imidazopyridine zolpidem and the triazolopyridazine CL 218872 appear to be respectively full and partial agonists with selectivity for the BDZ_1 receptor sub-type which may functionally correlate with a greater sedative effect

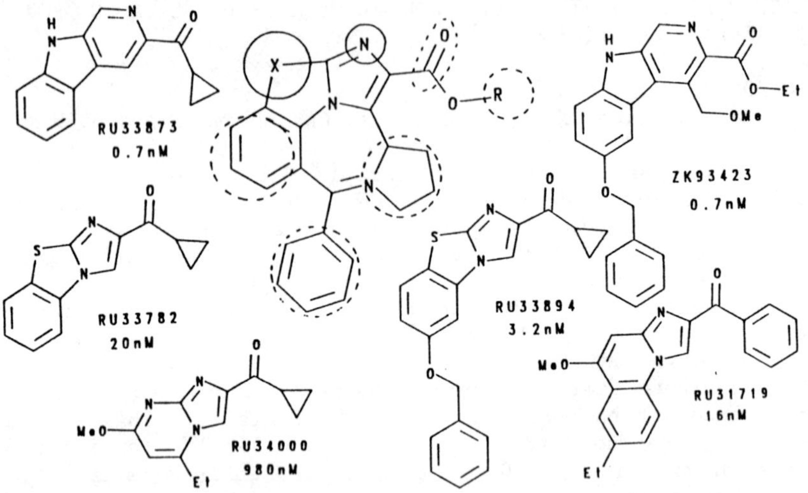

Fig. 1: Examples of non-BDZ ligands for BDZ receptors (agonists – right, inverse agonists – left) with IC$_{50}$ values for 3H-flunitrazepam binding. A pharmacophore for BDZ receptors (centre) shows areas affecting affinity (solid lines) and those also affecting efficacy (dashed lines).

superimposed on the classical BDZ profile. SR 95195, a positional isomer of CL 218872, shows inverse agonist properties.

By comparison of the structures of different series of ligands and structure-activity relationships within series, a pharmacophore has been proposed to account for the different efficacies of compounds from all these apparently diverse chemical structures (Fig.1). The proposed pharmacophore has been further tested by showing that the same chemical modifications of regions of each molecule that are proposed to interact with the same region of the receptor do induce similar changes in efficacy.

REFERENCES

1. Blanchard, J.C. et al.: Pharmacological profile of new cyclopyrrolones (59037RP - 60503RP): Partial agonists for benzodiazepine receptors. Psychopharmacol. 96 suppl: 219, 1988.
2. Gardner, C.R.: Functional in vivo correlates of the benzodiazepine agonist – inverse agonist continuum. Prog. Neurobiol. 31: 425-476, 1988.
3. Gardner, C.R.: Imidazoquinolines and pyrimidines: Benzodiazepine receptor ligands with different separations of anxiolytic and CNS depressant effects. Psychopharmacol. 96 suppl: 16, 1988.
4. Gardner, C.R.: Interpretation of the behavioural effects of benzodiazepine receptor ligands. Drugs Fut. 14: 51-67, 1989.
5. Stephens, D.N. et al.: Benzodiazepine receptor partial agonists: ß-carbolines. Psychopharmacol. 96 suppl: 16, 1988.

PHARMACOLOGICAL PROFILE OF A NOVEL BENZODIAZEPINE INVERSE AGONIST, S-135, AS A MEMORY ENHANCER

KAZUO KAWASAKI and AKIRA MATSUSHITA
Division of Pharmacology, Shionogi Res. Labs., Shionogi & Co., Ltd., 5-12-4 Sagisu, Fukushima-ku, Osaka 553, Japan.

There is a line of evidence suggesting that a benzodiazepine (BDZ) inverse agonist might be a new category of memory enhancing drugs different from nootropics; (1) BDZ agonists can cause dementia syndrome like that inhumans with senile dementia[2]. (2) The pharmacological action of pentylenetetrazol formerly prescribed for patients with senile dementia[5], is selectively potentiated by inverse agonists. (3) CGS8216, a partial inverse agonist, is reported to show a vigilance enhancing effect in humans[1]. (4) Release of acetylcholine is shown to be decreased by BDZ agonists[3]. Based on these findings we have tried to examine the pharmacological characteristics of several BDZ inverse agonists with different intrinsic activity including S-135, 85-0507, CGS8216 and β-carbolines, and to clarify the correlation between intrinsic activity as an inverse agonist and pharmacological effect as a memory enhancer.

Methods and Materials

The following pharmacological methods were used for characterizing several compounds as inverse agonists; proconvulsant activity test in combination with pentylenetetrazol in mice, crossed extensor reflex model in rats[4] and in vitro binding experiments which have been already published elsewhere[6]. Further evaluations were done in animals with impaired learning/memory process, which were produced by several agents (scopolamine, cycloheximide, CO_2 inhalation, diazepam, pentobarbital, a NMDA antagonist or electroconvulsive shock) or basal forebrain lesion. Water & radial maze and passive avoidance behavioral paradigms were used for detecting learning/memory function. Guinea-pig hippocampal slice preparations were used for examining effects of inverse agonists on the long termpotentiation (LTP). In intact animals, effects on EEG level and period of memory consolidation[7] were examined. The content of extracellular acetylcholine was measured in the hippocampus and cerebral cortex of rats. BDZ inverse agonists used here were S-135, CGS8216, β-carbolines (β-CCE, β-CCM, DMCM, FG7142) and 85-0507 (our novel imidazoquinoline derivative).

Results and Discussion

According to our methods the order of intrinsic activities of several inverse agonists examined here is as follows; DMCM > β-CCM > FG7142 > S-135 ≒ β-CCE > 85-0507 > CGS8216. In the passive avoidance behavioural paradigms of rats and mice, S-135 could improve learning/memory deficit elicited by scopolamine, cycloheximide, diazepam, pentobarbital, CO_2 inhalation or basal forebrain lesion but not that by a NMDA antagonist or electroconvulsive shock. S-135 was the most effective when it was administered before acquisition. In addition to improvement of some agents- or lesion-induced amnesia S-135 enhanced the memory consolidation in normal mice. S-135 alsoaugmented LTP in the hippocampal slices and this effect could be reduced by a NMDA antagonist. These results suggest that S-135 can positively influence the learning/memory process by acting on BDZ receptors. Our previous findings[6] demonstrate that uptake of 2-deoxyglucose in the hippocampus and cerebral cortex, which are closely related to learning/memory function, is increased by S-135 and conversely decreased by diazepam. In these two areas, EEG arousal was observed and also the extracellular concentration of acetylcholine was increased following S-135 suggesting activation of cholinergic function. In this sense, uptake of glucose is increased by S-135[6] in the basal magnocellular nucleus, which has cholinergic neurones innervating to the hippocampus and cerebral cortex, and they have an important role to regulate learning/memory function. It is suggested that S-135 can improve learning/memory impairment possibly by acting directly on the hippocampus and/or the cerebral cortex, or indirectly via acting on cholinergic neurones in the basal magnocellular nucleus.

In reserpine-induced hypomotility, tetrabenazine-induced ptosis and despair tests all inverse agonists tested here were effective. These pharmacological actions are characteristic of antidepressants.

EEG activation and an increase in the spontaneous motor activity could be observed after administration of all inverse agonists. These effects might be in accordance with vigilance enhancing effect of CGS8216 in humans[1]. Although spontaneous motor activity is increased by inverse agonists as well as amphetamine or caffeine, the pattern of increase is quite different. We have also obtained data that S-135 but not 85-507 can diminish ataxia or sleep produced by barbiturates.

In this paper we showed S-135 can improve dysfunction of learning/memory process in some animal models, and it also can prolong the periods of memory consolidation and augment LTP in the hippocampus. These results suggest that inverse agonists with intrinsic activity ($\geq$CGS8216 and $\leq \beta$-CCE)could be a new category of memory enhancing drug for senile dementia of Alzheimer type and could also be used as antidepressants with different characters from conventional antidepressants (tricyclic antidepressants ormonoamine oxidase inhibitors). We will discuss the possible correlation ofthe intrinsic activity and pharmacological activity of each inverse agonist as a memory enhancer, an antidepressant or a vigilance enhancer.

References

1. Bieck, P.R., (1984): Clin. Neuropharmacol., 7:Suppl. 1, 674.
2. Block, R.I. et al., (1985): Exp. Aging Res., 11:151-155.
3. Consolo, S. et al., (1975): In Mechanism of Action of Benzodiazepines, E. Costa and P. Greengard, eds., pp. 63, Raven Press, New york.
4. Kawasaki, K. and Matsushita, A., (1983): Jap. J. Pharmacol., 33:694-697.5.
   Leckman, J. et al., (1971): J. Clinical Pharmacol., 11:301-303.
6. Matsushita, A. et al., (1988): Prog. Neuro-Psychopharmacol. & Biol. Psychiat., 12:951-966.
7. Platel, A. and Porsolt, R.D., (1982): Psychopharmacol., 78:346-352.

SIGNIFICANCE OF GENETIC POLYMORPHISM AND SELECTIVE P450 INTERACTIONS IN PSYCHOPHARMACOLOGY

L.F. GRAM, K. BRØSEN, E. SKJELBO and S. SINDRUP
Department of Clinical Pharmacology, Institute of Medical Biology, Odense University, School of Medicine, Odense, DENMARK.

Pronounced interindividual variations in steady-state kinetics were described for the tricyclic antidepressants more than 20 years ago (1), and subsequently also for several neuroleptics. It was also shown nearly 20 years ago that neuroleptics are potent inhibitors of the oxidative metabolism of tricyclic antidepressants (2). Research within the last 10-15 years has revealed that these observations both are linked to the cytochrome P450 oxygenase of the liver.

DRUG OXIDATION, P450 ISOZYMES AND POLYMORPHISMS

The human liver P450 oxygenase is an assembly of isozymes, probably 30-60 different, with the same catalytic moiety but with different protein structure, resulting in a certain degree of substrate or regioselective oxidation of xenobiotics such as a variety of drugs. Within the last 10-12 years, it has been shown that at least two of the human liver P450 isozymes exhibit genetic polymorphism, i.e. a functional variability showing Mendelian inheritance with a bi- or trimodal distribution of phenotypes (3). These polymorphisms are named according to the substrates used to examine the oxidation via that particular P450 isozyme. For the sparteine/debrisoquine oxidation polymorphism (related to the isozyme P450IID6), 6-10% of European populations and 0.5-1% of East Asian populations oxidize the test substances extremely slowly (poor metabolizers, PM), whereas the remaining majority (extensive metabolizers, EM) have a much faster, although varying, rate of oxidation (3). Molecular studies have shown that there is a failing expression of the gene (isozyme) in sparteine/debrisoquine PM. For another polymorphism, related to a different P450 isozyme (P450IIC8), the mephenytoin oxidation polymorphism, the PM frequency is 2-3% in Europe and 20-25% in East Asia (3).

PSYCHOTROPIC DRUGS AND DRUG OXIDATION POLYMORPHISMS

All major classes of psychotropic drugs are predominantly eliminated by oxidation. For several tricyclic antidepressants (imipramine, desipramine, amitriptyline, nortriptyline, clomipramine) and some neuroleptics (perphenazine, thioridazine), it has been shown that the rate limiting hydroxylation is mediated via the sparteine/debrisoquine oxygenase. Sparteine PM thus have low clearance and develop very high steady-state levels on standard doses (4). For imipramine, our group has recently shown that the demethylation (leading to formation of desipramine) is partly mediated via the mephenytoin oxygenase (data to be published). Mephenytoin PM thus have a low ability to demethylate imipramine.

From a clinical point of view, the pharmacokinetic variability resulting from the sparteine/debrisoquine polymorphism, clearly exceeds the therapeutic index for both the tricyclic antidepressants and neuroleptics affected. Since clinical effect measurements are not suited for dose adjustments, phenotype testing might become an important supplement to or replacement for drug level monitoring.

The substrate selectivity of the sparteine/debrisoquine oxygenase points to specific and predictable drug-drug interactions. Besides the inhibitory effect of neuroleptics on hydroxylation of tricyclic antidepressants documented in several studies through the past 15-20 years (2,4), quinidine has been shown to be an extremely potent inhibitor of P450IID6, and recent reports suggest that some of the selective 5HT-reuptake inhibitors may also be both substrates and inhibitors of P450IID6.

REFERENCES

1. Gram, L.F. Metabolism of tricyclic antidepressants. A review. Dan. Med. Bull. 21:218-231, 1974.
2. Gram, L.F. and Fredricson Overø K. Drug Interaction: Inhibitory effect of neuroleptics on metabolism of tricyclic antidepressants in man. Br. Med. J.1:463-465, 1972.
3. Alvan, G., Balant, L.P, Bechtel, P. et al. (eds.). European Consensus Conference on Pharmacogenetics, Commission EEC, Luxembourg 1990, pp. 210.
4. Dahl, S.G. and Gram, L.F. (eds.). Clinical Pharmacology in Psychiatry. From Molecular Studies to Clinical Reality. Springer Verlag, Heidelberg 1989, pp. 330.

MONITORING NEUROLEPTIC DRUG LEVELS: TIME FOR INTRODUCTION INTO CLINICAL ROUTINE?

D.L. GARVER
Psychiatry and Behavioral Neurobiology, University of Alabama at Birmingham, Birmingham, AL, USA

A series of eleven prospective, predetermined fixed-dose studies relating neuroleptic drug level in plasma to antipsychotic response have been reported during the past decade. These studies delineate a generally consistent pattern with respect to the "left arm" of the plasma drug level-antipsychotic response relationship: increasing drug levels appear, within limits, to be associated with improving antipsychotic response. The effective drug level at which 50% of maximal response occurs can be estimated from these studies to be less than 0.2 ng/ml for fluphenazine, between 4 and 6 ng/ml for haloperidol, and about 1.0 ng/ml for thiothixene.

In contrast, a relatively inconsistent picture emerges with respect to response with higher levels of these high potency neuroleptic drugs. In attempting to evaluate this "right arm" of the plasma drug level-response relationship, two studies of patients receiving fluphenazine show diminished antipsychotic response at higher plasma fluphenazine levels. Three of six relevant studies with haloperidol similarly show diminished response at high haloperidol levels; the two remaining haloperidol studies suggest instead continued antipsychotic response at the higher haloperidol levels. One study designed to describe the upper portion of the thiothixene plasma level-response curve suggests continued response at high levels of thiothixene and active metabolites.

These studies relating plasma levels of neuroleptic to antipsychotic response are further confounded by the type of neuroleptic assay used. Some studies, using chemical assays, monitored only the parent neuroleptic; some studies included select metabolites. Other studies used neuroleptic radioreceptor binding assays, monitoring not only parent neuroleptic, but also active metabolites found in plasma. The results from the two different types of assays (chemical vs radioreceptor) have been found to yield fundamentally different "right arms" of the plasma neuroleptic level-response curve on the same patient populations: chemical assays often suggest diminished response at higher plasma neuroleptic levels, while radioreceptor assays suggest continued maximal antipsychotic response at highest total drug concentrations.

Several studies have also suggested that monitoring of neuroleptic drug concentrations in compartments other than in total plasma may provide the basis for clearer relationships of neuroleptic levels and response. In seven of eight such studies, superiority of free, cerebrospinal fluid (CSF) or erythrocyte concentrations of neuroleptic to that of simple total plasma neuroleptic levels in the same patients was documented. Variance between neuroleptic levels and antipsychotic response was reduced by 12.0% by the use of free, CSF or erythrocyte neuroleptic concentrations rather than plasma neuroleptic concentrations ($p < 0.04$).

Clearly, unresolved methodological difficulties in the choice of an assay (chemical or radioreceptor) and in the choice of tissue in which to measure the drug (total plasma vs. free, CSF or erythrocyte) confound our present day understanding of the relationship of neuroleptic drug levels to antipsychotic response. Even when such issues are resolved, we are left with uncertainty of whether such relationships (which have generally been defined within the first two to four weeks of neuroleptic treatment) also apply during neuroleptic treatment four or more weeks after drug initiation. No systematic studies have addressed the issue of whether such putative neuroleptic level-response relationships persist in the course of more chronic therapy. Preliminary data relevant to this problem suggest a progressively poorer relationship of drug level and response as time on neuroleptic is extended from two to four to six weeks.

Finally, it need be noted that no controlled studies adjusting dose of neuroleptic to achieve putative therapeutic ranges have been reported to date. That such adjustment could achieve therapeutic neuroleptic levels and that such therapeutic levels would improve antipsychotic response remains untested.

Though there is promise that drug level-response relationships can be clarified for some of the neuroleptic drugs, and additional promise that neuroleptic drug levels can be used as a guide for dose adjustment for optimal therapeutic response, there is presently no justification for routine clinical monitoring for dosage adjustment of any neuroleptic drug except for research purposes.

REFERENCES
1. Bigelow, L.B. et al. Absence of relationship of serum haloperidol concentration and clinical response in chronic schizophrenia: A fixed dose study. Psychopharm. Bull. 21:66-68, 1985.
2. Casper, R. et al. Phenothiazine levels in plasma and red blood cells. Arch. Gen. Psychiat. 37:301-305, 1980.
3. Cohen, B.M. et al. Neuroleptic blood levels and therapeutic effect. Psychopharmacology 70:191-193, 1980.
4. Dysken, M.W. et al. Fluphenazine pharmacokinetics and therapeutic response. Psychopharmacology 73:205-210, 1981.
5. Garver, D.L. Neuroleptic drug levels and antipsychotic effects: A difficult correlation; Potential advantage of free (or derivative) versus total plasma levels. J. Clin. Psychopharm. 9:277-281, 1989.
6. Linkowski, P. et al. Haloperidol plasma levels and clinical response in paranoid schizophrenics. Europ. Arch. Psychiat. Neurol. Sci. 234:231-236, 1984.
7. Mavroidis, M.L. et al. Fluphenazine plasma levels and clinical response. J. Clin. Psychiat. 45:370-373, 1984.
8. Mavriodis, M.L. et al. Clinical relevance of thiothixene plasma levels. J. Clin. Psychopharm. 155-157, 1984.
9. Mavroidis, M.L. et al. Clinical response and plasma haloperidol levels in schizophrenia. Psychopharmacology 81:354-356, 1983.
10. Potkin, S.G. et al. Does a therapeutic window for plasma haloperidol exist? Preliminary Chinese data. Psychopharm. Bull. 24:59-61, 1985.
11. Smith, R.C. et al. Haloperidol and thioridazine drug levels and clinical response in schizophrenia: Comparison of gas-liquid chromatography and radioreceptor assays. Psychopharm. Bull. 21:52-59, 1985.
12. Smith, R.C. et al. Haloperidol plasma levels and prolactin response as predictors of clinical improvement in schizophrenia: chemical vs. radioreceptor plasma level assay. Arch. Gen. Psychiat. 41:1044-1049, 1984.
13. Tang, S.W. et al. Total and free plasma neuroleptic levels in schizophrenic patients. Psychiatry Res. 13:285-93, 1984.
14. VanPutten, T. et al. Plasma levels of thiothixene by radioreceptor assay: Clinical usefulness. Psychopharmacology 79:40-44, 1983.
15. VanPutten, T. et al. Plasma levels of haloperidol and clinical response. Psychopharm. Bull. 21:69-72, 1985.
16. Wistedt, B. et al. Plasma haloperidol levels and clinical response in acute schizophrenia. Nord. Psykiat. Tids. 9-13, 1984.
17. Wode-Helgodt, B. et al. Clinical effects and drug concentrations in plasma and cerebrospinal fluid in psychiatric patients treated with fixed doses of chlorpromazine. Acta. Psychiatr. Scand. 58:149-173, 1978.

PREDICTING THERAPEUTIC OUTCOME FROM EARLY PHARMACOKINETIC MEASUREMENTS OF NEUROLEPTICS

W. GAEBEL, B. MÜLLER-OERLINGHAUSEN and J. SCHLEY
Psychiatrische Klinik und Poliklinik der Freien Universität Berlin, Eschenallee 3, D-1000 Berlin 19, FRG

Findings on the relationship between steady-state neuroleptic blood levels and treatment outcome are controversial: Linear, curvilinear and no relationships have been reported (5). Given a systematic relationship between blood levels and pharmacodynamics, early pharmacokinetic measurements from test dose approaches should be helpful in clinical decision-making concerning the right drug/dose for the right patient. From own previous research (2) we aimed at replicating our finding, that pharmacokinetic differences after a single test dose of perazine are predictive of treatment outcome after 28 days of oral drug administration in schizophrenia.

SUBJECT AND METHOD

Thirty-six acutely admitted schizophrenics (ICD-9) were included in a 28-day open treatment study with perazine. 2/3 of the sample were male, mean age was 30,4 (19-65) years, mean weight was 69,5 (50-150) kg, age at illness onset was 23,7 (14-36) years, 31% were first admissions. An oral test dose (TD) of perazine (150mg) was given after washout at the beginning of the study. Treatment response after 28 days was defined as a minimum 66% decrease of the initial schizophrenia-specific score (thought disturbance, activation, hostile suspiciousness) of the BPRS (3). Blood (serum) levels of parent drug (PER) and its main (inactive) metabolite desmethylperazine (DMP) were assessed 2 hours after TD (peak level) by TLC.

RESULTS

20 (56%) of the patients were responders (R), 16 (44%) were non-responders (NR). After correcting for extreme values (box-plots), the following results were obtained from a 2x2-ANCOVA (Table 1). The covariate weight did not contribute significantly to the overall results. Although NR-women had the highest PER-levels (45,8 ng/ml), for PER there was only a significant main effect for sex, but no sex x response interaction as in our previous study (2). For DMP however, a significant response effect was obtained according to our previous findings, whereas the quotient DMP/PER again was not significantly related to treatment outcome. The correlation between PER and DMP was $r=.72$, $p=.001$.

TABLE 1: 2x2 ANCOVA (WEIGHT, SEX x RESPONSE) FOR PER, DMP AND DMP/PER

	PER* MEAN (ng/ml)	F	p	DMP** MEAN (ng/ml)	F	p	DMP/PER*** MEAN	F	p
R	22.3	0.6	.46	4.8	4.6	.04	0.2	1.3	.26
NR	25.6			9.3			0.3		
MALE	17.0	5.0	.03	6.5	0.1	.80	0.3	4.0	.06
FEMALE	36.2			7.8			0.1		

*N=34 **N=35 ***N=33

DISCUSSION

The results replicate in part our previous findings. Accordingly, clinical response takes place in R despite of their either equal or even lower early blood levels of parent drug compared to NR. This underlines the importance of a responder-specific sensitivity to drugs (6), if differences in protein-binding between R and NR are ruled out. However, this interpretation relies on the predictive validity of early peak blood levels concerning steady-state blood levels (1). On the other hand, the higher level of the (inactive) metabolite DMP in NR reveals, that altered drug metabolism could be a possible reason for clinical nonresponse (4). For sex, however, despite of being an intervening variable in the relationship between metabolite (DMP) and parent drug (PER), a reliable impact on drug response via early pharmacokinetics could not be confirmed.

REFERENCES

1. Davis, et al. (1974): In Phenothiazines and structurally related drugs, J.S. Forrest, C.J. Carr and E. Usdin, eds., pp., 433-443, Raven Press, New York.

2. Gaebel, et al. (1988): Pharmacopsychiatry, 21: 384-386.

3. Overall, J.E., and Gorham, D.R. (1962): Psychol. Rep., 10: 799-603.

4. Sakurai, et al. (1980): Arch. Gen. Psychiat., 37: 1057-1062.

5. Simpson, G.M., and Yadalam, K. (1985): J. Clin. Psychiatry, 46: 22-28.

6. VanPutten et al. (1981): Psychol. Med., 11: 729-734.

THERAPEUTIC DRUG MONITORING OF ANTIDEPRESSANTS IN PRACTICE

Sheldon H. Preskorn, M.D.
Psychiatric Research Institute, Department of Psychiatry, University of Kansas School of Medicine and Veterans Affairs Medical Center, Wichita KS.

There are five major reasons for employing TDM: (1) to assess compliance, (2) to improve efficacy, (3) to guard against toxicity, (4) to reduce cost, and (5) to avoid medical-legal problems. There are seven factors which determine whether TDM will offer any advantage over dose titration based on response: (1) small therapeutic index, (2) large interindividual variability in metabolism, (3) delayed onset of action, (4) difficult early determination of efficacy, (5) difficult early detection of toxicity, (6) serious toxicity concerns, and (7) well-defined concentration: response relationships with regard to beneficial and toxic effects.

The number and diversity of medications with proven antidepressant properties has expanded such that a single statement about the value of therapeutic drug monitoring (TDM) cannot be made. Instead, recommendations must be made for each class as defined by structure, mechanism, and pharmacology: (a) tricyclic antidepressants (TCAs), (b) phenylproplyamides (e.g., fluoxetine), (c) triazolopyridines (e.g., trazodone), (d) aminoketones (e.g., bupropion), (e) monoamine oxidase inhibitors (MAOIs), and (f) azapirones (e.g., buspirone).

TRICYCLIC ANTIDEPRESSANTS (TCAs)

While the early research effort on TDM of TCAs focused on antidepressant efficacy, the value is as much with avoidance of toxicity as with improving efficacy. Generally, antidepressant response is poor below a minimum TCA plasma level threshold of 100 ng/ml and begins to plateau by an upper threshold of 300 ng/ml (nortriptyline is an exception having an optimal range of 50 to 150 ng/ml). Above 300 and 450 ng/ml respectively, there is a 13-fold and a 37-fold increase in the risk of TCA-induced delirium relative to the risk within the therapeutic range. Unfortunately, the prodrome of the delirium can present as a worsening of the depressive disorder leading the clinician to either increase the dose or add another medication (e.g., neuroleptic). Both of these steps will increase the toxicity. Above 1000 ng/ml, patients routinely develop slowing of intracardiac conduction which can lead to arrhythmias and sudden death. Due to the large intraindividual variability in TCA elimination rates, subtherapeutic, therapeutic, and toxic TCA plasma levels will occur in different patients receiving the same dose of the same TCAs. The only way to determine the optimal dose for a given patient is to measure the TCA plasma level.

PHENYLPROPLYAMIDES (e.g., fluoxetine)

Fluoxetine is the only representative of this class currently marketed. TDM of fluoxetine is unlikely to be clinically helpful because: (a) the apparent wide safety margin, and (b) the absence of a dose-response curve for antidepressant efficacy. Although the database is limited, two studies have failed to show a relationship between antidepressant efficacy and plasma levels of fluoxetine and/or desmethlyfluoxetine.

TRIAZOLOPYRIDINES (e.g.,trazodone)

Like fluoxetine, the known pharmacology and the available but limited database suggest that TDM has limited value with this class of medication. Trazodone has a wide safety margin. Its short half-life also makes TDM studies difficult.

AMINOKETONES (e.g.,bupropion)

There is both efficacy and toxicity reasons to suspect that TDM of bupropion and its metabolites will have clinical utility. First, plasma levels of bupropion and metabolites have been correlated to antidepressant response. In two studies (n=61 and 15), maximum response was observed at bupropion plasma levels of 50-100 ng/ml. Unfortunately, these studies did not measure plasma levels of the metabolites which under state conditions can be several times higher than the parent drug. In a subsequent study, Golden and colleagues found that high plasma levels of the metabolites were associated with poorer outcome. Finally, several lines of evidence suggest that seizure risk may be a function of plasma levels of bupropion and/or its metabolites: (a) seizure risk is a function of daily dose, (b) most seizures occur within a few hours of taking a dose, (c) seizures most often occur shortly after a dose increase, and (d) anorexic/bulimics with lean body mass appear to have an increased seizure risk relative to patients with other psychiatric diagnoses.

MONOAMINE OXIDASE INHIBITORS

While TDM of MAOI plasma levels has not been extensively studied, researchers have looked at the relationship between the degree of MAO inhibition and antidepressant response. These studies have primarily focused on the platelet as a model to infer the degree of brain MAO inhibition achieved during MAOI therapy. Unfortunately, there is evidence that the brain and platelet MAO activity are not correlated one to one. Yet, studies have suggested that optimal antidepressant response occurs when there is at least 80% inhibition of basal platelet MAO activity.

AZAPIRONES (e.g., buspirone)

Currently, buspirone is the only marketed azapirone and is approved only for the treatment of anxiety disorders. However, there are ongoing clinical trial programs with buspirone and several other azapirone to establish whether they have antidepressant properties. Preliminary results appear promising. Like fluoxetine and trazodone, the known pharmacology of these medications (i.e., wide safety margin and short half-life) suggest that TDM will have limited value.

References are available on request.

THE ROLE OF PHARMACOKINETICS AND DRUG LEVEL MONITORING IN THE CLINICAL DEVELOPMENT OF NEW PSYCHOTROPIC DRUGS

Paolo Lucio MORSELLI
Department of Clinical Research, Synthelabo Recherche, Paris 75013, France

The development of basic pharmacokinetics has led to an improved understanding of the pharmacodynamic profile of many therapeutic agents, the development of human pharmacokinetics has contributed to rationalize the therapeutic approach and to optimize the therapeutic potential of many drugs thus permitting a better benefit/risk ratio. Considering the different phases of development of new drugs, pharmacokinetics had and still have a very important role to play.

- The evaluation of the safety of the new drug by determining the maximum tolerated dose after single increasing dose and during repeated administrations for at least 2 to 4 weeks.

- The characterization of the pharmacokinetic profile of the new drug after single and repeated doses.

- The definition of the possible existence of a dose/response curve for pharmacodynamic events as well as of the relationships between doses, concentrations and effects.

- The definition of the pharmacokinetic profile in volunteers together with the above mentioned parameters is of a paramount importance for a correct choice of the dose and of the dosing intervals in patients.

In fact over the last 20 years, kinetic studies in healthy volunteers have been one of the pivotal moment in the dynamic process of discoveries and acquisition of new information. It is well known that different physiological and psychological conditions may have a significant effect on either drug kinetics or receptor sensitivity.

Since the final response depends on the mutual interactions between these two main variables, being impossible to know a priori the receptor status, we should try to acquire at least some information on other variables : drug's concentrations and disposition rates. Furthermore age related differences in drug responses have frequently a pharmacokinetic basis and an extensive pharmacokinetic information may avoid later the occurence of toxic effects.

Drug level monitoring during Phase II and III controlled studies is also very useful because on the one hand it permits an objective evaluation of the patient's compliance and it may help in explaining anomalous results, and on the other hand it may permit the identification of therapeutic and toxic tresholds.

During late Phase III open label trials, the monitoring of drug blood concentrations may again be very useful in assessing compliance, in identifying possible pharmacokinetic drug interactions and in understanding paradoxical responses.

Regular drug monitoring during intermediate and long term studies may be very helpful for the assessment of possible tachiphylaxis phenomena.

In conclusion the definition of the pharmacokinetic profile of new therapeutic agents during drug development as well as the monitoring of drug concentrations in biological fluids are hence a very necessary step towards a better definition of the new drug therapeutic potential. They also permit a more rational utilization of the new drug leading to an improved benefit/risk ratio.

FUTURE UTILIZATION OF PHARMACOKINETIC INFORMATION IN PSYCHIATRY

B.MÜLLER-OERLINGHAUSEN
Dept.of Psychiatry,Laboratory of Clinical Psychopharmacology,
Free University of Berlin,Berlin(West),Germany

Although a vast body of information exists on the pharmacokinetics of psychotropic drugs the everyday therapeutic practice in psychiatry appears not to be guided essentially by sound clinical-pharmacological principles.Cases of fatalities related to inadvertent overdosing of psychiatric patients and sometimes resulting into malpractice suits illustrate this situation.(Preskorn,1989;Müller-Oerlinghausen,unpublished findings)Negative attitudes towards the clinical significance of individual pharmacokinetic data are partly due to the fact that the scientific discussion for a long time had centered exclusively on the potential relationship between blood drug levels and therapeutic efficacy. Furthermore,clinicians are not always sufficiently aware of the many difficulties and pitfalls in interpreting data on blood levels of neuroleptics or antidepressants.It has also been emphasized by several authors that e.g. in the area of neuroletic treatment no clear-cut dosage-effect relationships seem to exist.(Baldessarini and Davis,1980),which might possibly due to a curvilinear correlation between drug blood level and the occupancy of dopamine receptors.(Farde et.al.,1988).In the future further PET studies will probably help us to a better understanding,how dose,concentration in the central compartment,and effect are connected to each other,- at least as regards classical neuroleptic compounds. Hopefully,they may also shed more light on the clinical significance of the inter-and intraindividually varying metabolic patterns of neuroleptic drugs,e.g.if administered as either oral or sustained -release preparations.The consideration of chronopharmaco-dynamic and-kinetic aspects of psychotropic drug administration(ref.Nakano,1989) may also allow us to understand and control more satisfactorily the still puzzling variability of drug response in psychiatric patients.

However,even if a "therapeutic window"can not be defined with sufficient certainty for various drugs,the intelligent use of pharmacokinetic information can definitely increase the safety of drug treatment in psychiatry.This aspect will gain particular importance in various risk populations,such as elderly,possibly treatment-refractory,depressed patients with a high probability of multimorbidity,long-term medication, and polypharmacy including the combined use of antidepressants and neuroleptics.E.g.,recent findings by AMÜP-a national collaborative drug surveillance project on more than 10,000 patients-demonstrated a sixfold increased risk of toxic delirium in elderly psychiatric patients;on the other hand,several authors have shown a relationship between the occurrence of toxic delirium and high blood levels of tricyclic antidepressants.(Ref.Preskorn,1989)

Efforts should be taken to improve the general knowledge of psychiatrists on the pharmacokinetics of their most important therapeutic tools. Only against a background of improved professional competence will the assessment of more sophisticated parameters such as the genetic metabolizer phenotype,linear/nonlinear kinetics,metabolic ratios,protein binding or alpha1-acid glycoprotein concentration etc.result into a truly optimized pharmacotherapy,i.e. maximal therapeutic efficacy combined with the lowest possible risk of adverse drug reactions.Better training in clinical pharmacology and/or close cooperation with clinical pharmacologists are,therefore,required in clinical psychiatry as in other medical disciplines.

REFERENCES

Baldessarini,R.J.,and Davis,J.M.(1980):Psychiatry Res.,3:115-122
Farde,L.,et.al.(1988):Arch.Gen.Psychiat.,5:71-76
Nakano,S.(1989):InChronopharmacology.Cellular and biochemical interactions. B.Lemmer,ed.,pp267-280.Marcel Dekker,Inc.,New York,Basel.
Preskorn,S.H.,(1989): In Clinical Pharmacology in Psychiatry.From molecular studies to clinical reality,S.G.Dahl and L.F.Gram,eds.,pp.237-243. Springer-Verlag,Berlin,Heidelberg,New York

ASPECTS OF ANIMAL EXPERIMENTS FOR EVALUATION OF COGNITIVE ENHANCERS

H. Kuribara and S. Tadokoro
Division for Behavior Analysis, Behavior Research Institute, Gunma University School of Medicine, Maebashi 371, Japan

Cognitive function is considered to include mainly learning and memory processes. Although many behavioral procedures have been applied to study the cognitive function of animals, and to evaluate drugs that may enhance the cognition, there is no standard method for these purposes. Here, we would like to point out several problems in the animal experiments, particularly regarding passive avoidance response as a sample, for the estimation of cognitive function in rodents, and in the preclinical evaluation of the cognitive enhancers.

When an animal is put into a novel situation, it may exhibit behavioral changes. The changes are commonly considered to reflect cognition for an adaptation to the situation. However, since the behavior is a final product of the complicated interaction between the whole body and the experimental conditions, cognition as well as many other factors affect the behavior as shown in Tabel 1. The performance observed is extremely diverse depending on the conditions of both animal and experimental sides.

Table 1. Factors that may affect animal behaviors.

Animal side	Ability of cognition Species, strains and colony differences Breeding condition Antecedent operation Sensory function Motility Motivation Emotionality etc
Experimental side	Apparatus Type of behavior Task, and its training schedule Type of stimulus, and its intensity Data analysis etc

One of the typical samples is the results in Mongolian gerbils. Mongolian gerbils demonstrate extremely pooer performance than mice and rats in the passive avoidance situation, requiring a number of trainings to reach a critical level of latency time, and showing a fractuation in the latency time in the retention sessions (1). In contrast, Mongolian gerbils show the best performance in the discrete avoidance situation among them (2, 3). Thus, the result obtained from a single test is probably insufficient in rodents to estimate the cognitive function. It is also important to study the correlation between the results obtained from the multiple tests.

For a purpose of preclinical evaluation of cognitive enhancers, a certain treatment including chamical, surgical and physical operations, or aging is generally applied to induce impairment of the brain function. Scopolamine, for an instance, has been frequently used as a typical chemical that disturbs the passive avoidance response in rodents. In fact, when up to 0.5 mg/kg of scopolamine is administered before the training session, it increases the number of trainings to reach a critical level of latency time in the acquisition session. Such the treatment also shortens the response latency time when the performance is observed 24 hr or later after the training. In contrast, the same doses of scopolamine hardly shorten the response latency when it is administered immediately after the training, or before the retention session. A similar result is commonly produced by various drugs such as general depressants, anxiolytics etc. Furthermore, a clear relationship can not be confirmed between the disturbed performance and the histopathological or biochemical changes in the brain. Thus, a confirmation is always necessary whether the behavioral change is induced specifically by the alteration in the cognition.

In an animal experiment for evaluation of cognitive enhancers, the test drug has sometimes been administered just before the brain treatment which may disturb the performance. However, the results obtained from such the procedure may reflect a protective effect of the drug on the brain dysfunction, and may be inappropriate to estimate the effect on the cognitive function. It is rather required to administer the test drug to the animals that have been comfirmed to exhibit a long-lasting and spontaneously irreversible disturbance of the performance. If the disturbed performances are improved in the multiple tests, the drug is expected as a cognitive enhancer. The time relation between the brain treatment and drug administration is also a basic factor in the preclinical evaluation of cognitive enhancers.

REFERENCES

1. Tadokoro, S. et al. Methodological problems on learning and memory tests in rodents from the view points of behavioral toxicology. In Fujii, T. and Adams, P.M. (Eds.), Functional Teratogenesis: Functional Effects on the Offspring after Parental Drug Exposure. Teikyo University Press, Tokyo, pp. 53-67, 1987.
2. Kuribara, H. and Tadokoro, S. Effects of psychotropic drugs on conditioned avoidance response in Mongolian gerbils (Meriones unguiculatus): Comparison with Wistar rats and dd mice. Pharmacol. Biochem. Behav. 23: 1013-1018, 1984.
3. Umezu, T. et al. Acquisition process and effects of psychoactive drugs on discrete shuttle avoidance response in Mongolian gerbils (Meriones unguiculatus). Japan. J. Pharmacol. 47: 245-252, 1988.

COWORKERS: T. Umezu, S. Fujiwara, T. Saito, H. Yasuda, Y. Hiraga

LONG TERM TREATMENT WITH ACETYL-L-CARNITINE REDUCES AGE-DEPENDENT IMPAIRMENT OF COGNITION

L. ANGELUCCI*, O. GHIRARDI**, M.T. RAMACCI** and A. IMPERATO*
Farmacologia 2a*, Faculty of Medicine, University of Rome "La Sapienza"
Institute for Research on Senescence**, Sigma Tau, Pomezia, Italy.

Acetyl-l-carnitine (ALCAR) is the acetylic derivative of L-carnitine, a natural substance that acts as a carrier of fatty acids across the inner mitochondrial membrane for subsequent β-oxidation. Many reports support the hypothesis that ALCAR is likely to have an action in energy-producing reactions as well as in complex biochemical reactions related to the structural function of the phospholipid component, this being especially true in the central nervous system. Because ALCAR and the enzymes that take part in its biosynthesis are present in several brain areas, ALCAR has been assumed to fulfil a regulating role of neuronal transmission. ALCAR crosses the blood-brain barrier and exerts central cholinergic effects, increasing the amplitude of evoked potentials. An ACh/ALCAR relationship has been observed "in vitro" where ALCAR increases the ACh formation.

Our group in Rome has carried out studies of the effects of long term treatments with ALCAR in various strains of rats; here we report the results on some cognitive activities and their putative cholinergic counterparts, both of which are age-dependently impaired.

ALCAR AND COGNITIVE FUNCTIONS IN THE AGED RAT

Aging in the rat is characterized by specific deficits in learning and memory, quite similar to those producible by experimental hippocampal lesions in young rats, evidenced by procedures of discrimination, as well as by performance in spatial orientation tasks. These cognitive deficits are strongly reminiscent of those occurring in patients with senile dementia of the Alzheimer type. Female Wistar rats 16 months old, treated with ALCAR (75 mg/kg/day in drinking water) for 110 days, compared with age matched controls, exhibited a higher capacity of discrimination learning in a test in which food reinforcement was given to lever pressing in presence of a light on. Similarly treated animals, compared with their controls, showed a better performance in a temporal discrimination test (DRL-6sec), consisting in the faster acquiring of a number of non rewarded responses lower than the rewarded ones, and lower than the non rewarded responses in controls.

Sixty-six 18 month old male Sprague Dawley rats were classified by means of the cluster analysis in two groups: "good" (71 per cent) and "poor" (29 per cent) performers in the Morris water maze, and half of each group were randomly assigned to an 8 month treatment with ALCAR

(100 mg/kg/day in drinking water), the other half acting as control. At the age of 24 months the surviving animals free of pathologies were retested in the maze. "Poor" performers treated with ALCAR exhibited an enrichment in their learning higher than "poor" performers control, reaching a level equivalent to that of "good" performers in which the improving effect of ALCAR treatment was less marked compared with "poor" performers. Sixty per cent of all rats maintained their characteristic as "good" or "poor" passing from the selection to the retesting; however any worsening in performance occurred only in the control population.

Because poor learning of light discrimination, temporal discrimination and spatial orientation task in aged rats is to be attributed to attentional deficit, perseveration phenomenon and inability in utilization of external cues, respectively, which are typical of impairments of the hippocampal function and of cholinergic systems, the benefit of ALCAR treatment might be ascribed to the preservation of this function against the degenerative process of normal aging.

ALCAR AND THE CHOLINERGIC ACTIVITY IN THE HIPPOCAMPUS OF THE AGED RAT

Age-dependent changes in the cholinergic innervation of the hippocampus while very modest with regard to ACh and Ch-acetylase concentrations, mostly consist, functionally, in a great reduction in basal and stimulated release of ACh, and, anatomically, in an increase in muscarinic M_1 and a decrease in M_2 receptors. These impairments are reminiscent of the cholinergic impairment described in senile dementia of the Alzheimer type, to which are ascribed the cognitive deficits quintessential in this pathology. The effect of long term treatment with ALCAR (75 mg/kg/day in drinking water) for six months in Wistar, Sprague-Dawley and Fischer 344 rats, aged 24-30 months, was evaluated from the point of view of the responsiveness of the cholinergic synapsis to pharmacological stimuli, with transcerebral microdialysis in the freely moving animal. Compared with age-matched controls, in treated animals, exhibiting a greater basal release of ACh, a greater increase in ACh release was produced by the M receptor blocker atropine as well by the M_1 blocker pirenzepine. This indicates that ALCAR might reduce the age-dependent loss of M receptors, which is in fitting with the finding that long term treatment with ALCAR has a sparing effect on hippocampal pyramidal cells. Even more likely, ALCAR, because of its role in metabolism might preserve the chemical requisites of the synaptic membrane.

Data obtained in the above experimentation are supportive of a study of the effects of long term ALCAR treatment in pathological or age-dependent conditions characterized by cognitive impairment.

PHARMACO-EEG AND BRAIN MAPPING IN COGNITIVE ENHANCING DRUGS

B. SALETU, J. GRÜNBERGER, P. ANDERER
Department of Psychiatry, School of Medicine, University of Vienna, Austria

Normal and – even more so – pathological aging is neurophysiologically characterized by an increase of delta/theta activity and of superimposed fast activities, a decrease of alpha-activity as well as by a slowing of the centroid of the total EEG activity (1). These alterations may be due to deficits in the vigilance-regulatory systems. According to Head vigilance is defined as the availability and grade of organization of man's adaptability, which in turn is dependent on the dynamic state of the neuronal network. The latter can be measured objectively and quantitatively by the EEG. Disturbance of vigilance may be regarded as the "common pathway" in the pathogenesis of dementias of different etiologies. It may be hypothesized that nootropic treatment should induce oppositional changes in brain function as found during aging. Indeed, in the last 2 decades we demonstrated that cognition enhancing drugs produce exactly such vigilance-promoting changes (1).

METHODS

In acute and subacute human gerontopsychopharmacological studies 10 - 20 elderly normal healthy subjects in the age range of 60 - 80 years were included in double-blind, placebo-controlled, cross-over studies. They usually received in random order placebo, 3 doses of an experimental drug and a reference compound. Pharmaco-EEG and brain mapping as well as psychometric tests measuring noopsychic, thymopsychic and psychophysiological variables were carried out before as well as 1, 2, 4, 6 and 8 hours post drug administration (2).

Therapeutic studies involved patients with dementias of different etiologies (SDAT, MID, alcoholic and uremic OPS). In studies concerning brain protective effects against an experimentally-induced hypoxic hypoxidosis normal healthy young volunteers were included.

RESULTS

Cognition enhancing drugs produced in various double-blind, placebo-controlled pharmaco-EEG and brain mapping studies significant changes in brain function of elderlies

(1). They were characterized by a decrease of slow activities, increase of alpha or alpha adjacent/beta activities, an acceleration of the centroid of the slow activities as well of the centroid of the total power spectrum and eventually an augmentation of total power. These neurophysiological findings indicate an improvement of vigilance.

Such changes were found after representatives of co-dergocrine-type compounds (CDM, nicergoline), piracetam-type compounds (piracetam, etiracetam, aniracetam, tenilsetam); vincamine-type compounds (vincamine, vinconate, SL76100, SL76188); cholinergic compounds (DUP 996); alpha-adrenergic agonists (adrafinil, modafinil); vasodilators and hemorheological agents (buflomedil, cinnarizine, ifenprodil, tinofedrine, hexobendine and its combination with ethophylline and ethamivan - Instenon forte[R]); antianoxic agents like Duxil[R] (an almitrine/raubasine combination); vitamin-type compounds (xantinol-nicotinate, pyritinol); antidepressants (fluvoxamine, fluoxetine, moclobemid) and Actovegin[R], a standardized deprotenized hemoderivative as well as the anticonvulsant milacemide. The neurophysiological alterations were associated with improvement of noopsychic and partly also of thymopsychic variables.

Searching for a model to proof brain protection of antihypoxidotics in humans, an experimentally-induced cerebral hypoxic hypoxidoses was utilized whereby we could demonstrate that effective antihypoxidotic/nootropic drugs can attenuate the deterioration in vigilance. Brain protective qualities were also substantiated at the behavioral level as psychometric deterioration during hypoxia was dose dependently attenuated.

Finally, in several therapeutic studies we demonstrated that treatment of dementias of different etiologies with cognition enhancing drugs can lead to improvement of psychopathology and psychometric performance which is based on improvement of vigilance as reflected in pharmaco-EEG and EEG-brain mapping. Drugs investigated in such manner include nicergoline, xantinol-nicotinate, piridoxilate, EMD 21657 (a piritinol derivative), modafinil and oxiracetam.

REFERENCES
1. Saletu, B. (1989): Mod.Probl. Pharmacopsychiatry, 23: 43-55; 2. Saletu, B. et al. (1987): Meth.Find.expl.clin. Pharmacol., 9: 385-408;

NEW CHOLINESTERASE INHIBITORS FOR TREATMENT OF ALZHEIMER DISEASE

EZIO GIACOBINI[1] AND ROBERT BECKER[2]
Depts. [1]Pharmacology and [2]Psychiatry, Southern Illinois University School of Medicine, Springfield, IL 62794-9230 USA

An ideal cholinesterase inhibitors (ChEI) suitable for symptomatic treatment of memory and cognitive impairment should satisfy the following requirements: a) produce a long-term acetylcholinesterase (AChE) inhibition in brain with a steady-state of increased cortical acetylcholine (ACh); b) not inhibit ACh synthesis or release in nerve endings; c) and produce only mild side effects at therapeutic doses (1). Based on our experimental results in animals we have proposed two new ChEI for experimental therapy of Alzheimer Disease (AD), heptyl-physostigmine (heptyl-Phy) (Fig. 1A), a physostigmine (Phy) derivative, and metrifonate (MTF) (Fig. 1B), a slow release formulation (1).

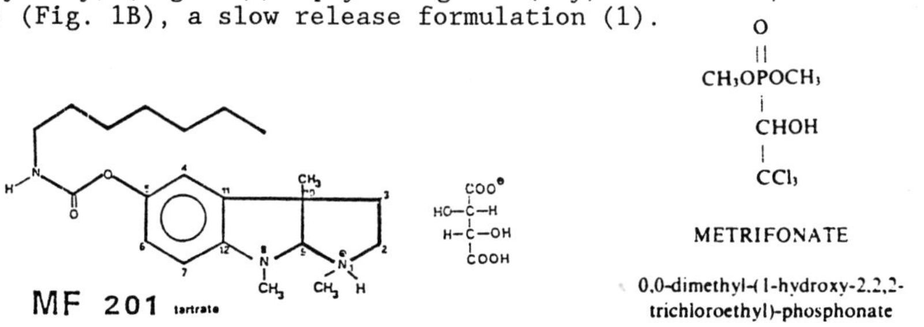

FIG. 1: Chemical structure of heptyl-physostigmine [(MF-201, heptastigmine) Mediolanum Farm., Milan, Italy] (A) and metrifonate (B).

a. <u>Metrifonate</u>. Metrifonate (Fig. 1B) is an organophosphorus ChEI with a duration of inhibition of brain cholinesterase (ChE) four times longer than Phy (1). In contrast to Phy it is not a directly acting inhibitor of ChE but requires non-enzymatic metabolism to form the active compound, dichlorvos (2,2-dichlorovinyl dimethyl phosphate). The maximal concentration of the active drug which reaches the brain is only around 2%. This is a safety mechanism that, together with the slow reversibility of inhibition, explains the long-lasting effect and the minimal adverse effects. Becker et al. (2) performed a study of a multiple dose trial of MTF over a prolonged period of time in humans. They administered MTF to 20 AD patients. Patients were given, under open conditions, single oral doses of MTF, 2.5, 5, 7.5 and 15 mg/kg/week. A statistically significant improvement in the AD Assessment Scale (ADAS) scores was observed with the 5 mg/kg/week dose. Maximal improvement on the ADAS was associated with a mean 55.9% (± 12.6% standard deviation) activity level of red blood cell (RBC) AChE. Over 80% inhibition of plasma and RBC ChE was achieved with only minor side effects (Table I). Cholinesterase inhibition in the CSF of two patients was 37% and 47.5%, 24 hrs after a second dose of 5 mg/kg/week of MTF separated by 7 days from the first dose.

Table I: Comparison of Clinical Trials of Four ChEI on AD Patients and Normal Volunteers (V)

Drug	Route	Dose (mg/kg)	% Plasma BuChE Inhib. (60 min)	% CSF AChE Inhib.	Side Effects	n	Subjects
Phy	oral	.06	24	--	++	12	AD
	i.v.	.01-.02	12-25	--	+++	20	AD
	i.c.v.	.001	5	85 (60 min)	0	3	AD
Heptyl-Phy	oral	.6	40	--	(+)	10	V
THA	oral	.4-3	25-30	--	+++	18	AD
MTF	oral	2.5-5	32-80	37-47 (24 hrs)	(+)	20	AD

b. <u>Analogues of Physostigmine</u>. The heptyl-physostigmine (heptyl-Phy) (C8) - derivative (Fig. 1A), produces an increase of ACh levels in brain and behavioral modifications suggesting a possible therapeutic use. The toxicity (LD_{50}) of heptyl-Phy (35 mg/kg) is about 60 times lower than that of Phy (0.6 mg/kg).

In human volunteers, 40 mg of a single oral dose of heptyl-Phy produced 40% plasma butyrylcholinesterase (BuChE) inhibition at 1 hr and 17.7% at 6 hrs (Table I). Red blood cell AChE was 46% and 30% inhibited at the same time points (3). No side effects were recorded. The results suggest that heptyl-Phy produces different duration of effects on AChE and BuChE. This could explain the low level of peripheral side effects mainly mediated by BuChE inhibition seen with this compound, as compared to Phy and THA. Using Phy or THA, in humans, we find that only a maximum 25-30% (Table I) inhibition of ChE can be achieved due to the appearance of side effects. The efficacy of THA and Phy is limited to the rapid reversibility of enzyme inhibition resulting in a short duration of the effect of the drug and poor therapeutic action (1). The necessity of designing new ChEI with different properties and effects than those presently available is apparent.

REFERENCES
1. Becker R., Giacobini, E.: Mechanisms of cholinesterase inhibition in senile dementia of the Alzheimer type: clinical, pharmacological and therapeutic aspects. Drug Devel. Res. 12:163-195, 1988.
2. Becker R.E., Colliver J., Elble R., Feldman E., Giacobini E., Kumar V., Markwell S., Moriearty P., Parks R., Shillcutt S.D., Unni L., Vicari S., Womack C., Zec R.F.: Effects of metrifonate, a long-acting cholinesterase inhibitor - in Alzheimer disease: report of an open trial. Drug Devel. Res. (In Press), 1990.
3. Unni L., Becker R.E., Hutt V., Bruno P.: Inhibition of acetylcholinesterase and butyrylcholinesterase after oral administration of heptastigmine in healthy volunteers. Intl. Contr. Pharmacology (In Press), 1990.

NICOTINE AS A COGNITIVE ENHANCER

D.M. Warburton.
Department of Psychology, Reading University, Reading, RG6 2AL, UNITED KINGDOM.

In the processing of information, an essential aspect is attention. In a vigilance test, nicotine tablets reduced the vigilance decrement which occurred over time in the placebo condition (7). The same effects were found in non-smokers, light smokers and heavy smokers. Similarly, performance on a rapid visual information processing task in both speed and accuracy above by nicotine, given to both smokers and non-smokers (6). Another type of attention task is performance under conditions of distraction, such as the Stroop Test. Nicotine reduced the size of the Stroop effect in this study in both deprived smokers and non-smokers (3). Thus, there was no evidence of tolerance to the effects of nicotine.

Information storage consists of input of the information, registration of the information in immediate memory and consolidation of the information in longer term memory. In four studies, both nicotine tablets and smoking improved immediate memory (5). Nicotine tablets also improved longer term recall, but had no effect on recall, which showed that nicotine was facilitating the input of information to storage but had no direct effect on retrieval (5).

Research with scopolamine on these same tasks (6) suggests that nicotine is acts on cholinergic pathways, which ascend to the cortex, releases acetylcholine which produces cortical desynchronization (4). The beneficial effects of nicotine on information processing can be explained by it producing and maintaining that cortical state (2). More recent research has linked Alzheimer's Disease with damage to the cholinergic pathways from the nucleus basalis of Meynert to the cortex.

Consequently, we have been very interested to know whether nicotine would have any effect on patients who are in the early stages of the disease. In a study in collaboration with the Institute of Psychiatry in London, the effects of subcutaneous doses of nicotine on information processing performance of patients with senile dementia of the Alzheimer type (SDAT) were examined (1).

Doses of nicotine produced a dose-related improvement in performance in the detection of signals in the rapid visual information processing task by SDAT patients and they approached the performance of the normal elderly. The equivalent data for reaction time show that nicotine doses produce improvements in reaction time in the SDAT patients in comparison with the baseline and placebo conditions. Nicotine also produced a dose-related improvement in the critical flicker fusion test. A higher resolution of flashes can be seen as improved cortical functioning. The result of this improved cortical functioning is an amelioration of the cognitive deficits in SDAT patients.

The improved information processing by nicotine in normal subjects and patients results from the sustained release of acetylcholine at the cortex, either by enhancing the activity in the ascending cholinergic pathway or acting presynaptically at the cortex. Thus, nicotine reduces fluctuations in electrocortical arousal. Consequently, there are not the lapses and variations in information processing that occur in normal subjects and, even more so, in the patients (3).

These data are particularly interesting for understanding smoking and for the use of nicotine and related compounds as cognitive enhancers with clinical populations.

REFERENCES

1. Sahakian, B., et al. (1989): Brit. J. Psychiat. 154: 797-800.

2. Warburton, D.M. (1989) Jap. J. Psychopharmacology, 9: 245-256.

3. Warburton, D.M. (1990): In Nicotine Psychopharmacology, S. Wonnacott, M.A.H. Russell and I.P. Stolerman, eds., pp. 77-111, Oxford University Press, Oxford.

4. Warburton, D.M. and Wesnes, K. (1979): In Electrophysiological Effects of Nicotine, A. Rémond and C. Izard, eds., pp. 183-200, Elsevier, Amsterdam.

5. Warburton, D.M., et al., (1986): Psychopharmacology, 89: 55-59.

6. Wesnes, K., and Warburton, D.M. (1984): Psychopharmacology, 82: 147-150.

7. Wesnes, K., Warburton, D.M. and Matz, B. (1983): Neuropsychobiology., 9: 41-44.

NEURONAL PHOSPHOLIPID ABNORMALITIES IN ALZHEIMER'S DISEASE: THERAPEUTIC OPPORTUNITIES.

J.H. Growdon*, I. Lopez Gonzalez-Coviella**, J. K. Blusztajn***, R.J. Wurtman**.
*Massachusetts General Hospital, Boston, MA.;
**Massachusetts Institute of Technology, Cambridge, MA; and
***Boston University, Boston, MA. U.S.A.

Discovery of neurochemical abnormalities in brains of demented subjects may suggest leads for developing treatments to enhance cognitive function. Abnormalities in the metabolism of phospholipid (PL) components of neuronal membranes can account for cell death in AD. In addition to giving physical shape and support, neuronal membranes are instrumental in regulating the internal milieu of cells, supporting the configuration of transmitter receptors, and housing transmembrane proteins such as the A4 peptide. Anything that alters the physical or metabolic properties of PLs in neuronal membranes therefore is likely to disrupt vital neuronal functions. In order to study the pathophysiology of neuronal dysfunction and identify potential therapeutic opportunities, we measured concentrations of glycerophosphocholine (GPC) and glycerophosphoethanolamine (GPE), the metabolites of two major membrane classes, phosphatidylcholine and phosphatidylethanolamine respectively, in cortical areas 20 and 40 and in cerebellar cortex and caudate of brains obtained at autopsy from patients with Alzheimer's disease (AD) Down's syndrome (DS) and age-matched control subjects.

METHODS

Brain tissue was obtained from the Massachusetts Alzheimer's Disease Research Center brain bank. All AD cases had characteristic clinical histories and met neuropathological criteria for the diagnosis of AD. Control brains were from subjects who died without clinical evidence of neurological or psychiatric illnesses, and whose brains were normal upon neuropathological examination. All DS brains showed severe histopathological changes characteristic of AD. The ages at death and times from death to autopsy were similar in all groups. Biochemical analyses were performed on samples taken from the following brain regions: Temporal cortex (area 20), parietal cortex (area 40), lateral cerebellar cortex, and caudate nucleus. Brain samples were weighed and extracted in 20 volumes of chloroform/methanol mixture. The phases were separated by centrifugation, transferred to separate tubes, and dried under a vacuum. The aqueous phase of the brain extract was reconstituted in water, filtered, and aliquots subjected to assay by HPLC procedures.

RESULTS

Comparison of the postmortem concentrations of metabolites of PE and PC revealed significant differences between AD, and DS and control subjects. GPC levels were significantly increased 1.7 to 2.5-fold (Figure 1) in AD brains relative to control brains in all 4 regions examined; similar significant differences were found between AD and DS patients. No significant differences between control subjects and DS patients were detected. Similarly, GPE levels were significantly increased in AD patients relative to control subjects and DS patients. No significant differences between control subjects and DS patients were detected.

Figure 1. GPC levels were significantly increased in areas 20, 40, caudate (CP) and cerebellum (CC) of AD brains compared to DS and control subjects.

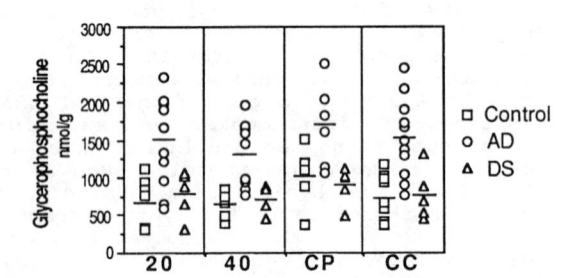

DISCUSSION

These data confirm and extend previous reports (1-5) based upon 31-P NMR spectroscopy, that phosphodiesters (GPC and GPE levels) are significantly elevated in brains of AD patients. These data demonstrate that altered PL metabolism in brain is characteristic of AD but is not detected in DS. This is an important pathologic distinction between AD and DS brains. These data also suggest that abnormal membrane PL metabolism may be a central phathophysiological feature of AD because levels of GPC and GPE were increased in all brain regions irrespective of AD histopathology. These data complement reports of membrane abnormalities affecting cells both within and outside the central nervous system in AD, and raise the possibility of a systemic defect in PL metabolism. Regardless of whether abnormalities in PL metabolism are the primary lesion in AD, or represent secondary manifestations of the disease, these observations suggest that treatments designed to stabilize neuronal membranes and normalize PL metabolism would be rational neuropharmacological approaches to treating AD.

REFERENCES

1. Barany et al., (1985): Lancet 1:517.
2. Miatto et al., (1986): Can. J. Neurol. Sci. 13:535-539.
3. Miatto et al., (1989): In Phospholipids in the Nervous System, NG Bazan, LA Horrocks and G. Toffano, eds., pp. 243-250. Livian Press, Padua.
4. Pettegrew et al., (1984): Neurology 34 (suppl 1):281
5. Pettegrew et al., (1988): Arch. Neurol. 45:1093-1096

EVOLUTION OF AMPHETAMINE PSYCHOSES, CONCEPT AND COURSE

M. SATO
Department of Psychiatry, Tohoku University Medical School, Sendai, Miyagi, JAPAN

A discrepancy of the concept of methamphetamine (MAP) psychosis between Japan and other countries often produces some problems for discussion about clinical relevance of the data obtained from MAP model of schizophrenia.

CLINICAL FEATURES OF MAP PSYCHOSIS

A transverse clinical feature of the MAP psychosis reported for these 4 decades in Japan appears coincident with that described by Connell(1): "the clinical picture is primarily a paranoid psychosis with ideas of reference, delusion of persecution, auditory and visual hallucinations, in a setting of clear consciousness. In fact, 92% of 131 cases (5), 90 % of 82 cases (4) and 73 % of 192 cases (3) showed abundant paranoid psychotic delusions frequently accompanied by auditory hallucination, bizarre ideas, e.g., delusions of being controlled, thought broadcasting, thought insertion and thought withdrawal. Thus, the clinical feature includes some of Schneider's first rank symptoms or active phase of schizophrenic disorders in DSM-III and indistinguishable from schizophrenic disorders by the transverse feature.

CLINICAL COURSE

Clinical course of the psychotic state of MAP psychosis established in Japan differs basically from that described by Connell in the duration of the paranoid psychotic state after MAP withdrawal. Tatetsu et al. reported that 14.4 % of 131 inpatients with intravenous MAP abusers with psychotic state did not recover from the symptoms within 5 years after MAP withdrawal, whereas Connell reported 42 oral amphetamine abusers with psychotic features and concluded that patients with AMP psychosis recover within a week unless there is a demonstrable cause for the continuance of symptoms. However, at least 12 reports on MAP psychosis in Japan since 1945 indicate a prolonged psychotic state after MAP withdrawal: more than 20 days and 2 years in 31 and 10 % of 74 cases (2), more than 1 month in 18% of 82 cases (4) and in 13 % of 192 cases (3). These evidence show that prolonged psychotic state, unfit for Connell's concept, is included into the MAP psychosis.

RELAPSE OF PARANOID PSYCHOTIC STATE

Prompt recurrence of the psychotic features, almost identical to the initial psychotic episode, has been reported following re-use of MAP (4) or psychological stress (3) after several months or years of remitted interval. The recurrence may be occured by a single dose of less than the initial injection of MAP, and is prevented by the pretreatment with antipsychotics (4). These evidence may suggest a long-lasting vulnerability to the paranoid psychotic state similar to that of schizophrenic disorders.

In animal experiments, lasting behavioral sensitization to MAP, cocaine and footshock stress has been confirmed after chronic MAP. In addition to increased release of striatal dopamine in response to catecholamine agonists, recent preliminary study showed an increased uptake of 11C-MAP in the striatum and hypothalamus in rats sensitized to MAP (Hishinuma et al. in press), suggesting a lasting change in peresynaptic membrane including dopamine and MAP uptake complex. These experimental data also support the concept of MAP psychosis that the psychotic state may develop and prolong on the base of MAP-induced lasting vulnerability.

MAP PSYCHOSIS AS A VULNERABILITY MODEL OF SCHIZOPHRENIA

Recent longitudinal investigations of schizophrenia have shown that a majority of patients with schizophrenia have an undulating course. Moreover, Kane reviewed the recent studies on relapse of schizophrenic symptoms, and indicated that about 75 % of fully remitted patients have relapse of schizophrenic symptoms within 2 years after discontinuation of antipsychotics. Together with the fact that full remission can be achieved in about 30 % of schizophrenic patients, an increasing awareness has emerged to the classical view since Meyer A. that a lasting vulnerability to schizophrenic symptoms consists the schizophrenia. The MAP psychosis appears to be an ideal model to investigate biological aspect of the vulnerability in schizophrenia.

REFERENCES
1. Connell P.H. Amphetamine Psychosis. Oxford University Press, London, 1958.
2. Hayashi S. Wake-amine addiction (in Japn). Sogo-igaku, 12: 656-661, 1955.
3. Konuma K. Multiphasic clinical types of methamphetamine psychosis and its dependence(in Japn). Psychiat. Neurol. Japn., 86: 315-339, 1984.
4. Sato M. et al. Acute exacerbation of paranoid psychotic state after long-term abstinence in patients with previous methamphetamine psychosis. Biol. Psychiatry, 18: 429-440, 1983
5. Tatetsu M. et al. The Methamphetamine Psychosis. Igaku-syoin, Tokyo, 1956.

MECHANISMS OF STIMULANT AND STRESS SENSITIZATION: WHERE TO LOOK

SEYMOUR M. ANTELMAN AND ANTHONY R. CAGGIULA
Depts. of Psychiatry and Psychology, Univ.of Pittsburgh

Sensitization refers to the ability of a strong stimulus to increase the subsequent response to that same, or a different agent. The sensitizing stimulus can be coincident with the augmented response, or it can precede the behavioral or physiological measurement by periods ranging from days to years. The impact of the sensitizing stimulus can not only endure but also grow with the passage of time (Antelman, 1988).

Most of the current work on drug-induced sensitization is focused on the stimulants amphetamine (AM) and cocaine (COC). This emphasis is based on the effectiveness of stimulants in inducing a psychosis which shows a progressive sensitization and is similar to paranoid schizophrenia (Robinson and Becker, 1986). Not unexpectedly, efforts to identify the mechanisms of this sensitization have concentrated on the specific pharmacological properties of stimulants as they affect brain dopamine (DA) activity and thus have emphasized changes in autoreceptor sensitivity or release (Robinson and Becker, 1986).

Although important information has accrued regarding DA function using this approach, the search for mechanisms of sensitization will undoubtedly also benefit --indeed depend-- on the adoption of a broader perspective that incorporates features of sensitization that are not restricted to DA systems, stimulants or even drugs.

Thus, sensitization is extremely widespread, cutting across drug categorizations (e.g., stimulants, antidepressants, neuroleptics, anxiolytics, anxiogenics, opioids, gonadal and pituitary hormones, lymphokines, industrial toxins, etc;), transmitters (DA, norepinephrine, serotonin and GABA), and bodily systems (nervous, endocrine and immune) (Antelman, 1988).

Moreover, the ability of drugs to induce long term sensitization to subsequent treatment with the same or other agents can be mimicked by non-pharmacological stressors. These include immobilization, footshock, needle jab, saline injection, tail pinch and others (Antelman, 1988). Furthermore, there exists a bidirectional interchangeability between these stressors and AM in the ability to induce long-term sensitization, since earlier exposure to an environmental stressor sensitizes the organisms response to later AM, and, conversely, a single experience with AM also induces a growing and persistent sensitization to subsequent stress (Antelman 1988). Our original reports of this work have received widespread support from both behavioral and neurochemical studies and have been extended to cocaine, morphine and D-Ala 2-Met-5-enkephalinamide (Robinson and Becker, 1986; Antelman, 1988 for review). Essentially, they have opened up a whole new area of research.

The heterogeneous nature of the pharmacological properties of agents able to induce sensitization indicates that it is due to something they share rather than their pharmacological distinctions. In addition, the apparent interchangeability of drugs and stressors in inducing sensitization suggests strongly that the ability of drugs to precipitate such effects depends more on the fact that they represent foreign/stressful agents than on their pharmacological properties.

The foregoing suggests that DA sensitization may be one manifestation of a more basic phenomenon that is induced by mechanisms responsive to a variety of exteroceptive and interoceptive stressors and that have wide access to all physiological systems, including brain DA. One common feature of these sensitization-inducing agents is their ability to activate the hypothalamic-pituitary-adrenocortical system (HPA). This system exhibits long-term sensitization to stressful stimuli (Caggiula et al, 1989) and is capable, in turn, of inducing long-term changes in a variety of other systems through its ability to influence gene transcription and mRNA translation. Indeed, the possibility that such changes may be the basis for sensitization is suggested by the finding that long-term sensitization of vitellogenin mRNA induction can be triggered *in vitro* across multiple generations of cell division by estrogen (summarized in Antelman, 1988). This finding also clearly indicates that sensitization does not depend on neural mediation.

Finally, although sensitization is typically induced by multiple drug exposures, it does not depend on such a regime, but can be shown to grow with the passage of time from a single exposure. Thus candidate mechanisms must be able to account for this growth process.
Supported by MH24114(SMA), MH42530(SMA) and BNS-8909487(ARC)

1. Antelman, S.M. (1988): **Drug Development Research**, 14:1-30.

2. Caggiula, A.R., et al., (1989): **Psychopharmacology**, 99:233-237.

3. Robinson, T.E., and Becker, J.B. (1986): **Brain Res. Revs.**, 11:157-198.

MECHANISM OF METHAMPHETAMINE-INDUCED BEHAVIORAL SENSITIZATION

K. AKIYAMA, T. HAMAMURA, H. UJIKE, A. KANZAKI and S. OTSUKI
Department of Neuropsychiatry, Okayama University Medical School, Okayama 700, Japan.

It is well documented that abuse of psychostimulants such as amphetamine or methamphetamine (MAP) by humans leads to psychotic symptoms which are hardly distinguished from that of schizophrenia. This chronological change in the clinical feature of the response to MAP suggests an evolution of the brain dysfunction which is progressively produced by repetition of MAP use. Once developed, the MAP-induced paranoid state readily recurs with a minimum dose of MAP reuse even after a long-term abstinence period without florid psychotic symptoms.

Repeated administration of MAP in animals causes a progressive augmentation of locomotion and stereotyped behavior. Such behavioral sensitization or reverse tolerance has been well established as an animal model of susceptibility to exacerbation of MAP-induced paranoid psychosis. The present study focuses on our recent behavioral and neurochemical data in the behavioral sensitization in rodents.

Male Sprague Dawley rats were used. Daily administration of MAP (4 mg/kg) for 14 days results in augmented response of stereotypy. Intense stereotypy, which was otherwise induced by a MAP challenge after abstinence, was abolished in the animals receiving co-administration of MAP plus SCH-23390 (a selective D_1 antagonist) or YM-09151-2 (a selective D_2 antagonist), implying that stimulation of both D_1 and D_2 receptors is indispensable for the formation of behavioral sensitization (3).

The efflux of dopamine and its metabolites (DOPAC and HVA) was examined in the striatal perfusates from animals chronically treated with MAP using _in vivo_ microdialysis. The degree to which dopamine efflux increased following a challenge of either MAP or cocaine was significantly greater in the MAP-treated animals than the control. Conversely, the degree to which DOPAC efflux decreased was significantly greater in the MAP-treated animals than the control (2). It was also demonstrated that the striatal dopamine efflux was enhanced in animals sensitized by chronic cocaine administration in response to a challenge of MAP as well as cocaine (1). No matter what psychostimulant (MAP or cocaine) was previously pretreated, dopamine efflux was greater following a challenge of MAP than cocaine. These lines of evidence indicate that the function of dopamine uptake sites on which cocaine acts may somehow be changed and may lead to an enhanced release of dopamine in cross reverse tolerance between MAP and cocaine.

Considering the fact that D_1 receptors and a substantial number of D_2 receptors are localized on neurons receiving projections from mesotelencephalic system, a question arises as to whether a postsynaptic mechanism may be involved in the formation of behavioral sensitization.

To test this hypothesis, the effect of co-administration of SCH-23390 or YM-09151-2 prior to each MAP injection on dopamine efflux in the striatal perfusates was investigated. After abstinence period of three months, a challenge of 4 mg/kg of MAP alone produced augmented stereotypy in the MAP-group, but not in the control, SCH-23390 + MAP, or YM-09151-2 + MAP groups. In parallel with the behavioral observation, the degree to which the dopamine efflux increased following the MAP challenge was significantly greater in the MAP group than the control, SCH-23390 + MAP or YM-09151-2 + MAP groups. While dopamine efflux did not differ significantly in intensity between the control and YM-09151-2 + MAP group, it was slightly, but significantly, greater in the SCH-23390 + MAP group than the control. These results suggest not only the long-lasting susceptibility to enhanced dopamine efflux, but also that blockade of any subtype of postsynaptic dopamine receptors during chronic MAP administration prevents the susceptibility to enhanced dopamine efflux which is associated with the behavioral sensitization.

Transsynaptic neural circuits via postsynaptic dopamine receptors might, therefore, play an important role for the formation of MAP-induced behavioral sensitization. It is well known that D_1 receptors are densely localized on axonal terminals of striatal nigral neuron which correspond to the substantia nigra pars reticulata. We recently demonstrated that D_1 receptor increased long-lastingly in the lateral part of the substantia nigra pars reticulata. This finding may reflect some aspect of the presumed plasticity in transsynaptic neural circuits, and explain the discrepancy between the complete prophylactic effect on behavioral sensitization and partial inhibitory effect on dopamine efflux by SCH-23390.

In conclusion, it is strongly suggested that enhanced dopamine release in response to a challenge of MAP to the previously sensitized animals underlies cross behavioral sensitization between MAP and cocaine. Such susceptibility to enhanced dopamine release may be directly associated with some dysfunction of the extracellular Na-dependent carrier which mediates dopamine uptake and release. However, the apparent preventive role of the selective D_1 antagonist and D_2 antagonist in the behavioral sensitization and accompanying dopamine releasability indicates that some plastic change in transsynaptic neural circuits may occur during the formation of behavioral sensitization.

REFERENCES

1. Akimoto K. et al. Enhanced extracellular dopamine level may be the fundamental neuropharmacological basis of cross-behavioral sensitization between methamphetamine and cocaine - an in vivo dialysis study in freely moving rats. Brain Res. 507;344-346, 1990.
2. Kazahaya Y. et al. Subchronic methamphetamine treatment enhances methamphetamine- or cocaine-induced dopamine efflux in vivo. Biol. Psychiatry 25:903-912, 1989.
3. Ujike H. et al. Effects of selective D-1 and D-2 dopamine antagonists on development of methamphetamine induced behavioral sensitization. Psychopharmacol. 98;89-92, 1989.

COCAINE-INDUCED PSYCHOSIS: COMPARISON WITH AMPHETAMINE

E.H. ELLINWOOD and T. LEE
Departments of Psychiatry and Pharmacology, Duke University Medical Center, Durham, N.C., U.S.A.

Both cocaine and amphetamine psychosis are frequently contrasted with functional psychoses such as paranoid schizophrenia. Amphetamine psychosis in the 1950's and 60's was often misdiagnosed as paranoid schizophrenia. The relative incidence of full-blown paranoid psychoses in cocaine users has not been as prevalent as it was with amphetamine users. As we will discuss, cocaine, more frequently than amphetamine induces an early onset of a hyper reactive state in which the individual appears to be reacting to illusional and hallucinatory phenomena without undergoing: 1) the more entrenched evolution of exploratory suspiciousness, 2) the more intense development of stereotyped behaviors and 3) the evolution of delusional constricted thinking that is associated with amphetamine psychosis (4,6). Kraepelin (7) mentions that "Catatonic states may further suddenly appear in each period of dementia precox....but, lastly the catatonic symptoms may be present in the morbid picture in all possible grades and groupings." Bleuler (4), points out that in examining the "catatonic" manifestations and their parallels with paranoid manifestations, it appeared that stereotypy might be a common mode in both conditions. Thus, the associated sustained attitudes and thinking modes could well be common to catatonic paranoid functional psychoses as well as to the stimulant induced psychosis. Bleuler (1) listed a variety of movement, postural, attitudinal and thinking stereotyped disorders noted in catatonic schizophrenia, but which also appeared in other schizophrenic forms. We (5) have described the contribution of the behavioral pattern manifested at the time of initial amphetamine injection with its topography and development of stereotypy that develops with chronic stimulant intoxication. These initial behavioral patterns reflect 1) learned behaviors, 2) species specific arousal behaviors, and 3) novel behaviors reflecting unique environmental circumstances prevailing at the time of drug administration. Even though learned or contingent behaviors may become incorporated into the stereotyped patterns, including self-administration operants with high chronic doses, behavioral patterns associated with stimulant arousal and species specific behaviors eventually supercede learned responses to the point that only a remnant of the environmentally contingent behavior remains.

Bleuler (2) wrote "Kraepelin called attention to the fact that in cases where the capacity for planned pursuit of definite goals is disturbed, secondary drives may assert themselves in the absence of inhibitions provided by new aims, the patient will continue whatever activity they had been practicing hitherto."

Cocaine, rather than amphetamine, abusers may have less intense evolution of stereotyped, ingrained, psychotic behaviors for a variety of reasons including: 1) the greater necessity of remaining contingently related to the environment with cocaine abuse, and 2) the types of individuals using cocaine in the current epidemic differ. The longer half-life of amphetamine allows for greater isolation from relevant human contact. Because cocaine has a much shorter half-life, individuals must repeatedly administer cocaine in order to sustain a long duration binge. On the other hand, amphetamine with its longer half-life permits infrequent administration to maintain binges over a period of days. In a previous time, amphetamine was much more readily available and did not require demanding, environmentally contingent, drug-seeking skills. Finally, many individuals developed isolated patterns of bizarre stereotyped behavior and thinking because they spent long periods of time alone in their homes. Since the cocaine addict must maintain a relationship with the environment to obtain the drug, psychotic-like responses tend to be more environmentally relevant, i.e., they develop hallucinations and delusional-like attitudes about the police, or people coming to shoot them, etc. In contrast, many amphetamine addicts develop much more bizarre, internally developed stereotyped delusions. The ready availability of amphetamine in the 50's and 60's also allowed a large number of vulnerable schizoid and schizo-affective patients to obtain the drug. The residual delusional behavior in amphetamine psychotics also appeared to be more entrenched and was also precipitated by stress or a subsequent low-dose of stimulant (7,8).

People with cocaine psychosis appear to have a greater hyper reactivity to the environment including aggressive responses to other individuals, and acting on sudden impulses often in a violent or homicidal way. In contrast to animal paradigms of long-term chronic cocaine administration, these behaviors have a greater similarity to serotonergic-like syndromes, including hallucinatory-like states, see Castellani et al. 1985. The underlying neurotransmitter and neurophysiological basis for these differences are reviewed and contrasted between amphetamine and cocaine.

REFERENCES

1. Bleuer, E. (1924): Textbook of Psychiatry, Macmillan, New York.
2. Bleuler, E. (1950): Dementia Praecox or the Group of Schizophrenias, Allen & Unwin, London.
3. Castellani, S., et al. (1985): Drug-induced Psychosis: Neurobiological Mechanisms. In Substance Abuse and Psychopathology, A.I. Alterman, ed., pp. 173-210. Plenum Press, New York.
4. Ellinwood, E.H. (1974): Amphetamine Model Psychosis: the Relationships to Schizophrenia. In Biologicald Mechanisms of Schizophrenia and Schizophrenia-like Pychoses H. Mitsuda and T. Fukuda, eds., pp 89-96. Igaku Shoin Ltd., Tokyo
5. Ellinwood, E.H., Jr. and Kilbey, M.M. (1975): Amphetamine Stereotypy: the Influence of Environmental Factors and Prepotent Behavioral Patterns on its Topography and Development. Biol Psychiat., 10(1):3-16.
6. Ellinwood, E.H., Jr., and Kilbey, M.M. (1977): Chronic Stimulant Intoxication Models of Psychosis. In Animal Models in Psychiatry and Neurology, Hanin and E. Usdin, eds., pp 61-74. Pergamon Press, New York
7. Kraepelin, E. (1971): Dementia Praexoc and Paraphrenia. Tr. Barclay, R.M. and Robertson, G.M., Robert Krieger Publishing Company, Huntingtdon, New York.
8. Sato, M. et al. (1983): Acute Exacerbation of Paranoid Psychotic State after Long-Term Abstinence in Patients with Previous Methamphetamine Psychosis. Biol. Psychiat. 18(4):429-440.
9. Tatetsu, S. (1972) Methamphetamine Psychosis In Current Concepts on Amphetamine Abuse, Ellinwood, E.H., Jr., Cohen S., eds. pp. 159-161, U.S. Govt Printing Office, Wash, DC.

MECHANISMS OF COCAINE-INDUCED SENSITIZATION

P.W. KALIVAS, P. DUFFY and J. D. STEKETEE
Department of Veterinary Pharmacology, Washington State University, Pullman, WA, U.S.A

Daily administration of cocaine to rodents produces a progressive elevation in motor stimulation, and when the daily injections are discontinued the motor stimulant response to a subsequent acute cocaine injection remains augmented for months afterward. Although behavioral sensitization to daily cocaine injections has been repeatedly demonstrated, the neuroanatomical and cellular substrates mediating this phenomenon are ill-defined. Because the acute motor stimulant effect of cocaine appears to result from the blockade of dopamine reuptake in the nucleus accumbens, research has focused on alterations in mesolimbic dopamine transmission as a possible mechanism for cocaine-induced behavioral sensitization. Based upon this postulate, a number of laboratories have attempted to measure changes in dopamine release in the nucleus accumbens or striatum following daily cocaine administration using intracranial dialysis. The majority of laboratories have found that daily cocaine administration resulted in an augmentation in acute cocaine-induced release of dopamine in these axon terminal fields (1,6,7; however, see 3). While these studies argue that enhanced dopamine release into the nucleus accumbens and/or striatum may mediate behavioral sensitization to cocaine, the mechanism by which dopamine release is augmented remains unknown. The three possibilities currently being experimentally evaluated by laboratories around the world are, 1) alterations in the presynaptic regulation of dopamine release at the axon terminal, 2) alterations in regulation of the dopamine cell bodies to modify action potential generation, and thereby alter terminal field dopamine release, and 3) alterations in afferents to the presynaptic terminal or dopamine neurons.

The focus in our laboratory has been on the postulate that intracellular or afferent regulation of the A10 dopamine neurons is altered following daily cocaine administration, and that this produces an alteration in impulse generation that elicits a greater release of dopamine in the terminal field. One possibility is that the inhibitory regulation of dopamine neurons may be diminished such that the neurons are more easily stimulated in cocaine-sensitized rats. The two most well characterized inhibitory regulators of dopaminergic impulse generation are activation of the D_2 autoreceptor and $GABA_B$ receptor. Activation of either of these receptors hyperpolarizes dopamine cells by coupling with a pertusis-toxin sensitive G protein to increase potassium conductance (4). Based upon the role of these G proteins in the inhibitory regulation of dopamine neurons, rats were pretreated with pertussis toxin (0.5 µg) into the A10 region. This resulted in a marked reduction (40%) in Gi and Go content in the A10 region, and an increase in the level of dopamine metabolites in the A10 region and nucleus accumbens by 48 hrs after injection. However, by 7 days after pertussis toxin administration dopamine metabolite content had returned to control levels. On day 14 after administration, rats were injected with cocaine (15 mg/kg, ip). Motor behavior and extracellular dopamine content in the nucleus accumbens were monitored simultaneously by conducting in vivo dialysis in a photocell apparatus. Rats pretreated with pertussis toxin demonstrated a marked sensitization compared to saline pretreated rats in both motor behavior and extracellular dopamine content. This argues that a disruption of inhibitory regulation of dopamine neurons is sufficient to elicit behavioral sensitization. This conclusion is consistent with the electrophysiological studies from the laboratory of White and coworkers (2). They observed that following daily cocaine, dopamine neurons were less responsive to the autoreceptor-induced inhibition, and more spontaneously active cells/track were observed. Also, in tissue slices prepared from the A10 dopamine region, potassium was less effective at releasing dopamine when the slices were obtained from rats pretreated with daily cocaine (15 mg/kg, ip X 3 days) compared to those pretreated with daily saline (5). The decrease in depolarization-induced release of somatodendritic dopamine would result in less autoreceptor activation, thereby increasing the excitability of the neurons.

In conclusion, recent studies point to three mechanisms whereby inhibitory regulation of dopamine neurons can be altered to enhance the excitability of the cells and promote behavioral sensitization. 1) A desensitization of D_2 autoreceptors. 2) An uncoupling of D_2 and/or $GABA_B$ receptors from potassium channels. 3) A decrease in depolarization-induced somatodendritic dopamine release, resulting in a decrease in D_2 autoreceptor inhibition.

1. Akiyama, et al., (1989): Br. Res.,
2. Henry, et al., (1989): J. Pharmacol. Exp. Ther., 251: 833-839.
3. Hurd, et al., (1989): Br. Res.,
4. Lacey, et al., (1988): J. Physiol., 401: 437-453.
5. Kalivas and Duffy (1988): J. Neurochem., 50: 1498-1504.
6. Kalivas and Duffy (1990): Synapse, 5: 48-58.
7. Pan et al., (1989): Soc. Neurosci. Abst., 15: 434.5.

ANATOMY AND PHARMACOLOGY OF COCAINE-INDUCED BEHAVIORAL SENSITIZATION

R.M. POST, S.R.B. WEISS and A. PERT
Biological Psychiatry Branch, National Institute of Mental Health,
Bethesda, Maryland, U.S.A.

While acute administration of cocaine can be associated with a variety of neuropsychiatric sequelae, chronic administration of cocaine and related psychomotor stimulants are more likely associated with profound psychiatric syndromes including states resembling mania, dysphoric mania, and a paranoid schizophreniform psychosis (2). The acute positive signs and symptoms resembling hypomania evolve into negative dysphoric symptomatology: sociability to intrusiveness, energy to disorganization and insomnia, vigilance to anxiety and paranoia, hyperactivity to stereotypy and punding, and social forcefulness to aggression and violence. As such, chronic psychomotor stimulant administration may be an interesting model for dysphoric mania and paranoid psychosis.

Repeated psychomotor stimulant administration in animals results in increased rather than decreased responsivity, manifest as hyperactivity and stereotypy, which are perhaps analogous to increasing psychiatric dysfunction noted in the clinical syndromes (3). This behavioral sensitization response in animals is related to both dose and number of repetitions of stimulant administration as well as to environmental context. For example, a single low dose of cocaine (10 mg/kg) does not produce behavioral sensitization while multiple low doses will. Alternatively, in a paradigm that we are currently studying, a single high dose of cocaine (40 mg/kg), compared to saline, will produce an increased response to a low-dose challenge with cocaine (10 mg/kg) the next day. In this latter paradigm, the behavioral sensitization can be shown to depend on environmental context, such that only the rats treated and tested with cocaine in the same environment (4) demonstrate an enhanced response. Animals that receive the identical dose of cocaine (40 mg/kg), but experience the cocaine hyperactivity in a different environment from the test cage do not demonstrate cocaine-induced behavioral sensitization (CIBS) to a cocaine challenge in the test environment. Pretreatment with neuroleptics on day 1, when rats receive the conditioning cocaine injection (40 mg/kg), blocks the development of CIBS, while neuroleptic pretreatment on day-two, prior to the low-dose challenge, is unable to block the expression of CIBS. The neuroleptic-induced dysjunction in the blockade of development, but not expression, of CIBS suggests a differential role of dopamine in these two phases of sensitization similar to what has been described for other neurotransmitters in model systems of learning and memory, such as LTP and kindling. These data may also offer a novel perspective on neuroleptic non-responsiveness. To the extent that the sensitization model is relevant, the data suggest the importance of early rather than late treatment intervention with neuroleptics. It is also of interest that a benzodiazepine, diazepam, and the α-2 agonist clonidine are capable of blocking both the development and expression of CIBS; related agents (clonazepam and clonidine) have been used to treat refractory mania. The antimanic anticonvulsant carbamazepine does not block either the development or expression of CIBS in the paradigm described above, although it partially inhibits peak stereotypy to repeated high-dose cocaine (40 mg/kg), and markedly inhibits the development of cocaine-induced seizures and their associated lethality (5,6).

We have attempted to dissect the neuroanatomical substrates involved in CIBS. In the one-day high-dose paradigm we have found that selective depletions of approximately 65% of dopamine in the nucleus accumbens will block CIBS. In addition, both electrolytic lesions and dopamine-selective depletions in the amygdala will block the phenomenon. Since the nucleus accumbens is thought to be involved in sensory motor integration and in the motor activating and rewarding effects of cocaine, we surmise that this substrate is critical for the motor programs of CIBS while the amygdala may be important for conveying the environmental context-dependent information for the conditioned component of CIBS. Preliminary data in collaboration with David Fontana suggest that amygdala lesions are not sufficient to block CIBS induced by multiple high doses of cocaine, suggesting the possibility that different neural substrates become involved with different induction paradigms. In this case, repeated cocaine administration may allow coding of the CIBS in an amygdala-independent fashion similar to that involved in "habit" memory. Habit memory is dependent solely on striatal pathways and does not require amygdala-hippocampal participation, which is necessary in representational memory (1).

Thus, dopaminergic substrates, particularly those in nucleus accumbens and amygdala, appear to be involved in some aspects of cocaine-induced behavioral sensitization and may be pertinent to the evolution of a variety of neuropsychiatric syndromes.

REFERENCES

1. Mishkin, M. and Appenzeller, T.: Sci. Am. 256:80-89.
2. Post, R.M. and Weiss, S.R.B. (1989): J. Clin. Psychiatry 50: 23-30.
3. Post, R.M., Weiss, S.R.B. and Pert, A. (1988): In Mesocorticolimbic Dopamine System, P.W. Kalivas and C.B. Nemeroff, eds., pp. 292-308. New York Academy of Science, New York
4. Weiss, S.R.B., et al., (1989): Pharmacol. Biochem. Behav. 34:655-661.
5. Weiss, S.R.B., et al., (1989): Brain Res. 497:72-79
6. Weiss, S.R.B., et al., (1990): Neuropsychopharmacology (in press).

CORTICOTROPIN-RELEASING FACTOR: PRECLINICAL AND CLINICAL STUDIES

C.B. NEMEROFF[*], G. BISSETTE[*], M.J. OWENS[*], M.A. VARGAS[*], C. PIHOKER[*], K.R.R. KRISHNAN[*], S.T. CAIN[*], and C. BANKI[**]
[*]Department of Psychiatry, Duke University Medical Center, Durham, NC; [**]Regional Neuropsychiatric Hospital, Nagykallo, Hungary

INTRODUCTION
Since elucidation of the structure of corticotropin-releasing factor (CRF) (10), considerable information has accrued concerning a role for the peptide in the regulation of pituitary-adrenal activity. In addition to its neuroendocrine role, it is now evident that CRF plays an important role as a neuroregulator in extra-hypothalamic brain areas and plays a preeminent role in coordinating the stress response. Recently obtained data provide support for a role for CRF in the pathophysiology of several neuropsychiatric disorders including major depression, anxiety disorders and Alzheimer's disease.

BASIC STUDIES
CRF and high affinity CRF binding sites are heterogeneously distributed in the mammalian central nervous system (CNS). Ca^{2+}-dependent CRF release from brain slices is stimulated by depolarizing concentrations of K^+. Electrophysiological studies have revealed that application of CRF to certain CNS neurons produces marked alterations in neuronal firing rates. These findings, taken together, support the hypothesis that CRF functions as a neurotransmitter in the CNS. We have recently reviewed these findings (9).
Considerable data support the hypothesis that CRF is the major physiological regulator of ACTH secretion from the anterior pituitary. When rats are exposed to acute or chronic stress, CRF concentrations in the median eminence are markedly reduced (4), presumably due to enhanced release required to activate the pituitary-adrenal axis. In contrast, concentrations of CRF in the locus coeruleus are markedly increased after acute or chronic stress. Acute treatment with the triazolobenzodiazepines, alprazolam or adinazolam produced opposite effects on CRF concentrations than stress, i.e. an increase in the median eminence and a decrease in the locus coeruleus (8). Furthermore when CRF is injected intracerebroventricularly (ICV) or directly into the locus coeruleus, it produces marked anxiogenic effects (3). This concatenation of findings raises the possibility that CRF plays a role in the pathophysiology of anxiety and affective disorders.

CLINICAL STUDIES
We have measured the cerebrospinal fluid (CSF) concentration of CRF in drug-free patients with major depression, schizophrenia, dementia and normal controls. In several studies the CSF concentration of CRF has been found to be elevated in drug-free depressed patients when compared to each of these groups (2). Like hypercortisolemia, CRF hypersecretion as evidenced by elevated CSF CRF levels is state-dependent.

Evidence for CRF hypersecretion comes from measurement of CRF receptor number and affinity in post-mortem tissue from suicide victims. If CRF is chronically hypersecreted in depressed patients, CRF receptors should exhibit a reduction in number, so-called receptor down-regulation. We observed a reduced number of CRF receptors in prefrontal cortex of suicide victims (7).

When CRF is administered intravenously to depressed patients, especially dexamethasone suppression test (DST) non-suppressors, a blunted ACTH response is observed when compared to the response of the normal controls (6). We have suggested that CRF receptor down-regulation in the adenohypophysis may contribute to the blunted ACTH response to CRF in depression.

In Alzheimer's disease, the concentrations of CRF in several cerebrocortical areas and the caudate are markedly reduced (1,5). Not suprisingly, CRF receptor number is markedly increased in response to the apparent reduction in synaptic availability of CRF (5).

CONCLUSIONS

It is evident that CRF plays a seminal role in the stress response and moreover likely plays a role in the pathophysiology of affective disorders, anxiety disorders and Alzheimer's disease. In depression CRF appears to be hypersecreted resulting in hyperactivity of the pituitary-adrenal axis and in down-regulation of CRF receptor number in the cerebral cortex and perhaps in the adenohypophysis. In Alzheimer's disease, CRF neurons appear to degenerate and CRF receptor number is increased. Development of lipophillic CRF receptor antagonists may allow positron emission tomography to be used to diagnostically distinguish Alzheimer's disease and depressive pseudodementia, as well as yielding novel antidepressants or anxiolytic compounds.

ACKNOWLEDGEMENTS

We are grateful to Ward Virts for preparation of this manuscript. Supported by NIMH MH-42088.

REFERENCES
1. Bissette, et al. (1985): J.Amer. Med. Ass'n. 245:3067-3069.
2. Bissette, G. and Nemeroff, C.B. (1990): In Corticotropin-Releasing Factor: Basic and Clinical Studies of a Neuropeptide, E.B. DeSouza and C.B. Nemeroff, eds., pp. 327-334. CRC Press, Inc., Boca Raton, FL.
3. Butler, et al. (1990): J. Neurosci., 10:176-183.
4. Chappel, et al. (1986): J. Neurosci., 6:2908-2914.
5. DeSouza, et al. (1986): Nature, 319:593-595.
6. Evans, et al. (1989): In Neuropeptides in Psychiatry, C.B. Nemeroff, Ed. (in press). APA Press, Washington, D.C.
7. Nemeroff, et al. (1988): Arch. Gen. Psychiat., 45:577-579.
8. Owens, M.J., Bissette, G. and Nemeroff, C.B. (1989): Synapse, 4:196-202.
9. Owens, M.J. and Nemeroff, C.B. (1990): In Corticotropin-Releasing Factor: Basic and Clinical Studies of a Peptide, E.B. DeSouza and C.B. Nemeroff, eds., pp.107-114. CRC Press, Inc., Boca Raton, FL.
10. Vale, et al. (1981): Science, 213:1394-1397.

NEURAL CIRCUITS MEDIATING INHIBITION OF THE HYPOTHALAMO-PITUITARY-ADRENOCORTICAL AXIS

J.P. HERMAN and S.J. WATSON
Mental Health Research Institute, University of Michigan, Ann Arbor, MI, U.S.A.

Activation of the hypothalamo-pituitary-adrenocortical axis (HPA) is modulated by neuronal input impinging on the primary effector corticotropin-releasing factor (CRF) and arginine vasopressin (AVP) neurons in the hypothalamic paraventricular nucleus (PVN). Recent data indicate that the hippocampal formation appears to tonically inhibit HPA activation, as demonstrated by marked increases in CRF and AVP mRNA expression in the parvocellular PVN following hippocampal ablation (1). The circuitry involved in conveying hippocampal inhibitory effects is not presently known, and is believed to be multisynaptic. Several possible pathways are illustrated in FIG. 1, including: 1) hippocampal-hypothalmic projections, travelling in the medial corticohypothalamic tract (MCHT) and relaying to PVN via medial-basal hypothalamic nuclei, or 2) hippocampal-forebrain projections, travelling via the fornix (FX) and relaying in the lateral septum (LS) or bed nucleus of the stria terminalis. (BNST).

METHODS

To further define critical limbic-HPA circuits, selective lesions were made to brain regions defining specific circuits, including electrolytic destruction of the MCHT (MCHT-X) and FX (FX-X). Based on the results of these experiments, additional lesions of the LS (LS-X) and BNST (BNST-X) were made using ibotenic acid, an excitatory neurotoxin which preferentially kills neuronal cell bodies at the injection site. All experimental groups were compared with data from animals receiving sham lesions. Effects of lesions on the HPA axis was assayed via deter-

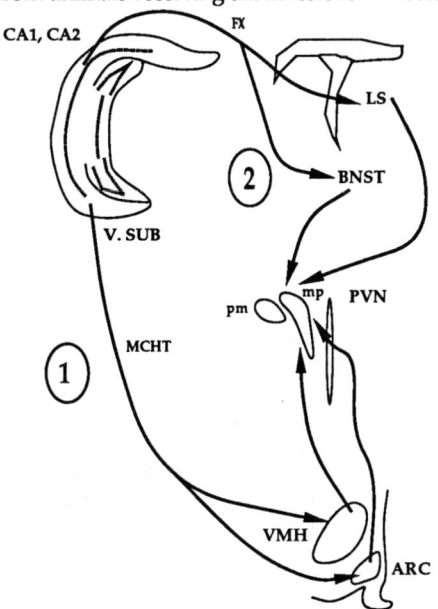

FIG. 1: Simplified diagram of potential circuits connecting the hippocampus with CRF-containing neurons in the medial parvocellular PVN. Circuit 1: hippocampal outflow relays in the medial basal hypothalamus (ventromedial (VMH) and arcuate (ARC) nuclei via the medial corticohypothalamic tract (MCHT). Circuit 2: hippocampal outflow relays in the forebrain (lateral septum (LS) and/or bed nucleus of the stria terminalis (BNST) via the fornix (FX). CA1, CA2: cornu ammonis 1 and 2; V. SUB: ventral subiculum.

minations of CRF mRNA levels in the PVN by semi-quantitative in situ hybridization histochemical analysis, as previously described (1). 35-S labeled cRNA probes directed against the peptide coding region and 3'-UT of the proCRF mRNA were employed in this study. For comparison across experiments, data are expressed as percentage of sham-lesion values.

RESULTS AND DISCUSSION

The data are summarized in FIG. 2. Comparison of the MCHT-X and FX-X groups clearly show that the fornix, which contains axons of hippocampal neurons projecting through forebrain and medial-basal hypothalmis structures, is necessary for normal expression of PVN CRF mRNA. However, the MCHT, which contains hippocampal-hypothalamic axons only, does not

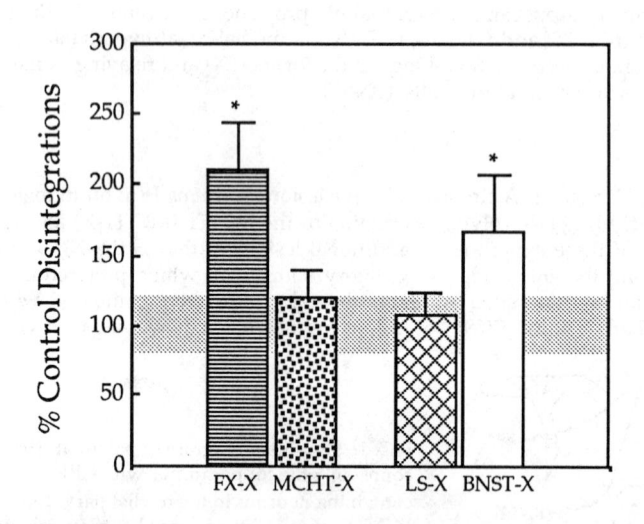

FIG.2. Effects of FX-X, MCHT-X, LS-X and BNST-X on PVN CRF mRNA content. Both FX-X and BNST-X cause significant increases in CRF mRNA relative to controls. Shaded area represents average standard error of the mean across groups.

seem to convey such information. By subtraction, these data indicate that the FX comprizes one part of an essential hippocampal-PVN inhibitory circuit, and that inhibition appears to be mediated via relays in forebrain nuclei.

Results of pathway lesions clearly suggested the LS or BNST as likely hippocamus-PVN relay structures. To assess this possibility, selective lesions were made to cell bodies in these region utilizing ibotenic acid. As can be appreciated from FIG. 2, BNST lesions significantly increased PVN CRF mRNA expression, whereas LS-X treated rats showed no differences from control rats. These data strongly implicate the BNST as an important regulatory element in PVN CRF mRNA expression, and suggest that hippocampal effects on the HPA axis may in part involve a multisynaptic pathway including the BNST.

Supported by NS08267 (JPH) and MH422251 (SJW).

(1) J.P. Herman et al, Evidence for hippocampal regulation of neuroendocrine neurons of the hypothalamo-pituitary-adrenocortical axis. J. Neurosci. 9, 3072-3028 (1989)

NEUROTENSIN INVOLVEMENT IN THE ACTION OF ANTIPSYCHOTIC DRUGS AND THE PATHOGENESIS OF SCHIZOPHRENIA
G. Bissette, B. Levant and C.B. Nemeroff
Departments of Psychiatry and Pharmacology, Duke University Medical Center, Durham, N.C. 27710, U.S.A.

Neurotensin (NT), a mammalian tridecapeptide, is found heterogeneously distributed in the CNS with relatively high concentrations in the hypothalamus as well as extra-hypothalamic brain regions such as the caudate nucleus, nucleus accumbens and medial pre-frontal cortex. NT was first isolated in 1973 (1) and has since been extensively investigated. The gene for NT has recently been cloned (2), specific high-affinity receptors for NT have been characterized (3) and several putative neurotransmitter criteria have been reported (See (8) for review). As these mesolimbicocortical projections are currently hypothesized to be one of the major anatomic loci involved in the pathophysiology of schizophrenia, the presence of NT in these regions provides an impetus to study NT-DA interactions.

Previous data from our laboratory has indicated that centrally administered NT can increase the dopamine turnover in several DA terminal regions (4). Moreover, NT injected directly into the nucleus accumbens blocks the DA-mediated increase in locomotor behavior after psychostimulants that increase DA synaptic availability (5). When NT is applied directly to the nucleus accumbens, it blocks the locomotor hyperactivity induced by direct injection of DA into the nucleus accumbens or systemically administered psychostimulants (6). NT increases the release of dopamine in the nucleus accumbens when applied directly to the VTA DA cell bodies with concomitant increases in locomotor activity (7). Thus, the behavioral effect of NT on either the VTA dopamine cell bodies or the nucleus accumbens DA terminals opposes the effect of DA injected in the same region. These data are concordant with other pharmacological and behavioral data that indicate similarities between centrally injected NT and antipsychotic drugs. These include effects in a conditioned avoidance paradigm, decreases in spontaneous locomotor behavior and hypothermia (8).

The chronic administration of several classes of clinically effective antipsychotic drugs increases NT concentrations in DA terminal regions (9) and this effect is observed within 16 hours of a single injection of haloperidol (10). Clinically inactive phenothiazines are ineffective in this regard. Moreover, the (-) isomer of butaclamol which is not a DA receptor antagonist, has no effect on CNS NT concentrations, while the active (+) isomer is quite effective in increasing NT concentrations (11). Destruction of DA neurons with 6-hydroxy dopamine does not alter the ability of antipsychotic drugs to increase NT concentrations (12). There is no tolerance to the effects of haloperidol on NT concentrations, and withdrawal of chronic antipsychotic drugs leads to a significant decrease in NT concentrations in the regions where NT is increased during treatment (13). Recent work in our laboratory has indicated that sigma receptor antagonists, which also include many antipsychotic drugs, can also increase NT concentrations in these brain regions (14). Thus the anatomic site for the ability of neuroleptic drugs to alter NT concentrations is apparently post-synaptic to the DA neuron, and mediated through neurons containing receptors for DA or sigma receptors.

Clinical evidence for the involvement of endogenous NT in patients with schizophrenia comes from studies of measurement of cerebrospinal fluid (CSF) concentrations of NT. In several studies, patients with schizophrenia have been reported to exhibit decreased CSF concentrations of NT, and some studies have demonstrated increases in CSF concentrations of NT after neuroleptic treatment (15,16). A recent study has reported that a population of psychotic patients with lower CSF NT concentrations do not respond to lithium treatment, but do respond to antipsychotic drugs (17). Post-mortem studies have not demonstrated any marked regional differences in NT concentrations in schizophrenics, though we did observe a marked increase in prefrontal cortex (18). However, the effects of antipsychotic drug treatment on endogenous NT levels may obscure group differences, although drugs are usually withdrawn for two weeks before CSF withdrawal.

While these data strongly support an interaction between NT and DA in the actions of antipsychotic drugs and possibly some of the symptoms of schizophrenia, direct testing of this hypothesis awaits clinical trials of a neurotensin receptor agonist that can cross the blood-brain barrier. Efforts are currently underway to realize this vision. (Supported by NIMH MH-39415.)

REFERENCES
1. Carraway, RE and SE Leeman. (1973): J. Biol. Chem. 248:6854-6861.
2. Kislauskis, E. et al. (1988): J. Biol. Chem. 263:4963-4968.
3. Checler, F. et al. (1986): Eur. J. Pharmacol 126:239-244.
4. Widerlov, E. et al. (1982): J. Pharmacol. Exp. Ther. 222:1-6.
5. Nemeroff, C.B. et al. (1983): J. Pharmacol. Exp. Ther. 225:337-345.
6. Kalivas, P.W. et al. (1983): Neuroscience 8:495-505.
7. Kalivas, P.W. et al. (1984): Neuroscience 11:919-930.
8. Levant, B. and Nemeroff, C.B. (1988): In The Neuroendocrinology of Mood, D. Ganten and D. Pfaff, eds., pp. 231-262. Springer-Verlag, Inc., Berlin.
9. Kilts, C.D. et al. (1988): Biochem. Pharmacol. 37:1547-1554.
10. Govoni, S. et al. (1980): J. Pharmacol. Exp. Ther. 215:413-417.
11. Bissette, G. et al. (1988): Neuropsychopharmacology 1:329-335.
12. Bissette, G. et al. (1988): Soc. Neurosci. Abst. 14:1211.
13. Radke, J.M. et al. (1989): Brain Res. 480:178-183.
14. Levant and Nemeroff. (1989): J. Pharmacol. Exp. Ther. (in press).
15. Widerlov, E. et al. (1982): Am. J. Psychiatry 139:1122-1126.
16. Lindstom, L.H. et al. (1988): Schizophrenia Res. 1:55-59.
17. Bissette, G. et al. (1989): Soc. Neurosci. Abst. 15:1122.
18. Nemeroff, C.B. et al. (1983) Science 221:972-975.

THE RELATIONSHIP BETWEEN STRUCTURAL BRAIN IMAGING, LIMBIC HPA ACTIVITY AND CSF CRF AND CATECHOLAMINE METABOLITES IN AFFECTIVE DISORDERS AND SCHIZOPHRENIA

S.C. RISCH*, R.J. LEWINE*, R.D. JEWART*, N.H. KALIN**, M. STIPETIC*, E.D. RISBY*, M.B. ECCARD*, J. CAUDLE*, W.E. POLLARD*, and M. BRUMMER*

*Emory University School of Medicine, Atlanta, Georgia; **University of Wisconsin School of Medicine, Madison, Wisconsin

Structural brain abnormalities, including alterations in ventricular to brain ratio (VBR) and asymmetries in brain anatomy, have been reported in affective disorder (3) and schizophrenic patients(1). In addition, alterations in CSF neurochemistry (7), neuropeptides, and in hypothalamic pituitary adrenal (HPA) function have also been widely reported in affective disorder and schizophrenic patients. However, to date, there have been relatively few studies of the relationship between structural brain alterations and brain function as reflected in CSF and HPA measures (2,5,6).

Our group has been prospectively studying the relationship between indices of structural brain anatomy (as defined by magnetic resonance imaging) and CSF neurotransmitter metabolites (HVA, MHPG, 5-HIAA), CSF neuropeptides (ACTH and CRF) and HPA function (24 hour urinary-free cortisol) in affective disorder patients (n = 21), schizophrenic patients, (n = 20) and in normal controls (n = 92).

Our preliminary data are consistent with a trend towards a decreased mean VBR in depressed patients (7.60) and an increased mean VBR in schizophrenic patients (9.52) as compared with normal controls (8.42) F = 2.58, p = .08. Our results reveal no significant differences in CSF MHPG, HVA, or 5-HIAA among patients with depression, schizophrenia, and normal controls. Our data replicate previous reports by Nemeroff and colleagues (4) of elevations in CSF CRF in depressed patients (78.4 ± 33.7, n = 18) as compared with schizophrenic patients (57.2 ± 26.9, n = 14) and normal controls (56.8 ± 32.2, n = 69), p = 04. In addition, our data replicate the frequently reported increased 24 hour urinary-free cortisol secretion in depressed patients as compared with schizophrenic patients or normal controls.

Our data, to date, reveal no significant relationships between mean VBR and either HPA activity or CSF HVA, MHPG, 5-HIAA, CRF or ACTH in affective disorder patients, schizophrenic patients, or normal controls. These data will be expanded to a larger subject number and the relationship between other measurements of brain structure and of other CSF indices will also be reported. To date, however, our data are consistent with the hypothesis that brain structural alterations may not cross-sectionally closely correlate with either CSF chemistry or HPA activity in depressed or schizophrenic patients.

REFERENCES

1. Coffman, J.A. and Nasrallah, H.A. (1986): Magnetic resonance brain imaging in schizophrenia. In: The Neurology of Schizophrenia. H.A. Nasrallah and D.R. Weinberger, eds., pp. 251-266. Elsevier Science Publishing Co., Inc., Amsterdam.
2. Houston J.P. et al., (1986): Cerebrospinal fluid HVA, central brain atrophy, and clinical state in schizophrenia. Psychiatry Research. 19:207-214.
3. Nasrallah H.A., Coffman J.A., Olson S.C., (1989): Structural brain-imaging findings in affective disorders: an overview. Journal of Neuropsychiatry. 1:21-26.
4. Nemeroff C., et al, (1984): Elevated concentrations of corticotropin-releasing factor-immunoreactivity in depressed patients. Science. 226:1342.
5. Potkin G., et al, (1983): Low CSF 5-hydroxyindoleacetic acid in schizophrenic patients with enlarged cerebral ventricles. Am. J. Psychiatry. 140(1):21-25.
6. Rao V.P., et al, (1989): Neuroanatomical changes and hypothalamo-pituitary-adrenal axis abnormalities. Biol. Psychiatry. 26:729-732.
7. van Kammen D.P., Peters J., van Kammen, W.B., (1986): Cerebrospinal fluid studies of monoamine metabolism in schizophrenia. Schizophrenia. 9:81-97.

THE ROLE OF CRH SYSTEMS IN MEDIATING PSYCHOPATHOLOGY:
ANIMAL MODELS

N.H. Kalin, L.K. Takahashi, and S.E. Shelton
Department of Psychiatry, University of Wisconsin, Madison,
WI, U.S.A.

INTRODUCTION

Evidence from clinical studies implicates alterations of HPA function in psychiatric patients. These abnormalities have been most completely characterized in depressed patients and have revealed: 1) hypersecretion of ACTH and cortisol, 2) dysregulation of diurnal rhythms of peripheral pituitary-adrenal hormones, 3) resistance to dexamethasone suppression, 4) blunted CRH-induced ACTH secretion, and 5) increased CSF concentrations of CRH.

Basic neurobiological studies have demonstrated that CRH-containing neurons and receptors are located not only in hypothalamus but also in other extrahypothalamic regions which may be of importance in mediating stress-induced autonomic and behavioral responses. Our laboratory has been engaged in a series of studies exploring the hypothesis that dysregulation of CRH systems in extrahypothalamic brain regions mediates maladaptive responses to stress.

RESULTS AND CONCLUSIONS

In studies with rats, we have demonstrated that ICV administration of CRH enhances shock-induced freezing behavior. Freezing is of interest because it is an adaptive reponse to threat and the amount of freezing an animal engages in indexes its degree of fearfulness. Consistent with this finding, ICV administration of the CRH antagonist, alpha-helical CRH(9-41), reduces shock-induced freezing. The CRH antagonist also reduces the occurrence of freezing behavior when rats are returned to an environment in which they received shock 24 hours earlier. This finding is of importance because it implicates CRH systems in mediating the behavioral response to nonpainful or psychological aspects of stress. These effects are mediated by brain CRH systems since the peripheral administration of these compounds does not affect freezing behavior.

To examine the generality of these effects we used another more naturalistic paradigm in which rats were exposed to an open field that contained a protective enclosure. When first placed in this situation, rats spent long periods of time in the protective enclosure and as they became more confident that the environment was safe gradually began to explore the open field. As expected, CRH increased the amount of time rats spent in the protective enclosure, whereas the CRH antagonist reduced the amount of time rats spent in the enclosure and increased their tendency to explore the environment. Taken together with the freezing studies, these experiments strongly implicate endogenous CRH systems in mediating a variety of stress-induced behaviors.

We have also studied the effects of CRH manipulations on the behavior of rhesus monkeys. These studies are of importance because they provide a closer link to modeling the function of CRH systems in humans. In addition, well established models of psychopathology have been established in the rhesus monkey. When administered in low doses to infant monkeys undergoing brief separation from their mothers, ICV-CRH resulted in decreased locomotion and increased freezing. These changes were also accompanied by a CRH-induced increase in ACTH concentrations which was greater than those that occurred when animals were administered vehicle prior to separation. Studies with the CRH antagonist have yielded less consistent results than those we observed when the antagonist was administered to rats. In other experiments we administered higher doses of CRH to adult animals and observed that these animals engaged in lying down and huddling behaviors. These findings are of considerable interest since huddling and lying down are behaviors characteristic of despairing monkeys. In summary, using animal models, our work implicates endogenous CRH systems in mediating adaptive responses to stress and suggests that dysregulation of CRH systems may be involved in mediating psychopathological stress responses in humans.

INTERLEUKIN-1 RECEPTORS IN THE BRAIN-ENDOCRINE-IMMUNE AXIS

Errol B. De Souza*, Toshihiro Takao* and Daniel E. Tracey**
*Laboratory of Neurobiology, Addiction Research Center, National Institute on Drug Abuse, Baltimore, MD 21224; **Hypersensitivity Diseases Research, The Upjohn Company, Kalamazoo, MI 49007

The cytokine interleukin-1 (IL-1), is one of the key mediators of immunological and pathological responses to stress, infection and antigenic challenge (6). IL-1 also has a variety of effects in brain including induction of fever, alteration of slow-wave sleep (6) and alteration of neuroendocrine activity. With regard to its neuroendocrine actions, administration of IL-1 stimulates the hypothalamic-pituitary-adrenocortical axis (1,3,9,12,13) and inhibits the hypothalamic-pituitary-gonadal axis (4,7,8). While there is some controversy regarding the precise site(s) of action of IL-1, direct effects of IL-1 have been reported on corticotropin-releasing factor (CRF) (1,9,12) and gonadotropin releasing hormone (8) release from hypothalamus, adrenocorticotropin secretion from the pituitary (2,13) and steroid production in the testis (4,7). The potential sites of action of IL-1 in the brain-endocrine-immune axis were examined by measuring the binding of ^{125}I-labeled recombinant human IL-1α (^{125}I-IL-1α) to cell membranes from mouse pituitary (11), hippocampus (5) and testis (10) and AtT-20 mouse pituitary cell line (11). In addition, the precise localization of the IL-1 binding sites in the tissues was examined using autoradiographic procedures.

KINETIC AND PHARMACOLOGICAL CHARACTERISTICS OF IL-1 RECEPTORS

The binding of ^{125}I-IL-1α was saturable, reversible, and of high affinity with K_D values of 50-100 pM and B_{max} values of approximately 11 (testis), 9 (pituitary), 8 (AtT-20) and 3 (hippocampus) fmol/mg protein. ^{125}I-IL-1α binding was specifically inhibited by recombinant human IL-1α, recombinant human IL-1β and a weak IL-1β analog, IL-1β+, in parallel with their relative bioactivities in the T cell comitogenesis assay, but not by unrelated peptides such as CRF and tumor necrosis factor (TNF) (rank order of potency: IL-1α~IL-1β > IL-1β+ >> CRF~TNF). The characteristics of ^{125}I-IL-1α binding in brain and endocrine tissues were similar to the properties of IL-1 receptors in the well-characterized EL-4 6.1 mouse thymoma cell line.

AUTORADIOGRAPHIC DISTRIBUTION IF IL-1 RECEPTORS

Autoradiographic localization of ^{125}I-IL-1α binding sites revealed low densities of receptors throughout the brain, with highest densities present in the dentate gyrus of the hippocampus and in choroid plexus. In the pituitary gland, IL-1 binding sites were localized in the anterior lobe; there was an absence of binding in the neurointermediate lobe. IL-1 receptors were heterogeneously distributed in testis with highest densities present in the luminal border of the epididymis and interstitial areas of the testis.

DISCUSSION

These studies demonstrating the characteristics and localization of IL-1 receptors in the brain-endocrine-immune axis with properties similar to the well-characterized EL-4 IL-1 receptors further substantiate that brain, pituitary and testicular sites of action may all be important in mediating the effects of IL-1 on neuroendocrine function. Stress, infection and inflammation are often accompanied by increased IL-1 production and by increased hypothalamic-pituitary-adrenocortical hormone secretion and by inhibition of reproductive function. In view of the presence of IL-1 in brain, in plasma and in testicular tissue, it is tempting to speculate on a role for IL-1 in mediating some of these stress-induced effects on neuroendocrine function. Furthermore, it is of interest to determine the role of IL-1 in the brain-endocrine-immune axis in neuropsychiatric disorders that show altered neuroendocrine activity.

REFERENCES

1. Berkenbosch, F. et al. Corticotropin-releasing factor-producing neurons in the rat activated by interleukin-1. Science 238:524-526, 1987.
2. Bernton, E.W. et al. Release of multiple hormones by a direct action of interleukin-1 on pituitary cells. Science 238:519-521, 1987.
3. Besedovsky, H. et al. Immunoregulatory feedback between interleukin-1 and glucocorticoid hormones. Science 233:652-655, 1986.
4. Calkins, J.H. et al. Interleukin-1 inhibits Leydig cell steroidogenesis in primary culture. Endocrinology 123:1605-1610, 1988.
5. De Souza, E.B., Takao, T., and Tracey, D.E. Interleukin-1 receptors in mouse brain. Int. Neuroendocrine Cong. Abstr. 1990.
6. Dinarello, C.A. Biology of interleukin-1. FASEB J. 2:108-115, 1988.
7. Fauser, B.C.J.M., Galway, A.B., and Hsueh, A.J.W. Inhibitory actions of interleukin-1β on steroidogenesis in primary cultures of neonatal rat testicular cells. Acta Endocrinol. 120:401-408, 1989.
8. Rivier, C. and Vale, W. In the rat, interleukin-1α acts at the level of the brain and the gonads to interfere with gonadotropin and sex steroid secretion. Endocrinology 124:2105-2109, 1989.
9. Sapolsky, R. et al. Interleukin-1 stimulates the secretion of hypothalamic corticotropin-releasing factor. Science 238:522-523, 1987.
10. Takao, T. et al. Identification of interleukin-1 receptors in mouse testis. Endocrinology 127: (in press), 1990.
11. Tracey, D.E. and De Souza, E.B. Identification of interleukin-1 receptors in mouse pituitary cell membranes and AtT-20 pituitary tumor cells. Soc. Neurosci. Abstr. 14:1052, 1988.
12. Uenara, A., Gillis, S, and Arimura, A. Effects of interleukin-1 on hormone release from normal rat pituitary cells in primary culture. Neuroendocrinology 45:343-347, 1987.
13. Woloski, B.M.R.N.J. et al. Corticotropin-releasing activity of monokines. Science 230:1035-1037, 1985.

CONTROLLED STUDIES OF THE PHARMACOLOGY OF CHILD AND ADOLESCENT MOOD DISORDERS

N.D. RYAN
Department of Psychiatry, University of Pittsburgh, Pittsburgh, PA, U.S.A.

Multiple lines of evidence demonstrate a strong relationship between juvenile and adult forms of major depressive disorder including similar clinical picture, familial transmission, longitudinal clinical course within childhood similar to the adult pattern, and sleep and neuroendocrine findings in part paralleling adult findings. Nevertheless, controlled studies demonstrating therapeutic efficacy of heterocyclic antidepressants in children and adolescents have thus far been elusive.

"Open label" (or plasma level/response) studies depend on the large plasma level variation seen in humans when given a fixed (weight adjusted) dose of tricyclic antidepressants, examining the relationship between plasma level and clinical outcome within individuals.

In prepubertal children, open label studies have strongly indicated efficacy of imipramine, one suggesting a therapeutic "window" of 125–225 ng/ml (4), and another suggesting that there was a threshold effect with levels over 150 ng/ml required but without an upper range, typical of adult plasma levels studies of this compound (5).

In adolescents, results are less clear. In one study, 34 outpatient adolescents were treated with imipramine titrated to 5 mg/kg/day as limited by side effects achieving a mean dose of 4.5 mg/kg/day (6). That study failed to demonstrate a plasma level/response relationship. Another study of imipramine given to inpatient adolescents failed to find a statistically significant therapeutic threshold though there was an almost statistically significant trend for higher plasma levels to respond better (7).

Double-blind placebo-controlled studies are the definitive study. In prepubertal children results of medication/placebo studies are mixed. One group has reported very interesting data on a small sample suggesting that medication superiority to placebo is found among dexamethasone non-suppressing prepubertal children (4). Two other studies, one of imipramine (5) and another of nortriptyline (1) found no difference between medication and placebo. A possible confound is the frequent high rate of placebo responders in younger children.

In adolescents, two medication/placebo studies have been completed, one (3) using amitriptyline and a second using nortriptyline (2) titrated to therapeutic plasma levels. Both failed to find differences in response rate between medication and placebo.

The author's ongoing study of amitriptyline versus placebo in non-bipolar adolescent major depression is, at the time of the first interim analysis after entering 25 subjects, 20 of which were randomized, entirely negative using either of several continuous or dichotomous outcome measures (see Fig 1). This study consists of a two-week single-blind placebo washout period followed by an eight week double blind medication period during which adolescents are titrated to 5.0 mg/kg/day of amitriptyline or placebo as limited only by side effects.

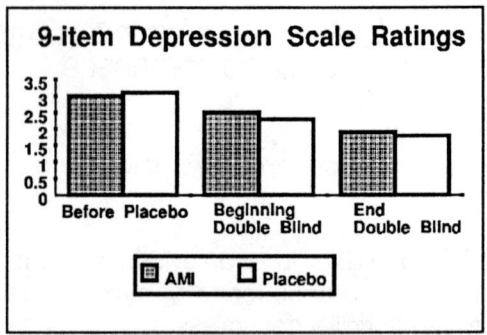

Figure 1

The total sample size in all controlled studies of tricyclic antidepressants in youth is to date very small. It is possible that tricyclics may yet prove relatively efficacious in that age group. Alternatively, subgroups of youth with major depression may be found in which the cyclic antidepressants are efficacious. However, it is possible that brain maturation effects (e.g. the development of noradrenergic systems into the third decade of life), changes in the ketosteroid hormonal milieu of the brain with development, inclusion of a relatively large number of youth who will turn out to be bipolar and thus may have a poor response to tricyclics, or choice of heterocyclic agent or dosage to test may be responsible for the lack of demonstrable efficacy to date. To test these, and other hypotheses, studies with serotonergic agents and non-heterocyclic antidepressants are indicated.

1. Geller, et al., (1989a): Psychopharmacol. Bull., 25:101-108.
2. Geller, B.: (1989b): A double-blind placebo-controlled study of nortriptyline in adolescents with major depression. NCDEU annual meeting. (Abstract)
3. Kramer, A.D. and Feiguine, R.J., (1981): J.Am. Acad. Child Psychiatry., 20:636-644.
4. Preskorn, et al., (1987): Psychopharmacol. Bull., 23:128-133.
5. Puig-Antich, et al., (1987): Arch. Gen. Psychiatry., 44:81-89.
6. Ryan, et al., (1986): Acta Psychiatr. Scand., 73:275-288.
7. Strober, M.: (1989): Effects of imipramine, lithium, and fluoxetine in the treatment of adolescent major depression. NCDEU annual meeting. (Abstract)

ALPRAZOLAM EFFECTS IN CHILDREN AND ADOLESCENTS WITH ANXIETY DISORDERS

J.G. SIMEON**, H.B. FERGUSON**, V. KNOTT**, N. ROBERTS**, C. DUBOIS*
and D. WIGGINS*
Royal Ottawa Hospital*, Department of Psychiatry**, University of
Ottawa, School of Medicine, Ottawa, Ontario, Canada.

    A variety of psychotropic drugs have been used to treat anxiety disorders in children. Benzodiazepines have been used in many different child psychiatry disorders, as well as in nonpsychiatric medical conditions in children. Clinical indications of benzodiazepines in child psychiatry are, however, not clearly established; childhood anxiety disorders are possible indications, and sleep disorders probable indications. Unfortunately, systematic studies and research data of anxiolytics in child psychiatry are very limited.
    Alprazolam, a newer benzodiazepine, has been shown to be effective and safe in the treatment of adult anxiety disorders. The aim of this study was to investigate the clinical efficacy, cognitive and EEG effects, and safety of alprazolam in the treatment of childhood and adolescent anxiety disorders. In this double-blind, placebo-controlled trial, alprazolam was given to 30 children 8.4 to 16.9 years old (mean, 12.6 years) with overanxious or avoidant disorders. Patients received placebo for one week, then alprazolam or placebo for four weeks; medication was then tapered over a one-week period, followed by one week of placebo. A follow-up assessment was done four weeks after the drug trial was completed. Evaluations included clinical, laboratory, cognitive, and quantitative EEG measurement. Clinical assessments included the Clinical Global Impressions Scale, the Brief Psychiatric Rating Scale for Children, Anxiety Rating Scale for Children, and parent, teacher and self-rating scales. Initial daily dose of alprazolam was 0.25 mg or 0.50 mg depending on body weight (40 kg). Dosages were individually titrated; average maximal daily dosage was 1.57 mg.
    On admission to the study the degree of global illness was rated as severe in three patients, marked in nine patients, and moderate in 18 patients. With alprazolam, improvements in the overanxious (N = 13) and the avoidant (N = 4) groups were very much in one patient, much in seven patients, minimal in seven patients, and no change in two patients. With placebo, improvements in the overanxious (N = 8) and avoidant (N = 5) groups were very much in one patient, much in four patients, minimal in three patients, no change in three patients, and worse in one patient. One patient did not complete this phase of the study.

On a clinical global rating, alprazolam appeared superior to placebo, but the differences did not reach statistical significance. The clinical global improvements were rated on a scale as no change (4), minimally improved (3), much improved (2), or very much improved (1). In the overanxious group (N = 13) alprazolam showed a slightly greater mean improvement than the placebo group (N = 8) - 2.69 versus 2.85. Following the tapering and post-drug placebo phases (Day 42) the alprazolam group showed a slight relapse (2.9), while the placebo group continued to improved (2.42). With alprazolam, the avoidant disorder group (N = 4) showed a mean clinical global improvement greater than that for the placebo group (N = 5) - 2.50 versus 3.00. Following the tapering and the post-drug placebo phases the alprazolam group showed a relapse (3.00), while the placebo group showed no further change (3.00). Self-ratings also indicated improvements of worry and negative-peer factors, suggesting greater changes with alprazolam than with placebo. Relative to baseline EEG, acute alprazolam administration significantly increased beta power in the right occiptal lead, and chronic administration increased beta power in both leads. These EEG data are compatible with those in adults. Analyses of a memory search task revealed that the placebo group showed evidence of decreasing cognitive efficacy relative to the alprazolam group. On other cognitive measures there were no differences between the alprazolam and placebo groups. Alprazolam was well tolerated, and adverse effects were few, mild, and transient.

The clinical results of this trial showed a strong treatment effect in both alprazolam and placebo groups. The data suggest that alprazolam may be more useful in avoidant disorders. The signifiance of the clinical data is limited by the small number of patients, the relatively low drug dosages, and short duration of drug administration. The role for alprazolam in specific child and adolescent disorders (overanxious, avoidant, separation anxiety, panic) should be evaluated in further controlled studies.

NEW PHARMACOTHERAPIES IN INFANTILE AUTISM

H.NARUSE*, M.TAKESADA**, T.HAYASHI***, Y.NAKANE****, K.YAMAZAKI*****
Dept. of Pediatrics, Kyorin Univ.*, Childrens Hosp. of Osaka City**, National Center of Neurology and Psychiatry***, Dept. of Psychiatry, Nagasaki Univ.****, Dept. of Psychiatry, Tokai Univ.*****

Many papers regarding to biochemical changes in infantile autism have suggested the existence of changes of metabolism of amines. However, these metabolic changes are not so marked and might be covered by many other factors. Therefore, we started a new experiment using "stable isotope labelled compounds" for investigating the metabolic changes of aromatic amino acids and these derivatives. The study could show interesting findings which might suggest the decreased turn over of catecholamines and serotonin in the brain of some autistic children. Based on the hypothesis, we started new treatments and found significant effect.

I. BIOCHEMICAL FINDINGS
[METHODS AND SUBJECTS]
Deuterated tryptophane (Trp-d5, Trp-d2). Deuterated phenylalanine (Phe-d5) and carbon13 (13C) labelled phenylalanine (Phe-13C6) were orally given to the patients. Labelled and non labelled compounds such as Phe, Tyr, Typ in blood and phenylethylamine, tyramine, tryptamine, serotonin, p-OH-Phenylacetate, VMA and HVM in urine were exactly measured by means of selected ion monitering using negative ion chemical ionization method.(T. Hayashi et al.) Ten cases of infantile autism were the subjects of the study.

[RESULTS]
Concerning the changes of labelled aromatic amino acid in blood, three different patterns were observed.
1) In three patients, transport of Phe-d5 or Trp-d5 from intestine into blood were disturbed significantly.
2) In four patients, only synthesis of labelled tyrosine in the blood was disturbed significantly.
3) Three cases did not show any abnormal patterns of labelled-phe, -trp and -tyr.

Labelled compounds in urine were determined in only limitted cases. Decreased excretion of labelled serotonin were observed in two cases, and also decreased excretion of 13C-labelled tyramine and p-OH-phenylacetate were ovserved in other two cases.

Based on these results and on some other reports, we postulated that there might be decreased synthesis of catecholamine and serotonin in the brain of some autistic children.

II. CLINICAL PHARMACOLOGICAL FINDINGS

1) INTRODUCTION OF THE PRECURSOR TREATMENT

Based on the assumption, H.N.& M.T. have started a new treatment with very low dosis of L-DOPA and 5HTP and found significant improvement of clinical symptoms of autistic patients. However, a small portion of the patient showed more agitated symptoms which could be interpreted as the over stimulation. Therefore, the clinical effect of R-tetrahydrobiopterine (RTHBP) was studied, because O. Hayaishi and his coworkers reported that RTHBP could enhance the synthesis of serotonin and catecholamine in the rat brain.

2) CLINICAL EFFECT OF RTHBP

Pure RTHBP, synthesized by Suntory Co., were provided for the clinical usage. After obtaining marked clinical effect in a preliminary trial with seventeen cases of autistic children, a double blind trial of RTHBP in the early phase II was conducted. R-THBP and the inactive placebo were given to 84 cases of typical autistic children for three monthes and the changes of clinical symptoms were analyzed in a double blind way. Clinical symptoms were checked by a rating scale for abnormal behaviors of children which was developed by the "Study Group on Behavioral Disorders of Children" in Japan. A fixed-flexible method was applied and the active drug was given per as at a dosage of 1.0-3.0 mg/kg/day in the form of a granule containing 2.5% RTHBP.

General improvement rating of RTHBP group at the 12th week was clearly superior to that of the placebo group ($p<0.05$) and marked effect was observed in the group under the age of 5 years. Clinical improvement was most significant in a cluster of the rating scale for "Autistic Behaviors" which seemed to be the core symptoms of the disease.

A open trial of RTHBP was performed with 99 cases of autistic patients and mentally retarded children. Medication were continued for 6 months in 7 different hospitals and detailed analyses concerning the clinical changes and adverse reaction due to RTHBP were achieved. Finally, the third phase study with 138 cases in 33 different institutions was organized by M.Nagahata and H.Kazamatsuri. The results of these studies were consistent with that of DBT and no serious adverse reaction was observed through all these clinical studies.

Bases on these studies, it will be concluded that RTHBP seems to be effective for improving the core symptoms of infantile autism in some patients. However, the drug have no effect in some patients and the further analysis concerning the responder and non-responder will be very important in order to investigate the bioligical basis of the disease.

REFERENCES

1. Naruse,H. et al. Therapeutic effect of tetrahydrobiopterin in infantile autism. Proceedings of the Japan Academy. 63(6):231-233, 1987.

2. Hayashi,T. et al. Sensitive determination of deuterated and non deutrated phenylalanine and tyrosine in human plasma by combined GC-negative ion chemical ionization MS. J. Chromatogr. 380(5):239-245,1986.

PHARMACOTHERAPY OF BEHAVIOR DISORDERS

R. KLEIN

Department of Psychiatry, Columbia University, and New York State Psychiatric Institute, New York, NY, U.S.A.

Since the advent of DSM-II, American nosology has been explicit in its formulation of two separate behavior disorders, hyperactivity and a conduct disorder syndrome. The DSM-II had a major influence on pharmacological research in hyperactive children. In contrast, conduct disorders have been virtually ignored.

Pharmacotherapy of the Hyperactivity Syndrome (ADHD)
Several classes of compounds were examined in ADHD over the past two decades: neuroleptics (thioridazine, chlorpromazine, haloperidol), psychostimulants (dextroamphetamine, levoamphetamine, methylphenidate, and magnesium pemoline), antidepressants (imipramine, tranylcypromine). Not only has the overall clinical efficacy of these agents been studied, but much work has been done to assess their effect on important behavioral domains that are not definitional diagnostic signs, such as social behaviors such as mother/child interactions, peer/peer interaction, teacher/child interaction (2). The demonstration of positive drug effects on interpersonal interaction has had a positive impact on attitudes towards drug treatment of the hyperactivity syndrome. The evidence concerning the claim that long-term stimulant treatment induces growth retardation is contradictory. However, the weight of the evidence supports the phenomenon. Importantly, this side effect appears limited to the period of active treatment and eventual height does not appear compromised (3).

Pharmacotherapy of Conduct Disorders
Conduct disorders differ in clinical presentation from the hyperactivity syndrome by encompassing antisocial behavior (such as stealing, truanting, vandalism), and aggression.

Methylphenidate. Methylphenidate has been compared to placebo in a small study of children classified as hyperactive or conduct disordered, based on cluster analysis (5). A larger percentage of children in the hyperactive cluster (90%) responded to methylphenidate than in the conduct disorder cluster (57%). These results are interpreted as documenting the greater efficacy of methylphenidate for hyperactivity than conduct disorders. However, the differences are not significant.
The other placebo study of methylphenidate in conduct disorder is our own investigation in a large group of 7-14 year olds diagnosed according to DSM-III. Two major clinical observations emanate from

the study. First children with pure conduct disorder are exceedingly rare among referred cases. Conduct disorders almost always have a history of hyperactivity. Second, methylphenidate is an effective treatment for conduct disorders, regardless of the cooccurrance of hyperactivity. Multiple aspects of dysfunction, including clear-cut antisocial behavior, were ameliorated by methylphenidate.

Lithium/Haloperidol. The first systematic drug study of well-diagnosed non-psychotic children with aggressive conduct disorder compared haloperidol, lithium, and placebo in hospitalized 5-13 year olds (1). Lithium doses ranged from 150 to 2000 mg/d, mEq/l serum levels from .32 to 1.8 (means, 1450 mg/d, and .99 mEq/l). The two compounds did not differ and both were significantly better than placebo in reducing hyperactivity, aggression, and hostility. Global ratings of clinical improvement also indicated a marked advantage for the active treatments. The lithium effect was felt to be qualitatively superior to that induced by haloperidol. However, three recent investigations of lithium in children and adolescents with conduct disorders (two inpatient (4), one outpatient) have failed to observe a significant beneficial effect in these youngsters.

Conclusion

Recent investigations have documented the positive impact of stimulant treatment on multiple functional domains of hyperactive children. Long-term effects on growth have not been found.

Conduct disorders represent an extremely important childhood condition, with a poor long-term prognosis, entailing much disadvantage to the individual and cost to the community. If the progression from early conduct disorder to later delinquency can be interrupted, it will have tremendous beneficial social implications. The treatment of conduct disorders is an area of great neglect. There are some data indicating that psychopharmacology can play a role in the amelioration of the symptoms of conduct disorder. The short-term efficacy of methylphenidate on antisocial behaviors is impressive, but that of lithium is now in question.

References

1. Campbell, M., et al. (1984): Arch. Gen. Psychiat., 41:650-656.

2. Klein, R.G. (1987): In Psychopharmacology: The Third Generation of Progress. H.Y. Meltzer, ed., pp. 1215-1224. Raven Press, New York.

3. Klein, R.G., and Mannuzza, S. (1988): Arch. Gen. Psychiat., 45:1131-1134.

4. Rifkin, A., et al. Psychopharm. Bull., (in press).

5. Taylor, E., et al. (1986): Br. J. Psychiat., 149:768-777.

LITHIUM IN AGGRESSIVE CHILDREN WITH CONDUCT DISORDER

M. CAMPBELL[*], A.M. SMALL[*], M.V. PADRON-GAYOL[*], J.J. LOCASCIO[*], V. KAFANTARIS[*] and J.E. OVERALL[**]
[*]Psychiatry, NYU Medical Center, New York, NY; [**]Psychiatry and Behavioral Sciences, University of Texas Medical School at Houston, Houston, TX, U.S.A.

Symptoms of severe aggressiveness directed against others and explosiveness are displayed in various psychiatric disorders in children of both normal and subnormal intelligence. In children under 12 years of age the most common reason for referral to a psychiatric clinic and admission to a psychiatric inpatient unit is conduct disorder, with these target symptoms (13). Because of failure to respond to a variety of treatment modalities many of these children are referred to residential treatment centers where they may remain for a prolonged time. In adolescence and young adulthood, this type of child will frequently become a substance abuser and/or engage in antisocial and criminal behavior. There is little systematic research in the area of psychopharmacology involving this population (for review, see 2). Stimulants, diphenylhydantoin and phenobarbital fail to control severe aggressiveness (1,14). Carbamazepine is not infrequently being administered to children with these behavioral problems but its efficacy and safety has not been critically assessed (for review, see 6). Haloperidol is effective (1,4,15), but its long-term administration is associated with tardive or withdrawal dyskinesias (5). Furthermore, there is some evidence that haloperidol affects adversely performance in the laboratory even when administered only for a period of four weeks (10), and patients experience significantly more side effects with this drug as compared to placebo (4). Lithium carbonate is reported to have antiaggressive properties in the absence of sedative effects (1,3,8,12). However, the onset of therapeutic effects may require 2 to 4 weeks: in a recent report involving aggressive adolescents, lithium did not differ from placebo when given over a period of 2 weeks, under double-blind conditions (11). Furthermore, it appears that aggressiveness is reduced when accompanied by angry affect and explosiveness (1,3,4,8). We systematically studied the efficacy and safety of lithium carbonate in those children (1,4). In a double-blind and placebo controlled comparison of lithium and haloperidol, involving 61 hospitalized children, ages 5.2 to 12.9 years, both drugs were significantly superior to placebo in reducing target symptoms (4).

SUBJECTS AND METHODS

Subjects were inpatients in Bellevue Hospital Center; all met the criteria for Conduct Disorder, Aggressive Type (9) and had a profile of severe aggressiveness and explosiveness. Their intellectual functioning was within normal range. After a two-week placebo baseline period, subjects were randomly assigned to lithium or placebo for 6 weeks, followed by a two-week post-treatment placebo period. The study was double-blind. The children were rated by multiple trained raters on several rating instruments in a variety of settings at fixed intervals and specified times. Behavioral assessments were conducted at week one and two of the placebo baseline period, four and six weeks after start of treatment, and at the end of the two-week post-treatment placebo period.

RESULTS

This is a preliminary report of this ongoing clinical trial. At the present time, 45 subjects, 42 males and 3 females, ages 5.12 to 11.95 years (mean 9.5; S.D.= 1.8; median 10.0) completed the study. They underwent careful clinical and laboratory monitoring. Optimal daily doses of lithium ranged from 600 to 1,800 mg (mean, 1,252; median 1,200; mean serum level 1.12 mEq/L). Most common side effects were vomiting, stomachache, nausea, headache, and tremor of hands, in most cases above therapeutic doses, during the period of dosage regulation. In addition, 7 of the 23 children who were assigned to lithium, gained more than 1 kg during the 6-week treatment. Lithium was significantly superior to placebo as rated on the Children's Psychiatric Rating Scales (CPRS)(7). For CPRS items assessing "fighting with peers," "bullying," and "temper outbursts" significant ($0.01 < p < 0.07$) condition X time interactions were found indicating sharper declines in ratings during treatment periods for lithium as opposed to placebo.

ACKNOWLEDGMENT: This work was supported in part by National Institute of Mental Health Grants MH-40177 (Dr. Campbell) and 1 T32 MH-18915 (Dr. Campbell and Dr. Kafantaris).

REFERENCES

1. Campbell, M., Cohen, I.L., and Small, A.M. (1982): Drugs in aggressive behavior. Amer. Acad. Child Psychiat., 212:107-117.
2. Campbell, M., and Spencer, E.K. (1988): Psychopharmacology in child and adolescent psychiatry: A review of the past five years. Am. Acad. Child Adol. Psychiat., 27:269-279.
3. Campbell, M., et al. (1972): Lithium and chlorpromazine: A controlled crossover study of hyperactive severely disturbed young children. J. Aut. Childh. Schizo., 2: 234-263.
4. Campbell, M., et al. (1984): Behavioral efficacy of haloperidol and lithium carbonate: A comparison in hospitalized aggressive children with conduct disorder. Arch. Gen. Psychiat., 41:650-656.
5. Campbell, M., et al. (1988): Tardive and withdrawal dyskinesia in autistic children: A prospective study. Psychopharmacol. Bull., 24:251-255.
6. Campbell, M., Malone, R.P., and Kafantaris, V. (in press): In Advances in Treatment of Child Psychiatry Disorders, J. G. Simeon and H.G. Ferguson (eds.), Human Sciences Press, New York.
7. Children's Psychiatric Rating Scale. (1985): Psychopharm. Bull. 21:765-770.
8. DeLong, G.R. and Aldershof, A.L. Long-term experience with lithium treatment in childhood: Correlation with clinical diagnosis. J. Amer. Acad. Child Adol. Psychiat., 26(3):389-394, 1987.
9. Diagnostic and Statistical Manual of Mental Disorders (DSM-III), 3rd Edition (1980), American Psychiatric Association, Washington, D.C.
10. Platt, J.E. et al. (1984): Cognitive effects of lithium carbonate and haloperidol in treatment-resistant aggressive children. Arch. Gen. Psychiat., 41:657-662.
11. Rifkin, A., et al. (1990): Lithium in adolescents with conduct disorder. Psychopharm. Bull., 26.
12. Sheard, M.H. et al. (1976): The effect of lithium on impulsive aggressive behavior in man. Amer. J. Psychiat., 133(12):1409-1413.
13. Stewart, M.A., et al. (1980): Aggressive conduct disorder of children: The clinical picture. J. Nerv. Ment. Dis., 168:604-610.
14. Stores, G. (1978): Antiepileptics (anticonvulsants). In Pediatric Psychopharmacology. The Use of Behavior Modifying Drugs in Children, J.S. Werry, (ed.), p. 274. Brunner/Mazel, New York.
15. Werry, J.S. and Aman, M.G. (1975): Methylphenidate and haloperidol in children. Arch. Gen. Psychiat., 32:790-795, 1975.

CONTROLLED STUDY OF LITHIUM FOR MOOD AND SUBSTANCE DEPENDENCY
    DISORDERS IN ADOLESCENCE

B. GELLER*, J.S. WILLIAMS*, T.B. COOPER**, and D.L. GRAHAM*
William S. Hall Psychiatric Institute-University of South Carolina
School of Medicine, Columbia, SC.* College of Physicians and Surgeons,
Columbia University, New York, NY**, U.S.A.

   This investigation was just initiated. It is the first controlled study of lithium treatment of adolescents dually diagnosed with substance use and mood disorders. We are communicating early in the work in order to inform other investigators of the methodological issues in the hope that this will encourage the development of further work in this area.
   There has been widespread use of lithium in adolescents since the 1950's, when it became available. Two large reports include a review of 190 cases of lithium use in children and adolescents and another of 196 cases (3,12). Most reports have been of mood disordered patients. The few studies have been difficult to interpret due to the inclusion of heterogeneous diagnostic groups with respect to type of mood disorder; small numbers of subjects; not reporting dose or serum level; or lacking rigorous assessment. Thus, despite the long span of time during which lithium has been widely used in adolescents, there is not yet a single well-designed double-blind placebo-controlled study, with an adequate number of subjects in a homogeneous sample, for any mood disorder in teenagers. There is also not a single systematic double-blind placebo-controlled study of lithium for adolescent substance use disorders (7). Studies of lithium use in adult populations who have drug/alcohol dependency range from the recent encouraging report of lithium effectiveness for cyclothymic cocaine abusers (albeit from a small, open trial) (6) to the most recent controlled study which reported poor outcome of lithium treatment for alcohol dependency regardless of depression (4). Importantly, the studies of lithium treatment of substance use disordered adults are not entirely relevant to the adolescent age group because treatment was not begun at the time of or soon after the onset of the disorder.
   Although it would have been ideal to have begun our investigation of dually diagnosed teenagers after studying lithium for each disorder separately, we decided not to do this for the following reasons: Both mood and substance use disorders are important risk factors for adolescents and young adults who have attempted or completed suicide (2,5). Also, the onset of mood disorders has occurred at a younger age over the past decades, which coincides temporally with a dramatic increase in the rate of suicide among teenagers during the past two decades (9,11). Given the evidence for significant morbidity and mortality for both of these diagnoses and the lack of any proven treatments, we decided that delaying a study of lithium treatment for the dually diagnosed was unwarranted.

METHODS AND RESULTS

Subjects were males and females 12-18 years old who met DSM-III-R criteria for substance dependency disorder and criteria for bipolar disorder except for the substance use exclusionary criteria. They were also included if they had major depressive disorder with at least one of the adolescent predictors of future bipolarity (1,10). This was a stratified random assignment double-blind placebo-controlled 12 week protocol which included a two week single-blind placebo-washout phase and a ten week double-blind placebo-controlled phase. In addition to scheduled weekly monitoring, random urine drug/alcohol assays and random serum lithium levels were also obtained on a weekly basis. Random specimens were collected in the subjects' homes. All subjects were outpatients. Steady state serum lithium levels of 0.9-1.3 mEq/L were obtained by predicting the dose from a baseline serum lithium level drawn 24 hours after a single 600 mg dose, utilizing a nomogram (8). Early findings will be presented at the C.I.N.P meeting in 1990.

ACKNOWLEDGEMENT: Supported by NIDA grant R01 DA 04844 to Dr. Geller.

REFERENCES

1. Akiskal, H.S. et al., (1983), Bipolar outcome in the course of depressive illness. J Affective Disord. 5:115-128.
2. Brent, D.A. et al., (1988), Risk factors for adolescent suicide. Arch Gen Psychiatry. 45:581-588.
3. DeLong, G.R. and Aldershof, A.L., (1987), Long-term experience with lithium treatment in childhood: correlation with clinical diagnosis. J Am Acad Child Adol Psychiatry. 26:389-394.
4. Dorus, W. et al., (1989), Lithium treatment of depressed and nondepressed alcoholics. J Am Med Assoc. 262:1646-1652.
5. Fowler, R.C. et al., (1986), San Diego suicide study. II. Substance abuse in young cases. Arch Gen Psychiatry. 43:962-965.
6. Gawin, F.H. and Kleber, H.D., (1984), Cocaine abuse treatment: open pilot trial with desipramine and lithium carbonate. Arch Gen Psychiatry. 41:903-909.
7. Geller, B. (1988), In: Adolescent Drug Abuse: Analyses of Treatment Research. National Institute on Drug Abuse Research Monograph Series, E.R. Rahdert, J. Grabowski, eds., pp. 94-112. DHHS Pub. No. (ADM) 88-1523, Washington, DC.
8. Geller, B. and Fetner, H., (1989), (ltr) Children's 24-hour serum lithium level after a single dose predicts initial dose and steady-state plasma level. J Clin Psychopharmacol. 9:155.
9. Gershon, E.S. et al., (1987), Birth-cohort changes in manic depressive disorders in relatives of bipolar and schizoaffective patients. Arch Gen Psychiatry. 44:314-319.
10. Strober, M. and Carlson, G., (1982), Bipolar illness in adolescents with major depression - clinical, genetic, and psychopharmacologic predictors in a three-to four-year prospective follow-up investigation. Arch Gen Psychiatry. 39:549-555.
11. Suicide - United States, 1970-1980, (1985), MMWR CDC DHHS, 34:353-7.
12. Youngerman, J. and Canino, I.A., (1978), Lithium carbonate use in children and adolescents. Arch Gen Psychiatry. 35:216-224.

LOW DOSE NEUROLEPTICS FOR NONPSYCHOTIC DISEASES IN PSYCHIATRY

W. Pöldinger
Department of Psychiatry, University, Basel, Switzerland

Beside the antipsychotic effect some neuroleptics like chlorprothixene, sulpiride, levomepromazine and thioridazine show an antidepressive activity.

These neuroleptics with an antidepressive efficacy are well known for additive antidepressive therapy. They are specially used for additive therapy of suicidal behaviour, anxiety, psychomotor agitation, and insomnia.

On the other hand classical neuroleptics like flupenthixol exhibit an antidepressive potential when administered at low dose. Low dose neuroleptic therapy for the treatment of depressive syndromes is particularly widespread in Europe. Montgomery et al. investigated the effectiveness of flupenthixol-depot in a placebo-controlled study in reducing suicidal behaviour in patients with personality disorder and repeated suicidal attempts. The flupenthixol treated group showed a significant reduction in the number of suicidal acts as compared to the placebo group. In a follow-up investigation the author found flupenthixol-depot also effective in patients with recurrent brief depression.

Additionally, low dose flupenthixol, flupenthixol-decanoate and fluspirilene are increasingly prescribed for the treatment of depressive and psychosomatic syndromes by general practitioners.

This treatment regime, however, is not uncontested especially by psychiatrists and neurologists. In September 1989 in Stresa, Italy, this issue was discussed by psychiatrists and practitioners. At this occasion the results of controlled trials were presented, demonstrating the antidepressive and anxiolytic effectiveness of low-dose neuroleptics.

Extrapyramidal side effects were only very rare and mild.

Nevertheless, in view of possible risks practitioners and psychiatrists concluded that the treatment of nonpsychotic mental diseases with low dose neuroleptics should be limited by time and dosage.

Following syndromes or indications could possibly be treated with low dose neuroleptics:

- state of tension
- generalised anxiety
- mild depressive and depressive-anxiety syndromes
- psychosomatic diseases
- dysthymic disorders

Finally, experiences at the Psychiatric University Hospital, Basel, Switzerland, indicate that in bipolar depressed and manic disorder, the prophylactic effect of flupenthixol decanoate was similar to that of lithium salts.

References
Montgomery St. A., Montgomery D.: Pharmacological Prevention of Suicidal Behavior. J. Affect. Dis. 4, 291-298 (1982).
Montgomery St. A.: Niedrigdosierte Neuroleptika bei ängstlich-depressiven Zustandsbildern und psychosomatischen Erkrankungen. Kolloqium Stresa, 1989. TW Neurologie/Psychiatrie 3: Suppl. (1989).
Kielholz P., Terzani S., Pöldinger W.: The Long-Term Treatment of Periodical and Cyclic Depressions with Flupenthixol Decanoate. Int. Pharmacopsychiat. 14: 305-309 (1979)
Pöldinger W.: Niedrigdosierte Neuroleptika bei ängstlich-depressiven Zustandsbildern und psychosomatischen Erkrankungen. Kolloquium Stresa 1989. TW Neurologie/Psychiatrie 3: Suppl. (1989)

PREFERENTIAL DOPAMINE AUTORECEPTOR BLOCKADE: A POSSIBLE PHARMACOTHERAPEUTIC PRINCIPLE IN ANTIDEPRESSANT THERAPY

A. CARLSSON
Department of Pharmacology, University of Gothenburg, Gothenburg, Sweden

For a long time it has been recognized that neuroleptic agents can possess antidepressant properties. They have been suggested to be more effective in anxious, agitated and delusional patients with depression than in cases where psychomotor retardation is a dominating feature (3,6). An attractive hypothesis to explain these otherwise puzzling antidepressant properties is that these agents are capable of blocking dopaminergic autoreceptors preferentially. Animal experiments have demonstrated stimulating properties of low doses of neuroleptic agents, though generally within a narrow dose range (1). A preferential blockade of dopaminergic autoreceptors leads to an increased dopaminergic tone and thus to psychomotor stimulation.

The behavioral consequences of this preferential dopamine autoreceptor blockade are, however, not easy to study, mainly because of the narrow dose range in which they become manifest. We have had the opportunity to investigate this problem in some more detail, thanks to our discovery of a series of dopamine receptor antagonists with a more clearcut preference for the autoreceptors. The two most thoroughly investigated compounds with these properties are the N-mono and N-dipropyl derivatives of cis-(+)-(1S,2R)-5-methoxy-1-methyl-2-aminotetralin, also called (+)-AJ76 and (+)-UH-232, respectively. These agents cause mild psychomotor stimulation over a wide dose range in rats and mice. Since the former agent exhibits a somewhat higher preference for the autoreceptors than the latter, it produces a higher level of stimulation. However, in both cases the level of stimulation is much lower than for classical central stimulants such as amphetamine. When the doses are increased the degree of stimulation is not further elevated but may, in fact, be reduced, at least in the case of (+)-UH-232.

Biochemically these agents have been shown to stimulate the firing of dopaminergic neurons in the substantia nigra as well as the synthesis, release and metabolism of dopamine in the striatal nerve terminal regions. In this respect they do not differ from classical neuroleptics. However, whereas the latter cause psychomotor inhibition, the former, as mentioned, induce stimulation. This stimulation is obviously due to the increased release of dopamine, because it is effectively antagonized by a classical neuroleptic such as haloperidol. In vivo binding experiments using an aminotetralin derivative with dopamine (D-2) receptor agonist properties shows that both (+)-AJ-76 and (+)-UH-232 are capable of binding to postsynaptic dopamine receptors in higher dosage but they do so less completely than haloperidol. Thus the biochemical data demonstrate a clearcut difference between these novel antagonists and classical neuroleptics, which supports the view that their psychomotor stimulating action is due to preferential dopamine autoreceptor stimulation (4,5).

A most fascinating feature of these novel agents is that the degree of psychomotor stimulation is dependent on the baseline activity level. Thus, in animals with a low level of locomotor activity, which occurs if the animals have been habituated to their environment for about an hour, the degree of stimulation induced by these agents is much more pronounced than in animals actively exploring a new environment. Moreover, if the rats have an excessively high level of activity, induced by a directly or indirectly acting dopaminergic agonist, treatment with the novel agents will actually be inhibitory on locomotor activity. This dual, "normalizing" or "stabilizing" action is reminiscent of lithium and raises the question if this profile of activity could lead to both an antidepressant and antimanic effect. They might also prove beneficial in schizophrenia, perhaps especially with marked negative symptomatology, as well as in psychasthenic conditions and in drug abuse (2).

Our research group is still engaged in investigating the structure-activity relations for these preferential dopamine autoreceptor antagonists. Hopefully it will prove possible to start clinical trials with a representative of this new class of drugs in the not too distant future.

REFERENCES

1. Ahlenius, S. and Engel, J. (1971): Effects of small doses of haloperidol on timing behavior. J. Pharm. Pharmacol. 23:301-302.
2. Carlsson, A. (1988): The current status of the dopamine hypothesis of schizophrenia. With commentaries and author's reply. Neuropsychopharmacology, 1:179-203.
3. Jimerson, D.C. (1987): Role of dopamine mechanisms in the affective disorders. In Psychopharmacology: The Third Generation of Progress. H.Y. Meltzer ed., Raven Press., New York, pp. 505-511.
4. Svensson, K., Johansson, A.M., Magnusson, T. and Carlsson, A. (1986): (+)-AJ 76 and (+)-UH 232: Central stimulants acting as preferential dopamine autoreceptor antagonists. Naunyn-Schmiedeberg's Arch. Pharmacol., 334:234-245.
5. Svensson, K., Hjorth, S., Clark, D., Carlsson, A., Wikström, H., Andersson, B., Sanchez, D., Johansson, A.M., Arvidsson, L.-E., Hacksell, U. and Nilsson, J.L.G. (1986): (+)-UH 232 and (+)-UH-242: Novel stereoselective DA receptor antagonists with preferential action on autoreceptors. J. Neural Transm., 65:1-27.
6. Willner, P. (1985): Depression. A Psychobiological Synthesis. pp. 170-172. John Wiley & Sons, New York.

INDICATIONS FOR A LOW-DOSE NEUROLEPTIC THERAPY IN NON-PSYCHOTIC
PSYCHIATRIC DISEASES

H.J. MÖLLER
Department of Psychiatry of the University Bonn, D-5300 Bonn 1, FRG

The minor tranquilising effect of neuroleptics is well known since the development of these compounds. But this effect was neglected for a long time in the therapy of non-psychotic patients because of the favorable clinical profile of the benzodiazepines: potent anxiolytic power, excellent tolerability. However, in the last years the problem of benzodiazepine dependency was considered more and more intensively. Although the risk of dependency is comparatively low, the absolute figures are impressive because of the high rate of prescriptions. Especially this more critical view of the benzodiazepines stimulated the search for alternatives, and among these low-dose strategy of neuroleptics in non-psychotic patients exceeded any expectations.

During the last years several controlled studies demonstrated that low-dose therapy with neuroleptics is significantly superior to placebo and seems equally effective in comparison to benzodiazepines with respect to anxiolysis (compare the reviews by Möller (2), Hippius and Laakmann (1) and Tegeler (3)). Contrary to the expectations low-dose therapy with neuroleptics was tolerated very well, also with respect to extrapyramidal disturbances.

Principal indications for this therapy are anxiety, tension, depressive mood, vegetative or functional psychosomatic disturbances in the framework of non-psychotic disorders (reactions, neurotic disturbances, personality disturbances, psychosomatic disturbances).

However, the following specifications should be considered:

a) The acute panic attack should be stopped very effectively with benzodiazepines, for long-treatment of panic disorders antidepressants should be administered (especially imipramine or MAO inhibitors).

b) Compulsive disorders should be treated with clomipramine or similar antidepressants.

c) In case of psychosomatic disorders with prominent depressive mood application of antidepressants should be the therapy of first choice.

d) Treatment of first choice in neurotic depressions are the antidepressants.

Low-dose neuroleptic therapy is especially indicated in patients with a predisposition to addiction or a manifest alcohol or drug abuse. On the other hand, patients with an increased sensibility for extrapyramidal side-effects (e.g., patients with brain disorders, aged patients) and patients with manifest extrapyramidal disturbances will be preferably treated with benzodiazepines, not with neuroleptics.

A special question is whether oral preparations or depot-neuroleptics have to be preferred for this therapeutic regimen. In general, the patients in question here are compliant thus the depot-neuroleptic strategy does not seem necessary. On the other hand, treatment with depot-neuroleptics has some pharmacokinetic advantages.

To avoid the risk of tardive dyskinesia as far as possible the following rules should be followed:

a) Primary treatment should in general not exceed two to three months.

b) If careful withdrawal of the neuroleptic after this time leads to a deterioration of symptoms, treatment should be continued over the next three months but, if possible, using a lower dosage.

c) If after six months of treatment withdrawal of neuroleptics leads again to a deterioration, continuation of treatment is necessary in these seldom cases. But also for the future this treatment should be interrupted by withdrawals of neuroleptics or the neuroleptics should be replaced, if possible, by other medications, e.g. sedative antidepressants.

d) Careful clinical examinations should be performed according to a strict time-schedule to detect early signs of tardive dyskinesia. In case of such early signs treatment with neuroleptics has to be stopped.

REFERENCES

1. Hippius, H., and Laakmann, G. (1988): Therapie mit Neuroleptika - Niedrigdosierung. Perimed, Erlangen
2. Möller, H.J. (1986): Med. Klinik, 81: 385-388
3. Tegeler, J. (1988): In Therapie mit Neuroleptika - Niedrigdosierung, H. Hippius and G. Laakmann, eds., pp. 80-91. Perimed, Erlangen

NEUROLEPTICS IN THE TREATMENT OF ANXIETY

K. Achté
Department of Psychiatry, University of Helsinki, Finland

Small doses of neuroleptics can be used instead of hypnotics in patients who do not develop side effects, particularly when normal benzodiazepine doses are not sufficient or cannot be used. The response is individual, and relatively small doses of neuroleptics with a sedative effect are often sufficient.

Small doses of neuroleptics are needed in alcohol withdrawal. Neuroleptics are often extremely useful in borderline states and other personality disorders. The closer the disorder is to psychosis, the more useful the neuroleptics. They are also used in small doses for vomiting and hyperhidrosis, and in general anaesthesia to intensify the hypnotic effect. Various states of restlessness and agitation which are not psychotic are aften a good indication for the use of neuroleptics. Prolonged pain often responds to neuroleptics. In therapy-resistant depression, a small dose of a neuroleptic can be combined with antidepressants. In haemorrhagic shock neuroleptics are used to improve tissue perfusion.

However, in the control of anxiety the role of neuroleptics is essential. This will be discussed in more detail below.

In the 1960s and 1970s small doses of neuroleptics were used in Finland to treat anxiety disorders, but this practice is being abandoned. Many neuroleptics are sedative and they also have a hypnotic effect. There is no risk of tolerance associated with the use of neuroleptics, which are a possible alternative for patients who develop dependence on benzodiazepines. Anxiety is a common symptom in difficult personality disorders, and this type can be controlled by neuroleptics. In psychoses and senile dementia, psychomotor anxiety and agitation can be combined with aggressive behaviour. In such cases neuroleptics are often more effective than benzodiazepines.

Experience shows undisputably that neuroleptics are less effective - often ineffective - than benzodiazepines in the treatment of anxiety, and often produce difficult side-effects, such as hypotension, sedation without abating anxiety, tasikinesia, muscular restlessness and, above all, tardive dyskinesia.

Since anxiety is an unspecific symptom in many psychiatric disorders, it may be appropriate in individual cases to try neuroleptics, particularly if the ordinary use of benzodiazepines presents problems. I give small doses of neuroleptics at bedtime to anxious patients whose benzodiazepine dose I do not wish to increase unnecessarily, and if neuroleptics seem to help.

In psychotic syndromes, the clinician is often confronted with both anxiety and agitation. Anxiety is often a part of the syndrome and may be associated with sleep disorders, difficulties in concentration, lack of appetite and depressive symptoms (2). It is also common in various "borderline" personality disorders. These patients may benefit from neuroleptics.

There are three principal indications for the treatment of anxiety with neuroleptics (3):
1) anxiety in organic brain syndromes, including senile dementia
2) mild unspecific anxiety in cases with psychasthenia or mild depression
3) drug and alcohol abuse, acute toxic anxiety and withdrawal anxiety.

To summarize, neuroleptics are of some use for anxiety disorders related to organic brain syndromes and senile dementia. Neuroleptics are classically used the control of anxiety in psychotic, paranoid and schizophrenic states.

Patients receiving neuroleptics must be carefully monitored and side-effects followed. High doses may produce cognitive disorders and confusion in older patients. This risk is particularly increased if neuroleptics are used simultaneously with tricyclic antidepressants with anticholinergic effects. Somatic side-effects, such as increased intraocular pressure, dryness of the mouth, voiding difficulties and orthostatic disorders also limitthe use of neuroleptics, particularly in high doses in the elderly. The use of neuroleptics in the treatment of anxiety is contraindicated in states in which neuroleptics cause adverse effects or if some other group of drugs is more effective.

There is no clear contraindication to the use of neuroleptics in the treatment of anxiety, although they are not particularly effective. High doses should be avoided. The basic rule is to use small doses for only three months at a time. Again, medication should be stopped gradually (1).

REFERENCES

1. Achté, K. (1989): Treatment of anxiety disorders. In Many faces of panic disorder. Proceedings of the Symposium by the Section of Clinical Psychopathology of the World Psychiatric Association 1988, K. Achté, T. Tamminen, and R. Laaksonen, eds., pp. 102-111. Psychiatria Fennica Supplementum, Helsinki.

2. Forsman, A. (1988): The place of neuroleptic drugs in the pharmacological treatment of anxiety disorders. In Pharmacological Treatment of Anxiety. National Board of Health and Welfare, Drug Information Committee, Sweden, Uppsala.

3. Reich, J. (1986): The epidemiology of anxiety. J. Nerv. Ment.Dis., 174:129-136.

LOW DOSE NEUROLEPTANXIOLYSIS IN ANXIETY STATES

K.HEINRICH and E.LEHMANN
Department of Psychiatry,Heinrich-Heine-University,
Düsseldorf,F.R.G.

Benzodiazepines belong to the anxiolytics administered most frequently worldwide due to their wide therapeutic range and efficacy.The use of benzodiazepines increased nearly exponentially in the 70ties (1). The majority of benzodiapine prescriptions are given by general physicians and internal specialists, only approx.6% by psychiatrists or psychotherapeutists (2).
Especially the risks of addiction gave rise to appropriate warnings of such a wide, uncritical application of benzodiazepines.During the recent years low dose neuroleptics are therefore increasingly discussed as a pharmacotherapeutical alternative in the treatment of anxiety syndromes (3).
The clinical benefits of fluspirilene in anxiolysis were already observed in 1973. Later investigations with larger groups of probands confirmed these first reports.

As an advantage of this therapeutic procedure as apposed to a treatment with benzodiazepines it was pointed out that within the frame of neuroleptic therapy no disturbing sedation and no development of addiction must be apprehended.

The danger of extrapyramidal motoric, vegetative and endocrinological side-effects under antipsychotic dosage was insignificant under low dose neuroleptanxiolytic dosage.
In an experimental study of a total of 45 out-door anxiety patients suffering from organic- functional complaints and psychoreactive disorders, the effect of six weeks's treatment with 1.5 mg fluspirilene per week was compared with 6 mg bromazepam per day. The drugs were administered in a double blind double-dummy technique. To objectify the diagnosis the Minnesota Multiphasic Personality Inventory and a life history questionnaire were used. At the beginning of the study, as well as after 14,28 and 42 days the Hamilton Anxiety Scale was applied. In addition a global assessment of therapeutic effectiveness was made. It was demonstrated, that fluspirilene in six weeks of treatment was therapeutically superior to bromazepam (Table 1).

Table 1: Global therapeutic improvement after 42 days

	markedly improved and improved	slightly improved	unchanged and deteriorated
BROMAZEPAM	8	15	23
FLUSPIRILENE	16	6	22
TOTAL	24	21	45

$Chi^2 = 6.51; p\ 0.02$

The tolerance of fluspirilene was made the subject of a separate study. 1261 patients with anxiety and psychoreactive disorders received 1.5 mg fluspirilene per week for six weeks under controlled and open conditions.

Table 2: Side effects in 1261 patients under fluspirilene

	incidence	percentage
weight gain	74	5,87
tiredness	48	3,81
extrapyramidal disorders	42	3,33
dryness of the mouth	17	1,35
perspiration	10	0,79
vertigo	9	0,71
circulatory disorders	7	0,56
gastrointestinal symptoms	4	0,32
visual defects	4	0,32
unspecific reactions	11	0.87

Table 2 shows the frequencies of side effects we observed. All side effects had in common that they occured already within the first few weeks of treatment.

REFERENCES:
1. Hoffmeister,F. :Zur Pharmakologie der Benzo-und Thienodiazepine.In:Gegenwärtiger Wissensstand der Anwendung von Benzo- und Thienodiazepinen.Hrsg.v.d.Fed.Abt.d.Troponwerke Köln. PMI-Verlag,Frankfurt/Main 1982.
2. Ladewig,D.:Abusus von Benzodiazepin-Tranquilizern.Med. Welt 33,13o6-13o9,1982.
3. Lehmann,E., Hassel,P., Thörner,GW., Karras,W.:Alternatives Therapiekonzept zur Behandlung psychosomatischer Beschwerden.Fortschr.Med.4o,1o33-1o36,1984.

FLUPENTHIXOL-DECANOAT VERSUS FLUSPIRILEN IN ANXIOUS-DEPRESSIVE SYNDROMES: A DOUBLE-BLIND COMPARISON

M. OSTERHEIDER
Department of Psychiatry, University of Wuerzburg
(Head: Prof. Dr. H. Beckmann), Wuerzburg, FRG

Low dose neuroleptics are more often used in the past years in the treatment of anxious-depressive symptoms. The so-called "neuroleptanxiolysis" has sometimes been described as an alternative to benzodiazepines for example.
Flupenthixol (F)/Flupenthixoldecanoat (FD) and Fluspirilen (FLU) are the most often used drugs in this indication and in several studies since the early seventies their anxiolytic and antidepressant properties had been shown by several authors (2,3).
But nevertheless there is a risk of specific side effects - especially Tardive Dyskinesia (TD) - as has been pointed out in recent studies (1,4).

SUBJECT AND METHOD

With a special focus on the different side effect profiles we carried out a study comparing FD and FLU in their effectiveness on anxiety and depression.
In a randomised, doubleblind-design 60 outpatients (M/F; 18 - 60 y.) with diagnoses of anxiety neurosis (ICD 300.0) and neurotic depression (ICD 300.4) were treated with either FD 10 mg/2 weekly or F 1.5 mg/weekly.
Efficacy was determined by the Hamilton scales for depression (HRSD) and anxiety (HRSA). The HRSD-score at the beginning had to be ≥ 20, evaluation time was 8 weeks. Psychopathometric evaluation was done by using CGI, D-S and STAI. Also different side effect rating scales were used: Akathisia (AKA)-scale, AIMS and WEBSTER-parkinsonian-scale.

RESULTS

According to the HRSD and HRSA an improvement is seen in both groups indicating good anxiolytic and antidepressant effects for both drugs. There were no statistically relevant group differences.
Also referring to the other rating scales there were only trends in differences; as for example in the CGI reflecting FD clinically more effective.

Only in the side effect ratings relevant differences had been observed, especially in the frequency of akathisia and abnormal involuntary movements, which - totally - are rare and not severe.

DISCUSSION

The data derived under these conditions were supportive to early studies in which the efficacy and safety of this treatment had been confirmed.
Finally the different effects of FD and F on anxiety and depression (item-analysis) will be discussed and a benfit-risk-ratio for application of low-dose neuroleptics in non-psychotic disorders will be done critically.

REFERENCES

1, Osterheider, M. et al. (1990):
   Pharmacopsychiat., (in press)
2. Pöldinger,W. et al. (1983):
   Neuropsychobiology, 10: 131 - 136
3. Rüther, E. and Hippius, H. (1982):
   MMW, 124: 683 - 684
4. Schmidt, L.G. (1989):
   Pharmacopsychiat. 22: 188 - 191

EFFICACY AND TOLERABILITY OF FLUPENTHIXOL-DEPOT IN THE TREATMENT OF DEPRESSIVE AND PSYCHOSOMATIC DISORDERS: A MULTICENTER TRIAL IN GENERAL PRACTICE.

G. Budde
Medical Department, Troponwerke GmbH & Co. KG, D-5000 Cologne 80, FRG

A number of uncontrolled as well as controlled studies indicate that flupenthixol in low-dose regimen is effective in syndromes with depression, anxiety and psychosomatic disorders. In view of the low compliance rate in depressed patients we evaluated the efficacy and tolerability of flupenthixol decanoate i.m. in an unselected collective of depressed patient in general practice.

SUBJECT AND METHOD

4772 patients aged 15-94 (mean age 53 years) entered the trial.
81.4 % showed depressive symptoms, 59.1 % suffered from anxiety, 25.8 % had a chronic nonorganic pain syndrome and 52.5 % manifested with a psychosomatic disorder. 34.5 % of the patients had more than 2 of the symdromes:
The subjects were treated with one injection of flupenthixol-depot every two weeks. A flexible dose of 6 to 14 mg was administered. The treatment was continued for 10 weeks and assessments were made before and after 2, 4, 6, 8 and 10 weeks of treatment.
50.8 % of the patients were pretreated with a variety of psychotropic drugs which were discontinued during the trial except in 12 % of the patients.
Therapeutic effect was rated on a 4-point-intensity-scale and a final global assessment about efficacy and tolerability was given by the investigating physician.

RESULTS

The mean dosage of flupenthixol-depot was 10 mg/14 days. In about 80 % the dosage was stable during the treatment.

Outcome:
There was a remission of symptoms in 25 % (pain) to 29 % (psychosomatic disorder) of the patients (depression and anxiety 27 %). Therapeutic benefit was seen in more than 90 % of the patients (tab. 1).
Unwanted effects:
9.2 % of the subjects developed side effects and the treatment had to be stopped in 2.5 %. The most frequent side effect was sedation, 2.0 % developed mild extrapyramidal signs (tab. 2).

table 1: FINAL GLOBAL ASSESSMENT OF EFFICACY (n = 4772)

remission	marked improvement	moderate improvement	unchanged deterioration discontinuation of treatment
1893	1882	536	461

Better treatment results were seen in patients

1) who were not pretreated with psychotropic drugs

2) with a duration of disease shorter than one year

3) younger than 60 years

4) with a lower dose than 0.5 ml = 10 mg flupenthixol decanoate

table 2: SIDE EFFECTS; POSSIBLY CORRELATED TO FLUPENTHIXOL

Kind of side effect	frequency (number of patients)	percentage
Extrapyramidal signs	94	2.07
akathisia	11	0.25
fatigue	97	2.09
dry mouth	41	0.89
vertigo	50	1.01
sweating	7	0.14
gastrointestinal disorders	74	1.61
weight gain	31	0.64
cardiac disorders	21	0.46
restlessness, nervousness	32	0.69
sleep disorders	13	0.30
impaired vision	6	0.11
local irritations(reactions)	11	0.23

CNS 5-HT NEURONS AND GLIAL S-100$_B$

Efrain C. Azmitia[1] and Patricia M. Whitaker-Azmitia[2]
1. Dept. Biol; NYU, New York, N.Y. 10003 2. Dept. Psych, State Univ. of N.Y., Stony Brook, N.Y. 11794.

Dissociated primary cultures of neurons and glial cells are used to demonstrate the existence of a 5-HT$_{1A}$ receptor-mediated releasable astrocytic-protein (S100$_{beta}$) which can stimulate the growth of serotonergic neurons. S-100$_{beta}$ is also a neuronotrophic factor for cortical neurons (10, 17). The functional interactions between CNS 5-HT neurons and glial S-100$_{beta}$ has implications for the etiology of Alzheimer's Disease.

SUBJECT AND METHOD

Primary neuronal microcultures are prepared from rat fetuses at 13 dg (1,2). In glial-suppressed cultures, FDUr is added after 48 h. Astrocytic primary cultures are grown from 1-3 day neonatal rat pups (14). High grade purified S-100$_B$ from human, calmodulin and anti-S-100 antibody are used (East Acres Biological). Neuronal growth of 5-HT cultures is assessed by high-affinity uptake of 50 nM ^{3}H-5-HT for 20 min at 37$_o$C (2). Morphometric analysis of 5-HT-immunoreactive neurons performed on 8-well glass culture chamber slides.

RESULTS

NGF, EGF, Insulin and S-100 in serial dilution,(10 ug/ml to 1 ng/ml) are added daily to primary cultures and only S-100 produced a stimulation (maximal 170% of control at 16 ng/ml). This stimulation was confirmed by morphometric analysis of 5-HT-immuno-reactive neurite length in cultures (147% of control at 3.2 ng/ml). Activity is predominately in the S-100$_b$ form compared to S-100$_a$ and not due its Ca^{++} binding property since calmodulin is without affect. The activity of S-100$_b$ is potentiated by the addition of 1mM 1,4-dithiothreitol, a protective agent for SH groups. S-100$_{beta}$ activity is seen in glial suppressed (FDUr treated) cultures.

S-100$_{beta}$ is a soluble astroglial specific protein in CNS (8). Primary astroglial cultures secrete a soluble protein which stimulates cultured 5-HT neurons (15). Astrocytes contain a high density of high-affinity 5-HT$_1$ receptors (13) which decreases in mature cultures (14). Stimulation with a specific 5-HT$_{1a}$ agonist (8-OH-DPAT or ipsapirone) results in an increased 5-HT growth factor activity. Application of a polyclonal antibody raised against human S-100 (dilution 1/10,000) blocked both the activity of 5-HT-glial media and of exogenously applied $S-100_b$. Our results indicate that 5-HT neurons can auto-regulate their own development by stimulation of $S-100_b$ from glial cells in culture and in vivo through a $5-HT_{1A}$ receptor. $S-100_b$ and 5-HT may act as trophic factors in concert on a variety of target cells.

DISCUSSION

Alzheimer's Disease is characterized by neurite tangles and plaque formation. Neurite tangles are rich in phosphorylated tau protein (11), a microtubules association protein protected from phosphorylation by $S-100_{beta}$ (4,5). In primate brain, plaques are rich in neurite containing 5-HT (9) and in astrocytes containing $S-100_{beta}$ (7). Furthermore, the receptor which releases S-100 from astrocytes, 5-HT-1A, is decreased in Alzheimer's brain (6,12). We propose that a primary cause of the neurodegenerative process in Alzheimer's is an inability to release $S-100_{beta}$ from astrocytes because of down regulation of the $5-HT_{1a}$ receptor. NSF 8812892 (ECA) and NINCDS 2539102 (PMW-A).

REFERENCES

1. Azmitia, E.C. and Whitaker-Azmitia, P.M. (1987): Neuroscience 20: 47-62.
2. Azmitia, E.C., Dolan, K. and Whitaker-Azmitia, P.M. (1990): Brain Res. In Press
3. Azmitia, E.C. (1990): In Methods in Neuroscience, Vol. 2: In Press. P.M. Conn, ed., Acad Press, CA.
4. Baudier, J. and Cole, R.D. (1987) J. Biol. Chem. 262: 17577-17583.
5. Baudier, J. et al, (1987): Biochem 26: 2886-2893.
6. Cross, A.J. and Deakin, J.F.W. (1985): Neurosci. Lett. 60: 261-265.
7. Griffin, W.S.T. et al, (1989): P.N.A.S. 86: 7611-7615.
8. Isobe, T. Takahasi, K. and Okuyama, T. (1984) J. Neurochem. 43: 1494-1496.
9. Kitt, C.A. et al. (1989): Synapse 3:12-18.
10. Kligman, D. and Marshak, D.R., (1985): P.N.A.S. 82: 7136-40.
11. Kosik, K., Joachim.C., and Selkoe, D. (1986) P.N.A.S. 83: 4044-4048.
12. Middlemiss, D.N. et al, (1986): J. Neurochem. 46:993-996.
13. Whitaker-Azmitia, P.M. (1988); In Astroglial Receptors, 107-123, H. Kimelberg, ed., Raven Press, N.Y.
14. Whitaker-Azmitia, P.M. and Azmitia, E.C. (1986): J.Neurochem. 46,1186-1189
15. Whitaker-Azmitia, P.M. and Azmitia, E.C., (1989): Brain Res. 497: 80-85.
16. Winningham-Major, F. et al, (1989): J.Cell .Biol. 91: 142-152.

ANALYSIS OF MOLECLULAR MECHANISMS UNDERLYING UP-REGURATION AT CEREBRAL MUSCARINIC RECEPTOR USING PRIMARY CULTURED CEREBRAL CORTICAL NEURONS

S.OHKUMA and K.KURIYAMA
Department of Pharmacology, Kyoto Prefectural University of Medicine, Kyoto 602, Japan

It is well known that chronic treatment with muscarinic antagonists induce the up-regulation of muscarinic receptors in a variety of organs and tissues. However, such alterations in muscarinic receptor was reported to be associated with the decreased responsiveness of phosphoinositide hydrolysis (PI turnover) to muscarinic stimulation, although exact mechanism underlying this phenomenon was not clear (3). In this study, we have investigated molecular mechanisms underlying these changes using mouse cerebral cortical neurons in primary culture following the exposure of neurons to atropine (10^{-8} M) for 5 days.

MATERIALS AND METHOD

Primary cultured neurons was prepared from 15 day old fetus of mouse according to the method previously described (4). Measurements of the [^{3}H]inositolphosphate formation, GTPase activity, and the bindings of [^{3}H]quinuclidinyl benzilate ([^{3}H]QNB) and [^{3}H]guanylylimido diphosphate ([^{3}H]GppNHp) to the particulate fraction of neurons were carried out according to the methods of Berridge et al.(1), Brandt et al. (2), Yamamura and Snyder (6) and Salomon and Rodbell (5), respectively.

RESULTS AND DISCUSSION

Exposure of neurons to atropine (10^{-8} M) for 5 days induced a

Fig.1 Effect of long-term (5 days) exposure to atropine (10^{-8} M) on calbachol-stimulated [^{3}H] inosotolphosphates accumulation in mouse cerebral cortical neurons in primary culture.
*p<0.05, **p<0.01, compared with each control value.

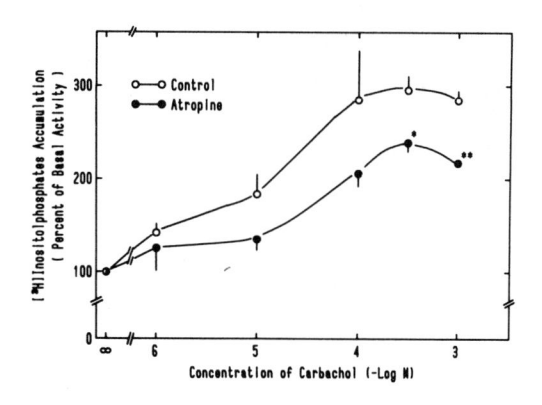

Table 1. Effect of long-term(5 days) exposure of mouse cerebral cortical neurons in primary culture to atropine(10^{-8}M) on [^{3}H]guanylylimido diphosphate(GppNHp) binding.

	[^{3}H]GppNHp binding	
	Kd (µM)	Bmax (pmol/mg protein)
Control	0.19 ± 0.02	39.61 ± 2.74
Atropine	0.23 ± 0.02	50.27 ± 2.84*

*p<0.05, compared with control.

significant increase of [^{3}H]QNB binding, which was due to the increase of Bmax value but not the change in Kd value. This increase in [^{3}H]QNB binding was completely abolished by the concomitant addition of cycloheximide with atropine, indicating that this increase in muscarinic receptor is attributed to the increase in newly synthesized receptor molecules. In primary cultured neurons exposed to atropine, the reduction of carbachol-stimulated PI turnover was observed in spite of the elevation of [^{3}H]QNB binding as reported in the brain in vivo (3). Furthermore, the reduced formation of [^{3}H]inositol phosphates in atropine-treated neurons was observed in the presence of GTPγs, a non-hydrolyzable GTP analogue (Fig.1). On the other hand, carbachol competition curve of [^{3}H]QNB binding was shifted to the right by the addition of GTP and GTPγS in both atropine-treated and non-treated cells, and the extent of this shift was found to be similar in both types of cells. Therefore, it was concluded that the treatment with atropine had no affect on the coupling between muscarinic receptors and GTP-binding protein (G protein). GTPase activity in atropine-treated cells determined in the presence and absence of carbachol was also elevated in comparison with those in non-treated neurons. In addition, the binding of [^{3}H]GppNHp to particulate fraction obtained from atropine-treated cells was significantly increased, which was due to the increase in Bmax value with no change in Kd value (Table 1). These results indicate that G protein, especially the α-subunit of G protein, increases during the occurrence of up-regulation of muscarinic receptors following a long-term exposure to atropine. On the other hand, the activity of membrane-bound phospholipase C in both types of cells was found to be unaltered. Based on these results, it may be concluded that the reduced responsiveness of PI turnover associated with the up-regulantion of muscarinic receptors is due to the deterioration of functional coupling between G protein and phospholipase C.

REFERENCES

1. Berridge, M.J., et al., (1982) : Biochem. J., 206 : 587-595.
2. Brandt, D.R., et al., (1983) : Biochemistry, 22 : 4357-4362.
3. Goodbar, L. and Bartifai, T. (1988) : Biochem. J., 250 : 727-734.
4. Ohkuma, S., et al., (1986) : Int. J. Dev. Neurosci., 4 : 383-395.
5. Salomon, Y. and Rodbell, M., (1975) : J. Biol. Chem., 250 : 7245-7250.
6. Yamamura, H.I. and Snyder, S.H., (1974) : Proc. Natl. Acad. Sci. U. S. A., 71 : 1725-1729.

DYNAMIC ASPECTS OF INOSITOL POLYPHOSPHATE METABOLISM IN CULTURED ADRENAL CHROMAFFIN CELLS.

NOBUYUKI SASAKAWA, TOSHIO NAKAKI and RYUICHI KATO
Department of Pharmacology, Keio University School of Medicine, 35 Shinanomachi, Shinjuku-ku, Tokyo, Japan.

It has been reported that inositol polyphosphates are generated by a signal transduction process comprising three main component : a receptor, a GTP-binding protein and phospholipase C.(1) However, it is still possible that changes in cytosolic calcium concentration have physiologically relevant effects on phospholipase C, and it remains controversial as to whether the activation of phospholipase C is consequence or forerunner of the rise in intracellular calcium concentration. In the present study, we have investigated the effects of various kind of agents on formation of inositol polyphosphates and cellular calcium uptake in cultured adrenal chromaffin cells.

MATERIALS AND METHODS

Chromaffin cells were isolated from fresh bovine adrenal medulla and were purified by differential plating (2). The cells were labelled with [^{3}H]inositol, used for experiments 5 days after plating and preincubated at 37 °C for 30 min in 10 mM LiCl-containing Locke's solution. Stimulants were added to the incubation mixture and the cells were incubated for various time. At the end of the incubation, inositol phosphates were extracted as described previously (3). Isomers of inositol polyphosphates were separated by H.P.L.C. according to the method of Balla et al. (4), who used a linear gradient (1% increase/min) of ammonium phosphate with monitoring of effluent radioactivity by an on-line flow detector (Packard Japan, Co. Ltd., Tokyo, Japan).

FIG.1: Time courses of the [^{3}H]InsP$_3$ accumulation and ^{45}Ca^{2+} uptake stimulated by High K$^+$, CCh or AngII.
The cells were preincubated with Locke's solution containing LiCl (10 mM) and bovine serum albumin (0.1%) for 20 min. Thereafter the cells were treated with or without stimulant for the indicated time period. [^{3}H]InsP$_3$ accumulation and cellular ^{45}Ca^{2+} uptake induced by several stimulants were determined. The basal values were subtracted from the data. High K$^+$, KCl (56 mM), CCh, carbamylcholine (300 µM), AngII, angiotensin II (10 µM).

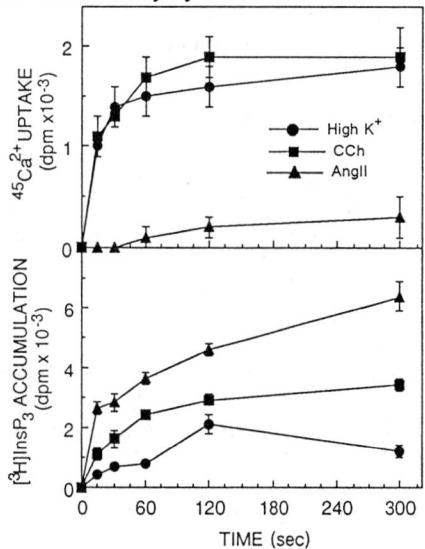

FIG. 2: Accumulation of [^{3}H]InsP$_3$, [^{3}H]InsP$_4$, [^{3}H]InsP$_5$ and [^{3}H]InsP$_6$ stimulated by nicotine for 15 sec. The concentrations of nicotine was 10 μM. The experiments were repeated twice and gave similar results.

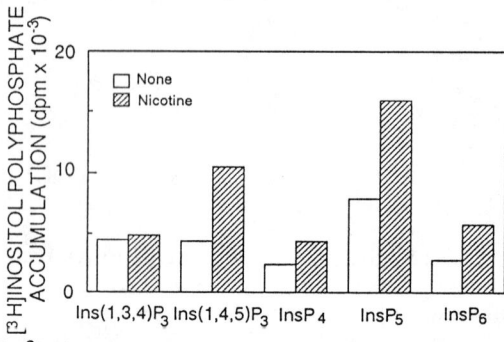

RESULTS

FIG.1 shows the time course of [^{3}H]inositol trisphosphate (InsP$_3$) accumulation and ^{45}Ca^{2+} uptake induced by several stimulants. When the [^{3}H]inositol-prelabelled cells were stimulated by high K$^+$, CCh or Ang II, a rapid accumulation of [^{3}H]InsP$_3$ was observed. At the same time, high K$^+$ or CCh induced rapid increases in ^{45}Ca^{2+} uptake, whereas AngII did not induce a significant ^{45}Ca^{2+} uptake. Stimulation with nicotine increased Ins(1,4,5)P$_3$ in the chromaffin cells (Fig. 2), consistent with previous reports (3). Nicotine induced a large increase in inositol pentakisphosphate (InsP$_5$). Inositol tetrakisphosphate (InsP$_4$) and inositol hexakisphosphate (InsP$_6$) was also increased with a lesser amount than InsP$_5$.

DISCUSSION

These results demonstrate the existence of two different mechanisms of InsP$_3$ formation, i.e. calcium uptake-dependent and -independent mechanisms, in chromaffin cells. Moreover, InsP$_5$ is rapidly increased by nicotine, a nicotinic agonist, in these cells. In chromaffin cells agonist-stimulated increase in Ins(1,4,5)P$_3$ is small.(3). In fact, InsP$_5$ is the most pronounced inositol phosphates identified so far in the chromaffin cells. A current hypothesis proposes that InsP$_5$ is formed by phosphorylation of InsP$_4$ (5). Alternatively, it is possible that InsP$_5$ is generated independently of InsP$_4$ formation, although more rigorous research is necessary for establishing this possibility. Although inositol pentakisphosphate-containing phospholipid has not been shown, it is possible that such phospholipids exist in plasma membranes.

REFERENCES

1. Berridge, M. J., and Irvine, R. F.: Inositol phosphates and cell signalling, Nature, 341 : 197-205, 1989.
2. Sasakawa, N. et al., (1989) : Stimulation by ATP of inositol trisphosphate accumulation and calcium mobilization in cultured adrenal chromaffin cells, J. Neurochem., 52 : 441-447.
3. Sasakawa, N. et al/, (1989) : Calcium uptake-dependent and -independent mechanisms of inositol trisphosphate formation in adrenal chromaffin cells: comparative studies with high K$^+$, carbamylcholine and angiotensin II, Cell. Signal., 1 : 75-84.
4. Balla, T. et al. : Metabolism of inositol 1,3,4-trisphosphate to a new tetrakisphosphate isomer in angiotensin-stimulated adrenal glomerulosa cells, J. Biol. Chem. 262 : 9952-9955, 1987.
5. Stephens, L. R. et al. : Synthesis of myo-inositol 1,3,4,5,6-pentakisphosphate from inositol phosphates generated by receptor activation, Biochem. J., 253 : 721-733, 1988.

ASSOCIATIVE COOPERATIVITY BETWEEN EXCITATORY AMINO ACID (EAA) RECEPTORS TO TRIGGER ARACHIDONIC ACID RELEASE FROM STRIATAL NEURONS IN CULTURE

J. BOCKAERT, J.P. PIN, K. OOMAGARI*, M. SEBBEN and A. DUMUIS
Centre CNRS-INSERM de Pharmacologie-Endocrinologie, Rue de la Cardonille, 34094 Montpellier Cedex 5, France, *Department of Psychiatry, Kyushu University School of Medicine, Fukuoka, Japan.

We have used striatal neurons in primary culture to study arachidonic acid (AA) release during EAA receptor stimulation. These cultures were generated in serum-free medium from 14-15 day old mouse embryos (1,7) and were tested after 6 and 13 days *in vitro* (DIV). They did not contain more than 7% of glial cells (1). After 10 DIV, the presence of differentiated synapses was confirmed by electron microscopy and immunostaining of synapsin I (7).

RESULTS AND DISCUSSION

Neurons of 6 or 13 DIV were incubated overnight with [3H]-AA. Cells were washed with a Krebs bicarbonate medium. After the final wash, the experimental agents were added in 2 ml Krebs bicarbonate buffer. In 6 DIV neurons, and in the absence of Mg^{++}, glutamate (Glu) and N-methyl-D-aspartate (NMDA) were able to release [3H]-AA (2). Kainate (KA) and quisqualate (QA) were totally inactive (2). The receptor involved in the Glu and NMDA effects was a typical NMDA receptor. Mg^{++} as well as a competitive (2-amino-5-phosphonovalerate) and a non-competitive (phencyclidine) antagonist of NMDA receptors blocked the Glu and NMDA effects.

An extensive analysis of [3H]-AA and its possible metabolites in extracellular medium by reverse phase HPLC indicates that only [3H]-AA was released. No detectable release of hydroxyeicosatetraenoic acids (HETEs) or prostaglandins could be found.

Increasing intraneuronal Ca^{++} concentrations with ionomycin also induced AA but not HETEs nor prostaglandin release. In contrast, increasing intracellular Ca^{++} concentration in glial cells induced the release of AA as well as the release of HETEs and prostaglandins. Therefore neurons, at least developed neurons in primary cultures, produced a very specific eicosanoid message : the AA.

In 13 DIV neurons, NMDA still produced AA release in the absence of Mg^{++}. In the presence of Mg^{++}, depolarization of neurons associated with NMDA receptor stimulation is needed to induce AA release. Depolarization can be obtained by specific activation of the quisqualate ionotropic (Qi) receptors by AMPA (DL-α-amino-3-hydroxy-5-methyl-4-isoxazole propionic acid). In the presence of Mg^{++}, NMDA or AMPA alone did not produced any

AA release. However, their association produces a full response. Similarly, in 13 DIV, stimulation of the other quisqualate receptors : the Qp (a metabotropic receptor coupled to phospholipase C) (6) by a specific agonist : ACPD (trans-1-amino-cyclopentyl-1,3-dicarboxylate) did not produce any AA release, whereas the association of Qp and Qi produced a full response.

During the stimulation of NMDA + Qi receptors, it is likely that the Mg^{++} blockade of NMDA channels is suppressed by the depolarization induced by Qi receptors and that Ca^{++} entry through NMDA receptors activates phospholipase A2 (PLA_2). During the stimulation of Qp + Qi receptors, the mechanisms of PLA_2 activation is still unknown. In striatal neurons compartimentalization of PLA_2, Ca^{++} entry, EAA receptors, is likely.

CONCLUSION

It must be pointed out that the association of Qi and NMDA receptor activation, as well as the association of Qi and Qp receptor activation produce, at least qualitatively, the same pattern signals : depolarisation, Na^+ entry, Ca^{++} mobilisation, protein-kinase C activation and then [3H]-AA release (2,4,5).

Finally, it has been proposed that AA could play an important role in synaptic plasticity, involving NMDA receptor activation. Williams and collaborators recently showed that AA may play a role in long term potentiation (LTP) genesis (8) and several groups have reported a blockade of LTP induction with inhibitor of PLA_2 (9). Since the association of non-NMDA receptor activation and post-synaptic excitation has also been shown to induce synaptic plasticity in the hippocampus (9) and in the cerebellum (3). Our results showing that neuronal excitation associated with Qp receptor activation is required for AA release, bring new evidence in favour of the involvement of Qi-Qp receptor association in plasticity events.

REFERENCES
1. Bockaert, J. et al. (1986) : J. Physiol. (Paris)., 81:219-227.
2. Dumuis, A. et al. (1988) : Nature, 336:68-70.
3. Kano, M. and Kato, M. (1987) : Nature, 325:276-279.
4. Manzoni, O. et al. (1990) : Neurosci. Lett., 109:146-151.
5. Nicoll, R.A., Kanes, J.A. and Malenka, R.C. (1988) : Neuron, 1:97-103.
6. Sladeczek, F., Récasens, M. and Bockaert, J. (1988) : Trends in Neurosci. 11:545-549.
7. Weiss, S. et al. (1986) : Proc. Natl. Acad. Sci. USA, 83:2238-2242.
8. Williams et al. (1989) : Nature, 341:739-742.
9. Okada, D., Yamagishi, S. and Sugiyama, H. (1989) : Neurosci. Lett. 100:141-146.

MECHANISMS OF DRUG PROTECTION AGAINST NEUROTOXICITY IN NEURONAL CELL CULTURES

P.J. PAUWELS AND J.E. LEYSEN
Department of Biochemical Pharmacology, Janssen Research Foundation, B-2340 Beerse, Belgium.

Dissociated neuronal cell cultures are an elegant system for investigating neurotoxic mechanisms and neuroprotection.

Under serum-free conditions, foetal brain neurons can be easily cultured. Neuronal cell death in neuronal cultures can be induced by activation of glutamate receptors, glucose deprivation, anoxia and mechanical insults. Cell culture methodology is useful in the quantitative characterization of these types of injury. The efflux into the culture medium of the cytosolic lactate dehydrogenase (LDH) is a reliable way to quantify neurotoxicity.

Glutamate neurotoxicity may be predominantly mediated by the activation of the NMDA subclass of glutamate receptors. It can be induced directly by exposure to exogenous glutamate, or indirectly during glucose deprivation, anoxia and mechanical insults, due to the release of endogenous NMDA agonists. Glutamate neurotoxicity in neuronal cultures is attenuated by competitive and non-competitive NMDA antagonists. This suggests that NMDA receptors are preferentially involved in the pathogenesis of hypoglycemia, trauma and hypoxia/ischemia.

Besides NMDA antagonists, Ca++ antagonists are a heterogenous group of compounds with special interest for neuroprotection. We are interested in the class IV Ca++ antagonist flunarizine. This compound shows neuroprotection in different _in vivo_ models of brain hypoxia, ischemia, epilepsy, metabolic intoxication and stroke (2). In neuronal cultures, flunarizine blocks neurotoxicity induced by the depolarizing agent veratridine (3). Flunarizine is without effect against glutamate neurotoxicity induced directly by exposure to exogenous glutamate. Flunarizine might provide its beneficial effect by increasing the threshold for depolarization. Under such condition, it can be expected that there will be less synaptic excitotoxic neurotransmitter release and glutamate receptor activation.

Recently, we investigated the neuroprotective effect of a novel benzothiazol derivative, sabeluzole. In pharmacological studies, the compound revealed antihypoxic and antiepileptic properties and was shown to improve memory and learning in rats, guinea-pigs and in healthy young and elderly volunteers (1). Serum-free cultures of neurons were prepared from the cerebral hemisferes of 17-day-old rat embryos, as described previously (3). Cultures were chronically treated with 0.1 % cyclodextrin or sabeluzole in 0.1 % cyclodextrin on days 1 and 4 in culture. On day 8 in culture, cultures were washed and incubated for 2 h in 0.2 ml chemically defined DMEM medium. Thereafter, the medium was sucked off and cultures were incubated in 0.2 ml chemically defined DMEM medium in the absence and the presence of 1 mM glutamate without sabeluzole. For quantitative assessment of the neuronal damage after 16 h, the efflux into the culture medium of the cytosolic LDH was measured as described previously (3). The total LDH activities in neuronal cultures were not altered after chronic sabeluzole-treatment. In control cultures, LDH released in the medium over 16 h constituted 5.9 % of total LDH activity, it reached 16.5 % in glutamate-exposed cultures. Cultures chronically treated with 0.1 µM sabeluzole showed almost no glutamate-induced released LDH (Table I).

Table I. Dose-response of chronic sabeluzole-treatment on released LDH in neuronal cultures.

	Sabeluzole treatment (µM)			
	control	0.03	0.1	1
	(7)	(3)	(7)	(2)
Trigger:	mean released LDH (%) ± S.D.			
basal	5.9 ± 1.2	4.8 ± 1.6	5.4 ± 1.1	5.8 ± 0.4
1 mM glutamate	16.5 ± 1.9	11.8 ± 2.2	7.7 ± 1.0	7.6 ± 1.1

No effect was observed on released LDH after acute treatment of 8-day-old cultures for 20 min with 1 µM sabeluzole followed by a drug-free period of 2 h. Hence, the resistance of neuronal cultures to glutamate was in contrast to NMDA antagonists only pronounced after chronic treatment with sabeluzole.

In conclusion, the neuronal culture model offers, as a simplified system for quantification of neurotoxicity, an easy tool to explore new cerebroprotective drugs.

REFERENCES

1. Clincke, G.H.G., and Tritsmans, L. (1987): In Current Research and Issues, vol. 2, Clinical and educational implications, P.E. Morris, R.N. Sykes, eds., pp. 211-216. M.M. Grunberg.
2. De Ryck, et al., (1989): Stroke, 20: 1383-1390.
3. Pauwels, et al., (1989): Mol. Pharmacol., 36: 525-531.

MONOAMINE OXIDASE (MAO) ACTIVITY AND MONOAMINE EFFECTS IN CEREBELLAR NEURONS AND ASTROCYTES.

L. PENG[1], X.M. Li[4], P.H. YU[4], B.H. JUURLINK[2], E. HERTZ[1], A.V. JUORIO[4] and L. HERTZ[1,3].
Departments of Pharmacology[1], Anatomy[2], and Anesthesia[3], and Neuropsychiatric Research Unit, Dept. of Psychiatry[4].
University of Saskatchewan,
Saskatoon, Sask.
S7N OWO, Canada.

Primary cultures of rodent cerebellar granule cells and of astrocytes have become an important tool for investigation of developmental, biochemical, and pharmacological characteristics of glutamatergic neurons and of their interactions with astrocytes. These cultures are generally obtained from the cerebellum of approximately 7-day-old rats or mice. To obtain a granule cell culture a cell suspension is seeded in dishes coated with polylysine or similar substrates (Chapter by Schousboe et al. in ref. 4). In our hands, relatively dense cultures (one 35 mm - dish culture/brain) can be grown for 2-3 weeks either at a partly depolarizing concentration of potassium chloride (24.5 mM) or at the usual KCl concentration in the medium (5.4 mM). The two types of granule cells cultures are relatively similar when observed by phase contrast microscopy. By electron microscopy it can be seen that the cells grown at the normal K^+ concentration show a very marked degeneration of specifically dendritic elements, whereas the synaptic vesicles (and the content of synaptophysin, determined by ELISA) are not affected (2). After culturing at the elevated K^+, cells look similar to cerebellar granule cells in vivo. In the neuronal cultures the number of astrocytes is kept low (below 5-10%) by the addition of the cytotoxic drug cytosine arabinoside.

Cerebellar astrocytes are obtained by seeding the cell suspension at a normal K^+ concentration in uncoated plastic dishes and omitting addition of cytosine arabinoside (chapter by Hertz et al in ref 4).

The ability to release glutamate in a transmitter-related manner, e.g., by exposure to a depolarizing concentration of K^+ in the presence of calcium has been studied by superfusion. The "resting" (5mM KCl) and "stimulated" (by 50 mM KCl) release of glutamate and aspartate is under our experimental conditions studied by continuous superfusion with a phosphate-buffered saline (PBS) containing 6 mM glucose and either no glutamine precursor or either glutamine (3) or alpha-ketoglutarate (2) as the glutamate precursor. Superfusion media with high and low KCl concentration are alternated during the superfusion. After at least 8 days in culture the stimulated release of glutamate from neurons grown at the elevated K^+ level ("transmitter-competent" neurons) amounts, in our hands, to about 5 nmol/min/mg protein without any precursor and to 10-15 nmol/min mg protein with either glutamate or alpha-ketoglutarate as a precursor. The stimulated releases of aspartate are 1/3 to 1/2 of these values in "transmitter-competent" cells. There is no "stimulated" release of either amino acid in "transmitter-incompetent" granule cells, i.e., cells grown at 5.4 mM K^+. Release of glutamate is also stimulated by an elevated KCl concentration in cerebellar astrocytes (after both 8 and 18 days in culture), but this response is not calcium-dependent.

The stimulated release of glutamate from neurons is inhibited by the presence of either serotonin (5-HT) or the trace amine phenylethylamine. In mature cultures of "transmitter-competent" granule cells (8 or 12 days in culture) the response is specific for the "stimulated" release, whereas the resting release is virtually unaffected. In 4-day-old-cultures (which do not yet show a potassium induced glutamate release), the glutamate release is dramatically decreased by these monoamines both in the presence and the absence of an elevated potassium concentration. In astrocytes both the "stimulated" and the resting release are decreased by serotonin or phenylethylamine to about the same level. This means that the actual inhibition becomes larger in the presence of an elevated potassium concentration than in its absence. The response is identical in younger (8-day-old) and in older (18-day-old) cells.

The activities of both MAO-A and MAO-B in young (i.e., at most 7 days in culture) neurons and astrocytes are similar to those in cerebellum in vivo (about 1.0 nmol/mgprotein/min) for MAO-A and 0.1 nmol/mg protein/min for MAO-B. In vivo both MAO-A and B activities increase 2 - 4 fold during the following week. This increase is mimicked both temporally and quantitatively in the cultured astrocytes, whereas the MAO activities remain virtually unaltered in "transmitter-competent" neurons during the entire life span (1). No information is available for "transmitter-incompetent" cells.

Binding studies have shown the presence of 5-HT$_2$ receptors in both intact "transmitter-competent" cerebellar granule cells and cerebellar astrocytes. The B$_{max}$ is identical in 8-day-old "transmitter-competent" neurons and in 3-week-old astrocytes ($\approx$150nmol/mol/mg protein). The K$_D$ values are 2-10 nM and appear to be slightly higher in the neurons than in the astrocytes. Downregulation of these receptors in the presence of the 5-HT$_2$ agonist ($\pm$)-1-(2,5-dimethoxy-4-iodophenyl)-2 amino propane in the medium during the culturing has up until now only been studied in neurons, where the B$_{max}$ value was decreased by about 20% after continuous presence of this drug during the culturing.

Thus, in "transmitter-competent" granule cell neurons an inhibitory effect of serotonin on glutamate release is present already after 4 days in culture. It is not known whether the neurons express serotonin receptors at this stage. This is well before the activities of MAO-A and B increase in vivo and in cultured astrocytes. In 8-12-day-old neurons the inhibition of the "resting" release has disappeared but the "stimulated" release (which now has developed) is strongly inhibited by serotonin. These changes occur at the same time as MAO activities increase in astrocytes. Presently no information is available about possible developmental changes in serotonin binding, MAO-A and B activities and serotonin effects on glutamate release in "transmitter-incompetent" granule cells.

In cerebellar astrocytes, serotonin effects remain unaltered during the period when MAO activities increase. No information is yet available about developmental alterations in serotonin binding.

These effects of serotonin are likely to be of importance for glutamate-mediated metabolic interaction between neurons and astrocytes. Thus, serotonin seems to affect interactions between neurons and astrocytes both during development (Azmitia and Whitaker-Azmitia, this meeting) and during function in the adult CNS.

References
1. Hertz, L. et al. Development of monoamine oxidase activity and monoamine effects on glutamate release in cerebellar neurons and astrocytes. Neurochem. Res. 14: 1039-1046, 1989.
2. Peng, L. et al. Development of cerebellar granule cells in the presence and absence of excess extracellular potassium - do the two culture systems provide means of distinguishing between events in transmitter-related and non-transmitter-related glutamate pools? Submitted for publication (Dev. Brain Res.), 1990.
3. Peng, L. et al. Utilization of alpha-ketoglutarate as a precursor for transmitter glutamate in cultured cerebellar granule cells. (Neurosci. Letts.), 1990.
4. Shahar, A. et al (eds.) A Dissection and Tissue Culture Manual of the Nervous System, Liss, New York, 1989.

FURTHER STUDIES ON SLEEP-WAKE REGULATION BY PROSTAGLANDINS D_2 AND E_2

OSAMU HAYAISHI
Director, Osaka Bioscience Institute, 6-2-4 Furuedai Suita, Osaka 565, Japan

Prostaglandin(PG) D_2 is unique among the prostaglandins in being present in high concentrations in the central nervous system of rats and other mammals including humans. It is biosynthesized and metabolized in the neurons and glia cells by specific enzymes, PGD_2 synthetase and PGD_2 dehydrogenase, respectively. The binding protein for prostaglandin D_2 was found mainly in the gray matter, namely, the neuron-rich areas, and is highly concentrated in certain specific regions such as the olfactory bulb, cerebral cortex, occipital cortex, hippocampus, hypothalamus, and preoptic area, thus indicating that PGD_2 may be involved in certain specific neural functions. Although the preoptic area has long been shown to be a center of sleep regulation by neuroanatomical and electrophysiological studies, the chemical mechanisms involved in the induction of sleep have not yet been elucidated. In 1982, we showed that when several nanomoles of PGD_2 were microinjected into the preoptic area of a rat under conditions of sleep deprivation, the amount of sleep was increased more than fivefold. The site of action was confined to the preoptic area. The effect was dose-dependent and specific for PGD_2.

Further studies with rats employing the more sophisticated continuous infusion sleep bioassay system revealed that the intracerebroventricular infusion of as little as one femtomole (10^{-15} mol) per second of PGD_2 was effective in inducing statistically significant amounts of excess sleep. Sleep induced by PGD_2 was indistinguishable from physiological sleep as judged by EEG, EMG, locomotor activities, body temperature, heart rate, and general behavior of the rat.

These studies were further extended and confirmed using the rhesus monkey, Macaca multta. Sleep induced by the infusion of PGD_2 into the lateral or third ventricle of a monkey during the day was indistinguishable from natural sleep on the basis of EEG, EMG, EOG, body temperature, heart rate, general behavior and power spectral data but was clearly different from sleep induced by the sleep-inducing drugs such as nitrazepam, a benzodiazepine derivative.

More recently, we found that either intracerebral microinjection or intraventricular infusion of picomolar amounts of prostaglandin E_2, a positional isomer of PGD_2, reduced the amount of diurnal sleep of rats. The effect of PGE_2 was dose-dependent and quite specific for PGE_2. When AH6809, a PGE_2 antagonist, was infused at a rate of 20 pmoles/min into the third ventricle of a rat during the night, the amount of slow wave sleep was increased by about 22% over the control, while REM sleep was increased by about 60%. These experiments indisputably show that PGE_2 is involved in the maintenance of the waking state under physiological conditions.

Because PGE_2 is known to be a pyrogenic agent and the center of temperature regulation is reportedly localized in the preoptic area, one wonders if the waking effect of PGE_2 is secondary to its pyrogenic activity. When PGE_2 was infused into the third ventricle of a rat in the amount of 10 pmol/min, the amount of sleep was decreased and the body temperature was elevated to a significant extent. As mentioned above, when AH6809 was infused, the amount of sleep was increased. But the body temperature was not affected at all. When both PGE_2 and AH6809 were infused, the effect on sleep was completely neutralized while the pyrogenic effect of PGE_2 was hardly inhibited by AH6809. These results are interpreted to mean that (1) the awaking effect of PGE was independent of the pyrogenic effect and (2) the PGE_2 receptors for sleep regulation and temperature regulation are probably different, one being sensitive to AH6809 and the other insensitive to this antagonist.

In order to determine the site of action of PGD_2 and PGE_2, we then employed the microdialysis technique originally developed by Ungerstedt in Sweden. The results clearly established that the site of action of the waking effect of PGE_2 is in the posterior hypothalamus close to the mamillary body. When PGE_2 was infused in the preoptic area, the brain temperature increased significantly while the effect on the amount of wakefulness was much smaller than the effect observed when PGE_2 was infused into the posterior hypothalamus. Under the latter conditions, the effect on brain temperature was almost insignificant. These results indicate that (1) the site of action of PGE_2 on waking activity is in or near the posterior hypothalamus and (2) the site of action of PGE_2 on the brain and body temperature is clearly different from that on wakefulness.

On the basis of these various lines of evidence regarding sleep- and wake-inducing experiments by intracerebroventricular infusion, microdialysis technique, autoradiographic studies and electrophysiological and pharmacological data, I would like to conceptualize the following central dogma as a current working hypothesis: Namely PGD_2 and E_2 are probably the ultimate endogenous sleep-regulating substances, one inducing sleep and the other, wakefulness, under physiological conditions in the rat and monkey. The sites of action of PGD_2 and E_2 are located in the sleep center near the preoptic area and in the wake center near the posterior hypothalamus, respectively. The balance of these two compounds in the sleep and wake centers appears to be responsible for maintaining the sleep-wake cycle.

FUNCTIONAL SITES OF CYCLOOXYGENASE PRODUCTS IN THE CNS

Y. WATANABE, Yu. WATANABE, K. MATSUMURA*, H. ONOE,
P.G. GILLBERG**, Y. KOYAMA, S. TSUBOKURA, AND O. HAYAISHI
Osaka Bioscience Institute, Osaka 565, *Department of Physiology, Osaka University Medical School, Osaka 530, Japan, and **Department of Neurology, University of Uppsala, Uppsala, Sweden.

Cyclooxygenase products (PGs and TX) exert various neurophysiological functions in the central nervous system. We have been investigating the active sites of prostaglandins in the CNS using immunohistochemical and autoradiographical techniques. Prostaglandin endoperoxide synthase (cyclooxygenase) is shown to be localized ubiquitously in the neurons and glias in the monkey brain by the use of a specific monoclonal antibody. The immunoreactivity is predominantly localized in the neurons, especially in the hippocampus, caudate nucleus and cerebral cortices, but it is very low in the cells of the cerebellum. Concerning the localization of each PG synthetic enzyme, only PGD synthase has been stuidied by using immunohistochemical technique. Urade et al. (1) reported that the immunoreactivity specific for PGD synthase was localized in almost all neurons in the weanling rats but in the limited number of neurons in the specific brain regions in the adult rats. Instead, the positive staining was mainly localized in the oligodendroglias in the adult rat brain. Most interesting point is whether PGE and PGF synthases are localized mainly in the neurons or glias, but their localization has not so far obtained.

The receptor sites of PGs have been investigated by the use of *in vitro* autoradiography coupled with quantitation by computerized image processing system. PG binding sites were localized in the gray matter and especially in the specific neuronal populations (nucleus) (2, 3), indicating that the receptors are present in the neurons or neuronal dendrites. This means that the precise study on the localization of receptors leads us to explore the functions of PGs in the CNS. Distinct localization of PGD_2, PGE_2, and $PGF_{2\alpha}$ receptors has been shown in the monkey preoptic area, hypothalamus, thalamus, hippocampus, and amygdala (4). Precise mapping has been performed of PGD_2 (6) and PGE_2 receptors in the rat brain, and of PGE_2 receptor (5) in the monkey diencephalon. The function of each PG has been shown in such nuclei through a variety of neurophysiological experiments (Table I).

Table I. Receptor Localization and Central Action of PGs

PGs	Localization	Action
PGD$_2$	mitral cell layer of olfactory bulb	modification of olfactory stimulus-response
	preoptic area	sleep induction
	arcuate n. of hypothal.	inhibition of LHRH release
	central gray of midbrain	biphasic effects on pain
	substantia gelatinosa of spinal cord	biphasic effects on pain
	Purkinje cell layer of cerebellum	modulation of neuro-transmitter action
PGE$_2$	anterior wall of the 3rd ventricle	hyperthermia(fever)
	supramamillary n.	promotion of wakefullness
	lateral hypothal. area	anorexia
	median eminence of hypothalamus	enhancement of LHRH release
	substantia gelatinosa of spinal cord	biphasic effects on pain
PGF$_{2\alpha}$	paraventricular and supraoptic nuclei of hypothalamus	enhancement of vasopressin and oxytocin release

(n. = nucleus, hypothal. = hypothalamus or hypothalamic)

More recently, we investigated the localization of PGI$_2$ and thromboxane receptors with PGD$_2$, PGE$_2$, and PGF$_{2\alpha}$ receptors in the monkey brain. Thromboxane receptor binding was negligible but [^{3}H]iloprost binding for PGI$_2$ receptor was concentrated in the caudoputamen, amygdaloid nuclei, and cingulate cortex. The function of PGI$_2$ in the caudoputamen will be also discussed.

REFERENCES
1. Urade, Y. et al. (1987) : J. Biol. Chem., 262:15132-15136.
2. Watanabe, Y. et al. (1983) : Proc. Natl. Acad. Sci. USA, 80:4542-4545.
3. Watanabe, Y. et al. (1986) : In Biomedical Imaging, O. Hayaishi and K. Torizuka, eds., pp. 227-238. Academic Press, New York.
4. Watanabe, Y. et al. (1989) : Brain Res., 478:143-148.
5. Watanabe, Yu. et al. (1988) : J. Neurosci., 8:2003-2010.
6. Yamashita, A. et al. (1983) : Proc. Natl. Acad. Sci. USA, 80:6114-6118.

LIPOXYGENASE METABOLITES AS MEDIATORS OF SYNAPTIC MODULATION

A. VOLTERRA

Department of Pharmacology, Center for Neurobiology and Behavior, Howard Hughes Medical Institute, Columbia University, New York N.Y. 10032, U.S.A.

Present address: Center of Neuropharmacology and Institute of Pharmacological Sciences, University of Milan, Via Balzaretti 9, 20133 Milan, Italy.

The neurotransmitters histamine, dopamine and the peptide Phe-Met-Arg-Phe-NH2 (FMRFa) cause pre-synaptic inhibition at many synapses in the nervous system of the marine mollusk Aplysia Californica. The common ionic mechanism of their inhibitory action lies in a combined down-modulation of a Ca^{++} conductance and up-modulation of a K^+ conductance (S-type K^+ conductance) of the presynaptic neuron, leading to reduced transmitter release from the synaptic terminals.

With the patch-clamp technique it has been studied the modulatory action of the peptide FMRFa on Aplysia sensory neurons at the molecular level of single S-type K^+ channels (S channels). Application of FMRFa to cell-attached patches brings to increased opening of the S channels (1). The peptide does not modulate S channel function directly, but via a second messenger system. A series of evidences leads to the conclusion that a metabolite of the 12-lipoxygenase pathway of arachidonic acid (possibly 12-hydroperoxyeicosatetraenoic acid, 12-HPETE) mediates FMRFa action. First, 5 and 12-lipoxygenase products are synthesized in response to FMRFa application; Second, the action of FMRFa is blocked by both phospholipase and lipoxygenase inhibitors; Third, 12-lipoxygenase products, and in particular 12-HPETE, effectively mimic FMRFa action (4).

Studies were carried out to assess how the arachidonic acid cascade in Aplysia sensory neurons is activated in response to FMRFa, finding that a Pertussis toxin-sensitive GTP binding protein is involved, probably coupling FMRFa receptor to phospholipase activation (5). Interestingly, this receptor-activated release of arachidonic acid is independent of increased intracellular Ca^{++} levels, as measured by the fluorescent dye Fura-2.

The next study was undertaken in order to understand the molecular mechanism of S channel modulation by 12-lipoxygenase metabolites. Among the possible mechanisms of ion channel modulation by second messengers, phosphorylation via kinase activation or direct second messenger-channel interaction have been described. To distinguish among these possibilities, cell-free patch experiments (where a small patch of membrane is excised from the remaining of the cell) have been performed. In particular, cell-free patches have been exposed to artificial media lacking high energy nucleotides (ATP and GTP) and S channel modulation by lipoxygenase metabolites evaluated. Since 12-HPETE is still effective when applied to isolated patches in these conditions, it has been concluded that phosphorylation/dephosphorylation reactions, GTP binding protein activation or cyclic nucleotides formation are not involved in the modulation of S channel function by 12-HPETE and a direct second messenger-channel interaction is conceivable. Moreover, the cell-free patch technique has allowed to test the efficacy of 12-HPETE in increasing S channel opening after application on either side of the cell membrane, finding that this metabolite is dramatically effective when applied to the outer side (3). Recently, Belardetti et al. (2) have shown that unidentified 12-HPETE derivatives (possibly hepoxilins) are as effective as 12-HPETE, but when applied to the inner side of the membrane. Therefore, S channel may be modulated by different 12-lipoxygenase products at different sites.

These studies implicate arachidonic acid metabolites among the mediators of synaptic modulation. However, eicosanoids differ from other second messengers in many aspects. An important one is that, due to their amphyphilic nature, they can cross the cell membrane and leave the cell in which they are generated to act on neighbouring cells. This phenomenon has been clearly demonstrated in the cross-talk between blood cells and vascular wall. The present data suggests that lipoxygenase metabolites may have a similar role in the nervous system. Therefore it will be of interest to check for an involvement of these metabolites in phenomena of synaptic plasticity in the C.N.S. (e.g. long-term potentiation) where a trans-synaptic communication has been postulated.

REFERENCES

1. Belardetti F., Kandel E.R. & Siegelbaum S.A., (1987): Nature, 325: 153-156
2. Belardetti F. et al., (1989): Neuron, 3: 497-505
3. Buttner N., Siegelbaum S.A. & Volterra A., (1989): Nature, 342: 553-555
4. Piomelli D. et al., (1987): Nature, 328: 38-43
5. Volterra A. & Siegelbaum S.A. (1988): Proc. Natn. Acad. Sci. U.S.A., 85: 7810-7814

LIPOXYGENATION OF ARACHIDONIC ACID (AA) IN RETINA

NICOLAS G. BAZAN
LSU Eye Center and Neuroscience Center, Louisiana State University Medical Center School of Medicine, New Orleans, LA USA

The retina comprises a network of synaptic circuitry in its neural part and a specialized layer of photoreceptor cells, rods and cones, containing the light signal transduction machinery. These cells interact with the retinal pigment epithelium (RPE), through continuous shedding and phagocytosis of outer segment tips. Here, some of the salient features of the AA cascade in the retina are summarized.

The free arachidonic acid pool As in brain, free AA in retina rapidly increases in response to anoxia (1). A rapid efflux of the fatty acid, as well as of other free polyunsaturated fatty acids, also occurs during *in vitro* incubation of the retina in the presence of albumin in the medium (1). Efflux may play an important role in the retina and in the nervous system in general as a signalling mechanism at low AA concentration, and may have a neuroprotective effect by preventing accumulation of fatty acids above certain concentrations. The enzyme arachidonoyl coenzyme A synthetase may function in the retina as a controlling step in the retention of AA by the retina (2) and RPE (3); moreover this enzyme may also control the availability of the fatty acid for the AA cascade (4).

Depolarization increases 12-HETE in retina An acylation/deacylation metabolic pathway of 12-HETE was observed in K^+-induced depolarization studies in rat retina (5). Depolarizing concentrations of K^+ may lead to Ca^{2+} influx, which in turn may result in phospholipase A_2 activation, followed by selective lipoxygenation (5,6).

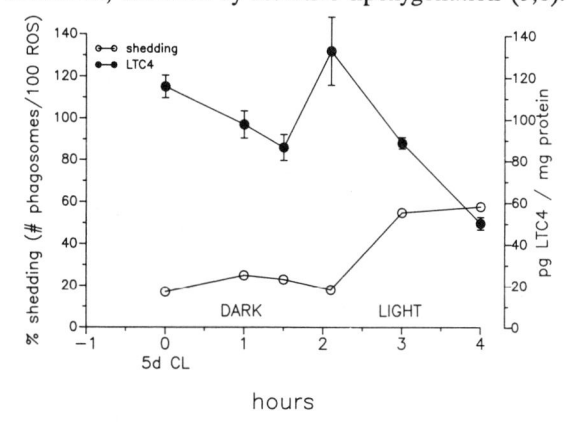

Figure 1. Massive shedding in Xenopus retina/RPE (open circles) after 5 days constant light, 2 h dark (time 0-2 h) and 2 h light (time 2-4 h). Time = 0 is the end of the constant light period. Shedding values are the means of 10-20 eyes and are expressed as percent shedding (number of phagosomes per 100 outer segments). Standard errors were less than 15% of the mean. LTC_4 values (filled circles) are means ± SE of 5-10 samples (5 RPE per sample) obtained from 4 independent experiments. A significant difference is seen in LTC_4 5 min after light onset (at time = 2 h) compared to 30 min before light onset and 1 and 2 h after light onset (p < 0.05, Student's t-test). From reference 8, with permission.

Leukotrienes in retina and RPE The 5-lipoxygenase reaction products are made in the frog retina and RPE (7). Synthesis of the sulfidopeptide leukotriene LTC_4 was stimulated by the ionophore A23187. This synthesis appears to occur in the neural retina. A relatively large amount of LTC_4 was found bound to rod outer segments, suggesting the presence of binding sites (7).

Lipoxygenation of arachidonic acid and shedding and phagocytosis of photoreceptors by RPE The leukotrienes LTB_4 and LTC_4 from RPE were studied in *Xenopus laevis* as a function of the photoreceptor shedding cycle (8). Leukotrienes mediate phagocytosis in other cell types. We found a rise in LTC_4 in the RPE immediately after the dark-to-light transition (Figure 1), followed by a decrease in LTC_4 during the time when the shed outer segments are ingested by the RPE. We are currently studying the role of second messengers derived from membrane lipids in photoreceptor/RPE interactions.

Concluding remarks The retina is an integral part of the central nervous system and represents an excellent model for the study of neuropharmacological agents, which can be applied either *in vivo* or *in vitro* to this natural tissue layer. The retina is readily accessible *in vivo* through the vitreous for administration of experimental compounds. The features of the AA cascade described here are now allowing the study of the effects of drugs on retinal function and the correlation of these effects with changes in biologically active eicosanoids. Retinal preparations also afford an experimental model for the study of drug effects on retinal diseases.

Acknowledgement
This work was supported by National Institutes of Health grant EY05121.

References
1. Aveldano, M.I., Bazan, N.G.: Displacement into incubation medium by albumin of highly unsaturated retina free fatty acids arising from membrane lipids. FEBS Lett. 40:53-56, 1974.
2. Reddy, T.S., Bazan, N.G. Synthesis of arachidonoyl coenzyme A and docosahexaenoyl coenzyme A in retina. Curr. Eye Res. 3:1225-1232, 1984.
3. Reddy, T.S., Bazan, N.G.: Synthesis of docosahexaenoyl-, arachidonoyl- and palmitoyl-coenzyme A in ocular tissues. Exp. Eye Res. 41:87-95, 1985.
4. Reddy, T.S., Bazan, N.G.: Kinetic properties of arachidonoyl-coenzyme A synthetase in rat brain microsomes. Arch. Biochem. Biophys. 226:125-133, 1983.
5. Birkle, D.L., Bazan, N.G.: Effects of K^+ depolarization on the synthesis of prostaglandins and hydroxyeicosatetra(5,8,11,14)enoic acid (HETE) in the rat retina. Evidence for esterification of 12-HETE in lipids. Biochim. Biophys. Acta 795:564-573, 1984.
6. Aveldano, M.I., Giusto, N.M., Bazan, N.G.: Polyunsaturated fatty acids of the retina. Prog. Lipid Res. 20:49-57, 1981.
7. Bazan, N.G., Bazan, H.E.P, Birkle, D.L., Rossowska, M.: Synthesis of leukotrienes in frog retina and retinal pigment epithelium. J. Neurosci. Res. 18:591-596, 1987.
8. Birkle, D.L., Rossowska, M., Woodland, J., Bazan, N.G. Increased levels of leukotriene C_2 in retinal pigment epithelium are correlated with early events in photoreceptor shedding in *Xenopus laevis*. Curr. Eye Res. 8:557-561, 1989.

PROSTAGLANDIN - HYPOTHALAMIC-PITUITARY-ADRENAL AXIS INTERACTION

A.A.MATHÉ*, M.THORÉN**, N.H.KALIN***, S.SHELTON***, P.BERGMAN*, and C.STENFORS*
Psychiatry* & Endocrinology**, Karolinska Institute, Stockholm, Psychiatry***, U. Wisconsin Medical School, Madison, WI.

Many experiments demonstrate intricate relationships between eicosanoids, in particular PGE, and the HPA axis hormones. Corticosteroids inhibit release of PGs, and in turn PGs (e.g., PGE), augment synthesis of corticosteroids and, depending on the experimental conditions, can enhance or inhibit release of ACTH from the pituitary. Moreover, under certain conditions (pregnancy and toxic shock) parallel steroid and eicosanoid increases are found. Further exploration of these issues was carried out by measuring plasma cortisol, ACTH, 11-deoxycortisol, and 15-keto-13,14-dihydro-PGE (determined as its bicyclic product, 11-deoxy-15-keto-13,14-dihydro-11B,16E-cyclo-PGE, PGEM) in a series of human and animal (Rhesus monkey) experiments.

METHODS AND RESULTS

I. DIURNAL STUDY
(a) Seven plasma samples (Q4hr) were collected from 5 human subjects. Cortisol showed a typical early am rise and an evening nadir. PGEM range of concentrations was 25-158 pg/ml. For each person, the PGEM mean of noon-midnight was higher than that of 02-08hr samples; the mean increase was 25%.
(b) Four monkeys were adapted to partial chair restraint and samples collected hourly for 48hr from indwelling venous catheters. Plasma ACTH and cortisol showed nadir at 18hr and zenith at 06 hr. Diurnal PGEM change was also apparent. However, compared to cortisol and ACTH, the time points of low and high PGEM were not as uniform between the animals. Late afternoon and early am samples showed a trend toward higher values. No correlations between plasma PGEM and cortisol or ACTH were found. The so far available data indicate that a diurnal PGE change may exist.

II. DEXAMETHASONE SUPPRESSION TEST (DST)
(a) Ten subjects referred for endocrinological evaluation received 1 mg dex orally at 23hr. Samples were drawn at 8 am preceding and on the day immediately following the drug. Mean±SEM cortisols decreased: 510 ± 77 to 108 ± 6 nmol/l, $p<0.001$, while PGEM increased: 157 ± 16 to $186\pm$ pg/ml, $p<0.05$.
(b) Seven monkeys were injected IM 150 ug/kg dex at 23hr. The sampling times were similar to those used in human DST. Cortisol was suppressed in all animals: 483 ± 146 to 69 ± 25 nmol/l, $p\ 0.001$. ACTH was also decreased: 45 ± 9 to 17 ± 2 pg/ml, $p<0.03$. PGEM changed from 88 ± 12 to 104 ± 13 pg/ml, $p=0.1$. Positive

correlations were found between pre-DST cortisol and both pre-DST PGEM (r=0.84, p<0.02) and post-DST PGEM (r=0.85, p<0.02). Pre- and post-PGEM were also correlated (r=0.7, p<0.05). Finally, baseline cortisols in the DST and the non-invasive stress experiments (cf IV.) were not different and were positively correlated. Analogous results were obtained for baseline PGEM.

III. METYRAPONE TEST

Ten patients undergoing diagnostic work-up were given metyrapone (an inhibitor of adrenal B-hydroxylase) 250-1,000 mg depending body weight, Q4hr for 20hr. Blood was drawn at 06, 08 and 18hr/day one and at 06hr/day two. Following metyrapone, cortisol decreased: 289±42 to 42±3 nmol/l, p<0.001. Plasma 11-deoxycortisol, not detectable before the test, was measurable in all patients (max 484 nmol/l). PGEM was also elevated. Baseline at -120 and 0 min: 115±12 and 121±11; ten and 22hr after the first metyrapone dose: 154±17 and 150±17 pg/ml, p<0.05.

IV. NON-INVASIVE STRESS

(a) Blood samples were taken by femoral venipuncture within 3 min of approaching the animal at times 0 and +30 min while the animal was manually restrained (n=7, single cage housed). There was a parallel increase in plasma PGEM, cortisol and ACTH. PGEM: 83±8 to 129±16, p<0.005; cortisol: 601±72 to 960±58 nmol/l, p<0.005; ACTH: 73±9 to 94±4, p<0.04. Pre-stress cortisol was correlated both to pre-PGEM (r=0.78, p<0.04) and to post-PGEM (r=0.79, p<0.04). Furthermore, pre-post PGEMs were also correlated (r=0.83, p<0.02).

(b) Plasma samples were obtained on 4 occasions, 1 week apart, counterbalanced for treatment and day. Baseline: animal taken from home cage and sampled immediately; +15 and +30 min: confined to a small cage for 15 and 30 min, respectively, before sampling; +60: confined for 30 min, returned home for 30 min and sampled. All three compounds were elevated at +15 and 30 min. PGEM: from 118±24 to 139±31 and 151±38 pg/ml, p<0.004; cortisol: from 499±27 to 706±30 and 863±36 nmol/l, p<0.001; ACTH: from 28±2 to 44±2 and 49±5 pg/ml, p<0.001. At 60 min ACTH returned to baseline, while cortisol and PGEM remained elevated. In contrast to other experiments, an increase in both PGEM and HPA axis hormones was observed.

COMMENT

The data indicate existence of two types of the HPA axis - eicosanoid relationships: (1) inhibitory/stimulatory regulatory mechanisms, exemplified by diurnal changes, dexamethasone test, metyrapone test, and CRH and ACTH challenge tests (presented elsewhere), and (2) a mechanism leading to parallel activation of HPA axis and eicosanoids, exemplified by non-invasive stress as well as electroconvulsive treatment (presented previously).

ACKNOWLEDGEMENT

We thank K. Renk for expert help. Supported by Karolinska Institute, Groschinsky Fund and Swedish Society of Medicine.

GUIDELINES TO ENSURE ANTIPANIC DRUGS ARE EFFECTIVE

H.G.M. WESTENBERG and J.A. DEN BOER
Department of Biological Psychiatry, Rudolf Magnus Institute, Academic Hospital, Utrecht, The Netherlands.

The syndrome panic disorder (PD), as now delineated in the Diagnostic and Statistical Manual of Mental Disorders 3rd Edition-Revised (DSM-IIIR), has been labeled previously with various names, depending on which symptom the investigator placed the main emphasis.
In the current definition of this syndrome primacy is given to the panic attack: discrete episodes of irrational anxiety attacks (periods of extreme fear) associated with a number of autonomic symptoms. Other components of this syndrome are anticipatory anxiety and phobic avoidance. In the current nomenclature of PD the emergence of agoraphobia is considered to be secondary to the occurrence of recurrent panic attacks.

TREATMENT OF PANIC ATTACKS.

Recent clinical research has highlighted the efficacy of antidepressants in the treatment of PD. The use of this class of drugs originates from the observation of Klein and Fink (1962), who reported that imipramine was effective in anxiety states. The patients in their study were rather heterogenous in respect to their clinical picture, but those patients that now would be classified as suffering from PD, responded favorably to imipramine. Today various studies have confirmed the efficacy of imipramine in the treatment of PD. Some investigators claim, however, that the alleged anti-panic efficacy of antidepressants must be considered as an epiphenomenon of the antidepressant efficacy of these drugs. They assert that the effects of antidepressants are globally patholytic rather than merely anti-panic and that these drugs may only be therapeutic in patients with "dysphoric mood".

PHARMACOLOGICAL DISSECTION OF THE EFFICACY.

A disadvantage of imipramine and other related antidepressants is, that they affect a host of neurotransmitter systems. Regarding their pharmacological main effects, the blockade of serotonin (5-HT) and/or noradrenaline (NA) into their respective presynaptic neurons is considered to comprise the site at which these drugs exert a significant proportion of their action. Most antidepressants, including imipramine, inhibit the uptake of both 5-HT and NA. These mixed pharmacological effects impede to link the different therapeutic features to certain psychopathological dimensions and to dissect and characterize these effects in terms of an underlying biological substrate.

To dissect the mixed effects of imipramine and to disentangle its different features (antidepressant vs. antipanic), we conducted a comparative study with two pharmacologically different antidepressants. The first drug, Fluvoxamine, is a potent 5-HT uptake inhibitor, with virtually no effect on other neuronal systems, while the second drug, Maprotiline, is a selective and potent NA uptake blocker. Both compounds have reported to be effective antidepressant drugs. If the effect of antidepressants in PD patients is rather patholytic or linked to the associated depressive symptoms, both drugs should be equally effective. To exclude the bias that improvement was mainly due to a possible effect on depressive symptoms, patients with major depression and patients with a high score on the Hamilton Depression Rating Scale (HDRS) were excluded.

RESULTS.

The results of this study indicated that Fluvoxamine is an effective drug in the treatment of patients with PD. The mean frequency of panic attacks decreased significantly from the third week of treatment. Anticipatory anxiety and phobic avoidance, as measured with different psychometric instruments, were also attenuated when treatment was ensued for several weeks. Maprotiline, on the other hand, was not effective in this respect, although it did have some effect on the associated depressive symptoms. It appeared to be entirely ineffective to block panic attacks and to mitigate phobic avoidance. At the onset of treatment no difference was seen as to the intensity of the associated depressive symptoms.

CONCLUSIONS.

The results of this study permit the following conclusions. Firstly, these data provide compelling evidence in favor of a specific pharmacological effect of some antidepressants in PD. Secondly, the outcome of this study provides circumstantial evidence as to the role of 5-HT in the mechanism of action of antidepressants in PD.
On the basis of this trial the guidelines will be discussed to ensure that drugs are efficacious in PD

REFERENCES

1. Klein, D.F. and Fink, M. (1962): Psychiatric reaction patterns to imipramine. **Am. J. Psychiatry**, 119:432-438.

GUIDELINES FOR INVESTIGATING ANTIDYSTHYMIC AND
ANTIDEPRESSANT DRUGS MUST TAKE EPIDEMIOLOGICAL DATA INTO
ACCOUNT

J. ANGST
Psychiatric University Hospital Zurich, Research
Department, Zurich, Switzerland

Recent research has given much attention to major
depressive disorder (MDD) and Dysthymia as if they were the
most frequent depressive categories. In general medical
settings, as shown by Wells et al. (1), minor depression
may be as relevant as major depression in terms of
physical, social and role functioning. Recurrent brief
depression (RBD) belongs to the spectrum of major
depressive syndromes in the community. Montgomery et al.
(2) found a high association between recurrent brief spells
of depression and suicide risk. Studies of the total
spectrum of depressive syndromes are very desirable.

A Swiss cohort studied prospectively from age 20 to 30 with
four semi-structured interviews (Angst et al. (3)) shows
that in the community about half of all treated depressives
of this age do not meet the criteria for MDD or dysthymia.
Two thirds of the remaining subjects suffer from recurrent
brief depression (RBD). RBD is defined by the symptomatic
criteria of a major depressive episode but characterized by
a short duration of a few days and a high recurrence
(usually at least once or twice per month over one year).
The rapid coming and going of depressed mood is associated
with equal suffering and subjective work impairment as in
major depression. In addition the rapid mood change is
frequently associated with a considerable risk of suicide
attempts. Longitudinally the diagnostic change from RBD to
major depression or vice versa is equally frequent. The
one-year pevalence of recurrent brief depression in the age
group of 20 to 30 is about 7% with a sex ratio f:m of 1.3.

Dysthymia defined by DSM-III-R has a one-year prevalence of
about 3%. It can follow major depressive episodes but
occurs also independently. Koscis and Frances (4) showed in
psychiatric outpatients that 95% of dysthymics meet the
symptomatic criteria for a major depressive syndrome. This
is confirmed by the Zurich data of the normal population.

The data suggest that MDD, dysthymia, and RBD are
characterized by an identical depressive syndrome and

differ only in their course pattern. Based on a threshold of criterial symptoms, the dichotomy into major and minor depressive syndromes is necessary. Both can be subclassified by course characteristics into congruent subgroups.

RBD and minor depression play a major role outside of psychiatric facilities. Both together characterize half of all treated depressives in the general population and are present in many subjects requiring but not receiving treatment. Systematic research on minor depressive syndromes on an operational level is missing to a great extent.

Epidemiological findings ought to be considered for drug studies especially in non-psychiatric settings. Contrary to MDD, dysthymia and RBD take a long-term course over one or more years. Patients suffering from these syndromes should be identified by interviews taking into account symptoms, course patterns of recurrences, and social consequences. Patients not meeting the threshold of 5 of 9 symptoms for major depressive syndromes according to DSM-III-R should be diagnosed as minor depressives and studied in their social impairment as well as major depressives. New data suggest that they should also be included as a subgroup in modern drug trials. Restricting drug trials mainly to MDD does not provide us with representative results for general practice.

A new task is the design of good drug studies in the field of dysthymia and recurrent brief depression because much longer treatment periods will be necessary in order to establish clinical efficacy.

REFERENCES

1. Wells, K.B., Stewart, A., Hays, R.D. et al.: The functioning and well-being of depressed patients. Results From the Medical Outcomes Study. JAMA. 262: 914-919, 1989.
2. Montgomery, S.A., Roy, D., Montgomery, D.B.: The prevention of recurrent suicidal acts. Br.J.Clin.Pharmacol 15: 183S-188S, 1983.
3. Angst, J., Dobler-Mikola A., Binder, J.: The Zurich Study. A prospective epidemiological study of depressive, neurotic and psychosomatic syndromes.
I. Problem, Methodology. Eur Arch Psychiatr Neurol Sci. 234: 13-20, 1984.
4. Koscis, J.H. and Frances, A.J.: A critical discussion of DSM-III dysthymic disorder. Am. J. Psychiatr. 144: 1534-1542, 1987.

GUIDELINES FOR THE EVALUATION OF BRIEF DEPRESSIONS AND THE SEPARATION FROM MAJOR DEPRESSION

S. A. MONTGOMERY, D. MONTGOMERY, D. BALDWIN
Dept. Psychiatry, St Mary's Hospital, London W2, UK

The main characteristic which separates brief depression from major depression is the very short duration of the episodes. In our series 81% of episodes of intermittent brief depression lasted four days or less. The depressions are abrupt in onset and mainly last 3 days whereas major depressions have a minimum duration of 2 weeks and mostly last much longer. The duration of intermittent brief depression are found in almost all cases to be a week or less. In our series 97% of episodes lasted a week or less and this is very close to the intermittent depression category in RDC which was perceived as representing chronic mild symptomatology. The duration criterion of a week or less is appropriate for a diagnosis of brief depression.

The main characteristic which separates the episodes of brief depression from minor depression dysthymia is the severity of the depressions. In our patients the brief depressions are quite severe with two thirds registered as moderate or severe on the MADRS. The severity of the episodes varies from one episode to the next. The suicidal attempt risk is high and appears to be related to the brief depressive episodes (Montgomery et al 1979,83) (2,3).

In clinical trials the episodes should be mainly of moderate or greater severity. At least one or two episodes in the previous three should satisfy a minimum entry criterion eg 22 on the MADRS. A principal measure of efficacy in medium term treatment would be a reduction of the mean severity of individual brief depressive episodes. In our experience almost all episodes of brief depression of moderate severity satisfy DSM III or DSMIIIR symptomatic criteria from major depression. Nevertheless the episode or episodes of brief depession of moderate severity should satisfy formal diagnostic criteria of major depression on DSMIIIR without duration. Adopting these criteria would exclude bipolar illness which is appropriate since in our experience manic or hypomanic episodes are rarte at 3-4% and most associated with individuals with a combined diagnosis of brief depression and major depression, the so-called combined depressions.

The criterion of a minimum recurrence rate is debated. The Zurich group (Angst & Dobler-Mikola 1985) (1) found occupational and social impairment in a normal population cohort clustered in those with at least monthly episodes of brief depression over a year which they suggest as a criterion for the illness. In our patients the median interval between episodes was eighteen days which suggests 20 episodes a year is the norm. However we found that the recurrences were not regular but erratic with 25% of individuals having an occasional interval of more than 4 weeks during close follow up. We also found retrospective recall of the number and nature of the episodes became less reliable beyond a three month period. For these reasons we recommend that a reasonable and sufficient requirement for the diagnosis of intermittent brief depression should be 3 episodes or more of brief depression over the previous three month period.

Since the individual episodes of intermittent brief depression are so short and available psychotropics take so long to work treatment of the acute episodes is not possible. It is more appropriate to adopt a prophylactic design in intermittent brief depression measuring efficacy by the reduction in the severity of the episodes, the number of episodes and the duration of the episodes over a two to three month period. In the absence of an established treatment an appropriate design would be a placebo controlled group comparison over a three month period.

REFERENCES

1. Angst J. and Dobler Mikola A. The Zurich study - a prospective epidemiological study of depressive neurotic and psychosomatic syndromes. IV Recurrent and nonrecurrent brief depression. Eur. Arch. Psychiat. Neur. Sci. 234: 408-416, 1985

2. Montgomery S., et al. Maintenance therapy in repeat suicidal behaviour: a placebo controlled trial. Proc. X Cong. IASP 227-229, 1979

3. Montgomery S.A. et al. The prevention of recurrent suicidal acts. Brit. J. clin. Pharmacol. 15: 183S-188S, 1983

METHODOLOGY AND APPLICATION OF LONG-TERM EFFICACY STUDIES FOR LONG-TERM ILLNESSES

J.M. DANION* and S. MONTGOMERY**
*Department of Psychiatry, Centre Hospitalier Universitaire, 67091 Strasbourg Cedex F, and **St Mary's Hospital Medical School, Praed Street, London W2 1NY, UK.

The efficacy of psychotropic drugs is primarily assessed by their ability to treat acute symptoms of psychiatric illnesses. However, the course of illnesses such as schizophrenia, mood disorders and anxiety is often chronic, with remissions, relapses and recurrences, and, in clinical practice, long-term treatment with psychotropic drug is the rule rather than the exception. Over the past decade, it has been recognized that long-term, controlled studies are required to demonstrate the long-term efficacy of a drug. Increasingly sophisticated methodological strategies have been applied to the design and interpretation of these clinical trials.

METHODOLOGICAL REQUIREMENTS

Placebo control. In most cases, placebo-controlled studies are the only scientifically valid means of establishing the long-term efficacy of a drug. When a well validated reference compound is available, the inclusion of a third group treated with this compound may provide a useful internal standard for checking the validity of the study. Reference-controlled studies without a placebo group are less useful because the sample size required to establish equivalent efficacy is far beyond the reach of most investigators.

Adequate sample size. Sufficient numbers of patients must be included to establish with confidence the difference between the placebo and drug responses. The size of the sample depends on the proportion of patients expected to have a reappearance of symptoms in both the placebo and the active drug groups during the study period. Thus, it is important to include patients expected to have a sufficient risk of relapse and to study them over a sufficient period of time : the longer the study period, the more relapses would be expected and the better the chances of testing long-term efficacy. However, too a long period, leading to poor compliance and a high drop-out rate, would compromise the ability of the trial to test efficacy. In most cases, a duration of about 12 months will be adequate. Adequate sample size becomes even more critical in determining the relative influence of multiple-treatment strategies within the same trial.

Response assessment. The return of symptoms and/or rehospitalization are usually the main criteria for assessing outcome. Since these criteria rely upon subjective judgments, which are influenced by many factors besides psychopathology levels, more objective and reliable criteria, such as predefined changes on specific rating scales, are needed. The level and length of remission at study, which may have an effect on treatment outcome, must also be fully described and quantified.

APPLICATION TO NEUROLEPTICS, ANTIDEPRESSANTS AND ANXIOLYTICS

Long-term neuroleptic treatment has proven of great value in treating chronic schizophrenia (1). In recent years, trials have shifted towards improving the benefit to risk ratio by reducing doses. Two major issues remain unsolved : how to improve deficit or residual symptoms of schizophrenia, and how far long-term neuroleptic treatment is truly prophylactic, in terms of preventing a new episode, as compared to suppressing continuously present symptoms.

Long-term antidepressant treatment of recurrent depression is the best example of the need to distinguish between maintenance treatment, to control an acute episode after the initial resolution of symptoms, and prophylactic treatment, to prevent new episodes of the illness. The inclusion of a symptom-free period of at least 4 months after the resolution of symptoms is required to make this distinction clear. A recent study of fluoxetine, applying this method, provided the strongest evidence so far available for the true prophylactic effect of an antidepressant in recurrent depression (2).

Due to the risk of dependence and abuse linked to the chronic administration of benzodiazepines, long-term treatment of anxiety is controversial and has been little studied. Whereas continuous benzodiazepine treatment lasting months and years is inappropriate, intermittent long-term therapy, i.e., treatment lasting a few weeks and then interrupted for several weeks or months, may be advisable in certain patients with generalized anxiety disorder, panic disorder and chronic physical illness. Long-term studies of new drugs and intermittent benzodiazepine therapy are clearly needed, with special emphasis on assessing the benefit to risk ratio (3).

REFERENCES
1. Kane J.M. , Lieberman J.A., (1987) : Maintenance pharmacotherapy in schizophrenia. In Psychopharmacology : the Third Generation of Progress, H.Y. Meltzer, ed, pp 1103-1109, Raven Press, New York.
2. Montgomery S. et al., (1988) : The prophylactic efficacy of fluoxetine in unipolar depression. Br. J. Psychiatry, 153 (suppl. 3) : 69-76.
3. Rickels K., (1987) : Anxiety therapy : potential value of long-term treatment. J. Clin. Psychiatry, 48 (suppl) : 1-11.

17th COLLEGIUM INTERNATIONALE NEURO-PSYCHOPHARMACOLOGICUM, 1990

For inquiries concerning the published papers, contact the following contributors:

M. E. Abreu, **12-7-5**
Nova Pharmaceutical Corporation
6200 Freeport Centre
Baltimore, Maryland 21224-2788

F. S. Abuzzahab, Sr., **12-11-1**
Department of Psychiatry, Pharmacology, and Family Practice
University of Minnesota
701 25th Avenue South, Suite 303
Minneapolis, Minnesota 55454-1490

Kalle Achté, **11-2-3, 14-13-4**
Department of Psychiatry
University of Helsinki
Lapinlahdentie
00180 Helsinki, Finland

Norio Akaike, **12-13-4, 13-11-1**
Department of Neurophysiology
Tohoku University School of Medicine
1-1 Seiryo-cho, Aoba-ku
Sendai 980, Japan

Kazufumi Akiyama, **14-10-3**
Department of Neuropsychiatry
Okayama University Medical School
Shikata-cho 2-5-1
Okayama 700, Japan

Larry D. Alphs, **12-9-3**
Department of Psychiatry
Cleveland Department of Veteran's Affairs Medical Center
10000 Brecksville Road
Brecksville, Ohio 44141

Luigi Amaducci, **13-16-6**
Department of Neurology and Psychiatry
University of Florence
Viale Morgagni, 85
Florence, Italy

Ray Ancill, **14-1-1**
Division of Geriatric Psychiatry
Department of Psychiatry
The University of British Columbia
Riverview Hospital
500 Lougheed Highway
Port Coquitlam, B. C., Canada

Edmund G. Anderson, **12-6-6**
Department of Pharmacology
University of Illinois at Chicago
835 S. Wolcott Avenue
Chicago, Illinois 60612

Luciano Angelucci, **14-9-2**
Farmacologia 2a, Faculty of Medicine
University of Rome "La Sapienza"
Piazzale A. Moro, 5
I-00185 Rome, Italy

Jules Angst, **PL-2, 14-6-2**
Research Department
Psychiatric University Hospital Zurich
P.O. Box 68
8029 Zurich, Switzerland

Seymour M. Antelman, **14-10-2**
Department of Psychiatry
Western Psychiatric Institute and Clinic
University of Pittsburgh
3811 O'Hara Street
Pittsburgh, Pennsylvania 15213

Heii Arai, **13-8-2**
Department of Psychiatry
Juntendo University School of Medicine
2-1-1 Hongo, Bunkyo-ku
Tokyo 113, Japan

Efrain C. Azmitia, **14-14-1**
Department of Biology
New York University
Washington Square East Main 1009
New York, New York 10003

Torgjorn Backström, **14-3-5**
Department of Obstetrics and Gynecology
Academic Hospital
S-751 85 Uppsala, Sweden

C. A. Barnes, **12-5-5**
Department of Psychology
University of Arizona
Psychology Building, Room 312
Tucson, Arizona 85721

Janine Barnes, 12-6-4
Postgraduate Pharmacology
University of Bradford
Richmond Road
Bradford, West Yorkshire, U.K.

Nicolas G. Bazan, 14-15-5
LSU Eye Center and Neuroscience Center
Louisiana State University Medical Center
  School of Medicine
2020 Gravier Street, Suite B
New Orleans, Louisiana 70112

Helmut Beckmann, 11-12-6
Department of Psychiatry
University of Würzburg
Füechsleinstrasse 15
8700 Würzburg, F.R.G.

Otto Benkert, 12-1-3
Department of Psychiatry
University of Mainz
Untere Zahlbacher Strasse 8
D-6500 Mainz, F.R.G.

Dorit Ben-Shachar, 11-5-5
Department of Pharmacology
Technion/Israel Institute of Technology
Ephron Street, POB 9649
Haifa, Israel

Giorgio Bignami, 14-6-2
Laboratory of Organ and System Pathophysiology
Istituto Superiore di Sanità
Viale Regina Elena, 299
I-00161 Roma, Italy

Michel Billiard, 11-10-4
Sleep and Wake Disorders Unit
Gui de Chauliac Hospital
Avenue Bertin Sans
34050 Montpellier, France

Jean-Claude Bisserbe, 11-7-6
INSERM U. 320
Centre Esquirol
C.H.U. Cote de Nacre
14033 Caen Cedex, France

Garth Bissette, 14-11-3
Department of Psychiatry
Duke University Medical Center
Box 3859
Durham, North Carolina 27710

Helmut Bittiger, 13-6-5
Research and Development Department
Pharmaceuticals Division
CIBA-GEIGY, Ltd.
4002 Basel, Switzerland

Douglas Blackwood, 13-15-4
Department of Psychiatry
Edinburgh University
Royal Edinburgh Hospital
Morningside Park
Edinburgh EH 10 5HF, Scotland

Robert J. Blanchard, 14-2-3
Department of Psychology and Bekesy Laboratory of
  Neurobiology
University of Hawaii
2430 Campus Road
Honolulu, Hawaii 96844

Avraham Bleich, 12-16-4
Mental Health Department
Medical Corps, I.D.F.
Military P.O. Box 02149
Haifa, Israel

Joël Bockaert, 14-14-4
CNRS-INSERM
Rue de la Cardonille
Montpellier, France

Alyson J. Bond, 12-8-3
Department of Psychiatry
Institute of Psychiatry
De Crespigny Park, Denmark Hill
London SE5 8AF, U.K.

Brigitta Bondy, 12-14-3
Department of Neurochemistry
Psychiatric Hospital
University of Munich
Nussbaumstrasse 7
D-8000 Munich 2, F.R.G.

Alexander Borbély, 12-10-3
Institute of Pharmacology
University of Zurich
Gloriastrasse 32
8006 Zurich, Switzerland

Richard Lewis Borison, 12-3-8
Psychiatry Service 116A-D
Downtown VA Medical Center
Augusta, Georgia 30910

A. L. Boutillier, **13-7-2**
Institute de Physiologie
Université Louis Pasteur
21, Rue René Descartes
67084 Strasbourg, France

Norman G. Bowery, **13-6-1**
Department of Pharmacology
The School of Pharmacy
29/39 Brunswixck Square
London WC1N 1AX, U.K.

Ian Brockington, **14-4-2**
Department of Psychiatry
University of Brimingham
Queen Elizabeth Hospital
Birmingham B15 2TH, U.K.

Martin J. Brodie, **12-12-4**
Epilepsy Research Unit
University Department of Medicine and Therapeutics
Western Infirmary
Glasgow G11 6NT, Scotland

Nicoletta Brunello, **12-7-2**
Center of Neuropharmacology
University of Milan
Via Balzaretti, 9
20133 Milan, Italy

Monte S. Buchsbaum, **13-2-5**
Department of Psychiatry and Human Behavior
University of California, Irvine
Room 164, Whitby Research Center
Irvine, California 92717

Gisela Budde, **14-13-7**
Medical Department
Troponwerke GmbH & Co. KG
Berliner Strasse 156
D-5000 Cologne 80, F.R.G.

Raimund Buller, **11-7-2**
Department of Psychiatry
University of Mainz
Untere Zahlbacher Strasse 8
D-6500 Mainz, F.R.G.

Brian Callingham, **12-3-2**
Department of Pharmacology
University of Cambridge
Tennis Court Road
Cambridge CB2 1QJ, U.K.

Magda Campbell, **14-12-5**
Department of Psychiatry
New York University School of Medicine
550 First Avenue
New York, New York 10016

Arvid Carlsson, **13-2-2, 14-13-2**
Department of Pharmacology
University of Gothenburg
Box 33031
S-400 33 Gothenburg, Sweden

Marc G. Caron, **11-12-1**
Department of Cell Biology
Duke University Medical Center
Durham, North Carolina 27710

Marilyn E. Carroll, **13-12-4**
Department of Psychiatry
University of Minnesota
Box 392 UMHC
625-C Diehl Hall
505 Essex Street, S.E.
Minneapolis, Minnesota 55455

Wen-Ho Chang, **14-5-4**
Laboratory of Biological Psychiatry
Taipei City Psychiatric Center
309 Sung-Te Road
Taipei, Taiwan 10510, R.O.C.

V. Chan-Palay, **13-8-5**
Department of Neurology
University Hospital
Frauenklinikstrasse 26
Zürich 8091, Switzerland

Timothy Cheek, **13-11-3**
Department of Zoology
University of Cambridge
Downing Street
Cambridge CB2 3EJ, U.K.

Dennis W. Choi, **13-11-6**
Department of Neurology H-3160
Stanford University Medical Center
Stanford, California 94305-5235

David M. Clark, **13-1-5**
Department of Psychiatry
University of Oxford
Warneford Hospital
Oxford OX3 7JX, U.K.

Anthony Clarke, **14-1-5**
Medical Department
Smith Kline Beecham Pharmaceuticals
SB House
Great West Road
Brentford, Middlesex, U.K.

Alessandra Concas, 13-5-4
Department of Experimental Biology
University of Cagliari
Via Palabanda, 12
09123 Cagliari (Sardinia), Italy

Carol Cotman, 12-5-1
Department of Psychobiology
University of California, Irvine
249 Steinhaus Hall
Irvine, California 92717

Timothy J. Crow, 13-2-1
Department of Psychiatry
Clinical Research Centre
Watford Road
Harrow, Middlesex, U.K.

Vincenzo Cuomo, 14-6-5
Institute of Pharmacology
University of Bari
Piazza G. Cesare, Policlinico
70124 Bari, Italy

S. G. Dahl, 11-4-5
Department of Pharmacology
University of Tromsø School of Medicine
Institute of Medical Biology
N-9001 Tromsø, Norway

Jean-Marie Danion, 14-16-5
Department of Psychiatry
Centre Hospitalier Universitaire
Hospices Civils
67091 Strasbourg Cedex, France

Mosé Da Prada, 11-5-3, 12-3-3
Pharmaceutical Research
F. Hoffmann-La Roche, Ltd.
124 Grenzacherstrasse
CH-4002 Basel, Switzerland

J. Davidson, 12-16-2
Department of Psychiatry
Duke University
Durham, North Carolina 27710

Claude de Montigny, 12-4-5, 12-15-4
Department of Psychiatry
McGill University
1033 Pine Avenue West #208
Montreal, Quebec, Canada H3A 1A1

Errol B. De Souza, 14-11-6
Neuroscience Branch
Neurobiology Laboratory
National Institute on Drug Abuse
Addiction Research Center
4940 Eastern Avenue, Building C
Baltimore, Maryland 21224

Harriet de Wit, 13-12-3
Department of Psychiatry
University of Chicago
5841 South Maryland Avenue
Chicago, Illinois 60637

Annette Dolphin, 13-11-5
Department of Pharmacology
St. Georges Hospital Medical School
Cranmer Terrace
London SW1 7ORE, U.K.

J. Guy Edwards, 13-14-5
Department of Psychiatry
Royal South Hants Hospital
Southampton SO9 4PE, U.K.

Arlene S. Eison, 11-11-2
Preclinical CNS Research
Bristol-Myers Squibb Company
5 Research Parkway
Wallingford, Connecticut 06492

Everett H. Ellinwood, 14-10-4
Departments of Psychiatry and Pharmacology
Duke University Medical Center
Box 3870
Durham, North Carolina 27710

Jürg Elsner, 14-6-3
Institute of Toxicology
Federal Institute of Technology and University Zurich
Schorenstrasse 16
CH-8603 Schwerzenbach, Switzerland

Hinderk M. Emrich, 12-12-5
Department of Psychiatry
Max Planck Institute for Psychiatry
Kraepelinstrasse 10
8000 Munich 40, F.R.G.

M. Endo, PL-5
Department of Pharmacology
Faculty of Medicine
University of Tokyo
Bunkyo-ku, Tokyo, Japan

Lars Farde, **11-8-5**
Department of Psychiatry and Psychology
Karolinska Institutet
P.O. Box 60500
S-104 01 Stockholm, Sweden

J. P. Feighner, **12-15-5**
Feighner Research Institute
La Mesa, California 92041

Sandra E. File, **14-2-4**
Psychopharmacology Research Unit
UMDS Guy's Hospital
London SE1 9RT, U.K.

Alan C. Foster, **11-15-4**
Neuroscience Research Centre
Terlings Park
Eastwick Road
Harlow, Essex CM20 2QR, U.K.

Walter Fratta, **13-5-5**
"B.B. Brodie" Department of Neuroscience
University of Cagliari
Via Porcell, 4
Cagliari, Italy

Tomoko Fujii, **14-6-4**
Department of Pharmacology
Teikyo University School of Medicine
2-11-1, Kaga, Itabashi-ku
Tokyo 173, Japan

Kjell Fuxe, **11-12-3**
Department of Histology and Neurobiology
Karolinska Institute
Box 60400
S-104 01 Stockholm, Sweden

Wolfgang Gaebel, **14-8-3**
Psychiatrische Klinik und Poliklinik
Freie Universität Berlin
Eschenallee 3
D-1000 Berlin 19, F.R.G.

Beat Gähwiler, **13-6-3**
Brain Research Institute
University of Zürich
August Forel-Strasse 1
CH-8029 Zürich, Switzerland

Colin Robert Gardner, **14-7-5**
Biological Research
Roussel Laboratories
Kingfisher Drive
Covingham, Swindon, Wiltshire, U.K.

David L. Garver, **14-8-2**
Department of Psychiatry and Behavioral
  Neurobiology
University of Alabama at Birmingham
UAB Station
Birmingham, Alabama 35294

Arne Geisler, **12-4-3**
Department of Pharmacology
University of Copenhagen
20, Juliane Maries Vej
2100 Copenhagen O, Denmark

Y. G. Gelders, **12-1-6**
Clinical R & D Department of Psychiatry
Janssen Research Foundation
Turnhoutseweg 30
2340 Beerse, Belgium

Barbara Geller, **14-12-6**
William S. Hall Psychiatric Institute
University of South Carolina School of Medicine
1800 Colonial Drive
Columbia, South Carolina 29208

David George, **14-2-5**
Laboratory of Clinical Studies
National Institute on Alcohol Abuse and Alcoholism
National Institutes of Health
9000 Rockville Pike
Bethesda, Maryland 20892

Frank George, **13-12-2**
NIDA Addiction Research Center
4940 Eastern Avenue
Baltimore, Maryland 21224

Jes Gerlach, **12-9-4**
Department P
Sct. Hans Hospital
4000 Roskilde DK, Denmark

Ezio Giacobini, **14-9-4**
Department of Pharmacology
Southern Illinois University School of Medicine
P.O. Box 19230
Springfield, Illinois 62794-9230

Earl Giller, **12-16-1**
Department of Psychiatry
University of Connecticut Health Center
Farmington Avenue
Farmington, Connecticut 06032

Gary B. Glavin, **13-5-2**
Pharmacology and Therapeutics and Surgery
University of Manitoba Faculty of Medicine
770 Bannatyne Avenue
Winnipeg, Manitoba, Canada

Vivette Glover, **14-4-3**
Department of Chemical Pathology
Queen Charlotte's and Chelsea Hospital
Goldhawk Road
London W6 0XG, U.K.

C. G. Gottfires, **13-8-3**
Department of Psychiatry and Neurochemistry
Gothenburg University
St. Jörgen's Hospital
S-422 03 Hisings Backa, Sweden

David Grahame-Smith, **PL-1**
MRC Unit and University Department of Clinical Pharmacology
Radcliffe Infirmary
Woodstock Road
Oxford OX2 6HE, U.K.

Lars F. Gram, **14-8-1**
Department of Clinical Pharmacology
Institute of Medical Biology
Odense University
J.B. Winsløws Vej 19
DK-5000 Odense C, Denmark

Roland Griffiths, **13-14-4**
Department of Psychiatry and Neuroscience
The John Hopkins University School of Medicine
720 Rutland Avenue
Baltimore, Maryland 21205

John H. Growdon, **14-9-6**
Department of Neurology
Massachusetts General Hospital
Fruit Street
Boston, Massachusetts 02114

Alessandro Guidotti, **14-7-3**
FIDIA Georgetown Institute for the Neurosciences
Georgetown University Medical School
3900 Reservoir Road, N.W.
Washington, DC 20007

Wilfried Gunther, **11-16-4**
Psychiatric University Hospital
Nussbaumstrasse 7
D-8000 Munich 2, F.R.G.

Helmut Haas, **12-7-3**
Department of Physiology
University of Mainz
Saarstrasse 21
D-65 Mainz, F.R.G.

Uriel Halbreich, **14-3-7**
Department of Psychiatry
State University of New York at Buffalo
Erie County Medical Center
462 Grider Street, K-Annex
Buffalo, New York 14215

Elizabeth Hampson, **14-3-6**
Department of Psychology
The Hospital for Sick Children
555 University Avenue
Toronto, Ontario, Canada

Toshiki Harada, **12-12-6**
Department of Neuropsychiatry
Okayama University Medical School
2-5-1 Shikata-cho
Okayama 700, Japan

Tsuneichi Hashimoto, **14-2-2**
Department of Pharmacology
Kyoto Prefectural University of Medicine
Kawaramachi-Hirokoji, Kamikyo-ku
Kyoto 602, Japan

Hiroshi Hatanaka, **11-6-2**
Division of Protein Biosynthesis
Institute for Protein Research
Osaka University
3-2 Yamadaoka
Suita-shi, Osaka 565, Japan

Osamu Hayaishi, **14-15-2**
Osaka Bioscience Institute
6-2-4 Furuedai
Suita, Osaka 565, Japan

Franz Hefti, **11-6-4**
Department of Gerontology
University of Southern California
Andrus Gerontology Center
University Park MC-0191
Los Angeles, California 90089-0191

S. Heinemann, **12-5-2**
Molecular Neurobiology Laboratory
The Salk Institute
P.O. Box 85800
San Diego, California 92138

K. Heinrich, **14-13-5**
Department of Psychiatry
Heinrich-Heine-University, Düsseldorf
Bergische Landstrasse 2
D-4000 Düsseldorf 12, F.R.G.

Hanfried Helmchen, **13-10-2**
*Psychiatrische Klinik und Poliklinik
Freie Universität Berlin
Universitätsklinikum Rudolf Virchow
Eschenallee 3
1000 Berlin 19, F.R.G.*

James Herman, **14-11-2**
*Department of Psychiatry
Mental Health Research Institute
205 Washtenaw Place
Ann Arbor, Michigan*

Paul L. Herrling, **12-9-5**
*Preclinical CNS Research Department
Sandoz Research Institute Berne Ltd.
115 Monbijoustrasse
3007 Berne, Switzerland*

Albert Herz, **13-4-2**
*Department of Neuropharmacology
Max Planck Institute for Psychiatry
Am Klopferspitz 18a
D-8033 Martinsried, F.R.G.*

Marvin I. Herz, **13-10-1**
*Department of Psychiatry
State University of New York at Buffalo
462 Grider Street
Buffalo, New York 14215*

Isabella J. Heuser, **12-2-4**
*Max Planck Institute for Psychiatry
Kraepelinstrasse 10
D-8000 Munich 40, F.R.G.*

Marcel Hibert, **11-4-4**
*Department of Chemistry
Merrell-Dow Research Institute
16 Rue d'Ankara
67000 Strasbourg, France*

Christoph Hiemke, **14-3-1**
*Department of Psychiatry
University of Mainz
Untere Zahlbacker Strasse 8
D-6500 Mainz, F.R.G.*

Ian Hindmarch, **11-10-2**
*Institute of Health and Safety
Robens Institute
University of Surrey
Guilford, Surrey GU2 5XH, U.K.*

Robert M. A. Hirschfeld, **13-1-1**
*Mood, Anxiety, and Personality Disorders Research Branch
National Institute of Mental Health
Parklawn Building, Room 10C24
5600 Fishers Lane
Rockville, Maryland 20857*

William Hoffman, **11-13-5**
*Psychiatry Service/116A-P, Portland Division
Portland Veterans Administration Medical Center
3710 S.W. U.S. Veterans Hospital Road
Portland, Oregon 97207*

Florian Holsboer, **PL-6**
*Max Planck Institute for Psychiatry
Kraepelinstrasse 2
D-8000 Munich 40, F.R.G.*

Edith Holsboer-Trachsler, **11-2-5**
*Department of Psychiatry
University of Basel
Wilhelm Klein-Strasse 27
CH-4025 Basel, Switzerland*

Philip S. Holzman, **12-14-2**
*Department of Psychology
Harvard University
33 Kirkland Street
Cambridge, Massachusetts 02138*

Tage Honoré, **11-15-5**
*CNS Discovery
Novo Nordisk CNS Division
Sydmarken 5
2860 Soeborg, Copenhagen, Denmark*

R. Horowski, **11-5-7**
*Schering Research Laboratories
Berlin/Bergkamen, F.R.G.*

Siegfried Hoyer, **13-8-1**
*Department of Pathochemistry and General Neurochemistry
University of Heidelberg
Im Neuenheimer Feld 220/221
Heidelberg, F.R.G.*

Osamu Inoue, **13-14-1**
*Division of Clinical Research
National Institute of Radiological Sciences
4-9-1 Anagawa
Chiba-shi 260, Japan*

Thomas Insel, **11-7-5**
Laboratory of Clinical Science
National Institute of Mental Health
P.O. Box 289
Poolesville, Maryland 20837

Jerome Jaffe, **13-4-4**
National Institute on Drug Abuse
5600 Fishers Lane
Rockville, Maryland 20857

Chris Johanson, **13-14-3**
Department of Psychiatry
Uniformed Services University of the Health Sciences
4301 Jones Bridge Road
Bethesda, Maryland 20814

E. Roy John, **13-2-4**
Department of Psychiatry
New York University Medical Center
550 First Avenue
New York, New York 10016

Lewis L. Judd, **13-1-6**
National Institute of Mental Health
5600 Fishers Lane
Rockville, Maryland 20857

Harold Kalant, **13-4-1**
Department of Pharmacology
University of Toronto
Medical Sciences Building
8 Taddle Creek Road
Toronto, Ontario, Canada M5S 1A8

Ned H. Kalin, **14-11-5**
Department of Psychiatry
University of Wisconsin Medical School
600 Highland Avenue
Madison, Wisconsin 53792

Peter Kalivas, **14-10-5**
Veterinary Pharmacology
Washington State University
Pullman, Washington 99164-6520

Werner Kalow, **14-5-1**
Department of Pharmacology
University of Toronto
8 Taddle Creek Road
Toronto, Ontario, Canada M5S 1A8

Shigenobu Kanba, **12-15-1**
Department of Neuropsychiatry
Keio University School of Medicine
35 Shinanomachi, Shinjuku-ku
Tokyo 160, Japan

John M. Kane, **11-13-1**
Department of Psychiatry
Hillside Hospital
Division of Long Island Jewish Medical Center
75-59 263rd Street
Glen Oaks, New York 11004

Hiroshi Kaneto, **13-4-5**
Department of Pharmacology
Faculty of Pharmaceutical Sciences
Nagasaki University
1-14 Bunkyo-machi
Nagasaki 852, Japan

Baruch I. Kanner, **13-7-6**
Department of Biochemistry
Hebrew University
Hadassah Medical School
P.O. Box 1172
Jerusalem 91010, Israel

Osamu Kanno, **11-10-6**
Department of Psychiatry
Teikyo University School of Medicine
2-11-1 Kaga Itabashi-ku
Tokyo 173, Japan

Ingvar Karlsson, **11-9-6**
Department of Psychiatry and Neurochemistry
St Jörgen Hospital
S-442 03 Hisings Backa, Sweden

Nobufumi Kawai, **13-7-5**
Department of Neurobiology
Tokyo Metropolitan Institute for Neurosciences
2-6 Musashidai
Fuchu-City, Tokyo, Japan

Kazuo Kawasaki, **14-7-6**
Department of Pharmacology
Shionogi Research Laboratories
Shionogi & Co., Ltd.
5-12-4 Sagisu, Fukushima-ku
Osaka 553, Japan

Hajime Kazamatsuri, **11-13-3**
Department of Psychiatry
Teikyo University School of Medicine
2-11-1 Kaga, Itabashiku
Tokyo 173, Japan

Terence M. Keane, **12-16-5**
National Center for PTSD, Boston
Boston VA Medical Center and Tufts University
 School of Medicine
150 South Huntington Avenue
Boston, Massachusetts 02130

Martin Barry Keller, **13-9-1**
Department of Psychiatry and Human Behavior
Brown University
Providence, Rhode Island 02912

Inayat Khan, **13-14-6**
World Health Organization
Avenue Appia
1211 Geneva 27, Switzerland

Sumant Khanna, **11-3-1**
Department of Psychiatry
National Institute of Mental Health and
 Neurosciences
P.O. Box 2900
Bangalore 560029, India

Paul Kielholz, **11-14-1**
Badweg 1
5707 Seengen, Switzerland

Akira Kishimoto, **12-12-3**
Department of Neuropsychiatry
Tottori University School of Medicine
36-1 Nishicho
683 Yonago, Japan

Donald F. Klein, **13-9-2**
Department of Psychiatry
Columbia University
College of Physicians and Surgeons
722 West 168th Street
New York, New York 10032

Rachel Klein, **14-12-4**
Department of Psychiatry
Columbia University
New York State Psychiatric Institute
722 West 168th Street
New York, New York 10032

Joel E. Kleinman, **11-16-6**
Clinical Brain Disorders Branch
National Institute of Mental Health
Room 500
2700 Martin Luther King, Jr., Avenue
Washington, DC 20032

Ora Kofman, **12-4-4**
Department of Behavioral Sciences
Beer Sheva Mental Health Center
Ben-Gurion University of the Negev
P.O. Box 4600
Beer Sheva, Israel

Kyuya Kogure, **11-15-1**
Department of Neurology
Institute of Brain Diseases
Tohoku University School of Medicine
1-1 Seiryo-machi, Aoba-ku
Sendai 980, Japan

Tatsuro Koike, **11-6-3**
Department of Natural Science
Saga Medical School
5-1-1 Nabeshima-machi
Saga 840-01, Japan

Stephen H. Koslow, **13-13-1**
Division of Basic Brain and Behavioral Sciences
National Institute of Mental Health
5600 Fishers Lane
Rockville, Maryland 20857

Athanasio Koukopoulos, **12-12-2**
Centro "Lucio Bini"
Via Crescenzio, 4
00193 Roma, Italy

Lee-Ming Kow, **14-3-2**
Department of Neurobiology and Behavior
The Rockefeller University
1230 York Avenue
New York, New York 10021

Tsukasa Koyama, **12-4-1**
Department of Psychiatry and Neurology
Hokkaido University School of Medicine
North 15, West 7
Sapporo 060, Japan

Jürgen-Christian Krieg, **12-14-4**
Clinical Institute
Max Planck Institute for Psychiatry
Kraepelinstrasse 10
D-8000 Munich 40, F.R.G.

Josef Krieglstein, **11-15-3**
Institut für Pharmakologie und Toxikologie
Ketzerbach 63
D-3550 Marburg, F.R.G.

Yoshio Kudo, **12-1-5**
Institute of Clinical Pharmacology
Aino Hospital
11-18 Takada-cho
Ibaraki City, Japan

R. Kumar, **14-4-1**
Department of Psychiatry
Institute of Psychiatry
De Crespigny Park, Denmark Hill
London SE5 8AF, U.K.

Hisashi Kuribara, 14-9-1
Division for Behavior Analysis
Behavior Research Institute
Gunma University School of Medicine
3-39-22 Showa-machi
Maebashi 371, Japan

Neil Kurtz, 11-9-3
CNS Medical Research
Miles, Inc., Pharmaceutical Division
400 Morgan Lane
West Haven, Connecticut 06516

Malcolm Lader, 11-11-5
Department of Psychiatry
Institute of Psychiatry
De Crespigny Park, Denmark Hill
London SE5 8AF, U.K.

Salomon Z. Langer, PL-4, 12-11-3
Department of Biology
Synthelabo Recherche (L.E.R.S.)
58 Rue de la Glacière
75013 Paris, France

Peretz Lavie, 12-16-6
Sleep Laboratory
Faculty of Medicine
Technion/Israel Institute of Technology
Haifa, Israel

Robert J. Lefkowitz, PL-3
Department of Medicine and Biochemistry
HHMI/Duke University Medical Center
Box 3821, Room 468, CARL Building
Durham, North Carolina 27710

Louis Lemberger, 12-11-4
Lilly Laboratory for Clinical Research
Eli Lilly and Company
Lilly Corporate Center
Indianapolis, Indiana 46285

Robert H. Lenox, 12-4-6
Neuroscience Research Unit
Department of Psychiatry
University of Vermont College of Medicine
Medical Alumni Building
Burlington, Vermont 05405

Brian Leonard, 12-11-6
Department of Pharmacology
University College
Galway, Ireland

Henrietta Leonard, 11-3-4
Child Psychiatry Branch
National Institute of Mental Health
Building 10, Room 6N240
9000 Rockville Pike
Bethesda, Maryland 20892

Bernard Lerer, 12-16-3
Department of Psychiatry
Yaacov Herzog Research Center
Hebrew University
P.O. Box 140
Jerusalem 91001, Israel

Josée Leysen, 12-6-3
Department of Biochemical Pharmacology
Janssen Research Foundation
Turnhoutseweg 30
2340 Beerse, Belgium

Jeffrey Lieberman, 13-10-5
Department of Research/Psychiatry
Hillside Hospital
Division of Long Island Jewish Medical Center
266th Street & 76th Avenue
Glen Oaks, New York 11004

Richard G. Lister, 14-2-1
Laboratory of Clinical Studies
National Institute on Alcohol Abuse and Alcoholism
9000 Rockville Pike
Bethesda, Maryland 20892

J. J. López-Ibor, Jr., 11-9-7
Department of Psychiatry
University of Alcala de Henares
Madrid, Spain

Wolfgang Maier, 12-4-1
Department of Psychiatry
University of Mainz
Untere Zahlbacher Strasse 8
D-6500 Mainz 1, F.R.G.

Stephen Marder, 13-10-4
Department of Psychiatry
Brentwood VA Medical Center/UCLA
B210, Room 15
11301 Wilshire Boulevard
Los Angeles, California 90073

Aleksander A. Mathé, 14-15-6
Department of Psychiatry
Karolinska Institute at St Göran's Hospital
S-112 81 Stockholm, Sweden

John C. Mazziotta, **13-13-2**
Reed Neurology
UCLA School of Medicine
710 Westwood Plaza
Los Angeles, California 90024

Joseph Meites, **12-2-3**
Department of Physiology
Michigan State University
East Lansing, Michigan 48823

Brian Stuart Meldrum, **13-3-1**
Department of Neurology
Institute of Psychiatry
De Crespigny Park, Denmark Hill
London SE5 8AF, U.K.

Herbert Y. Meltzer, **11-1-3, 12-9-2**
Biological Psychiatry/Department of Psychiatry
Case Western Reserve University School of Medicine
2040 Abington Road
Cleveland, Ohio 44106-5000

Julian Mendlewicz, **11-14-4, 13-15-2**
Department of Psychiatry
Free University of Brussels
Erasme Hospital
Route de Lennik 808
1070 Brussels, Belgium

Wallace B. Mendelson, **11-10-5**
Department of Psychiatry
State University of New York at Stony Brook
Health Sciences Center, T-10
Stony Brook, New York 11794-8101

Ronald Meyer, **12-5-4**
Developmental and Cell Biology
University of California
Irvine, California 92717

Bengt J. Meyerson, **14-3-4**
Department of Medical Pharmacology
Uppsala University
Box 593, Biomedicum
S-751 24 Uppsala, Sweden

Katsuhiko Mikoshiba, **13-15-6**
Division of Regulation of Macromolecular Function
Institute for Protein Research
3-2 Yamadaoka
Suita, Osaka, Japan

Masahiko Mikuni, **11-1-2**
Division of Mental Disorder Research
National Institute of Neuroscience, N.C.N.P.
4-1-1, Ogawahigashi
Kodaira, Tokyo 187, Japan

P. Mindus, **11-3-2**
Department of Psychology and Psychiatry
Karolinska Hospital
Box 60500
S-104 01 Stockholm, Sweden

Yasushi Mizuki, **12-1-2**
Department of Neuropsychiatry
Yamaguchi University School of Medicine
1144 Kogushi
Ube, Japan

Hanns Möhler, **14-7-1**
Institute of Pharmacology
University of Zurich
Gloriastrasse 32
8006 Zurich, Switzerland

Hans-Jürgen Möller, **14-13-3**
Department of Psychiatry
University of Bonn
Sigmund-Freud-Strasse 25
D-5300 Bonn 1, F.R.G.

Stuart Montgomery, **11-9-5, 12-11-5**
Department of Psychiatry
St. Mary's Hospital Medical School
Praed Street
London W2 1NY, U.K.

Paolo Lucio Morselli, **14-8-5**
Department of Clinical Research
Synthelabo Recherche (L.E.R.S.)
58 Rue de la Glacière
75013 Paris, France

Nobutaka Motohashi, **12-4-2**
Department of Neuropsychiatry
Yamanashi Medical College
1110 Shimogato, Tamaho
Yamanashi 409-38, Japan

Driss Moussaoui, **14-5-5**
Centre Psychiatrique Universitaire
Ibn Rochd, Bd Tarik Ibn Ziad
Casablanca, Morocco

B. Müller-Oerlinghausen, **14-8-6**
Department of Psychiatry/Laboratory of Clinical
  Psychopharmacology
Free University of Berlin
Eschenallee 3
D-1000 Berlin 19, F.R.G.

Mitsukuni Murasaki, **11-7-4**
Department of Psychiatry
Kitasato University School of Medicine
2-1-1 Asamizodai
Sagamihara, Japan

Dennis L. Murphy, **11-3-5**
Laboratory of Clinical Science
National Institute of Mental Health
National Institutes of Health
Building 10, Room 3D41
9000 Rockville Pike
Bethesda, Maryland 20892

Dieter Naber, **12-9-1**
Department of Psychiatry
University of Munich
Nussbaumstrasse 7
D-8000 Munich 2, F.R.G.

Toshiharu Nagatsu, **11-5-2**
Department of Biochemistry
Nagoya University School of Medicine
65 Tsurumai-cho, Showa-ku
Nagoya 466, Japan

Haruo Nagayama, **11-1-1**
Department of Neuropsychiatry
Medical College of Oita
Hasama-Machi
Oita-Gun Oita 879-56, Japan

Stefan Nahorski, **13-11-2**
Department of Pharmacology and Therapeutics
University of Leicester
Medical Sciences Building
University Road
Leicester, U.K.

Michio Nakagawara, **11-1-5**
Department of Neuropsychiatry
Yamanashi Medical College
1110 Shimogato
Tamaho, Yamanashi 409-38, Japan

Tsuneyuki Nakazawa, **11-3-3**
Tokyo Saiseikai Central Hospital
Mita 1-4-17, Minatoku
Tokyo 108, Japan

Hiroshi Naruse, **14-12-3**
Department of Pediatrics
Kyorin University
6-20-2 Shinkawa, Mitaka
Tokyo, Japan

Charles B. Nemeroff, **14-11-1**
Departments of Psychiatry and Pharmacology
Duke University Medical Center
Box 3859
Durham, North Carolina 27710

Michael E. Newman, **12-7-1**
Department of Psychiatry
Hebrew University
Yaacov Herzog Research Center
P.O. Box 140
Jerusalem 91001, Israel

Tsuyoshi Nishimura, **13-8-4**
Department of Neuropsychiatry
Osaka University Medical School
1-1-50 Fukushima
Osaka City, Japan

Anna-Lena Nordström, **11-13-4**
Department of Psychiatry and Psychology
Karolinska Institute
Karolinska Hospital
S-104 01 Stockholm, Sweden

Trevor R. Norman, **12-2-5**
Department of Psychiatry
University of Melbourne
Austin Hospital
Heidelberg, Victoria, Australia

Richard Alan North, **11-12-4**
Vollum Institute
Oregon Health Sciences University
3181 SW Sam Jackson Park Road
Portland, Oregon 97201-3098

David J. Nutt, **11-11-1**
Reckitt & Colman Psychopharmacology Unit
The School of Medical Sciences
University Walk
Bristol BS8 1TD, U.K.

Anna Lena Nyth, **13-8-7**
Departments of Psychiatry and Neurochemistry
Gothenburg University
St Jörgen's Hospital
S-422 03 Hisings Backa, Sweden

Sven Ove Ögren, **11-12-5**
CNS Research and Development
Astra Research Centre
S-151 85 Södertälje, Sweden

Seitaro Ohkuma, **14-14-2**
Department of Pharmacology
Kyoto Prefectural University of Medicine
Kawaramachi-Hirokoji, Kamikyo-ku
Kyoto 602, Japan

Yoshiyuki Ohmori, **13-6-2**
Department of Pharmacology
Kyoto Prefectural University of Medicine
Kawaramachi-Hirokoji, Kamikyo-ku
Kyoto 602, Japan

Tatsuro Ohta, **11-10-3**
Department of Psychiatry
Nagoya University School of Medicine
65 Tsuruma-cho, Showa-ku
Nagoya, Japan

Tadaharu Okano, **14-4-5**
Department of Psychiatry
Mie University School of Medicine
174, 2-Chome, Edobashi
Tsu-city, Mie, Japan

Berend Olivier, **12-8-1**
Department of Pharmacology
Duphar B.V.
P.O. Box 900
1380 DA Weesp, The Netherlands

John W. Olney, **12-13-2**
Department of Psychiatry
Washington University School of Medicine
4940 Audubon Avenue
St. Louis, Missouri 63110

Hans Rudolf Olpe, **13-6-4**
Research and Development Department,
   Pharmaceuticals Division
CIBA-GEIGY Ltd.
4002 Basel, Switzerland

Michael Osterheider, **14-13-6**
Department of Psychiatry
University of Würzburg
Fuechsleinstrasse 15
8700 Würzburg, F.R.G.

David G. C. Owens, **12-1-1**
Division of Psychiatry
Northwick Park Hospital and Clinical Research
   Centre
Watford Road
Harrow, Middlesex, U.K.

John E. Parsons, **11-15-2**
Department of Neurology
VA Medical Center
16111 Plummer
Sepulveda, California 91343

M. S. J. Pathy, **14-1-4**
Department of Geriatric Medicine
University of Wales College of Medicine
Heath Hospital
Cardiff, Wales, U.K.

Peter Pauwels, **14-14-5**
Department of Biochemical Pharmacology
Janssen Research Foundation
Turnhoutseweg 30
2340 Beerse, Belgium

Liang Peng, **14-14-6**
Department of Pharmacology
University of Saskatchewan
Saskatoon, Saskatchewan, Canada

Richard D. Penn, **13-6-6**
Department of Neurosurgery
Ruch Medical College
1653 West Congress Parkway
Chicago, Illinois 60612

Giancarlo Pepeu, **13-16-5**
Department of Preclinical and Clinical Pharmacology
University of Florence
Viale Morgagni, 65
50134 Florence, Italy

David Pickar, **11-16-3**
Section on Clinical Studies
Clinical Neuroscience Branch
National Institute of Mental Health
National Institutes of Health
Building 10, Room 4N214
9000 Rockville Pike
Bethesda, Maryland 20892

Per Plenge, **12-12-1**
Psychochemistry Institute
Rigshospitalet
Blegdamsvej 9
DK-2100, Copenhagen, Denmark

Walter Pöldinger, **11-2-6, 14-13-1**
Department of Psychiatry
University of Basel
Wilhelm Klein-Strasse 27
CH-4025 Basel, Switzerland

Robert M. Post, **14-10-6**
Biological Psychiatry Branch
National Institute of Mental Health
National Institutes of Health
Building 10, Room 3N212
9000 Rockville Pike
Bethesda, Maryland 20892

Steven G. Potkin, **11-8-2**
Department of Psychiatry
University of California, Irvine
101 City Drive South
Orange, California 92668

Sheldon Preskorn, **14-8-4**
Department of Psychiatry
Psychiatric Research Institute
Univesity of Kansas School of Medicine-Wichita
929 North St. Francis
Wichita, Kansas 67214

Leonid Prilipko, **11-14-3**
Division of Mental Health
World Health Organization
Avenue Appia
1211 Geneva 27, Switzerland

Alain J. Puech, **12-3-5**
Department of Clinical Pharmacology
Hôpital Pitiè-Salpêtrière
47, Bd de l'Hôpital
Paris 75013, France

James Quattrochi, **12-10-4**
Laboratory of Neurophysiology
Department of Psychiatry
Harvard Medical School
74 Fenwood Road
Boston, Massachusetts 02115

P. V. Rabins, **14-1-2**
Department of Psychiatry
Johns Hopkins University School of Medicine
725 North Wolfe Street
Baltimore, Maryland 21205

Michael J. Raleigh, **12-8-2**
Department of Psychiatry
UCLA School of Medicine
760 Westwood Plaza
Los Angeles, California 90024

Elliott Richelson, **12-15-3**
Departments of Psychiatry and Pharmacology
Mayo Clinic Jacksonville
4500 San Pablo Road
Jacksonville, Florida 32224

Peter Riederer, **11-5-1**
Psychiatrische Klinik und Poliklinik
Universitäts-Nervenklinik
Klinische Neurochemie
Füchsleinstrasse 15
D-8700 Würzburg, F.R.G.

Dieter Riemann, **12-10-5**
Department of Psychiatry
Central Institute of Mental Health
I5
6800 Mannheim, F.R.G.

S. Craig Risch, **14-11-4**
Department of Psychiatry
Emory University School of Medicine
Room 403
Uppergate Pavilion
1701 Uppergate Drive
Atlanta, Georgia 30306

Donald S. Robinson, **12-6-2**
CNS Clinical Research
Bristol-Myers Squibb Company
5 Research Parkway
Wallingford, Connecticut 06492

Thomas Roth, **11-10-1**
Sleep Disorders Center
Henry Ford Hospital
2921 West Grand Boulevard
Detroit, Michigan 48202

Neal Ryan, **14-12-1**
Child and Adolescent Depression Service
Western Psychiatric Institute and Clinic
University of Pittsburgh School of Medicine
3811 O'Hara Street
Pittsburgh, Pennsylvania 15213

Bernd Saletu, **11-16-2, 14-9-3**
Department of Psychiatry
Psychiatric University Clinic
University of Vienna School of Medicine
Wahringer Grutel 18-20
A-1090 Vienna, Austria

Elaine Sanders-Bush, **12-11-2**
Department of Pharmacology
Vanderbilt University School of Medicine
Nashville, Tennessee 37232

David J. Sanger, **11-11-3**
Department of Biology
Synthelabo Recherche (L.E.R.S.)
58 Rue de la Glacière
Paris 75013, France

Keisuke Sarai, **11-2-1**
Sarai Clinic
Kakuda Cho 8-47
Kitaku, Osaka City, Japan

Nobuyuku Sasakawa, **14-14-3**
Department of Pharmacology
Keio University School of Medicine
35 Shinanomachi, Shinjuku-ku
Tokyo, Japan

Mitsumoto Sato, **14-10-1**
Department of Psychiatry
Tohoku University Medical School
1-1 Seiryo-machi, Aoba-ku
Sendai/Miyagi, Japan

Dieter Schmidt, **13-3-5**
Department of Neurology
Free University
1000 Berlin 19
Spandaüer Damm 130, F.R.G.

Göran Sedvall, **11-8-1**
Department of Psychiatry and Psychology
Karolinska Institute
Karolinska Hospital
Box 60 500
S-104 01 Stockholm, Sweden

Philip Seeman, **11-12-2**
Department of Pharmacology and Psychiatry
University of Toronto
Medical Sciences Building
8 Taddlecreek Road
Toronto, Ontario, Canada M5S 1A8

Edward M. Sellers, **12-6-5**
Department of Pharmacology and Medicine/Clinical
  Psychopharmacology
University of Toronto/Addiction Research
  Foundation
33 Russell Street
Toronto, Ontario, Canada M5S 2S1

Akira Sengoku, **13-3-3**
Kansai Regional Epilepsy Center
Utano National Hospital
8 Ontoyama-cho, Narutaki
Ukyo, Kyoto, Japan

Haruo Shibuya, **13-2-3**
Department of Neuropsychiatry
Tokyo Medical and Dental University
1-5-45 Yushima, Bunkyu-ku
Tokyo, Japan

Makoto Shimizu, **12-2-2**
Department of Psychiatry
Jikei University School of Medicine
3-25-8 Nishi-Shinbashi, Minato-ku
Tokyo, Japan

Eric M. Shooter, **11-6-1**
Department of Neurobiology
Stanford University School of Medicine
Stanford, California 94305-5401

Ira Shoulson, **11-5-6**
Department of Neurology
University of Rochester Medical Center
601 Elmwood Avenue
Rochester, New York 14642

Jovan G. Simeon, **14-12-2**
Department of Psychiatry
Royal Ottawa Hospital
1145 Carling Avenue
Ottawa, Ontario, Canada

George M. Simpson, **11-13-6**
Department of Psychiatry
Medical College of PA/EPPI
3200 Henry Avenue
Philadelphia, Pennsylvania 19129

John Snaith, **12-3-6**
Clinical Development
CIBA-GEIGY
Klybeckstrasse
4002 Basel, Switzerland

D. G. Spencer, Jr., **11-9-2**
Central Project Management
Bayer AG
Pharmaceutical Research Center
Aprather Weg 18a
5600 Wuppertal 1, F.R.G.

Peter Spencer, **12-13-6**
Center for Research on Occupational and
  Environmental Toxicology
Oregon Health Sciences University
3181 S.W. Sam Jackson Park Road, L606
Portland, Oregon 97201

Stephen M. Stahl, **11-9-1**
Department of Psychiatry
University of California, San Diego
3350 La Jolla Village Drive, 116A
San Diego, California 92161

Axel Steiger, **12-10-6**
Department of Psychiatry
University of Freiburg
Hauptstrasse 5
7800 Freiburg, F.R.G.

Osamu Tajima, **12-15-2**
Department of Neuropsychiatry
Kyorin University School of Medicine
6-20-2, Shinkawa, Mitaka
Tokyo, Japan

Kohji Takada, 13-12-1
Preclinical Research Laboratories
Central Institute for Experimental Animals
1433 Nogawa, Miyamae
Kawasaki, Kanagawa, Japan

Saburo Takahashi, 14-5-3
Department of Psychiatry
Shiga University of Medical Science
Seta Tsukinowacho
Otsu, Japan

Masatoshi Tanaka, 13-5-1
Department of Pharmacology
Kurume University School of Medicine
Kurume 830, Japan

Leon Thal, 13-16-4
Department of Neurosciences
University of California, San Diego
3350 La Jolla Village Drive
San Diego, California 92161

William H. Theodore, 13-3-2
Clinical Epilepsy Section
National Institutes of Health
9000 Rockville Pike
Bethesda, Maryland 20892

John Tiller, 12-3-7
Department of Psychiatry
University of Melbourne
Royal Melbourne Hospital
Melbourne, Victoria, 3050 Australia

Hugh Tilson, 14-6-1
Neurotoxicology Division (MD-74B)
US Environmental Protection Agency
Research Triangle Park, North Carolina 27711

Arthur W. Toga, 13-13-3
Laboratory of Neuro Imaging
Department of Neurology
UCLA School of Medicine
710 Westwood Plaza
Los Angeles, California 90024

Jeroen A. D. M. Tonnaer, 13-5-6
Scientific Development Group
Organon International B.V.
P.O. Box 20, 5340 BH
Oss, The Netherlands

Michael Torello, 13-13-4
Department of Psychiatry and Psychology
The Ohio State University
473 West 12th Avenue
Columbus, Ohio 43210

Jörg Traber, 11-7-1
Institute for Neurobiology
Troponwerke
Berliner Strasse 156
D-5000 Cologne 80, F.R.G.

Lil Träskman-Bendz, 12-8-4
Department of Psychiatry
University Hospital
S-221 85 Lund, Sweden

Susan Treves, 13-11-4
Department of General Pathology
University
Via Borsari, 46
Ferrara, Italy

Fred W. Turek, 12-10-1
Department of Neurobiology and Physiology
Northwestern University
O.T. Hogan Hall
2153 Sheridan Road
Evanston, Illinois 60208

Michael B. Tyers, 12-6-1
Department of Neuropharmacology
Glaxo Group Research, Ltd.
Park Road
Ware, Hertfordshire, U.K.

Peter Tyrer, 11-7-3
Community Mental Health Unit
St. Charles' Hospital
Exmoor Street
London W10 6DZ, U.K.

Thomas Whitley Uhde, 11-11-4
Section on Anxiety and Affective Disorders
National Institute of Mental Health
National Institutes of Health
Building 10, Room 3S-239
9000 Rockville Pike
Bethesda, Maryland 20904

Christine Van Broeckhoven, 13-5-5
Department of Biochemistry
University of Antwerp (U.I.A.)
Universiteitsplein 1
B-2610 Antwerp, Belgium

Daniel P. van Kammen, 13-10-6
Department of Psychiatry
University of Pittsburgh School of Medicine
VA Medical Center
Highland Drive
Pittsburgh, Pennsylvania 15206

Theodore Van Putten, **13-10-3**
Department of Psychiatry
Veterans Administration Medical Center-Brentwood
 Division
11301 Wilshire Boulevard
Los Angeles, California 90073

J. M. van Ree, **13-4-3**
Department of Pharmacology
Rudolf Magnus Institute
Medical Faculty, University of Utrecht
Vondellaan 6
3521 GD Utrecht, The Netherlands

Guido Vantini, **13-6-3**
Department of Molecular Neurobiology
Fidia Research Laboratories
Via Ponte della Fabbrica, 3/A
Abano Terme, Italy

Marat E. Vartanian, **11-14-2**
National Mental Health Research Center
Zagorodnoe Shosse, 2
Moscow, U.S.S.R.

Matti Virkkunen, **12-8-5**
Psychiatric Clinic
Helsinki University
Central Hospital
Lapinlahdentie 00180
Helsinki 18, Finland

Andrea Volterra, **14-15-4**
Center for Neuropharmacology and Institute of
 Pharmacological Sciences
University of Milan
Via Balzaretti, 9
Milan 20133, Italy

John L. Waddington, **11-13-2**
Department of Clinical Pharmacology
Royal College of Surgeons in Ireland
St. Stephen's Green
Dublin 2, Ireland

Peter C. Waldmeier, **12-3-4, 12-7-4**
Research and Development Department
CIBA-GEIGY Ltd.
CH-4002 Basel, Switzerland

David M. Warburton, **14-9-5**
Department of Psychology
Reading University
Whiteknights
Reading RG6 2AL, U.K.

Yasuo Watanabe, **12-13-5**
Department of Pharmacology
Tokyo Medical College
6-1-1 Shinjuku, Shinjuku-ku
Tokyo 160, Japan

Yasuyoshi Watanabe, **14-15-3**
Department of Neuroscience
Osaka Bioscience Institute
6-2-4 Furuedai
Suita-shi, Osaka 565, Japan

Daniel R. Weinberger, **11-16-1**
Clinical Brain Disorders Branch
National Institute of Mental Health
2700 Martin Luther King, Jr., Avenue S.E.
Washington, DC 20032

Myrna M. Weissman, **13-1-2**
Department of Psychiatry
Columbia University College of Physicians and
 Surgeons
Box 14
722 West 168th Street
New York, New York 10032

Wolfgang Wesemann, **11-5-4**
Department of Neurochemistry
Physiological Chemistry
Hans-Meerwein-Strasse
D-3550 Marburg, F.R.G.

Gary L. Westbrook, **12-5-3**
Vollum Institute
Oregon Health Sciences University
3181 SW Sam Jackson Park Road
Portland, Oregon 97201

H. G. M. Westenberg, **14-16-1**
Department of Biological Psychiatry
Academic Hospital Utrecht
Heidelberglaan 100
3584 CX Utrecht, The Netherlands

Peter J. Whitehouse, **13-16-2**
Department of Neurology and Alzheimer Center
Case Western Reserve University
and
University Hospitals of Cleveland
2074 Abington Road
Cleveland, Ohio 44106

Frits-Axel Wiesel, **11-8-3**
Department of Psychiatry
Uppsala University
Ulleråker
S-750 17 Uppsala, Sweden

Bruno Will, 11-6-5
Département de Neurophysiologie et Biologie des
 Comportements
Centre de Neurochimie du C.N.R.S.
12 Rue Goethe
Strasbourg, France

Dean F. Wong, 11-8-4
Department of Radiology
Johns Hopkins Medical Institutions
Brady B1-07
600 North Wolfe Street
Baltimore, Maryland 21205

Kazuichi Yagi, 13-3-4
National Epilepsy Center
Shizuoka Higashi Hospital
886 Urushiyama
Shizuoka, Japan

Nariyoshi Yamaguchi, 13-14-2
Department of Neuropsychiatry
Kanazawa University School of Medicine
13-1 Takara-machi
Kanazawa, Ishikawa Prefecture 920, Japan

Toshiro Yamasaki, 11-8-7
Division of Clinical Research
National Institute of Radiological Sciences
9-1, Anagawa-4-chome
Chiba-city, Japan

Itaru Yamashita, 11-14-5
Department of Psychiatry
Hokkaido University School of Medicine
West 7, North 15
Sapporo 060, Hokkaido, Japan

Michael Zigmond, 13-5-3
Department of Behavioral Neuroscience
 and
Center for Neuroscience
University of Pittsburgh
Fifth and Ruskin Streets
Pittsburgh, Pennsylvania 15260

R. Suzanne Zukin, 13-7-4
Neuroscience Department
Albert Einstein College of Medicine
1300 Morris Park Avenue
Bronx, New York 10461

Stephen R. Zukin, 12-13-3
Departments of Psychiatry and Neuroscience
Albert Einstein College of Medicine
Room F111
1300 Morris Park Avenue
Bronx, New York 10461

Author Index

Abercrombie D, 382
Abreu ME, 245
Abuzzahab Sr FS, 277
Achermann P, 269
Achté K, 23,625
Ackenheil M, 315
Agnati LF, 126
Akaike N, 305,438
Akiyama K, 587
Akiyama N, 468
Allen C, 309
Allen R, 309
Alleva E, 543
Alling C, 253
Alms DR, 228
Alper K, 354
Alphs LD, 259,261
Alvir J, 434
Amaducci L, 494
Ancill RJ, 496
Andary JJ, 228
Anderer P, 166,575
Andersen J, 289
Anderson EG, 236
Andreason P, 168
Angelucci L, 573
Angst J, 3,657
Antelman SM, 585
Antonelli T, 126
Arai H, 412
Aravagiri M, 432
Arbilla S, 7
Attias Y, 334
Aymard N, 540
Azmitia EC, 633

Backhauss C, 158
Backhovens H, 482
Bäckström T, 520
Baillie D, 480
Bakker MHM, 160
Baldwin D, 97,659
Ballard LC, 141
Ballús C, 101
Bals-Kubik R, 370
Banger M, 514
Banki C, 595
Barnes CA, 224
Barnes JM, 232
Barnes NM, 232
Bathel F, 402
Bastani B, 17,259,261
Bates MD, 122

Bazan NG, 651
Becker R, 577
Beckmann H, 132
Belmaker RH, 211
Ben-Shachar D, 51
Bendahan A, 408
Beneke M, 95
Benkert O, 69,178
Bennett MVL, 404
Berger M, 273
Bergman P, 653
Bergmann K, 134
Berlin I, 198
Bernasconi R, 398
Berridge MJ, 442
Besset A, 108
Bettler B, 219
Bianchi E, 239
Biggio G, 384
Bignami G, 543
Bille A, 289
Billiard M, 108
Binder D, 271
Birnstiel S, 241
Bisserbe JC, 77
Bissette G, 595,599
Bittiger H, 398
Blackwood DHR, 480
Blanchard DC, 508
Blanchard RJ, 508
Bleich A, 332,334
Blier P, 213
Blusztajn JK, 581
Bockaert J, 639
Bond AJ, 251
Bondy B, 315
Bookstein F, 460
Borbély AA, 269
Borchardt D, 188
Borenstein M, 434
Borison RL, 204
Boulenger JP, 77
Boulter J, 219
Boutillier AL, 402
Bowery NG, 390
Boyer WF, 327
Bracco L, 494
Breeding W, 436
Brockington I, 528
Brodie J, 354
Brodie MJ, 295
Brøsen K, 559
Brown DA, 394
Brugger F, 396,398
Brummer M, 601

Brunello N, 239
Bruyland M, 482
Buchsbaum MS, 81,356
Budde G, 631
Buller R, 69
Bunney Jr WE, 81,356
Burgoyne RD, 442
Burrows GD, 190

Caggiula AR, 585
Cagiano R, 549
Cain ST, 595
Callingham BA, 192
Campbell IC, 526
Campbell M, 615
Cancro R, 354
Cantopher T, 474
Carlsson A, 350,621
Carlsson M, 350
Caron MG, 122
Carroll ME, 456
Carson S, 524
Casamenti F, 492
Casanova M, 164
Casey DE, 141
Caudle J, 601
Cavicchioli L, 488
Chan-Palay V, 418
Chang WH, 538
Checkley SA, 526
Cheek TR, 442
Chen GT, 460
Chen TY, 538
Chien CP, 538
Chiozzi P, 444
Choi DW, 448
Christison GW, 164
Clark DM, 344
Clarke A, 502
Clement H-W, 49
Clements JD, 220
Cohen RM, 168
Concas A, 384
Conde V, 101
Conti LH, 245
Cooper TB, 617
Costa J, 81
Costall B, 232
Costello DG, 245
Cotman CW, 217
Crow TJ, 348
Cruts M, 482
Cuomo V, 549

Dagan Y, 334
Dahl SG, 41
Danion JM, 661
Dannals RF, 85
Da Prada M, 47,194
Davidson J, 331
Davidson N, 408
Dearry A, 122
de Boer T, 388
De Mattei M, 444
Demeneix BA, 402
de Montigny C, 213,325
den Boer JA, 655
Deneris E, 219
de Salvia MA, 549
De Souza EB, 605
de Vry J, 93
de Winter G, 482
de Wit H, 454
Diemer N, 162
Dolev A, 332
Dolphin AC, 446
Domeney AM, 232
Dose M, 297
Dubois C, 609
Duffy P, 591
Dumuis A, 639
Duvoisin R, 219

Ebstein RP, 332
Eccard MB, 601
Edvardsen Ø, 41
Edwards JG, 474
Eison AS, 115
Eison MS, 115
Ellinwood EH, 589
Ellis J, 215
Elsner J, 545
Emrich HM, 297
Endo M, 9
Engel RR, 315
Enna SJ, 245
Ennis JT, 135
Ereshefsky L, 538
Ericksen L, 331
Erickson CA, 224
Eriksson L, 87
Ertl M, 315
Eskesen K, 162
Esnaud H, 281

Fadda P, 386
Falardeau P, 122
Farde L, 79,87,139
Feighner JP, 327
Ferguson HB, 609
Ferrey G, 540
File SE, 510

Fineberg N, 97
Fischhof PK, 166
Florijn WJ, 388
Foster AC, 160
Fratta W, 386
Fremau Jr RT, 122
Froestl W, 398
Fujii T, 547
Fusco M, 488
Fuxe K, 126

Gaebel W, 563
Gähwiler BH, 394
Galzin AM, 7
Gammans RE, 228
Gardner CR, 555
Garver DL, 561
Gasic G, 219
Geddes JW, 217
Geisler A, 209
Gelder M, 344
Gelders YG, 182
Geller B, 617
George DT, 512
George FR, 452
Gerhard U, 25
Gerlach J, 263
Gessa GL, 386
Gheuens J, 482
Ghiradi O, 573
Giacobini E, 577
Gillberg PG, 647
Giller Jr EL, 329
Giner J, 101
Gingrich JA, 122
Gjedde A, 85
Glavin GB, 380
Glazer WM, 426
Glover V, 530
Glue P, 113
Gottfries CG, 414,420
Graham D, 281
Graham DL, 617
Grahame-Smith DG, 1
Gram LF, 559
Gratz S, 143
Griffiths RR, 472
Grote CHR, 49
Growdon JH, 581
Grünberger J, 575
Guastella J, 408
Guenther W, 170
Guidotti A, 553
Guimón J, 101

Haas HL, 241
Haier R, 356

Hain CH, 311
Halaris A, 524
Halbreich U, 524
Hall H, 79
Hall R, 398
Halldin C, 79,87
Hamamura T, 587
Hampson E, 522
Hannah P, 530
Hansen AJ, 162
Hansen TE, 141
Harada T, 299
Haring R, 404
Harrison-Read PE, 174
Hartley DM, 448
Hartley M, 219
Hashimoto T, 506
Hatanaka H, 59
Hatzinger M, 25
Hausdorf A, 396
Hayaishi O, 645,647
Hayashi T, 611
Hefti F, 63
Heh C, 81
Heinemann S, 219
Heinrich K, 627
Heller AH, 95
Helmchen H, 428
Herman JP, 597
Hermans-Borgmeyer I, 219
Hermle L, 188
Herrling PL, 265
Hertz E, 643
Hertz L, 643
Herz A, 370
Herz MI, 426
Heuser IJ, 188
Heylen SLE, 182
Hibert M, 39
Hiemke C, 514
Higgins GA, 234
Hindmarch I, 105
Hippius H, 257
Hirsch D, 478
Hirschfeld RMA, 340
Hitchcott PK, 510
Hobi V, 25
Hobson JA, 271
Hoffman WF, 141
Hollman M, 219
Holsboer F, 11,275,317
Holsboer-Trachsler E, 25
Holzman P, 313
Honorato J, 101
Honore T, 162
Horinaka M, 547
Horowski R, 55
Hoyer S, 410
Hubbard A, 480

Huston E, 446
Hwu HG, 538

Iizuka R, 412
Imperato A, 573
Inaba T, 534
Inoue O, 466
Insel TR, 75
Ishida N, 536
Iwata T, 106

Jackson TR, 442
Jaffe JH, 374
Jahr CE, 220
Jann MW, 538
Janssen PAJ, 182
Javitt DC, 303
Jellinger K, 43
Jenkins SW, 228
Jensen HV, 289
Jewart RD, 601
Johanson CE, 470
John ER, 354
Johnson D, 219
Johnson-Cronk K, 432
Johnstone EC, 174
Judd LL, 346
Juorio AV, 643
Juurlink BH, 643

Kadri N, 540
Kafantaris V, 615
Kagaya A, 15
Kalant H, 368
Kalin NH, 601,603,653
Kalivas PW, 591
Kalow W, 534
Kamijima K, 321
Kaminer H, 338
Kanba S, 319
Kane J, 434
Kane JM, 134
Kaneto H, 376
Kanner BI, 408
Kanno O, 111
Kanzaki A, 587
Karkoutly C, 158
Karlsson G, 396,398
Karlsson I, 99
Kato F, 15
Kato H, 154
Kato R, 637
Kato T, 536
Katz M, 356
Kawai N, 406
Kawasaki K, 557
Kazamatsuri H, 111,137

Keane TM, 336
Keefe KA, 382
Keepers GA, 141
Keller MB, 422
Kelly ME, 232
Keppel-Hesselink J, 95
Keynan S, 408
Khan I, 476
Khanna S, 29
Kido H, 468
Kielholz P, 145
Kisby G, 309
Kishimoto A, 293
Kiyota Y, 468
Klebs K, 398
Klein DF, 424
Klein R, 613
Kleinman JE, 172
Knöpfel T, 394
Knott V, 609
Kofman O, 211
Kogure K, 154
Koike T, 61
Kolb C, 396
Kolyaskina GI, 146
Konicki PE, 168
Kornet M, 372
Koslow SH, 458
Kosten RT, 329
Koukopoulos A, 291
Kow L-M, 516
Koyama T, 152,205
Koyama Y, 647
Kraetz J, 196
Kreig J-C, 317
Krieglstein J, 158
Krishnan KRR, 595
Kroin JS, 400
Kubota Y, 468
Kudler H, 331
Kudo Y, 180
Kumar R, 526
Kuribara H, 571
Kuriyama K, 392,506,635
Kuroda Y, 15
Kurtz NM, 95
Kushner L, 404
Kwon K, 259

Lacey MG, 128
Lacomba C, 549
Lader M, 120
Lambert DG, 440
Langer SZ, 7,117,281
Larkin C, 135
Lauer CJ, 275,317
Lavie P, 334,338
Lawson CW, 113
Lebell M, 432

Lee T, 589
Lefkowitz RJ, 5
Lehmann E, 627
Lemberger L, 283
Lenane M, 35
Lenox RH, 215
Leon A, 488
Leonard BE, 287
Leonard HL, 35
Lerer B, 237,332,334
Lerma J, 404
Leshner AI, 458
Lester HA, 408
Lester RAJ, 220
Levant B, 599
Lewine RJ, 601
Leysen JE, 230,641
Li XM, 643
Lieberman J, 134,434
Linnoila M, 255,512
Links J, 85
Lippi A, 494
Lister RG, 504
Locascio JJ, 615
Loeffler JP, 402
Lofgren A, 482
Loo H, 540
Lopez Gonzalez-Coviella I, 581
López-Ibor Jr JJ, 101
Löschmann P-A, 55
Lottenberg S, 356
Ludolph AC, 309

Mabjeesh N, 408
Magolan JM, 400
Maier W, 311
Maitre L, 196,243
Malherbe P, 551
Mamelak A, 271
Marder SR, 430,432
Marks M, 526
Marshall JF, 81
Martelotta MC, 386
Martin J-J, 482
Mason JW, 329
Mathé AA, 653
Matsumoto K, 319
Matsumura K, 647
Matsushita A, 557
Mazziotta JC, 460
McAdam D, 436
McGuire MT, 249
McNaughton BL, 224
Meites J, 186
Meldolesi J, 444
Meldrum BS, 358
Mellerup ET, 289
Meltzer HY, 17,259,261

Mendelson WB, 109
Mendlewicz J, 150,478
Mercuri N, 128
Messina ME, 228
Meyer RL, 222
Meyerson BA, 31
Meyerson BJ, 518
Michelangeli F, 444
Mikoshiba K, 484
Mikuni M, 15
Mindus P, 31
Minelli G, 315
Miura S, 73
Mizuki Y, 176
Mizutani H, 506
Mohler H, 551
Möller HJ, 623
Montgomery D, 97,659
Montgomery SA, 97,285,659, 661
Moreton RB, 442
Mørk A, 209
Morselli PL, 567
Mos J, 247
Mostert MA, 426
Motohashi N, 207
Moussaoui D, 540
Mouton A, 436
Muir WJ, 480
Müller-Oerlinghausen B, 563, 569
Mundt C, 315
Muraki A, 205
Murasaki M, 73
Murphy DL, 37,75

Naber D, 257
Nagatsu T, 45
Nagayama H, 13
Nahorski SR, 440
Nakagawara M, 19
Nakajima T, 406
Nakaki T, 637
Nakane Y, 611
Nakazawa T, 33
Naruse H, 611
Nash JF, 17
Naylor RJ, 232
Nelson H, 408
Nelson N, 408
Nemeroff CB, 595,599
Newman ME, 237
Nishimura T, 416
Noguchi T, 536
Nomura J, 532
Nordahl T, 168
Nordström A-L, 79,87,139
Norman TR, 190
North RA, 128

Novacenko H, 434
Nutt DJ, 113
Nybäck H, 79
Nyth AL, 420

O'Callaghan E, 135
O'Connor W, 126
Odagaki Y, 205
Ögren SO, 130
Ohkuma S, 635
Öhman R, 253
Ohmori Y, 392
Ohta T, 106
Okano T, 532
Olafsson K, 289
Olivier B, 247
Olivieri S, 474
Olney JW, 301
Olpe H-R, 396,398
Omagari K, 639
Onoe H, 647
Osborne P, 126
O'Shea-Greenfield A, 219
Osterheider M, 629
O'Sullivan AJ, 442
Otsuki S, 587
Overall JE, 615
Owen RR, 168
Owens DGC, 174
Owens MJ, 595

Padron-Gayol MV, 615
Pallage V, 65
Papke R, 219
Parkinson Study Group, 53
Parsons JE, 156
Pathy MSJ, 500
Paulus E, 166
Paulus W, 43
Pauwels PJ, 641
Pearlson G, 85
Pelizzari CA, 460
Peng L, 643
Penn RD, 400
Pepeu G, 492
Perez J, 239
Perry BD, 329
Pert A, 593
Peters J, 436
Pfaff DW, 516
Pickar D, 168
Pigott TA, 37
Pihoker C, 595
Piletz J, 524
Pin JP, 639
Plenge P, 289
Podini P, 444
Poirier MF, 540

Pöldinger W, 27,619
Pollard WE, 601
Post RM, 593
Potkin S, 356
Potkin SG, 81
Pozza MF, 396,398
Pozzan T, 444
Prehn J, 158
Preskorn SH, 565
Prichep L, 354
Prilipko L, 148
Puech AJ, 198

Quattrochi J, 271

Rabins PV, 498
Racagni G, 239
Radian R, 408
Raleigh MJ, 249
Ramacci MT, 573
Ramirez LF, 259,261
Ramsey N, 372
Rapaport JL, 35
Ravert HT, 85
Redmond O, 135
Reginaldi D, 291
Regnéll G, 253
Renna G, 549
Rettew DC, 35
Reyntjens AJM, 182
Richards AL, 538
Richards GJ, 551
Richelson E, 323
Ried S, 366
Riederer P, 43
Riemann D, 273
Risby ED, 601
Risch SC, 601
Rist F, 311
Roberts N, 609
Robinson DS, 228
Rodriguez A, 101
Rogers S, 219
Rojansky N, 524
Rosenfeld AH, 346
Ross C, 85
Ross SM, 309
Roth T, 103
Rothe B, 275
Roy DN, 309
Runge I, 55
Ryan ND, 607

Safrany S, 440
Sakamoto H, 468
Saklad SR, 538

Saletu B, 166,575
Saltz B, 134
Sanders-Bush E, 279
Sandler M, 530
Sanger DJ, 117
Sanna E, 384
Sarai K, 21
Sasakawa N, 637
Sato M, 583
Satoh T, 444
Schleuning G, 315
Schley J, 563
Schmidt D, 366
Schreiber M, 17
Schreiber R, 93
Scott RH, 446
Sebben M, 639
Sedvall G, 79,87,139
Seeman P, 124
Seif el Nasr M, 158
Seino M, 364
Sellers EM, 234
Semple WE, 168
Sengoko A, 362
Senogles SE, 122
Serra M, 384
Shalev A, 334
Shaya E, 85
Sheard MA, 426
Sheardown MJ, 162
Shelton SE, 603,653
Shibasaki M, 536
Shibuya H, 352
Shibuya T, 307
Shimizu M, 184
Shippenberg TS, 370
Shooter EM, 57
Shouffani A, 408
Shoulson I, 53
Shrotriya RC, 228
Simeon JG, 609
Simonsson P, 253
Simpson GM, 143
Sindrup S, 559
Singer J, 81
Skjelbo E, 559
Small AM, 615
Smith R, 331
Snaith JA, 200
Snyder GL, 382
Sobell MB, 234
Sofic E, 43
Someya T, 536
Southwick S, 329
Spanagel R, 370
Spencer Jr DG, 93
Spencer PS, 309
Squalli A, 540
St. Clair DM, 480
Stack J, 135

Stahl SM, 91
Steiger A, 275
Stein R, 331
Steinmann MW, 396, 398
Steketee JD, 591
Stenfors C, 653
Stinissen P, 482
Stipetic M, 601
Stohler R, 25
Stricker EM, 382
Suddath R, 164
Swedo SE, 35
Sylte I, 41
Szymanski HV, 426

Tadokoro S, 571
Tafalla R, 356
Tafti M, 108
Tajima O, 321
Takada K, 450
Takahashi K, 15,438
Takahashi LK, 603
Takahashi S, 536
Takao T, 605
Takeda M, 416
Takenawa T, 406
Takesada M, 611
Tanaka M, 378
Tanaka T, 378
Tanganelli S, 126
Tateishi N, 305
Thal LJ, 490
Theodore WH, 360
Thompson SM, 394
Thorén M, 653
Tiller JWG, 202
Tilson HA, 541
Tinelli D, 239
Toffano G, 488
Toga AW, 462
Tondo L, 291
Tonnaer JADM, 388
Torello MW, 464
Torrey EF, 164
Traber J, 67,93
Tracey DE, 605
Träskman-Bendz L, 253
Treves S, 444
Tridgett R, 160
Tsubokura S, 647
Tsuda A, 378
Tundo A, 291
Tune L, 85
Turek FW, 267
Turski L, 55
Tyers MB, 226
Tyrer P, 71

Uchimura N, 128
Ueha T, 506
Uhde TW, 119
Ujike H, 587
Ulas J, 217
Ungerstedt U, 126

Valentino D, 460
Van Broeckhoven C, 478,482
Van Camp G, 482
Van Hul W, 482
van Kammen DP, 436
Van Putten T, 430,432
Van Ree JM, 372
Van Reeth O, 267
van Riezen H, 398
Vanden Bussche G, 182
Vandenberghe A, 482
Vannucchi MG, 492
Vantini G, 488
Vargas MA, 595
Vartanian ME, 146
Versteeg DHG, 388
Villa A, 444
Virkkunen M, 255
Volavka J, 354
Volterra A, 649
von Bardeleben U, 275
Von Euler G, 126

Wachtel H, 55
Waddington JL, 135
Wagner Jr HN, 85
Wakasa Y, 450
Waldmeier PC, 196,243
Walker M, 480
Wallis RA, 156
Warburton DM, 579
Wark H-J, 188
Wasterlain CG, 156
Watanabe H, 111
Watanabe Y, 307
Watanabe Y, 647
Watanabe Yu, 647
Watson SJ, 597
Wehnert A, 482
Weinberger DR, 164
Weiss JH, 448
Weiss SRB, 593
Weissman MM, 342
Wesemann W, 49
Westbrook GL, 220
Westenberg HGM, 655
Wetzel H, 178
Whitaker-Azmitia PM, 633
Whitehouse PJ, 486
Whitham EM, 440
Wicke L, 166

Wickland C, 267
Wieck A, 526
Wiedemann K, 178
Wiesel F-A, 83,139
Wiggins D, 609
Will B, 65
Williams J, 271
Williams JS, 617
Willis CL, 160
Wilson AA, 85
Wilson S, 113
Winslow JT, 75
Wirshing WC, 430,432
Wirz-Justice A, 25
Woerner M, 134,434
Wojcikiewicz RJH, 440

Wong DF, 85
Wooton JF, 446
Wu J, 81
Wurtman RJ, 581

Yagi G, 319
Yagi K, 364
Yamaguchi N, 468
Yamasaki T, 89,466
Yamashita I, 152,205
Yamazaki K, 611
Yanagita T, 450
Yao J, 436
Yeh EK, 538

Yehuda R, 329
Yokoo H, 378
Yoshida Y, 378
Youdim MBH, 51
Young T, 85
Yu PH, 643

Zbinden G, 545
Zharkovsky A, 510
Zigmond MJ, 382
Zivkovic B, 117
Zorzato F, 444
Zukin RS, 404
Zukin SR, 303

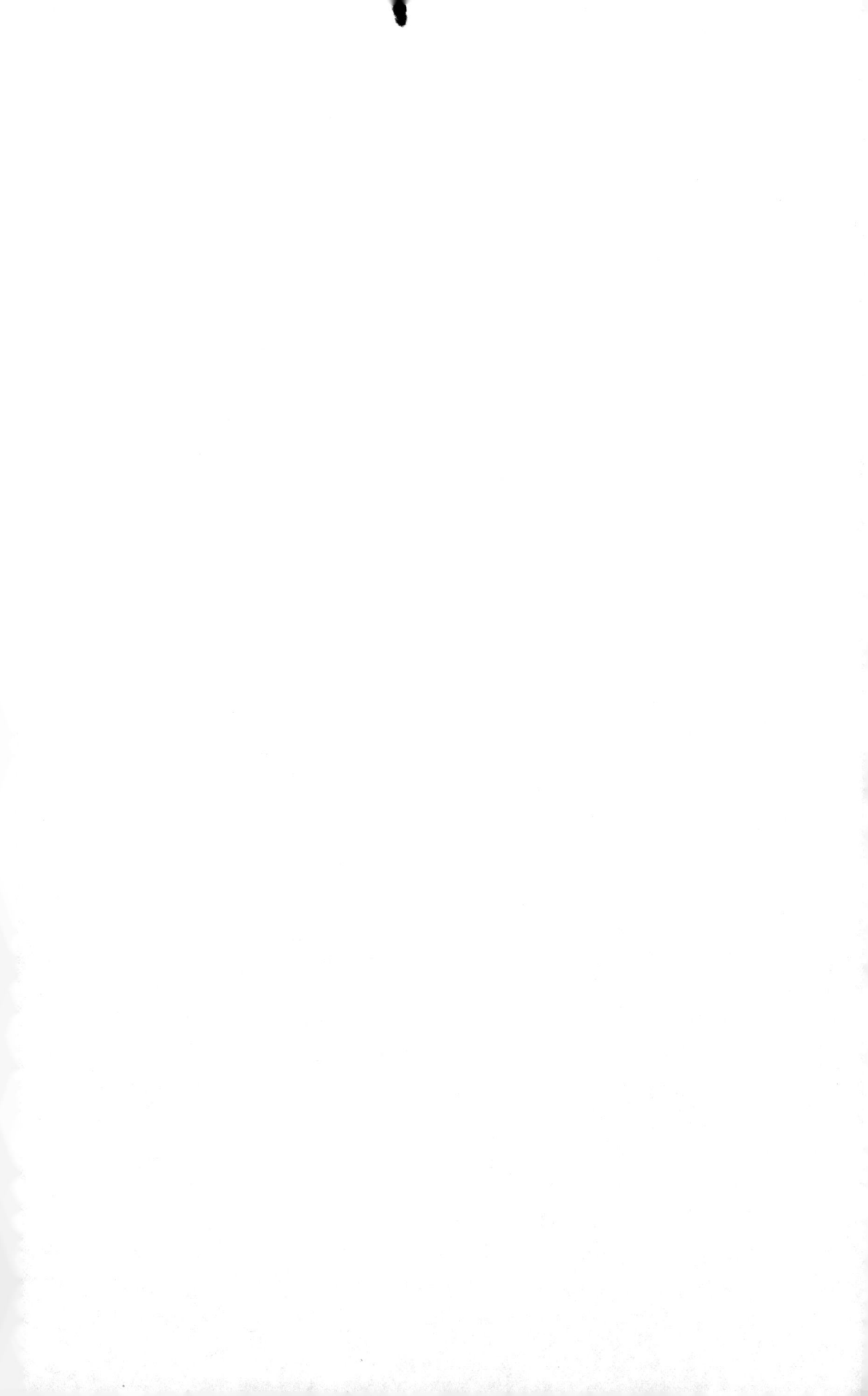